# TEXTBOOK OF ORTHOPAEDIC MEDICINE

1. Diagnosis of Soft Tissue Lesions

**Also by James Cyriax**

*Textbook of Orthopaedic Medicine, Volume II*
*Treatment by Manipulation, Massage and Injection*

*Osteopathy and Manipulation*
(1949; Crosby Lockwood)

*The Slipped Disc*
(1980; Scribner)

*Cervical Spondylosis*
(1971; Butterworths)

*Manipulation, Past and Present*
(1975; Heinemann)

# TEXTBOOK OF
# Orthopaedic Medicine

## VOLUME ONE

### Diagnosis of Soft Tissue Lesions

**JAMES CYRIAX**

*MD (Cantab), MRCP (Lond)*
*Honorary Consultant in Orthopaedic Medicine,*
*St Thomas's Hospital, London*
*Visiting Professor in Orthopaedic Medicine,*
*University of Rochester Medical Centre, New York*

*Eighth Edition*

Baillière Tindall
London Philadelphia Toronto Sydney Tokyo

*Baillière Tindall* 24–28 Oval Road
W. B. Saunders London NW1 7DX

The Curtis Center
Independence Square West
Philadelphia, PA 19106-3399, USA

55 Horner Avenue
Toronto, Ontario M8Z 4X6, Canada

Harcourt Brace Jovanovich
Group (Australia) Pty Ltd
30–52, Smidmore Street
Marrickville, NSW 2204, Australia

Harcourt Brace Jovanovich Japan Inc
Ichibancho Central Building, 22–1 Ichibancho
Chiyoda-ku, Tokyo 102, Japan



First published 1947 as
*Rheumatism and Soft Tissue Injuries*
Seventh edition 1978
Reprinted 1979, 1980, 1981
Eighth edition 1982
Reprinted 1988, 1989, 1991

Typeset by CCC
Printed in Great Britain by
Thomson Litho Ltd, East Kilbride, Scotland

**British Library Cataloguing in Publication Data**

Cyriax, James
Textbook of orthopaedic medicine.
Vol. 1: Diagnosis of soft tissue lesions.—8th ed.
1. Orthopedia
I. Title
617'3 RD731

ISBN 0-7020-0935-0

# CONTENTS

# LIST OF PLATES

# PREFACE

Orthopaedic medicine was born in 1929. Then, as an orthopaedic house surgeon, I saw a large number of patients whose radiographs revealed a variety of bony disorders. In these, a firm diagnosis was reached and crisp treatment was the rule. But I also saw many more in whom the X-ray appearances were negative or equivocal; about diagnosis and treatment in these cases there reigned a disturbing vagueness. After some months it dawned on me that no satisfactory method appeared to exist for testing the function of the radiotranslucent moving tissues. Realizing that here lay the crux of the clinician's dilemma, I set out to develop just such a system. This took me twelve years, though I can now explain the basic theory in as many minutes. I was then faced with scores of hitherto unrecognized disorders, for which treatment had to be found. It was not until twenty years ago that enough knowledge had been amassed for me to reach regularly a proper assessment in cases within the orthopaedic medical sphere.

The previous neglect of so large a section of human ills is remarkable, in that one of the commonest symptoms, ranking second only to neuroses and respiratory infection as a major cause of industrial disablement, is pain felt at a moving part of the body. Not all such symptoms stem from a local disorder, but a great many do, and everybody suffers from this kind of trouble at intervals throughout life. Thus, joints are sprained or become arthritic; muscles, tendons and ligaments are strained; bursae become inflamed. Nerve trunks, nerve roots and dura mater are liable to compression. Joints, especially spinal joints, are prone to internal derangement. These disorders of the moving parts of the body, so long neglected, deserve accurate diagnosis. Many require treatment by non-surgical orthopaedic measures, e.g. induction of local anaesthesia (which is also important diagnostically), infiltration with steroids, manipulation, traction or massage.

Who is to cater for this huge mass of patients? They wander from doctor to doctor, from one hospital department to another—finally visiting all sorts of lay healers—in the vain hope of finding the right man. Most of their disorders are not 'rheumatic' (although often misnamed so by the patient), since they are seldom concerned with rheumatic fever or rheumatoid arthritis, and they do not often call for surgery. Hence they are not the primary concern of the rheumatologist or the orthopaedic surgeon.

Orthopaedic medical disorders are the only major cause of human suffering and industrial sickness for which the National Health Service makes scarcely any provision. In consequence, many patients linger on in pain and off work (and, if they are athletes or sportsmen, off games) for indefinite periods, not for lack of the relevant medical knowledge, but for lack of doctors trained in the relevant discipline. This neglect has led to the eruption of numerous laymen into the void we have left gaping. Their number and success, together with the esteem in which the public holds them, serve to indicate the large numbers of people who have been compelled finally to look outside the ranks of the medical profession for relief, and have found it in lay hands.

But the picture has another side, for treatment without prior diagnosis entails great waste of time and money. Recourse to laymen, though it has its successes, involves many patients in repeated visits for futile treatment. Disorders easy to put right by the alternative measures of orthopaedic medicine are given routine manipulation in vain by enthusiastic laymen who, for lack of proper medical training, cannot know when or when not to apply their ministrations. This indefensible system is common knowledge; doctors and patients alike are aware that they must take their chance with unqualified people on their own initiative and at their own expense—all this at a time when the State has assumed responsibility for every type of medical care.

The hiatus must be closed on financial no less than on humanitarian grounds. If the Health Service can save itself money *and* help patients at the same time there seems little reason for delay.

In 1868 Sir James Paget gave a lecture on 'Cases that Bonesetters Cure', and his message was reinforced by Penny's criticisms on doctors' neglect in a paper 'On Bonesetting', published in the *British Medical Journal* in 1888. Yet the sad deficiency that they drew attention to persists little altered today. For the last forty years I have taken this hiatus seriously and the fruits of the work done have been set out in successive editions of this book.

The additions for the eighth edition include a review of the literature up to the end of 1981. Many of the facts that I had established clinically over the last thirty years have now been corroborated by recent and more objective studies. These are set out. Considerable trouble has been taken to establish when an observation was first made, so that research workers can be guided to the original record. It is remarkable how many discoveries, thought to be recent, were in fact first published during the nineteenth century. Chiropractice is discussed as comprehensively as in previous editions. It is clear that those who practise it are seeking to enlarge their sphere of action in the USA and Canada. A review of their assertions and advertising literature has therefore been added so that the medical profession becomes aware of the encroachment.

Orthopaedic medicine and orthopaedic surgery must not be thought of as in any way opposed. It is the very reverse: they complement each other. The existence of a physician within the orthopaedic team relieves surgeons of much non-surgical work for which few have much liking and none much time. Moreover, the decision on whether or not to operate may rest on the likely outcome of non-surgical measures. Who is better placed to assess that probability than the consultant practising the conservative approach? I know that this collaboration works smoothly and well; for this was the situation during my many years as orthopaedic physician at St Thomas's Hospital. An orthopaedic team comprising surgeon and physician covers the whole field within one department and ensures that each patient comes under the care of the appropriate expert; as Evarts pointed out in 1975 in his chairman's address to the Orthopaedic Section of the American Medical Association. In England, seventy-five years ago, orthopaedic surgery was branching off from general surgery to the accompaniment of some scoffing. Robert Jones was appointed to the first lectureship in orthopaedic surgery in 1909 but E. H. Arnold became 'instructor in orthopaedic surgery' at Yale University ten years before that. Just as it seemed redundant to a past generation to make a separate speciality of bone and joint surgery, so will the suggestion of a medical colleague to deal with the non-surgical aspects of the locomotor disorders meet with some resistance. Yet this division already exists in several other sections of medicine, e.g. neurologist and neurosurgeon, gastroenterologist and abdominal surgeon. The birth of a separate province will not be without pangs, though in fact it relieves surgeons of so much unwelcome non-surgical work. Resistance to new ideas is to be expected; it delays but does not affect the eventual outcome, since the needs of the sick have always proved paramount in the end. Already the cost to industry and the insurance companies of avoidable invalidism, added to the sum of overt public frustration, is leading to mounting pressure for the creation of the relevant speciality. It is only a question of time now before hospitals realize that they cannot afford to do without a consultant in orthopaedic medicine.

It has been my life's work to devise, and as far as possible to perfect, a method of clinical examination which leads to accurate diagnosis in locomotor disorders, enabling the physician to ignore the ubiquitous misleading phenomena of referred pain and referred tenderness. It consists of assessing in turn the function of each moving tissue, the positive and negative responses to selective tension forming a pattern. This pattern is then interpreted on the basis of applied anatomy. Logical conclusions of incontestable validity are drawn (but have roused much controversy). Since doctors receive little or no undergraduate tuition in how to examine the soft moving parts, they have been apt to look askance at such simple deductions, regarding them as more clear-cut than such obscure clinical material warrants. However, now that the basic research has been carried out, the stage is set for immediate impact on contemporary medical thought, diagnosis (since it is purely clinical and requires none of the apparatus that only hospitals possess) coming within the scope of every interested medical practitioner. At present the number of doctors and physiotherapists trained in this discipline remain so small that the methods of orthopaedic medicine are available to only a tiny fraction of all patients who need them.

Since displacements within the spinal joints are so common, and one aspect of orthopaedic medicine involves their reduction, I have become known as that odd and scarcely respectable phenomenon: a doctor who manipulates and, worse still, teaches these techniques (together with the indications and contra-indications) to physiotherapists. Nothing annoys me more; for, though true up to a point, it is a gross error in emphasis. I am a medical man who has spent his graduate days in elaborating clinical methods of examining the non-osseous moving parts (radiography takes care of the bones themselves). Based on these new concepts, I have gone on to as exact assessment as possible of the position, nature, size and stage of each soft tissue lesion. This has led to the discovery of scores of hitherto undescribed conditions within the sphere of orthopaedic medicine and of some outside it, e.g. irritation of the external aspect of the median nerve at the wrist (1942), and intermittent claudication in the buttock (1954). It has also led to a good deal of iconoclasm, 'sacroiliac strain' being debunked in 1941 and 'fibrositis' in 1948. The discal pathology of lumbago, regarded as a muscular affliction since 1904, was set out in 1945, together with the concept of pain arising from the dura mater. All these theories have been confirmed since by workers all over the world.

Logical extension of these clinical findings has led me to adapt, and where feasible improve upon, methods of treatment already in existence, but previously based either on empiricism or on false hypotheses. When no treatment existed, or the disorder had never been recognized, mere palliation was abandoned and methods of treatment were investigated in the light of our new-found diagnostic precision until, as far as possible, an effective measure was discovered. All successful manoeuvres were taught to our physiotherapists; for they were there to treat the patients, especially by the use of their hands. This is nothing new; the first record of the appointment of a teacher in bonesetting is contained in a ukase issued by the Tzar of Russia in 1655. Such delegation proved very satisfactory, since it enabled me to get on with my diagnostic work and carried the further advantage of affording physiotherapists a rewarding series of dramatic successes. On the one hand they were sent patients who had been found suitable for such procedures by a medical man; on the other patients were no longer asked to attend for ephemeral palliation that even today goes by the name of 'orthodox treatment'. (How could it ever be orthodox to treat a displacement by heat and exercises?) Neither was the patient left to the vagaries of fortune nor to the hits and misses of lay manipulators. Naturally, this policy enhanced students' interest in this part of their work. The good repute that manipulation by laymen enjoys from some people now began to be transferred to manual methods obtainable within the Health Service, with a corresponding increase in the esteem in which physiotherapists were held. Nevertheless manipulation, emotionally charged treatment though it is, has always provided only a minor part of the work, constituting merely one remedy called for by the major compulsion—an accurate diagnosis. Manipulation is easily learnt; diagnosis is not.

I did not invent massage, which has existed since time immemorial as an extension of the urge to rub a sore spot. Indeed, the first mention of a professor of physiotherapy dates from AD 585 when one was appointed under the Sui dynasty in China. I merely devised the method of giving deep massage penetrating to the lesion. I insisted that the structure at fault should alone be treated avoiding areas of normal tissue in the neighbourhood that happened to be the site of referred pain and tenderness. This turned out very fortunately; for, when the Medical Research Council allowed me hydrocortisone in 1952, the way to identify each lesion and the posture that made it easiest to palpate had already been established. It was thus merely a question of substituting the needle for the physiotherapist's finger. I did not invent manipulation or traction, both of which were practised by Hippocrates; a scamnum (bench for traction and reduction) made to his design and four hundred years old stands today in the Wellcome Historical Museum in London and a Turkish manuscript dated 1465 depicting spinal traction is preserved at the Louvre in Paris. My endeavour has been to codify the application of these measures, placing equal emphasis on 'when not' as on 'when', in an attempt to fit each into its due place in therapeutics.

In particular, I have tried to steer manipulation away from the lay notion of a panacea—the chief factor delaying its acceptance today. My only important discovery, on which the whole of this work rests, is the method of systematic examination of the moving parts by selective tension. By this means, precise diagnoses can be achieved in disorders of the radiotranslucent moving tissues. If in years to come I am to be remembered as an original worker at all, it is with this fundamental study that I should like posterity to link my name.

I would like to take this opportunity to thank Feliks Topolski for allowing me to reproduce his painting of my giving him an epidural injection as the frontispiece to this volume.

*August 1982* James Cyriax

CHAPTER 1

# GENERAL CONCEPTS

The disorders with which this book deals are universal. It is a rare individual indeed who does not suffer one or more lesions of his moving parts in the course of his life. Although diagnosis is considered difficult or impossible, it is in fact the reverse; it is merely a matter of applied anatomy. The function of every moving part has been established for years and clinical testing is no more than an informed, anatomical exercise. Function is assessed indirectly, like a series of simultaneous equations, and the pattern of movements—painful, painless; full range, limited range—elicited and interpreted in the light of the known behaviour of these tissues. Care is taken to avoid prejudice towards any particular hypothesis on the disorder likely to be present or on the causation of disease. The physical signs are paramount throughout. I have spent my life working out how best to ascertain the physical signs in soft tissue lesions and how to interpret the pattern thus brought to light. This devotion to physical signs is essential to the orthopaedic physician, for none of his patients dies in hospital and he is therefore denied the salutary discipline of the post-mortem room. Nor are X-rays of appreciable value when the radiotranslucent tissues are at fault, and in general other objective tests, e.g. on the blood, are of little assistance. Hence, he must take great trouble to be right, for contrary evidence is not often available to bring an error to his notice. Constant self-criticism is thus the hallmark of the orthopaedic physician, who has, with due humility, to approach the truth contained—better, perhaps, to say concealed—within each patient.

All pains have a source; the diagnosis names it. In visceral disease, abnormality is often difficult and sometimes impossible to demonstrate. With the moving parts the situation is reversed; function is obvious and easy to test clinically. A joint moves within certain known limits; a voluntary muscle contracts and relaxes to known effect. The examination of these structures thus presents little difficulty and interpretation of the findings is based on uncontroversial anatomical facts. The basis of this book is therefore a painstaking search for physical signs, positive and negative, and their interpretation on agreed grounds, unarguably valid. To my never-ending surprise this extreme simplicity has proved controversial and slow to gain acceptance.

## 'RHEUMATISM'

Nomenclature in medicine is important, for it is by words that we convey our meaning to others. 'Rheumatism' is a word often used by patients and doctors, but with many different meanings. To the layman it implies pain that he associates with the moving parts of the body, appearing for no clear reason. To some medical men it includes every disorder of the moving parts, whatever the cause—arthritis, tendinitis, tenosynovitis, ligamentous and muscle strain, post-traumatic adhesions and internal derangement, especially at the spinal joints. Others confine the term to the collagen diseases; yet others to chorea and rheumatic fever and its cardiac sequels. Hilton (1863) had already stated that the surgeon should not 'be satisfied, as is too frequently the case, with saying "Oh, this is rheumatism" (the favourite phantom)'.

The only useful way to employ 'rheumatism' is for the chorea–rheumatic fever group of diseases. Then it refers to well-defined clinical entities and has a clear aetiological significance. But when a variety of other disorders of diverse aetiologies is grouped together under this name the result is a logical morass. By common consent, arthritis is rheumatic; osteoarthrosis with a loose body, impaction of which is causing the symptoms, and neuropathic and pulmonary arthropathy are probably not; tuberculous and gouty arthritis are certainly not. Monarticular rheumatoid arthritis is rheumatic; the locally identical condition occurring in serum sickness is not, because its allergic origin is obvious. Gonococcal and Reiter's arthritis are rheumatic only so long as their urethral origin remains undetected. Tabes, localized neuritis or displaced fragments of intervertebral disc cause pain felt in muscles and joints; these conditions are regarded as rheumatic only when the true nature of the condition is overlooked. A familiar example is lumbago; until recently it was regarded to be the result of fibrositis caused by rheumatic toxins settling in the lumbar muscles; now that it is known to be caused by internal derangement of a lumbar joint it has ceased to be rheumatic. Tennis elbow and supraspinatus tendinitis were thought of as rheumatism of the elbow and shoulder only so long as the traumatic cause of these two types of tendinitis was not realized. When the aetiology of rheumatoid and spondylitic arthritis is ultimately discovered, these disorders also will cease to be caused by 'rheumatism'. The medical use of the word can then cease (apart from rheumatic fever). Thereafter 'rheumatic' would remain a useful evasion, but it would no longer carry any medical significance.

The word 'rheumatism' has another disadvantage. Since it is applied to all sorts of painful conditions, it means quite different things to different patients. Thus one patient may be deeply relieved to know that his pain is 'only rheumatism'; another is appalled, because a relation of his is crippled by 'rheumatism' in every joint.

For a detailed discussion on medical semantics, the reader is referred to Asher (1972).

## Primary Fibrositis

In this condition, pain and tenderness are experienced in the trunk. Since the trunk is covered by muscles, the patient complains of pain felt in the tissue he knows to lie there, i.e. the muscle. This provides no evidence that the pain arises from the muscle, and when resisted movement of the muscle alleged to be at fault proves strong and painless, the non-muscular origin of the pain becomes evident. In fact, primary fibrositis (the disorder, not the symptoms) is an imaginary disease. This has been amply borne out by post-mortem experience, for many pathologists have sought for evidence of 'fibrositis', and though almost every patient in the country has had this label applied to one or other of his symptoms, no evidence pointing to the real existence of primary fibrositis has ever come to light. Indeed, the conditions once ascribed to such inflammation in the soft structures of the body, e.g. acute torticollis, pleurodynia, lumbago, can be shown by proper interpretation of the physical signs to result from internal derangement of a spinal joint. 'Rheumatic' inflammation of the soft tissues was postulated as a pathological entity and the cause of lumbago by Sir William Gowers in 1904. He offered no evidence, but his bare statement was accepted for forty years until it was challenged for the first time in *The Lancet* and the *British Medical Journal* (Cyriax 1945, 1948, 1978). It had been my intention to omit this section from the present edition, since in England the battle against 'fibrositis' had been won. To my dismay, however, it has again reared its ugly head, this time on the other side of the Atlantic, figuring in titles of papers at various congresses in Canada and the USA. It has even been endowed with respectability by a review devoted to it in the *Bulletin on the Rheumatic Diseases* (1977). A further reason for debunking 'fibrositis' is the justification it offers for injections into the wrong spot, originally of a local anaesthetic solution, more recently of a steroid suspension. These are not wholly harmless; for Snell (1977) describes two cases of pneumothorax resulting from injections of hydrocortisone at a supposed trapezial lesion and Ritter and Tarala (1978) describe three more.

'Primary' fibrositis is in fact a secondary phenomenon. When the dura mater is compressed, usually via the posterior ligament by a protruding disc, pain is felt in the neighbourhood, but not necessarily at the site, of pressure. Within this painful area there is always a tender spot at a point where no lesion exists at all. It is a remarkable finding, but it does not mislead those who test the function of the tissue containing the tender spot. When such a spot is found in a structure, the function of which can be shown to be normal, its referred nature becomes evident. The irony of the situation lies in the fact that disc lesions, which do not result in inflammation of muscle but merely referred tenderness, are often called 'fibrositis', whereas when traumatic inflammation of fibrous tissue *is* present, e.g. in supraspinatus tendinitis, tennis elbow, a sprained ligament, this word is seldom used.

Various efforts have been made to relate referred tenderness to metabolites formed locally as the result of nervous impulses. That no such reaction occurs is clearly demonstrated by watching the changes in an area of referred tenderness during manipulative reduction of a displaced portion of cervical disc. At first, the patient has an area of tenderness which he fingers himself and regards as the source of his symptoms. As reduction of the displacement proceeds, this area

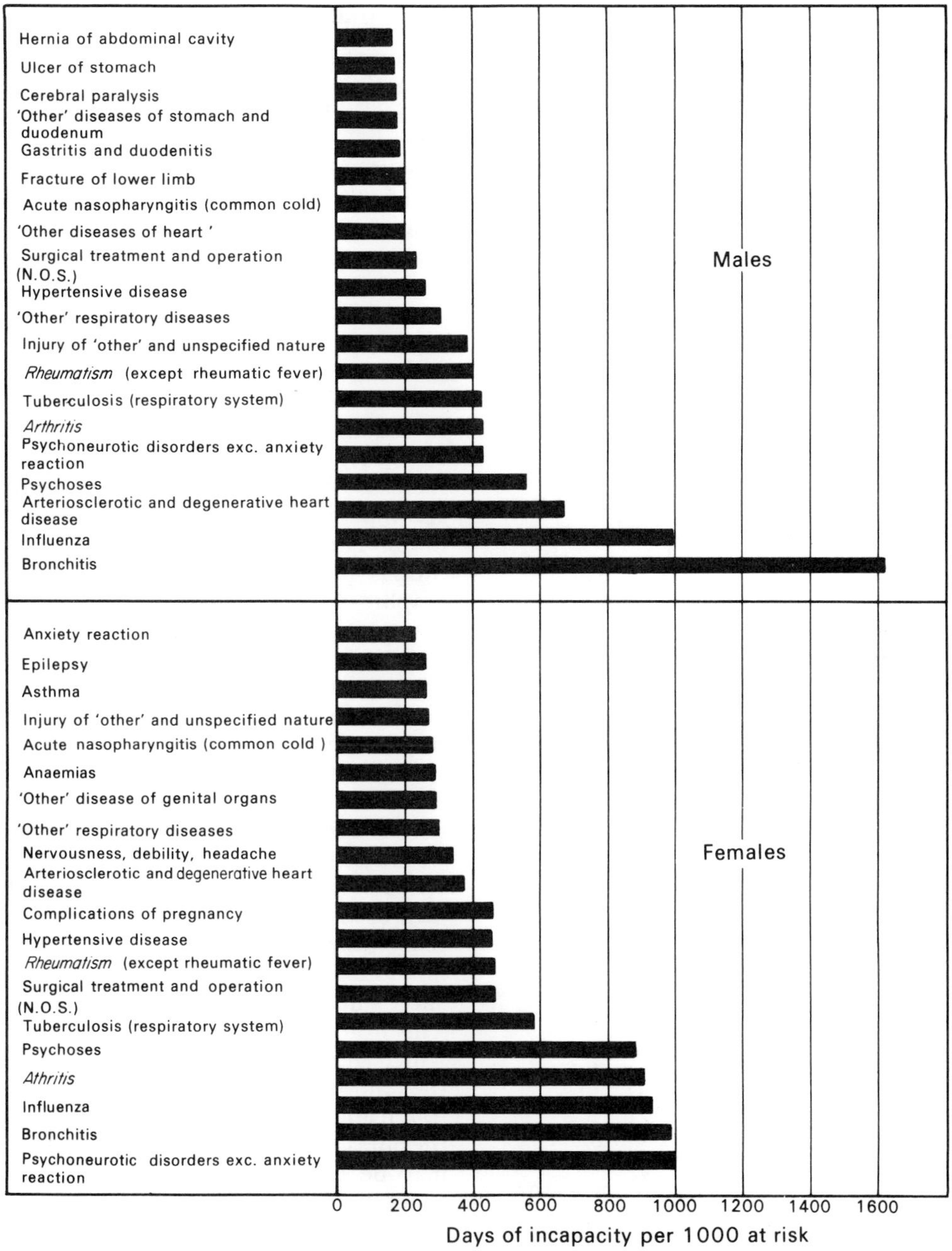


**Fig. 1.** Working days lost per thousand of the insured population (of equivalent 1951 age distribution) according to selected causes in Great Britain in 1961. Note that in man rheumatism and arthritis together are second only to respiratory disease, whereas in women they are the commonest cause of absence from work. The importance of back troubles has been emphasized by the Minister of Health (1967) who estimated that £100 million are lost on this account alone each year. Snider (1975) has already found that of all sums paid out in the USA for workmen's compensation, no less than 32% was for lumbar disorders. (*By courtesy of the Office of Health Economics*)

moves abruptly from place to place; as a rule, the pain and tenderness in the lower scapula area shift closer towards the midline and move upwards from the mid-thorax towards the lower neck. The tenderness follows the pain and, after a minor shift in the displaced fragment of disc, one tender spot disappears but is replaced by another in a fresh situation. Clearly, metabolites produced locally could not move from one muscle to another in a few seconds merely because the neck was manipulated. When a full and painless range of movement has been restored to the cervical joints the final tender point disappears.

Electromyography has shown that lower motor neurone lesions lead to fasciculation in the relevant muscles. It was once thought that this might explain the referred tenderness so frequently present in spinal nerve root compression. In sciatica the facts fit quite well, for the tenderness is usually found in the gluteal muscles (which are derived from the correct roots). But at the neck, in seventh cervical root compression, the tenderness lies in the trapezius, levator scapulae or spinatus muscles, none of which is supplied by this root. Electromyography reveals, as would be expected, that the scapular and vertebroscapular muscles are free from fasciculation in a disorder at this level; hence referred tenderness cannot be correlated with the muscular fasciculations due to partial denervation.

## Secondary Fibrositis

There is no important controversy about the existence of five categories of this disorder: traumatic, rheumatoid, infectious, parasitic and myositic.

### Traumatic Fibrositis

This may show itself as a painful scar. The cause may be overuse or a single strain. Perhaps the best example is a tennis elbow. A minor rupture occurs at the origin of the common extensor tendon from the lateral humeral epicondyle. Very little aching occurs at first, but, as the torn edges begin to unite and are pulled apart again each time the muscle is used, excess scar tissue is laid down in the healing breach. Within one to three weeks the elbow becomes quite painful from the development of chronic traumatic fibrositis at the site of the tear.

Scarring in an intercostal or in the gastrocnemius muscle, golfer's elbow, tendinitis at the shoulder, adherence of a ligament after a sprain, periarticular adhesions after an injury, capsular contracture after immobilization, crepitating tenosynovitis caused by overuse, olecranon bursitis after a blow, ischaemic contracture—all these and a number of similar conditions could be regarded as caused by post-traumatic fibrositis. But they are better described under their proper names.

### Rheumatoid Fibrositis

Rheumatic inflammation occurs, of course, in rheumatic fever and chorea. A similar type of inflammation has been found in rheumatoid arthritis. In the USA, Curtis and Pollard (1940) carried out biopsies on skin and muscle from patients with this disease and demonstrated small foci of round cells of the chronic inflammatory type. In 1942 Freund et al. demonstrated similar nodules on the nerve sheaths. In England, Gibson et al. (1946, 1948) confirmed these findings and further proved that they were absent in patients suffering from ankylosing spondylitis. They showed that local degenerative changes affected the axons and medullary sheaths of the nerves close to these lesions and also demonstrated an increase in the interstitial connective tissue accompanied by extreme thinning of the muscle fibres. These findings were again confirmed by Morrison et al. at Harvard in 1947. Electromyographic studies (Steinberg & Parry 1961) on patients with rheumatoid arthritis showed evidence of polymyositis in 85% of such cases. These changes bore no direct relation to the degree of muscular weakness or of wasting or to the use of steroid therapy.

Lately rheumatoid neuropathy has attracted increasing attention. This begins, most often in both lower limbs, with paraesthesia; later, motor weakness often supervenes. Patients with gross articular disease are liable to neuropathy; one-fifth of all such patients die within a year (Hart & Golding 1960; Steinberg 1960). There is thus no doubt that rheumatoid inflammation can affect a number of the fibrous tissues of the body. This fully accords with the clinical findings, which show that, in addition to the joint lesions, the tendon sheaths thicken, the tendons become rough and nodular (particularly in the palm) and the bursae swell and fill with fluid. 'The inference may be drawn that rheumatoid arthritis is a generalized affection of the fibrous tissues of the body in which the chief and most obvious incidence is on the capsule of the joints' (Cyriax 1947). Cox (1824) had already stated that 'it would appear that every texture of the body participates in the inflammation'.

### Infectious Fibrositis

Epidemic myalgia (Bornholm disease) is an infectious disease due to a virus which has been identified. It is characterized by fever, severe pain in the abdominal and thoracic muscles and speedy recovery.

### Parasitic Fibrositis

Infestation with *Trichinella spiralis* causes fever and painful swelling of the affected muscles; the overlying skin may become red; the tendons may also be invaded. The disease occurs about 10 days after eating infected pork. Active contraction of the affected muscle increases the pain. The symptoms and signs subside in some weeks, whereupon the patient becomes completely unaware of the foreign bodies in his muscles.

### Myositis

This is a diffuse inflammatory disease of muscle. There is no pain; the muscle wastes progressively and marked weakness develops, which can be halted only by steroid therapy. The affection is often bilateral and symmetrical and is seldom distinguishable from myopathy except by biopsy.

## Generalized Fibrositis

Rheumatoid arthritis is the only condition to which the term 'generalized fibrositis' properly applies. By contrast, the disorder to which this name is often given is disc lesions at several spinal levels. This may lead to considerable aching over part or the whole of the trunk—areas where muscular crepitus and fatty nodules are commonly detectable. Unrecognized osteitis deformans or ankylosing spondylitis is repeatedly called fibrositis. Snell (1977) describes two cases of pneumothorax created by injections of hydrocortisone intended to relieve 'fibrositis' of the trapezius.

Another disorder often called 'generalized fibrositis' is psychoneurotic pain. The idea of generalized fibrositis has led to such concepts as 'the psychological basis of rheumatism'—a notion in which the cart is put before the horse. Clearly, psychogenic pain is not rheumatism, and the discovery of the real cause should lead to revision of that ascription, not to an attempt to fuse two incompatible diagnoses.

## MUSCLE TONE

### Postural Tone

Feldberg (1951) points out that acetylcholine is released not only as a result of a nerve impulse, but also at a very low level when the muscle is at rest. So long as the mechanism for the destruction of acetylcholine is intact, the amount liberated is too small to cause muscular contraction and the electromyograph cannot therefore detect its presence. It is probable that this phenomenon is more marked in trained than untrained muscles; tone may well be affected by variation in the subliminal level of acetylcholine production. In mammals it appears that tone is served by what is now known as the small motor nerve fibre system. The anterior roots have long been known to contain a distinct group of small diameter fibres (Eccles & Sherrington 1930), as well as the large fibres. The function of these fibrils remained unknown until it was recently shown to serve the maintenance of sustained muscular contraction.

Kremer (1958) has summarized the results of Merton and his colleagues' work on the maintenance of postural tone, thus:

> A muscle is brought into action by motor impulses, but the degree of that contraction is estimated by sensory receptors in the muscle, and in the light of this information, called the 'feedback', it modifies the rate of motor discharge. It is true that visual information may modify the motor discharge, as may cutaneous impulses, but it is the muscle sense organs which play the major part in assessing or monitoring the performance of the muscles themselves.
>
> The muscle spindles are the sensory organs of muscles. They lie among the main muscle fibres, having the same attachments and therefore altering in size with contraction or relaxation of the muscle itself. It must be remembered that the poles of these muscle spindles are contractile and receive very fine-fibred efferent supply, the $\gamma$ fibres, whereas the main muscles receive large or $\alpha$ fibres. The reflex connections of the muscles are such that impulses set up by stretching the spindles excite the muscles' own motor neurones. Thus extension of the muscle results in an augmented contraction which tends to resist the extension. This is the stretch reflex of Liddell and Sherrington (1924). This has the properties of a closed loop self-regulating mechanism using information from the spindles to maintain a constant muscle length. It is clear that this has enormous advantages over a straight-through system in which posture is maintained by a steady stream of motor impulses without sensory modification or feedback, in that it automatically compensates for changes in load or for fatigue.
>
> This type of stretch reflex would maintain a fixed posture well, but it is clearly inflexible and needs modification for ease of changing muscle-lengths

while maintaining postural tone. This modification is carried out by means of the contractile poles of the muscle spindles. The sensory portion of the spindle lies between these poles, hence shortening the poles by impulses along the efferents will stretch the sensory spindle so that the stretch reflex will be activated just as if the muscle itself had been stretched. The muscle will then shorten reflexly until the increased rate of spindle discharge has been offset, and that will be when the muscle has shortened to the same extent as the contractile poles of the spindle.

Merton and his associates have named the loop mechanism of the simple stretch reflex the 'length-servo' mechanism and the modification next mentioned the 'follow-up servo'.

Joseph (1964) has shown that the maintenance of the upright position needs very little energy. The only muscles in constant action are the calf muscles and those over the maximum convexity of the trunk, i.e. mid-thorax; only slight activity can be detected in the lumbar and cervical regions. The knees are kept straight by the tautening of their posterior ligaments, not by quadriceps action. Provided the vertical dropped from the centre of gravity falls through the ankles, there is little difference between the energy consumption of a person erect or lying down, irrespective of different degrees of curvature of the spine.

## Athletic Tone

Electromyography has demonstrated that the concept of muscle tone as a state of slight neurogenic sustained muscular contraction is false. This is not surprising, for training increases what used to be called tone. Obviously, if use of a muscle caused it to relax less readily than before, training would defeat its own object and a highly trained runner would have to walk on tiptoe. Training clearly enhances the function of muscle, i.e. it contracts *and* relaxes more efficiently. Joseph (1964) states that it is difficult to eradicate the idea that a relaxed muscle still possesses tone. This idea was first put forward by Müller in 1838 and had proved most tenacious, in spite of clear demonstration by even the most delicate electromyography that no contracting motor units exist in relaxed muscle. Joseph suggests that the term 'muscle tone' should be abandoned and 'response to stretch' substituted. Hypertonic and hypotonic states would then refer to excessive or reduced stretch response respectively. He states that muscles which cannot be completely relaxed are contracting and should not be regarded as hypertonic. A spastic muscle is not just hypertonic; it is a muscle undergoing a continuous contraction easily demonstrated electromyographically.

This fact has an important practical bearing. For example, if a patient suffering from the thoracic outlet syndrome is given exercises to the elevator muscles of the scapulae, no advantage accrues; for however strengthened these muscles become, they relax perfectly as soon as voluntary contraction ceases and the scapulae then occupy the same position as before.

## Neurogenic Hypertonus

Muscular spasm secondary to painful lesions is unconnected with the hypertonus that accompanies neurological disease. In the former, when movement is limited at an arthritic joint a certain amount of mobility is painless, but at a constant point muscular spasm brings it to an abrupt stop and no forcing without anaesthesia can take it beyond this point. By contrast, neurogenic hypertonus results in an early resistance to passive stretching until, suddenly, the resistance of the muscles is overcome and a full range of painless movement is revealed. Initial resistance, later giving way, also occurs in hysteria.

## Cramp

This may result from hyperventilation, hypocalcaemia, tetanus, strychnine poisoning, salt deprivation or pyramidal lesions, and can be very painful. It is also common in healthy people, usually occurring only at night. The pain is in the calf, possibly in the foot also, the foot and toes becoming fixed in full flexion or full extension. The disorder is unconnected with tetany, but it is apt to affect the calf muscles on the same side as a past attack of sciatica and is a common sequel to a posterior radicotomy at the fifth lumbar or first sacral level. The fact that several muscles of one limb are affected in a coordinated way suggests a nervous aetiology; it may be due to a discharge of impulses from the spinal cord, analogous to the mechanism of epilepsy—a concept supported by the electromyographic studies of Norris et al. (1957) who regard the cramp as being initiated in the central nervous system. Certainly, in cramp, it is the muscles that hurt. Cramp does not spontaneously affect a muscle; it is brought on by a voluntary contraction. Hence patients soon discover that it is most quickly abolished by passively stretching the affected muscle.

## Muscle Spasm

The notion of 'fibrositis', with its emphasis on alleged primary disease of muscle, has led to further misconceptions. One is painful muscle spasm fixing a joint (Brown 1828). The spasm is thought to be primary, but it is merely called into being by a protective reflex originating elsewhere. Capener (1961) has lent his authority to the idea of painful muscle spasm in 'acute derangements of the lower spine'. In his view, the muscle spasm overshadows everything else and as soon as it is controlled the trouble begins to subside. The converse is the case, as can be proved by epidural local anaesthesia which cannot reach the lumbar muscles. When the disc displacement recedes, the pain, felt in the muscles but not originating from them, and muscle guarding abate together. This concept was finally proven by Conesa in 1976. He administered a muscle-relaxant (baclofen) to two hemiplegic patients with stiff and painful shoulders. The muscles relaxed but he found the range of passive movement and the pain on stretching the joint unchanged.

In orthopaedic disorders, the muscle spasm is secondary and is the result of, not the cause of, pain; it causes no symptoms of itself. It is only cramp and neurogenic spasms that hurt muscles. Muscle spasm is thought to require treatment, as evidenced by the many muscle relaxants that are advertised for the cure of lumbago, for example. Osteopaths attribute all sorts of dire diseases to vertebral muscle spasm. The treatment of muscle spasm is of the lesion to which it is secondary; it never of itself requires treatment in lesions of the moving parts.

The main function of muscle is to contract. This function is evoked by any important lesion in the vicinity of the muscle, whether it involves a moving tissue or not. For example, appendicitis or a perforated ulcer leads to spasm of the abdominal muscles, although this has no effect on the mobility of the viscus at fault. It is true that muscles spring readily into spasm to protect a moving part, but they also contract about lesions whose behaviour they cannot influence. Spasm is thus the reaction, indeed the only reaction of which a contractile structure is capable, to any lesion of sufficient severity in its neighbourhood. Although spasm (neurogenic apart) originally evolved as a protective mechanism, it is not always beneficial. It is clearly useful in acute arthritis, preventing movement at the joint; it is equally obviously harmful after the disorder has become chronic. If manipulation under anaesthesia does good, the spasm was clearly militating against recovery.

### Spasm in Arthritis

The muscles are *not* in constant spasm about an arthritic joint. When the joint is at rest in a neutral position, spasm is absent. It springs into being to prevent movement beyond a certain point and even then only one group of muscles contracts. When the capsule of the joint is stretched to a certain limit, involuntary spasm of the muscles that oppose that movement is elicited; the movement stops instantly. However often this movement is repeated, it always ceases at exactly the same point. If movement in a different direction is attempted, that too is restricted by spasm of another group of muscles. Such contraction of muscle is no more painful nor greater than if the patient had voluntarily used his muscles to arrest movement at that same point. For example, the muscle spasm that limits movement at the wrist in carpal fracture is no more intense than if the movement were stopped voluntarily. Moreover, at the extreme of the possible range, the pain is felt at the wrist, not in the upper forearm where the contracting bellies lie. It would have been reasonable to suppose that this muscle guarding would give them more to do; yet muscles waste about a damaged joint.

Another way to prove that it is not muscle spasm that hurts is to consider those joints that no muscle spans, e.g. acromio- and sternoclavicular and sacroiliac. Limitation of movement due to muscle spasm is now impossible; there is no muscle that can control movement. Yet stretching the joint hurts, as it does at any other arthritic joint. However, pain is not a necessary accompaniment of limitation of movement at a damaged joint. This is quite often the situation at an early osteoarthritic hip joint. Movement is restricted quite painlessly. Presumably, though the patient is unaware of it, the nociceptor system is sufficiently stimulated to provoke reflex muscle spasm.

Though muscle spasm in arthritis is protective, and in bacterial arthritis most beneficial, it is excessive in less grave articular disorders. For example, the marked traumatic arthritis in the knee after sprain of a ligament causes far more limitation of joint movement than is required merely to prevent further overstretching of the ligament. Indeed, there is no muscle at the knee which can limit the valgus mobility that would result in further stretching in medial ligament strain. The prompt abatement of the arthritis by a steroid applied at the point where the ligament is torn greatly hastens recovery. It is clear, therefore, that the arthritic reaction to the injury, and the consequent restriction of movement by muscle spasm, serve no useful purpose. The same may or may not apply to a chronic articular lesion. An adhesion may have formed and may prove incapable of rupture because of muscle spasm limiting the therapeutic movement. After rupture under anaesthesia, the joint remains mobile and painless. In this instance, the spasm is harmful. Yet in rheumatoid arthritis the same joint with the same degree of limitation of movement would flare up severely if anaesthesia were employed to abolish spasm and to permit manipulation. In this case the spasm is beneficial. When an abscess forms in the bone near a joint, arthritis with limited movement maintained by muscle spasm results. Such sympathetic arthritis serves no purpose, for no lesion of the joint exists at all. Immobility of the temporomandibular joint does not hasten the healing of a septic tooth socket. A similar situation exists in the lung, where commencing erosion of the ribs by a neoplasm may set up spasm of the pectoralis major muscle, such that the arm cannot be raised above the horizontal.

It is clear that the defences of the body cannot distinguish between lesions in which spasm is beneficial (e.g. bacterial and rheumatoid), in which it is useless (e.g. visceral) and in which it is harmful (e.g. post-traumatic adhesions). The lesion, whatever type it is, merely engenders spasm in neighbouring muscles, as a uniform reaction to various stimuli.

## Spasm in Bursitis

In bursitis, although limitation of movement occurs, involuntary muscle spasm is absent. For example, when the subdeltoid bursa is acutely inflamed, movement of the arm is so painful that the patient brings it to a halt by voluntarily contracting the relevant group of muscles. If he is asked to allow a little more movement disregarding pain, he can do so. This is a situation quite different from arthritis where the patient cannot be cajoled into permitting greater range, since this is limited by involuntary muscle spasm.

## Spasm in Internal Derangement

Internal derangement blocks a joint, partly mechanically, partly as a result of protective muscle spasm. This is beneficial when it prevents the ligamentous overstretching which would result if the blocked movement were forced, but a disadvantage when it impedes reduction of the displacement. When the meniscus is displaced at the knee, both mechanisms arise. The hamstrings go into beneficial spasm to prevent the ligamentous overstretching that full extension of the joint would produce; but this militates against manipulative reduction, which therefore has often to be carried out after the spasm has been abolished by general anaesthesia. The same applies in lumbago with considerable lateral deviation at the deranged spinal joint; side flexion towards the convex side is prevented by muscle guarding. Contraction is often on the painless side, thus proving that it is not the muscle that hurts. Lying down diminishes the compression strain on the lumbar joint and consequently the degree of protrusion. The list to one side visible on standing may therefore disappear so long as the patient remains recumbent. Manipulative reduction abolishes the pain and the deviation *pari passu.* This is quite a different situation from arthritis where, for example, the amount of limitation of movement at the knee or a tarsal joint is the same whether the patient bears weight on the joint or not. The patient whose lumbar spine tilts sideways may be told of his awkward posture and see it in a mirror, but he does not feel asymmetrical. The position which his lumbar spine adopts because of muscle contraction is involuntary and painless. In general, muscle spasm precludes treatment by forcing movement, and a safe principle is 'never manipulate against muscle spasm'. The exception is internal derangement when, despite muscle contraction, reduction is the doctor's first thought. The attempt, at least to start with, never consists of just forcing the joint in the limited direction.

## Spasm in Nerve Root Compression

Muscle spasm comes into play to protect the nerve roots from the third lumbar to the second sacral from painful stretching. This occurs only when the mobility of the dural sleeve of these five nerve roots is impaired. When the third lumbar nerve root loses its mobility, prone-lying knee flexion may be limited. When the other nerve roots are compressed, straight-leg raising is nearly always restricted. Spasm of the quadriceps or hamstring muscles is responsible; it is involuntary and painless. The pain on stretching originates from the nerve root, not the muscle.

This can be shown by lifting the straight leg as far as it will go; in sciatica, this hurts. The patient is then asked to bend his head forwards, and the sciatic pain is often sharply increased. Whereas the nerve root can be stretched via the dura mater by neck flexion, the hamstring muscles cannot.

Though straight-leg raising may have remained limited for many years, no contracture of the hamstring muscles results. Even in chronic cases, epidural local anaesthesia often restores a full range of straight-leg raising within a few minutes, by abolishing the sensitivity of the nerve root whence the stimulus to the hamstrings to contract originates.

## Spasm in Fracture and Dislocation

Spasm is constant about a recent fracture, immobilizing the broken ends, not necessarily in a good position. Reduction may prove impossible until the spasm is abolished. This can be accomplished by general anaesthesia, which inhibits the cerebral maintenance of muscle contraction, or by stopping the afferent impulses to which it is due, i.e. by local anaesthesia induced at the broken surfaces. Immobilization in a special position is often required, so that after reduction the broken piece is not pulled out of place again when muscle spasm returns after anaesthesia ceases.

Dislocation makes the muscles go into spasm and often prevents reduction, which has therefore to be carried out under general anaesthesia.

## Spasm in Partial Rupture of Muscle Belly

Partial rupture of a muscle belly causes localized spasm, protecting the breach from tension. This spasm is localized; for example, when some fibres of the gastrocnemius muscle are torn, the muscle shortens centrally only. In consequence, the foot can be moved down and up by contraction and relaxation of the unaffected upper and lower parts of the muscle, but full dorsiflexion is limited by the contracture and the patient has to walk on tiptoe for the first few days. In partial rupture of the quadriceps and hamstring muscles, prone-lying knee flexion or straight-leg raising is often limited by the muscle shortening owing to localized muscle spasm about the breach. This spasm does not hurt, but tension on the ruptured fibres, when exerted by passive stretching or resisted contraction of the damaged muscle, is painful.

When a tendon ruptures, the muscle belly does not go into spasm but, in due course, develops a contracture. No limitation of passive movement at the joint can result, although active movement may no longer be possible. Even if the belly shortens, since it is no longer attached to bone, the passive range at the joint remains unaltered.

## Muscle Spasm protecting the Dura Mater

The dura mater is stretched in flexion of the neck and is at its shortest in full extension. An early sign in meningism is limitation of neck flexion and Kernig's sign is merely another way of eliciting limitation of straight-leg raising. In severe meningitis intense muscle spasm fixes the neck in full extension, thereby relaxing the dura mater to the maximum. This, of course, does not help therapeutically. A minor manifestation of this phenomenon is thoracic or lumbar pain on flexion of the neck when the mobility of the dura mater is impaired by a posterocentral disc protrusion.

In lumbago, muscle spasm also comes into play to protect the lower extent of the dura mater from being stretched. In a posterocentral disc protrusion of any size, straight-leg raising is bilaterally limited by the hamstring muscles springing into involuntary contraction. This restriction protects the theca from pull via the sciatic nerve roots, but only when its mobility is impaired at a low lumbar level.

## Spasm in Sepsis

Sepsis in the region of a joint (e.g. staphylococcal olecranon bursitis) causes swelling and limited movement, the result of muscle spasm. Any inflammatory focus within the abdomen causes maintained spasm of all the anterior muscles. The board-like abdominal wall in peritonitis is the extreme example. Even a mere inflamed gland in the neck lying in contact with the scalene muscles may set up enough spasm to fix the neck in side flexion towards the painful side for a week or two. Such spasm has no virtue; the gland recovers at its own speed.

Spasm of unstriated muscle within the abdomen is of itself painful, as sufferers from biliary, renal or intestinal colic know well. Such intermittent contraction of the circular fibres provokes no secondary contraction of the abdominal muscles.

### Arterial Spasm

Damage to an artery leads to spasm of the circular coat but, as in spasm of the bronchioles, no pain is caused; it is a beneficial phenomenon which arrests the bleeding when the artery is cut or torn. However, it is dangerous when the artery is badly enough bruised to go into spasm while it is still intact. At the elbow, ischaemic contracture in the flexor muscles of the forearm results when the brachial artery is affected, usually after a supracondylar fracture of the humerus.

### Should Muscle Spasm be Treated?

Except in cramp, no. In the lesions with which this book deals, muscle spasm is a secondary phenomenon and its treatment is that of the primary disorder. No one treats by relaxants the muscle spasm due to appendicitis. Similarly, if arthritis or a degree of internal derangement can be abated, the protection given to the joint by the muscles becomes unnecessary. Muscle spasm takes care of itself; all that is necessary is to treat the lesion. This is important, since the wide vogue for relaxant drugs for 'rheumatism', 'fibrositis', lumbago, etc., is based on the fallacy of painful muscle spasm.

## Muscle Wasting

The bulk and strength of a muscle depends on three factors: use, nerve supply and the integrity of the joint it spans. The more the patient uses his muscles, the stronger they become. Disuse, especially immobilization in plaster, prevents a muscle working and quickly leads to wasting. If nerve conduction is impaired, a number of muscle fibres no longer contract since they receive no impulse; they waste. Use and a normal nerve supply do not suffice. For example, the gluteal and quadriceps muscles are given plenty of work by a man with a normal knee and osteoarthrosis of the hip, who walks about with a fairly good range of movement. Yet these muscles will have lost much of their bulk. The fact that the muscles waste unduly in rheumatoid arthritis has been noted for many years, and this wasting is much greater than the joint involvement warrants. Steinberg and Parry's (1961) electromyographic findings have demonstrated polymyositis in 85% of cases of established rheumatoid arthritis.

The integrity of the joint, even if the patient is unaware of any disease, is an important factor governing the state of the muscles. This is well illustrated by the following case. A man of 66 had spent six months in bed at the age of 40 with gonorrhoeal arthritis of the hip joint. The WR was negative. After apparent recovery he used the leg normally and stated that for 25 years he had walked as far as he liked without discomfort, apart from some feeling of tiredness in the thigh. He complained of some weeks' aching in the left thigh. Examination revealed gross wasting in quadriceps, gluteal and hamstring muscles, but, surprisingly, a full range of movement at the hip joint. However, his discomfort was produced by forcing rotation at the hip joint. X-ray examination revealed complete destruction of articular cartilage and large osteophytes (Plate XLV/2). A week later the pain ceased spontaneously.

This extreme instance of symptomless arthritis, accompanied by many years' full use of the muscles about the joint, shows how dependent muscle bulk is on the integrity of the joint as such. The wasting is not the result merely of disuse, because years of full function through the full range does not restore the muscle atrophy.

No structure of the body is so quickly altered by influences outside itself as muscle. Once a muscle has wasted considerably, even though no disease of the muscle itself has ever occurred, it may never regain full bulk. It is not uncommon, for example, to see, in a patient who had the meniscus removed, a full range of movement at the knee, which has given no trouble for years; yet the quadriceps muscle is noticeably and permanently wasted.

### Exercise and Exertion

When a patient is asked to 'take exercise', he thinks in terms of exertion. When he is asked to 'do exercises', he is more likely to think in terms of movement. 'Exercise' is an ambiguous term, which should not be used without further explanation when speaking to patients: otherwise, they are apt to do the wrong thing. From the therapeutic point of view, exercise and exertion are quite distinct, and often have contrary results. Consider a patient who has recently undergone meniscectomy. He now needs to restore the range of movement at his knee by *exercises*, i.e. gentle, voluntary increase in range each day. He also needs to strengthen his quadriceps muscles by *exercises*, i.e. exertion without weight-bearing at first, so as not to overstrain the joint. Were he to exert his knee joint and gently move his muscles, the result would be disastrous.

It is also an exercise to keep a joint still against

a force tending to move it, but the layman does not appreciate this. When a patient with a lumbar disc lesion without displacement is shown how to avoid recurrence by maintaining his lordosis by muscular effort, he is using his muscles to keep the joints motionless in a good position. In this way, the muscles are exercised and the joints are not. None of these differences is clear to patients, on account of the many interpretations of the word 'exercise'. Hence, many people with a stiff shoulder decide to dig, thus subjecting a painful joint to overuse and consequent increase in pain. By contrast, benefit may well follow gentle active movements of increasing amplitude without load. A footballer's knee muscles need exertion for final rehabilitation after injury, but no one (I hope) would make a patient bend to lift heavy weights in order to keep him free from lumbago. The lesion present and the aims of rehabilitation determine the type of exercise that is required.

## Limited Movement and Pain in Arthritis

By arthrosis is meant degenerative change without inflammation affecting a joint. Arthritis implies actual inflammation caused, for example, by recent trauma, bacteria, rheumatoid disease, allergy or deposition of crystals.

It is frequently taught and believed that in arthritis movement is necessarily limited in every direction. This is not so. For example, in early arthritis at the shoulder, lateral rotation may at first be the only movement to be limited, and even some time later medial rotation may be of full range, though painful. At the knee and elbow, in even moderately advanced arthritis, both rotations remain of full range and painless; gross arthritis often leaves the hip with a full range of lateral rotation; and arthritic talocalcanean joint fixes in full valgus. The idea that movement is necessarily limited in *every* direction in arthritis deserves revision, for it leads to long delay in reaching a correct diagnosis at those joints where the capsular pattern happens to be selective. It also prevents correct ascription in joints that are supported purely by ligaments and possess no muscles about them to control movement, e.g. the acromioclavicular or sacroiliac joints. Here, no limitation of movement can result however severe the arthritis, for muscle spasm limiting movement at a certain point cannot occur, since no such muscles exist.

It is also taught and believed that arthritis is visible radiographically. Advanced degeneration of a joint involving the bones does show, but in many instances this never happens. Even long-standing arthritis at the shoulder, for example, may produce no radiographic change at all. I have waited five years for an arthritic sacroiliac joint to show sclerosis, and in early gout, rheumatoid or Reiter's arthritis, the X-ray appearances are no help. Complete fixation of the lumbothoracic joints in spondylitis precedes visible ossification by many years, and spondylitic hips, even though movement is grossly limited during a flare, do not at first show any radiographic change. Traumatic arthritis at finger, elbow or knee, and even the meniscus displaced within the knee, are invisible on the X-ray photograph.

Arthritis is present when the capsular pattern (see Chapter 5) is found on clinical examination, whatever the X-ray and other ancillary examinations may or may not show.

Arthritis and arthrosis are often painful. Neither cartilage nor the synovial lining of a joint contains nerves, hence these tissues cannot be responsible for any pain. Especially at the hip, discomfort begins long before cartilage has become eroded and bone—a sentient structure—grinds against bone. The capsule of each joint and its supporting ligaments are well supplied with nerves. These are the structures responsible for pain on stretching and for limitation of movement in the capsular pattern. Except at joints like the knee and hip that contain ligaments within themselves, it is not possible to feel pain *in* a joint, only *at* a joint. It is from the capsule and ligaments that the impulses arise that make the individual aware of position, movement and pain.

### Menopausal Arthritis

I regard this term as a misnomer. Women develop a number of painful disorders at one joint or another, amongst other times, between the ages of 40 and 60. These disorders do not differ from the same conditions occurring at other ages, or in men. In fact, the commonest condition to which the label menopausal arthritis is erroneously applied is an impacted loose body in the knee joint.

In my view it is not reasonable to label a condition menopausal unless it occurs only in female patients at the climacteric, and I have been unable to identify any joint disease peculiar to this sex and this epoch.

## Hypogammaglobulinaemia and Rheumatoid Arthritis

A difficult situation has arisen with regard to rheumatoid arthritis. Webster et al. (1976) described five cases of rheumatoid arthritis of one to five years' standing, in three of which tenosynovitis was also present. The history of recurrent infections since adolescence led to suspicion of hypogammaglobulinaemia. This was found present and dramatic improvement followed gammaglobulin treatment. This is clearly a situation to which all doctors must now become alert.

## Polymyalgia Rheumatica (Arterica)

I am very doubtful if this term designates a real entity. It is most often used when the real lesion is arthritis at both shoulders of the monarticular rheumatoid type. Less often arteritis is present (Hutchinson 1890). Paulley's research (1977) has revealed that Ali Ibn Isa described a case a thousand years ago.

The patient is elderly and complains as a rule of stiffness in the neck and pain down both arms. The main objective finding is a high sedimentation rate. At that age, the neck movements are sure to be restricted. The limitation at both shoulders is not severe and passes unnoticed. In consequence a disorder easy to relieve remains apparently intractable because of a vague label.

If the cause is arteritis (Horton et al. 1932) and the sedimentation rate is over 50 mm in the first hour, cortisone must be started at once since one case in four otherwise develops irreversible blindness.

## Panniculitis

In middle-aged women, symmetrical fatty deposits develop, especially at the buttocks and thighs. They lie just under the skin, superficial to the muscles. If pain in the buttock or thigh arises in such a patient, the association of pain with the presence of sensitive deposits in the same area can be deceptive, but only if the examiner relies on palpation alone. If he finds, as might be expected, that some movement of the trunk or limb affects the pain, he knows that the pain arises from a moving part. Fat lying between skin and muscle cannot interfere with movement, as examination of the other limb—equally tender but painfless—will show. Nor can it give rise to referred pain, for it lies too superficially.

Relapsing non-suppurative nodular panniculitis (Weber-Christian disease) is, of course, a real entity. It is characterized by the periodic appearance of crops of tender subcutaneous fatty nodules with fever. This was regarded as an incurable disorder until Benson and Fowler (1964) found that oxyphenbutazone was effective in a dose of 200 mg three times a day for three days followed by 100 mg three times a day for a month.

# POROUS IMPLANTS

Porous bone substitutes have been elaborated on a basis of coral (Roy 1976). This has pores of uniform size, all communicating with interstices the same width as the holes. The channels are wide enough to admit blood cells. The coral was used as a mould and impregnated to form a reverse image. The coral was then dissolved away and replaced by an insoluble phosphate (Apatite). When this material was implanted in dogs' femora, bone grew not merely along the surface, but traversing the pores in the graft. It was found that, in dogs, when articular cartilage and subchondral bone were removed together and a porous implant then inserted, even the articular cartilage had begun to heal after some weeks. In monkeys, after four months, Apatite implants were found fixed by bony trabeculae, filling the pores.

It would now seem that we are in sight of causing regeneration of cartilage at osteoarthrotic joints and of elaborating prostheses of porous material which become fixed by bone growing into their substance.

Salter in Toronto showed that certain cells in bone appear able to form either bone, cartilage or fibrous scars, depending on the stimulus (1980). Continuous passive movement secured day and night by a machine ensured the development of new cartilage in 80% of post-operative cases.

## FILAMENTOUS CARBON

Another interesting development is carbon fibre; research on this is being carried out at Swansea University. It is wholly inert, provoking no reaction in the tissues, and has a much higher tensile strength than the toughest steel. It has already been used successfully in veterinary practice for replacing racehorses' torn ligaments. D. H. R. Jenkins of Cardiff had replaced the tendo Achilles of sheep with threads of carbon fibre. The animals bore weight within a few days and were running about normally within three weeks. Within six months, the carbon filaments had become incorporated within a new tendon. After a year, the threads had become buried in fibroblasts and a new tendon had formed. It thus turned out that the carbon prosthesis was needed only temporarily, being required only until it had been replaced by normal tendinous tissue. The experiment was repeated, this time with sheeps' cruciate ligament, with equal success. Two years ago, humans were used, and up until now (1978) instability due to cruciate and collateral overstretching have been treated with good result in forty cases.

CHAPTER 2

# TRAUMA TO SOFT TISSUES

## REST AND PAIN

An important landmark in medical history was the appearance, in 1863, of Hilton's book on the value of rest in the treatment of pain. This book has held sway over medical thought until recently, although perusal shows that nearly all the cases on which Hilton based his recommendations would now be recognized as tuberculous. When pain is due to bacterial inflammation, Hilton's advocacy of rest remains unchallenged and is today one of the main principles of medical treatment. When, however, somatic pain is caused by inflammation due to trauma, his ideas have required modification. When non-bacterial inflammation attacks the soft tissues that move, treatment by rest has been found to result in chronic disability later, although the symptoms may temporarily diminish. Hence, during the present century, treatment by rest has given way to therapeutic movement in many soft tissue lesions. Movement may be applied in various ways: the three main categories are (*a*) active and resisted exercises; (*b*) passive, especially forced, movement; and (*c*) deep massage.

Hilton spoke of pain generically, whereas inflammation causing pain is nowadays divided, from the point of view of treatment, into that which *is* caused and that which *is not* caused by bacteria. In either case it is pain and loss of function that the patient experiences; for the symptoms of, say, bacterial or rheumatoid or traumatic arthritis may be identical. Hence the patient cannot decide for himself whether his pain is due to a lesion requiring rest or movement for its alleviation. How can he understand that a sprained shoulder or ankle should be moved, but a sprained elbow or back rested? Indeed, a patient normally takes the view that pain is Nature's danger signal and regards any activity that causes pain as harmful. This theorizing is perfectly logical and sometimes correct; but sometimes it is not, even when it at first appears confirmed when avoidance of activity is found initially to ease the pain. Once more the false conclusion is reached that rest is the treatment of all pain. Only the medical man can decide whether the patient's symptoms arise from a lesion requiring treatment by rest or by movement. It depends on the diagnosis and is different for different joints and different tissues.

It is becoming increasingly clear that the reaction of the body to noxious stimuli, whatever their nature, is the same. Physical and chemical agents set up the same stereotyped inflammation as do bacteria. Menkin's series of experiments has left no doubt on this point.

The excessive reaction of tissues to an injury is conditioned by the overriding needs of a process designed to limit bacterial invasion. If there is to be only one pattern of response, it must be that suited to the graver of the two possible traumas. However, elaborate preparation for preventing the spread of bacteria is not only pointless after an aseptic injury, but is so excessive as to prove harmful in itself. The principle on which the treatment of recent post-traumatic inflammation is based is that the reaction of the body to an injury unaccompanied by infection is always too great. The most recent view of inflammation, now generally accepted, is that the noxious agent plays a smaller part in maintaining the defensive reaction than do the products elaborated by the injured tissues. These increase capillary permeability and encourage diapedesis of leucocytes: reactions of no advantage in an aseptic injury.

Obviously, local or distant oedema possesses no virtue in hastening the healing of a tear; on the contrary, since the tension it exerts causes pain and impedes movement, its effect must be damaging. Fluid in the joint obviously does no good either. The hindrance to movement set up by muscular spasm to the degree that often occurs is pointless. If the spasm were confined to protecting the torn structure from further overstretching it would be useful, but in fact it is great enough to cause more limitation of movement at the joint than is needed to fulfil this requirement. Apart from the synthesis of collagen, fibroblasts, new blood vessels, nerves and lymph channels grow in from adjacent intact structures. Union is accompanied by contracture. Tension within the granulation tissue lines the cells up along the direction of stress. Hence, during the healing of mobile tissues, excessive immobilization is harmful. It prevents the formation of a scar strong in the important directions by avoiding the strains leading to due orientation of fibrous tissue and also allows the scar to become unduly adherent, e.g. to bone. However, Rundles et al. made the surprising discovery that 2 mg of zinc sulphate taken three times a day led to marked acceleration of the union of wounds, especially in the speed of consolidation. This opens a way of so treating athletic injuries that sound union is obtainable in a shorter time. However, gastrointestinal bleeding has been described owing to erosion of the gastric mucosa (Moore 1978).

The rational basis for the use of movement in the treatment of recent injury still rests on the original work of Stearns (1940). Using a special technique, she watched the development of fibrous tissues under the microscope. Her main conclusion on the mechanics of the formation of scar tissue was that external mechanical factors, *not* a previous organization of the intercellular medium, were responsible for the development of the fibrillary network into orderly layers. Within four hours of applying a stimulus, an extensive network of fibrils was already visible round the fibroblasts; during the course of 48 hours this became dense enough to hide the cells almost completely; and in 12 days a heavy layer of fibrils had appeared. At first the fibrils developed at random, but later they acquired a definite arrangement, apparently as a direct result of the mechanical factors mentioned above. Of these factors, movement is obviously the most important; and equally obvious it is most effective and least likely to cause pain before the fibrils have developed an abnormal firm attachment to neighbouring structures. This was demonstrated afresh by Burri et al. (1978). Their photomicrographs show the medial collateral ligament of rabbits three weeks after division. When the leg was encased in plaster at once, the fibroblasts were shown to lie unevenly, pointing in all directions. When free mobility was encouraged from the onset, the fibres in the scar were arranged lengthwise as in a normal ligament. *Gentle passive movements do not detach fibrils from their proper formation at the healing breach but prevent their continued adherence at abnormal sites.* The fact that the fibrils rapidly spread in all directions provides a sufficient reason for beginning movements at the earliest possible moment; otherwise they develop into the strong fibrous scars (adhesions) that so often cause prolonged disability after a sprain.

Since the intensity of the inflammatory response to trauma leads to secondary effects that impair mobility, the immediate endeavour is to inhibit inflammation to the greatest degree possible, so as to facilitate early movement. A localized lesion is therefore infiltrated with triamcinolone as soon as the patient is seen. In diffuse lesions this approach is impractical and deep massage and passive movement have to be substituted, whereby the tissue is moved manually in imitation of its normal behaviour. Suffusion of tissues with blood and unwillingness of muscles to move are overcome passively. A haematoma or haemarthrosis calls for aspiration. Some ligaments, e.g. the coronary ligaments at the knee, can be kept moving adequately only by the physiotherapist's finger. The fact that bone and ligament move in relation to each other provides the way in which mobility is maintained; the agency is immaterial. It is the muscles about a joint, not the joint itself, that are differently affected by different types of movement; the ligament moves over the bone during a passive movement exactly as much as it does during an active movement of equal range, and it is no good giving exercises, i.e. treating the *muscle* for an *articular* lesion. If the joint can be quickly put right, the muscles do not have time to waste appreciably.

## SELF-PERPETUATING INFLAMMATION

Fibrous tissue appears capable of maintaining an inflammation, originally traumatic, as the result of a habit continuing long after the cause has ceased to operate. This is particularly apt to happen after minor injury to a tendon, the scar that forms remaining painful whenever tension is put upon it, perhaps for decades. Occasionally a ligament at the knee or ankle is affected in the same way. Tendinitis at the shoulder has no time limit and cases of 20 and more years' standing are not rare. It seems that the inflammatory reaction at the injured fibres continues, not merely during the period of healing, but for an indefinite period afterwards, maintained by the normal stresses to which such tissues are subject. This sustained phenomenon appears to be mediated by the prostaglandins. This set of hormones provokes inflammation and is found in exudates after burns, for example, and is present in fluid from blisters (Angaard et al. 1970). This fact also explains the good effect of indomethacin and aspirin in inflammatory disorders; both inhibit the synthesis of prostaglandin in the body. Curiously enough, the steroids have no effect on the production of prostaglandin. Yet, if this habit of chronic inflammation is broken for only a fortnight by inhibition at its exact site with a local steroid infiltration, the scar becomes painless and usually remains so. Obviously there has been no change in structure, only in a hitherto continuous hormonal process.

The same applies in rheumatoid arthritis. Patients are encountered who have had one or two joints chronically inflamed for years. A few injections into the joint serve to inhibit the rheumatoid inflammation. This may not return and the joint remains sign- and symptom-free for years. Again, nothing has been done to alter the bodily state that causes the inflammation in the joint capsule; the only result is the temporary cessation of a habit, which remains reversed.

Many lesions with which orthopaedic medicine deals are due to scarring that remains unwarrantedly painful, alternatively to rheumatoid inflammation. If, as seems evident, many such lesions are the result of a habit, an attempt to discover the mechanism of such a self-perpetuation would form an interesting piece of research.

## TREATMENT OF TRAUMATIC INFLAMMATION

The aim of treatment in non-specific inflammation of moving parts is the formation of a strong and *mobile* scar; of static parts, the attainment of strong *immobile* union. Thus, in the former case, healing must take place in the presence of movement: in the latter case, in the absence of movement. For a joint or a muscle, therefore, treatment is designed to reduce the normal reaction in the injured part to as small proportions as possible, the patient being encouraged to ignore whatever discomfort remains. In bone, on the contrary, firm union is encouraged by immobilization of the fracture, taking care that movement elsewhere is interfered with as little as possible.

## Minor Muscular Tears

The chief function of muscle is to contract; as it does so it broadens. The other function of muscle is to elongate; from the therapeutic point of view this movement appears less vital. Intramuscular scarring is apt to limit full broadening of a muscle. Treatment must therefore be directed chiefly to the maintenance of such mobility as allows full painless contraction of a muscle. Whereas active exercises cannot fail to secure the fullest possible stretching of any muscle—for this is a purely passive movement so far as the injured muscle is concerned—they may not be able to restore the full capacity to broaden, especially when a muscle spans a rigid part or is affected close to its bony attachment.

### Recent Injury

Normal movement of the uninjured part of a damaged muscle can usually be obtained by the immediate induction of local anaesthesia at the site of the lesion, since the cessation of impulses arising from the damaged area allows muscle spasm at each side of it to abate for the time being. The sooner this is done after a minor rupture the better; the injection is given when the diagnosis is made, followed by off-weight exercises.

Deep massage given transversely imitates its normal behaviour and restores the mobility of muscle towards broadening; it is therefore indicated in all recent muscular injuries and is begun the day after the infiltration. After-treatment follows; the limb is put into the position that best fully relaxes the muscle and voluntary or faradic contractions are carried out. This ensures movement of the muscle without tension on the healing breach such as might re-rupture the uniting fibres, and so ensures healing with full mobility.

### Established Scarring

Interference with mobility of moving tissues may arise from macroscopic or microscopic adhesions. It seems that the traumatic adhesions which form about a partial tear in a ligament are macroscopic; they bind the ligament down and part audibly when manipulatively ruptured. By contrast, the adhesions that diminish muscular

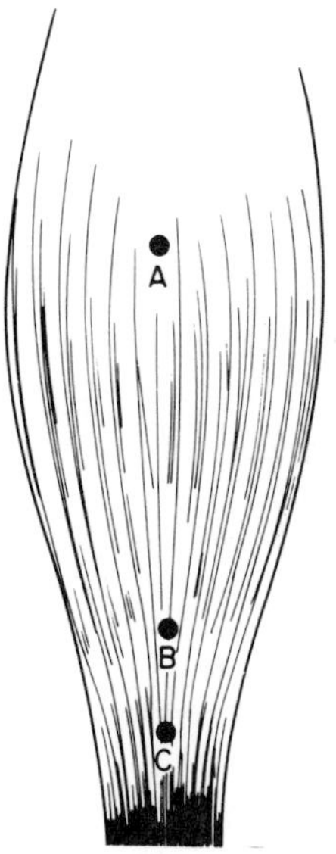


**Fig. 2.** Different sites of lesion in a muscle. At point *A*, treatment by active exercise, local anaesthesia and deep massage are all effective. At point *B*, treatment by local anaesthesia and deep massage are effective. At point *C*, only treatment by deep massage is effective.

mobility appear to be microscopic and to mat the fibres together. These cause pain when the muscle is called upon to contract, i.e. to broaden. Such adhesions also require manipulative rupture, not by stretching, which merely approximates the muscle fibres, but by teasing them apart with deep transverse massage; for it is not possible to broaden out muscles artificially in any other way. Active exercises or faradism with the muscle in the fully relaxed position broadens the muscle and serves to maintain the passive effect of the localized transverse friction.

The efficacy of treatment depends on the site of the lesion in the muscle belly (Fig. 2). If the minor rupture occurs in the centre of the belly, active exercises without resistance can restore the range of broadening, although they have this effect slowly. When the tear lies fairly close to the insertion of the muscle into tendon or bone, the local mobility towards broadening is diminished and active exercises become powerless, whereas transverse massage and local anaesthesia remain effective. When a muscle is affected very close to its insertion, the adjacent rigid structure markedly limits the increase in width possible and only massage can restore the range of broadening.

Gross scarring of a muscle is often unaccompanied by pain, for example in ischaemic or postseptic contracture, or when the belly adheres to the site of a fracture, or after division and suture during operation. In muscles, therefore, it is not so much diffuse fibrosis or one thick scar with normal tissues on either side of it that appears to cause symptoms, as localized areas of microscopic adhesion. The explanation is that small scars within the elastic tissue result in local variations in tension when the muscle contracts, with pain resulting from overstretching at the junction between normal and scar tissue. Such local variations in tension do not arise if the scar reaches right across the muscle belly or if the whole muscle is diffusely affected, e.g. in ischaemic contracture. The pull on the muscle is then evenly distributed.

Wyke (1976) has pointed out that muscle fibres themselves contain no nociceptor network. This runs with the blood vessels and it is thus only when the perivascular reticulum is stimulated that pain arises.

### Myosynovitis

This appears to be the best name for pain arising from a muscle as the result of overuse, with crepitus on movement. In severe cases, crepitus may be felt over a large extent of muscle belly (Cyriax 1941*b*). It occurs in the upper limb in the extensor muscles of the forearm. In the lower limb it is found in the tibialis anterior muscle only. Massage is quickly curative.

## Tendinous Lesions

Tendinous lesions have six sites: roughening of the gliding surfaces of a tendon in its sheath (tenosynovitis); painful scarring in the body of a tendon (tendinitis); painful scarring at a tenoperiosteal junction; painful scarring at the musculotendinous junction; primary thickening of a tendon sheath (tenovaginitis); a spindle-shaped enlargement of the tendon that jams in the sheath (the trigger phenomenon).

### Tenosynovitis

This is a primary lesion of the gliding surfaces of the external aspect of a tendon and the internal aspect of a tendon sheath. Pain is set up as the roughened surfaces move against each other; if the disorder is at all severe crepitus is clearly palpable. Fine crepitus results from tenosynovitis caused by overuse; coarse crepitus is due to rheumatoid disease or tuberculosis (not dealt with below).

The principle of treatment is to restore painless movement of the tendon within its sheath. This can be attained in three ways: (*a*) by injection of triamcinolone, (*b*) by slitting open the tendon sheath, and (*c*) by deep massage. Immobilization is the traditional treatment, but is slow to take effect, and splintage is so cumbersome and uncertain in its results that it should be forgotten. During friction, the inner aspect of the sheath is moved repeatedly to and fro across the external aspect of the tendon and the surfaces are smoothed off. The second method enlarges the sheath, so that it no longer fits the tendon, thus bringing about immediate cure. Since the gliding surfaces are no longer in contact, the roughening ceases to matter.

However, triamcinolone introduced into the plane between the tendon and its sheath is so quickly and uniformly effective that neither massage nor operation have much application today. Until well the patient must, so far as possible, avoid all activities that cause pain. Exercises are contraindicated, since the disorder is the result of over-exertion.

### Tendinitis

The function of tendons that do not possess a sheath is merely to transmit power from muscle belly to bone. For this purpose they must bear stress equally throughout their substance.

Strain occurs both at a tenoperiosteal junction and in the substance of a tendon. Minor rupture occurs at either site, leading to a small scar which often remains lastingly painful, as the result of voluntary movement imposing a series of pulls on the early fibroblasts. Each muscle contraction is apt to renew the rupture in the healing breach; later on, it further irritates the painful scar. Treatment consists of (*a*) disinflaming the painful scar by local steroid infiltration or (*b*) getting rid of the scar tissue by deep massage to the exact spot. The former is quicker, less painful and preferable, but reduction of inflammation is less radical than wearing down the scar by deep friction; hence the incidence of recurrence is higher.

*Athletes and Steroid Infiltrations.* Rupture of the tendo Achillis has occurred after steroid infiltration, but is the result of mistaken technique; the injection should be given along the surface of the tendon, not into it. Be this as it may, athletes are becoming increasingly wary of these injections, and with justification, since animal experiments by Wrenn et al. (1954) showed weakened union on oral steroid administration. As a result, the deep friction techniques that were devised in the 1930s have recently come back into favour in sports practice.

### Tenovaginitis

This is a primary lesion of the tendon sheath, usually with considerable thickening. It may follow repeated strains but is often apparently causeless. In rare instances, rheumatoid disease, gout, gonorrhoea or xanthomatosis is responsible. Crepitus never occurs in this condition.

In non-specific tenovaginitis, triamcinolone, deep massage or incision of the tendon sheath are curative, but again the steroid is preferable for its simplicity and speed. One or two infiltrations suffice. Till well, the patient should avoid exerting the affected tendon.

### Localized Tendinous Swelling

Any of the digital flexor tendons may develop a rounded swelling on its course in the palm or within the carpal tunnel. It may engage and become fixed within a constricted part of its sheath—the trigger phenomenon—or press on an adjacent nerve.

## Sprains at a Joint

The function of a joint capsule is to hold the bone ends together while allowing free movement at the joint. Ligaments reinforce the capsule at points of special stress; they have a large range of movement over bone, which has to be maintained after a sprain. Ligaments are not appreciably elastic; hence overstretching leads to permanent laxity, which in due course becomes painless. Those ligaments, the tension on which is not controlled by muscles, are particularly liable to such lengthening with consequent instability of the joint.

### Recent Articular Sprain

The principles of treatment depend on whether movement at a joint is, or is not, controlled by muscle.

*Joints at which Movement is under Voluntary Control.* As soon as the patient is seen a steroid should be injected at the site of the ligamentous or capsular lesion. Traumatic inflammation is thus reduced and so far as possible structural and reflex changes are prevented. There is considerable after-pain for 12 to 24 hours, requiring analgesics. Next day, if there is oedema, effleurage diminishes swelling and pain, thereby lessening both local and voluntary obstruction to movement. If the sprained point lies within reach of the physiotherapist's finger, a short period of friction then moves the damaged structure to and fro over subjacent bone. Since there is no question of breaking down strong scars but merely of preventing young fibroblasts from forming unwanted points of adherence, the deep massage need last only a minute or two and should be as gentle as is compatible with securing adequate movement of the damaged tissue. The physiotherapist then puts the injured joint or joints through the greatest possible range of movement without causing appreciable pain.

Before hydrocortisone existed, the best immediate treatment was to induce local anaesthesia at the lesion. It did not affect the local response to trauma, but enabled the patient to move the part better for two hours and temporarily abolished the afferent impulses that set up reflex oedema, fluid in the joint, muscle spasm, etc. Physiotherapy to the lesion followed the next day (as above).

*Joints at which Movement is not under Voluntary Control.* The important joints are the acromioclavicular, sternoclavicular, sacroiliac, sacrococcygeal, symphysis pubis, cruciate ligaments at the knee and inferior tibiofibular ligament. Since no muscles span the joint effectively, healing in the absence of enough movement need not be feared. Adhesions limiting movement cannot form since the patient cannot use his muscles to keep the joint too still. On the contrary, such capsular and ligamentous overstretching as may have taken place is permanent, although it does not necessarily cause symptoms. The principle of treatment is thus to avoid movement, as far as possible, by protection of the joint and to combat the traumatic inflammation by local infiltration with triamcinolone. Meanwhile the joint is kept as still as possible.

Under this regimen, recovery takes only a few days. Painful chronic laxity can be converted into painless laxity by local infiltration with triamcinolone suspension. Minor laxity is compatible with excellent function as long as the pain is abolished.

### Chronic Ligamentous Sprain

In such cases, adhesions have been allowed to form because of inadequate movement in the acute stage; they now limit the play of the ligament over bone, and each time the patient uses his joint vigorously, he resprains the adherent ligament. The object of treatment is restoration of full, painless mobility. Forced movement ruptures adhesions about a joint and is curative; carried out gently it stretches the adhesion to no purpose. However, there are three sites where manipulative rupture of adhesions is impossible and the attempt harmful: at the coronary ligaments, at the ligaments of the wrist and at the deltoid ligament of the ankle. In the first two, deep massage is quickly curative, but the deltoid ligament requires relief from tension and infiltration with triamcinolone.

## Internal Derangement of Joints

This is far commoner than was formerly supposed. At the knee joint, apart from the well-known subluxation of a torn meniscus, another type of internal derangement caused by an impacted loose body, has lately been recognized as of frequent occurrence (Cyriax 1954; Helfet 1963). At the elbow and wrist joints internal derangement is not uncommon. Moreover, a large number of obscure pains in the trunk and limbs are now known to result from displacements within the intervertebral joints, apart from fully developed brachial root pain and sciatica.

There is another variety of internal derangement against which the reader must be warned—the 'nipped synovial fringe' at the vertebral facet joints, dear to osteopaths. Synovial membrane contains no nerves, so the patient would suffer no discomfort if it were pinched.

Treatment varies from joint to joint, but in essence is:

1. Inducing the displaced intra-articular structure to return to its bed. For this purpose manipulation, usually during traction, is often required and may yield an immediate happy result. At the spinal joints reduction by sustained traction provides an alternative.
2. Once obtained, the maintenance of reduction is equally important; for in all disorders caused by loose body formation within a joint the liability to recurrence is pronounced. The avoidance of certain activities, postural training or retentive apparatus may be required.
3. Removal of the loose fragment. This is the normal procedure at the knee, less often at other peripheral joints. It is called for in young people in whom the loose body has an osseous nucleus whereby its position can be ascertained

radiologically. At the spinal joints, if reduction proves impracticable and the symptoms warrant, removal is indicated.

4. Chemolysis. The enzyme chymopapain metabolizes cartilage and intra-articular injection leads to its being eaten away.

## DIMETHYL SULPHOXIDE

Great hopes were raised in 1965 by the discovery that a well-known industrial solvent, dimethyl sulphoxide, when placed on a patient's skin, penetrated, carrying drugs dissolved in it. This raised visions of introducing procaine or hydrocortisone into the area of, say, a strained ligament at the knee or ankle merely by applying the appropriate solution at the site. It was quickly discovered that the solvent was toxic to eyes in experimental animals and the death of one patient was reported after the use of dimethyl sulphoxide for a sprained ankle. The Food and Drugs Committee in the USA forbade its use on human beings, but the restrictions were relaxed in September 1968, short-term topical use being regarded as 'reasonably safe'. Now the same Committee has reported that the solvent has a low toxicity and that 13 licences have been granted to test it on human beings (Pani 1974). It is available as Fluvet DMSO to veterinary surgeons.

## PHONOPHORESIS

Ultrasonic waves were shown by Griffin and Touchstone (1963) to drive the entire molecule of hydrocortisone through a pig's skin. The steroid could be recovered from underlying muscle to a depth of 6 cm. In 1975 Kleinkort and Wood reported excellent results in disorders like tennis elbow and subdeltoid bursitis, of which 63% were relieved when a 1% strength of hydrocortisone was used, rising to 95% when a 10% ointment was substituted. Treatment was given daily for a week, each session lasting six to nine minutes. However, other experiments on human limbs just before amputation have shown that transcutaneous passage by this means led to accumulation of heavy metals just beneath the skin. In any case, there may be a considerable difference in result between phonophoresis aimed say, all over the shoulder region and accurately beamed at the distal end of the supraspinatus tendon or at a localized area of subdeltoid bursa. So restricted an objective may enable a small area of tissue to be treated intensively for a very short time, without danger to the skin. Another of their indications is rheumatoid arthritis of the fingers, where the capsule of the joint lies subcutaneously.

A separate proposal is to inject the steroid suspension in the ordinary way and follow it at once by ultrasonic therapy. This might prevent the tendency to relapse some months later. Further research is clearly required.

## HYDROCORTISONE WITH ULTRA-SOUND

In 1981 Searle said: 'For some time I have considered the possibility of using a medicated gel as a coupling agent for use with the ultrasonic beam for the relief of those lesions which are least likely to respond to specific physiotherapeutic treatment. High on that list is bursitis which benefits from skilled injection therapy, but which does not respond to the ministrations of the physiotherapist.

I therefore made enquiries and discovered that a certain medicated gel was being widely used in certain hospitals and clinics in this country and on the Continent. This gel contains 20 mg of corticosteroids.

I wrote to Dr Cyriax asking for his opinion and he replied to suggest that I obtained an ultrasonic gel containing 10% hydrocortisone BP. This I have been able to obtain from the chemist.

Although I have not yet given this treatment a fair trial the results so far have been quite exciting. I have selected four patients with bursitis at the shoulder, one patient with supraspinatus tendinitis and one young man with a minor tear of the quadriceps muscle.

The technique I have used is to give 0.75 $Wcm^2$ for four minutes, pulsed 1:1, using a 1.5 meg transducer. Each patient was given one treatment; only the man with the muscle lesion was given massage as well as ultra-sound. The patients were asked to come back one week later. The muscle tear and the supraspinatus tendon were symptom-free and those with bursitis were greatly improved and were given a second similar treatment. Only one of those required a third treatment.

It seems that this method may revolutionize some of the treatments of soft tissue lesions and perhaps other members will try the same technique and report on their results.'

## CHYMORAL

This oral proteolytic enzyme has been used over the past 10 years to increase the speed of recovery after athletic injury. The published reports have been largely favourable. This was confirmed by a double-blind trial conducted on footballers by Buck and Phillips (1970). Two tablets of Chymoral were taken four times daily before meals for four to six days after the injury. The conclusion drawn from study of over 100 patients was a shortening of the recovery time by 1.3 days for haematomas and 2.4 days for sprains: a reduction by about a quarter of the control time-span.

## CHOICE OF STEROID

My experience with arthritis at the shoulder has been that a few do not respond to intra-articular hydrocortisone, whereas virtually all do well on triamcinolone. Moreover, the discomfort that follows all injections of steroid material into a joint is much less both in degree and duration when triamcinolone is used. The same applies to the tendons at the shoulder and knee, to the ligaments at knee and tarsus, to the subdeltoid bursa and the plantar fascia. Again, in tennis elbow, an injection of hydrocortisone into the epicondylar tendon provokes quite severe pain for two days. By contrast, the reaction to triamcinolone is not severe and lasts only 12 hours. The suspension containing 10 mg/ml is to be preferred to that containing 40 mg; subsequent tendinous ruptures have been reported with the stronger solution.

Macrogol, the vehicle in which prednisone is suspended, was shown by Brånemark et al. (1967) to have a low molecular weight, and thus no circulatory effect on the synovial tissue with which it lies in contact. When sorbitol, which has a high molecular weight, was employed as the suspending medium, circulatory arrest followed the injection into normal rabbits' knees.

Triamcinolone acetonide is suspended in Tween, which unfortunately has a high molecular weight. Nevertheless, I have found it most suited to orthopaedic medical practice. This suitability does not extend to triamcinolone hexacetonide, which causes up to several days after-pain and gives less satisfactory results.

It would appear that methylprednisolone is the steroid best tolerated by the arachnoid membrane and it is recommended by American authors for intrathecal injection.

CHAPTER 3

# REFERRED PAIN

It is important that referred pains should be designated as such, for the phrase invites the question—referred from where? When a referred pain has by common consent been given a name, e.g. sciatica, it is easy to suppose that a diagnosis has been reached. In consequence, the search for the origin of the pain ceases. Realization that 'sciatica' describes a symptom, common to many lesions placed at the upper part of the fourth lumbar to second sacral segments, avoids this error. Recognition that a pain, even if it has been given a name, is referred is essential to any organized search for its origin.

The chief obstacle to correct diagnosis in painful conditions is the fact that the symptom is often felt at a distance from its source. Diffusion of pain is a phenomenon common to all aspects of medicine, but in the strictly medical and surgical fields the pain is usually accompanied by constitutional signs that help to identify the lesion or at least give rise to unequivocal signs of disease. In the disorders of soft tissues and joints with which the orthopaedic physician deals the complaint is often merely of pain, local and general signs being conspicuously absent. The diagnosis in such cases turns on the assessment of the site and nature of the pain and the manner in which it is projected and elicited—in other words, on a clear understanding of 'referred pain' and of the conditions favouring reference. Moreover, this knowledge enables an otherwise misleading phenomenon to be turned to diagnostic advantage. In deep-seated soft tissue lesions the symptoms are often very deceptive and, taken at their face value, lead to incorrect diagnosis and treatment applied in the wrong place. Such symptoms are particularly common among patients sent to the orthopaedic physician.

Pain felt elsewhere than at its true site is termed 'referred'. Familiar examples are pain in the shoulder accompanying diaphragmatic disorders, pain in the knee in arthritis of the hip, the sacral pains of childbirth, pain in one or both arms in angina pectoris and testicular pain felt in the lower back.

Wyke (1976) stated that the site of a symptom is located by the sensory cortex which detects where it is felt. The fact that it is painful is determined by the cells in the supra-orbital part of the frontal lobes. This explains why the patient's emotional state influences the degree to which a sensation may be regarded as painful. Wyke points out that this concept was first propounded by Darwin in 1794. The memory of a pain is retained in the temporal lobes. He has found that it is not the severity of a pain but the length of time that it lasted that determines whether it can be recollected afterwards. (He therefore advises those who carry out a painful treatment to inflict one moment's severe pain rather than employ a gentler measure continuing for a longer time.)

Referred pain is an error in perception. This was well known to John Hunter who explained it as a disorder occurring in the mind (1835 edition, vol. 1, p. 363). But this was forgotten and referred pain became known as 'neuritis' or 'fibrositis' until the fact that it was an error in perception was pointed out again (Cyriax 1941*b*; Lewis 1942). On all previous occasions in the patient's lifetime, a stimulus reaching certain cells in the sensory cortex has meant to him that damage was being inflicted on a certain area of skin. When the same cells receive a painful stimulus arising from a deep-seated structure, naturally the sensorium interprets this impulse on a basis of past experience, i.e. refers the pain to the area of skin connected with those particular cortical cells, but with the important difference that the pain is felt deeply, not in the skin itself. Hitherto, all painful stimuli reaching the cortex have arisen by an external agency affecting primarily the skin—the tissue of which an individual is most aware. When, for the first time, pain arises from a structure within the body, the cortical cells 'feel' the pain at the area whence it has always arisen before, i.e. in the relevant dermatome: the dermatome corresponding to the segment that contains the lesion. The distance the pain can travel from its source is dependent upon the size of the dermatome. The curious situation thus arises that the shape of the dermatome determines the extent of the distal radiation of pain; yet, the sensory cortex correctly interprets the stimulus as having a deep origin, not in the skin itself. Thus the extent of the sensation depends on this interpretation—or more often misinterpretation—by the sensory cortex.

The crucial experiment in this sphere was made by Sir Thomas Lewis in the autumn of 1936. Wishing to investigate muscular pain, he injected an irritant deeply into the lower lumbar region. He found that a diffuse pain running down the lower limb resulted and that the subject experienced little or no discomfort at the site of the injection. In 1938, Kellgren published the results of a systematic examination of the phenomena of referred pain, showing them to radiate segmentally and not to cross the midline.

Until this time, wide radiation of pain had been regarded as evidence of involvement of nerves, whereas this research showed that many soft tissues could be the source of diffuse symptoms. Thus, to approach the problem of referred pain with an open mind, the reader must consciously divest himself of the idea that projection of pain necessarily follows a nerve. This idea has proved most tenacious, in spite of experimental proof that the pain is merely interpreted by the cerebrum as occupying part or the whole of an embryological segment. It has presented the chief obstacle to a logical approach to the problems arising when the origin of a diffuse pain is sought. The source of this confusion may be that the nerve supply to all structures is distributed on a segmental basis. This arrangement by no means warrants the notion that pains are projected down nerves.

There are many relevant clinical phenomena which any doctor can investigate for himself. One of the most common and obvious is tennis elbow. When pain from this lesion diffuses so far as the hand, it is nearly always felt in the long and ring fingers. No single nerve runs from the elbow with such a distribution, whereas this area represents the distal part of the seventh cervical segment. Rarely the pain is referred to the ring and little fingers; yet it is inconceivable that a lesion at the *lateral* humeral epicondyle could affect the ulnar nerve. Again, down what nerve can pain diffuse from the subdeltoid bursa or the supraspinatus tendon to the arm and forearm? How can a posterior cervical pain radiate to the area supplied by the trigeminal nerve in the forehead? What nerve stretches from the heart or diaphragm to the arm, from the appendix to the umbilical area, from the shoulder joint to the wrist, from the sacroiliac ligaments to the heel?

It might be argued that an axon reflex is involved and that sensory fibres carry the impulses to the cord, whence they are projected down the limb. Proof that this is not so is the fact that section of the supposed efferent trunk to this reflex does not affect reference of pain. Even amputation distal to the focus from which the pain starts is without effect, pains being felt to run along an absent limb, because *the cells corresponding to it in the sensory cortex remain*, and it is here that the stimulus spreads. Destruction of the ganglion of the trigeminal nerve, for example, does not affect the patient's capacity to perceive pain in the forehead referred from the cervical joints. Myocardial and diaphragmatic pains are projected down an absent upper limb and referred pain may occur in an area rendered anaesthetic from a peripheral nerve palsy. This finding was confirmed by Harman (1951) who found anginal pain in the arm to be unaltered by a brachial plexus block. Sciatica occurs in an absent limb, because the source of the pain lies at a low lumbar joint and the pathway from there to the cerebrum is in no way altered by amputation of the lower limb.

It has been suggested that root pain and referred pain are in some way different. This is not so; for pressure exerted on a nerve root leads to pain extending along the relevant dermatome and pain arising in any other tissue deeply placed at the proximal end of a segment also sets up pain felt in any part of the relevant dermatome. There is thus no difference in the nature or the extent of the pain, merely in which movements evoke it. Of course, paraesthesia does not appear unless a nerve root is affected and severe pain of sudden onset is more characteristic of root pain. However, the fact remains that the extent of the pain is no different when it originates at a nerve root than when it arises in some other tissue derived from the same segment.

## THE SEGMENTS

Fig. 3 gives a general impression of the embryological origin of the skin (dermatomes) but does not allow for the overlap. This is so considerable that division of one posterior spinal root causes little interference with cutaneous sensibility, and the changes after the division of two adjacent thoracic roots are sometimes barely perceptible. The figure does no more than indicate the general type of arrangement. Clinical diagnosis demands a much more accurate delineation of the area of each dermatome.

When the fetus is a month old, division into about 40 segments starts. The final 10 are coccygeal and by a fortnight later all but two of these have disappeared. In due course each segment becomes differentiated into dermatome (skin), myotome (muscles and other soft tissues) and sclerotome (bone and fibrous septa). The extent of the relevant dermatome governs the distance that pain arising from any point in the myotome may travel distally. Since the dermatome often projects further distally than the myotome, pain may be felt to occupy an area more extensive than the myotome in which it arises. For example, the pain of supraspinatus tendinitis may reach the radial border of the hand, whereas the fifth cervical myotome does not extend below the elbow. By contrast, in some places the myotome extends further proximally than the dermatome. For example the fourth cervical dermatome ends at the shoulder; this is therefore where pain arising from the diaphragm (C4) is felt, although the muscle itself occupies the lower thorax. The scapula and its muscles, and one division of each of the pectoral muscles at the front of the trunk, form part of the fifth cervical myotome lying between thoracic skin and thoracic ribs. However, the scapula and its muscles, and one division of each of the pectoral muscles at the front of the trunk, form part of the fifth cervical myotome lying between thoracic skin and thoracic ribs. The latissimus dorsi muscles (C7 and 8) reach the iliac crest. These overlapping and discontinuous areas make it impossible to draw accurate maps of the myotomes.

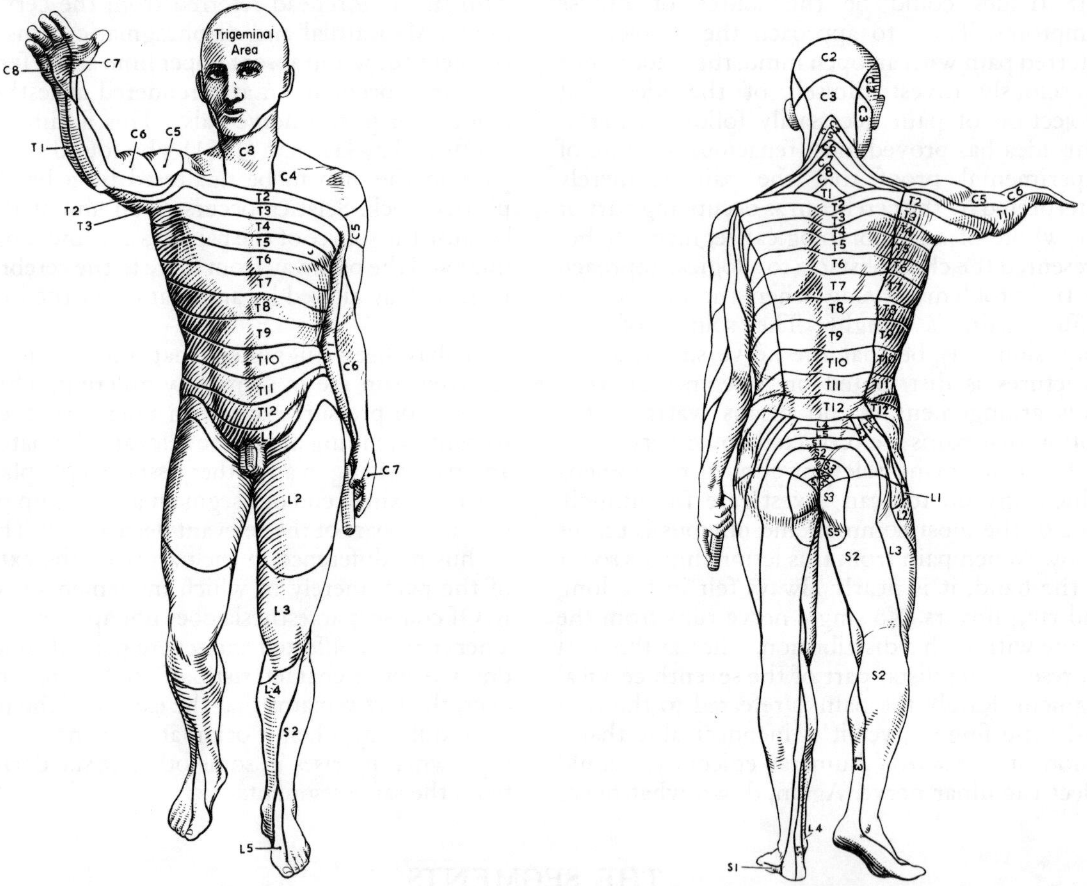


**Fig. 3.** The dermatomes. Anterior and posterior views of the embryological segmentation of the skin. Note how the circular arrangement at the trunk has suffered deformation at the lower cervical and lower lumbar regions where the dermatomes have been drawn out into the limbs. These diagrams give an adequate impression of the general arrangement but do not allow for the considerable overlap. Only the central portion of each dermatome is outlined.

## Dermatomes

These vary somewhat in shape from person to person. Judging by the distribution of paraesthesia in known root lesions in the neck, there are marked individual discrepancies. If, for example, patients with a cervical disc lesion leading to a seventh root paresis (as judged by the pattern of muscular weakness) are questioned about the site of the pins and needles that they experience in their fingers, a few state that all five digits are affected; some all four fingers but not the thumb; most the index, long and ring fingers; some the index and long finger; some the long and ring fingers; and some only the index or only the long finger. Yet in each case the pattern of muscle weakness shows that the seventh cervical root is compressed. Hence, one must infer that the distal cutaneous area supplied by one nerve root is very variable. One reason for this variability was put forward by Schwartz (1956). At cervical laminectomy he noticed twigs running to join the posterior root of the adjacent segment. He therefore dissected 13 normal necks and found such anastomotic rootlets in each. The sixth and seventh roots were those most often connected.

In 1933, Foerster mapped out the dermatomes afresh. The reader will note that his maps agree much more closely with clinical findings than do the charts found in standard neurological textbooks (see Fig. 3). They give merely a general outline of the central part of many of the skin segments. Since the outline of a pain is so often used by the orthopaedic physician to single out the segment containing the lesion, he needs a much more accurate chart of the contours of each overlapping dermatome. In previous editions I have contented myself with reproducing Foerster's diagrams. In this edition, I have permitted myself a few amendments, in those cases where clinical findings have consistently shown a minor discrepancy.

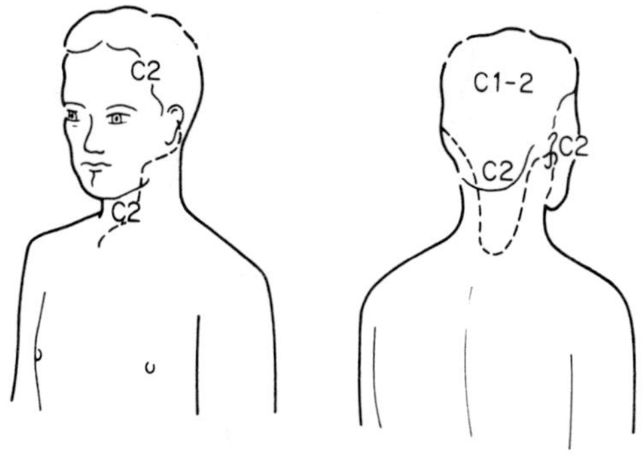


**Fig. 4.** Second cervical dermatome.

*Cervical 1 and 2.* The scalp, the central part of the front and back of the neck, the side of the head, the upper half of the ear, the cheek and upper lip (Fig. 4).

*Cervical 3.* The entire neck, the lower mandibular area, the chin and the lower half of the ear (Fig. 5).

*Cervical 4.* The shoulder area, the front of the upper chest, the lower half of the neck (Fig. 6).

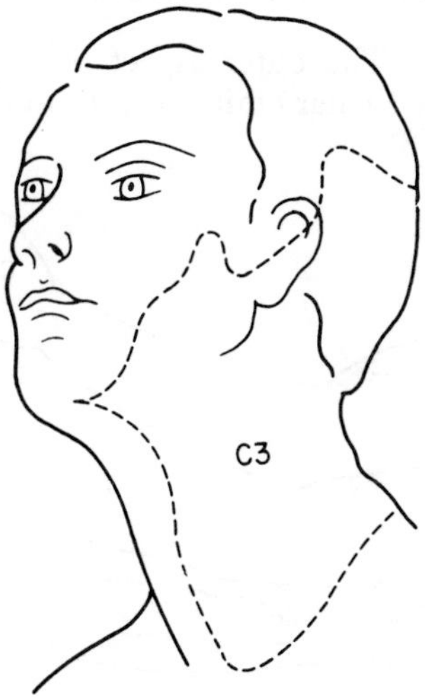


**Fig. 5.** Third cervical dermatome.

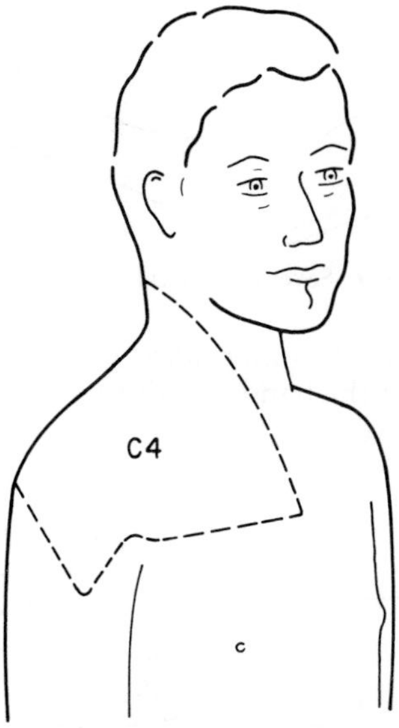


**Fig. 6.** Fourth cervical dermatome.

*Cervical 5.* The shoulder, the front of the arm, the forearm as far as the base of the thumb (Fig. 7).

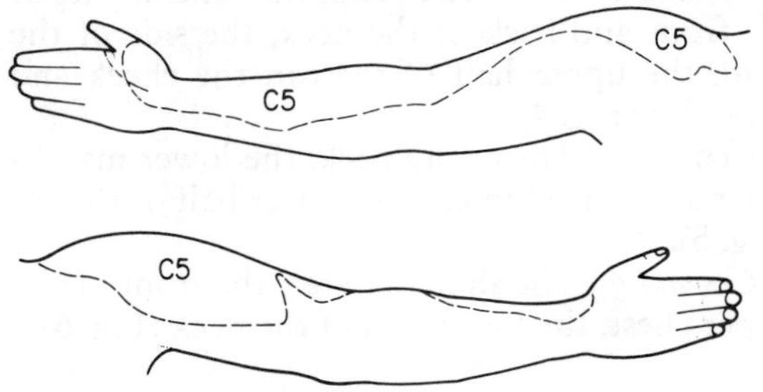


**Fig. 7.** Fifth cervical dermatome.

*Cervical 6.* The outer aspect of the arm and forearm, the thenar eminence, thumb and index finger (Fig. 8).

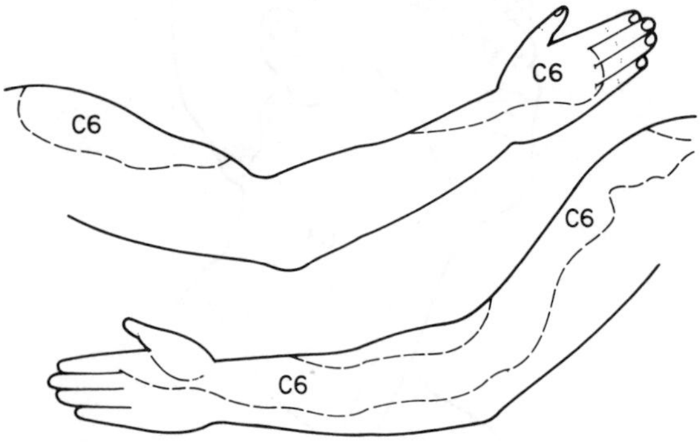


**Fig. 8.** Sixth cervical dermatome.

*Cervical 7.* The back of the arm and forearm to the index, long and ring fingers (Fig. 9).

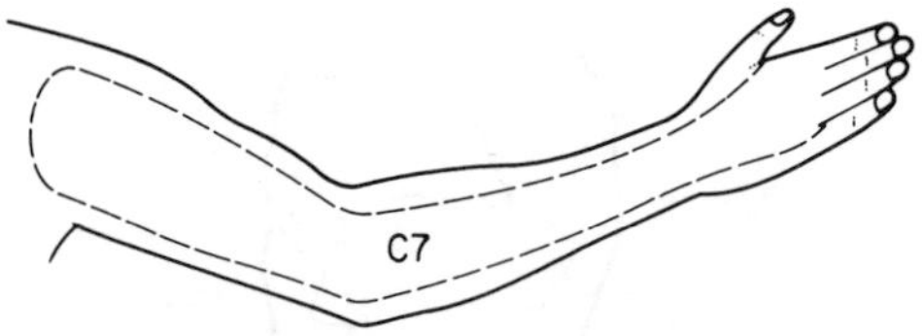


**Fig. 9.** Seventh cervical dermatome.

*Cervical 8.* The inner aspect of the forearm, the inner half of the hand, the third, fourth and fifth digits (Fig. 10).

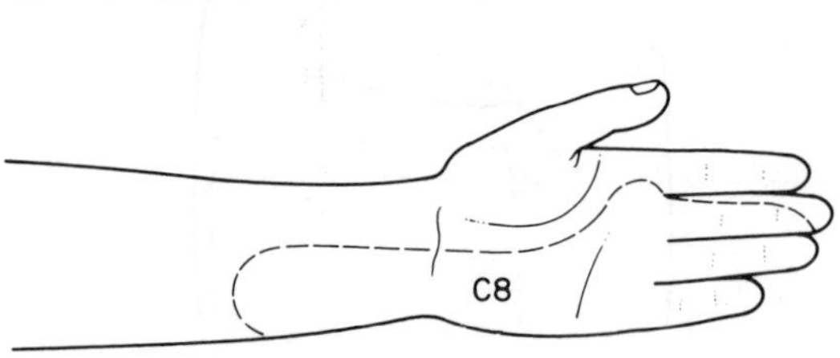


**Fig. 10.** Eighth cervical dermatome.

*Thoracic 1.* The inner side of the forearm as far as the wrist. The upper margin of the dermatome is uncertain (Fig. 11).

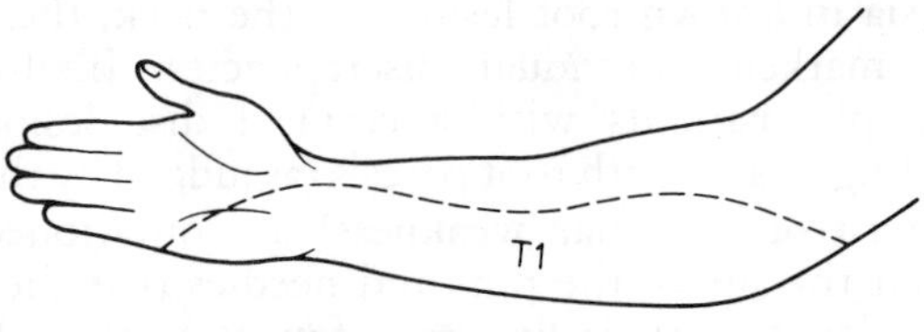


**Fig. 11.** First thoracic dermatome.

*Thoracic 2.* A Y-shaped area stretching from the inner condyle of the humerus up the arm and then dividing into two areas reaching to the sternum anteriorly and the vertebral border of the scapula behind (Fig. 12).

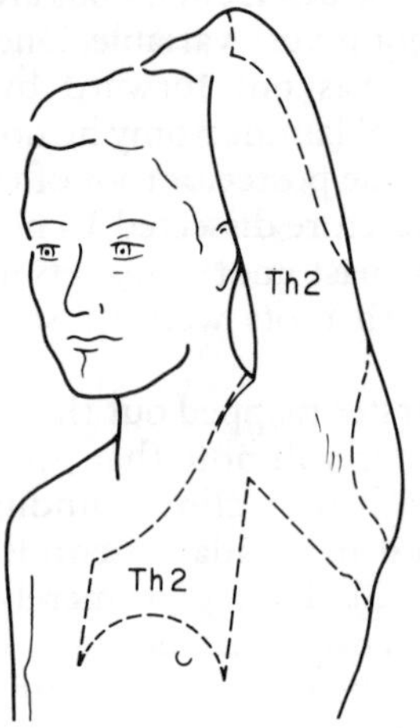


**Fig. 12.** Second thoracic dermatome.

*Thoracic 3.* An area on the front of the chest, and a triangular patch in the axilla (Fig. 13).

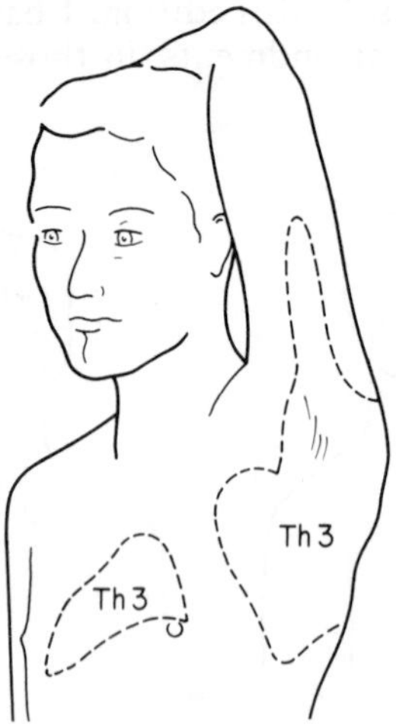


**Fig. 13.** Third thoracic dermatome.

*Thoracic 4, 5 and 6.* These encircle the trunk reaching the level of the nipple (Figs 14, 15).

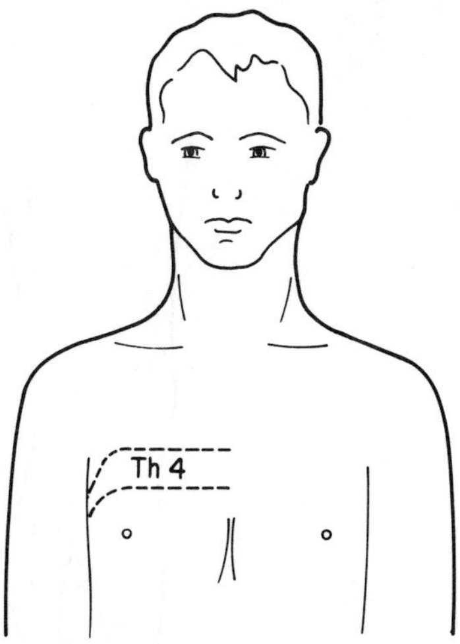


**Fig. 14.** Fourth thoracic dermatome.

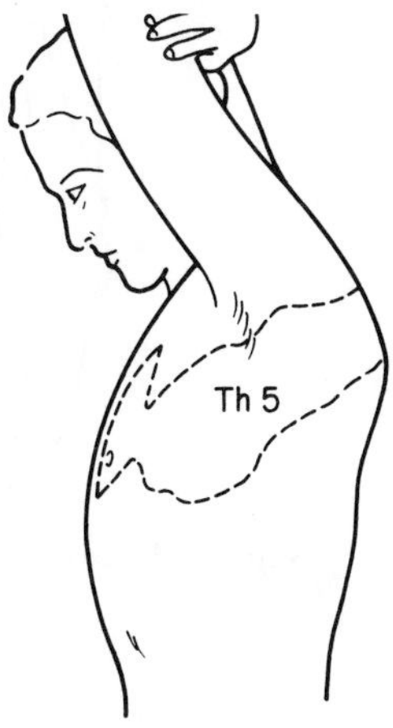


**Fig. 15.** Fifth thoracic dermatome.

*Thoracic 7 and 8.* These encircle the trunk reaching to the lower costal margin.

*Thoracic 9, 10 and 11.* These encircle the trunk reaching the level of the umbilicus (Fig. 16).

*Thoracic 12.* Uncertain. (Probably reaches to the groin and the area between the femoral trochanter and the iliac crest.)

*Lumbar 1.* The lower abdomen and groin; the lumbar region from the second to fourth vertebrae; the upper and outer aspect of the buttock (Fig. 17).

*Lumbar 2.* Two discontinuous areas. The lower lumbar region and upper buttock (Fig. 18). The whole of the front of the thigh (Fig. 19).

*Lumbar 3.* Two discontinuous areas. The upper buttock (Fig. 18). The inner aspect and the front

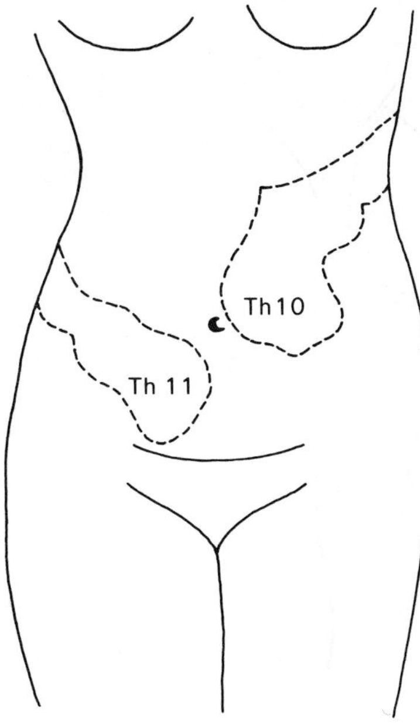


**Fig. 16.** The tenth and eleventh thoracic dermatomes.

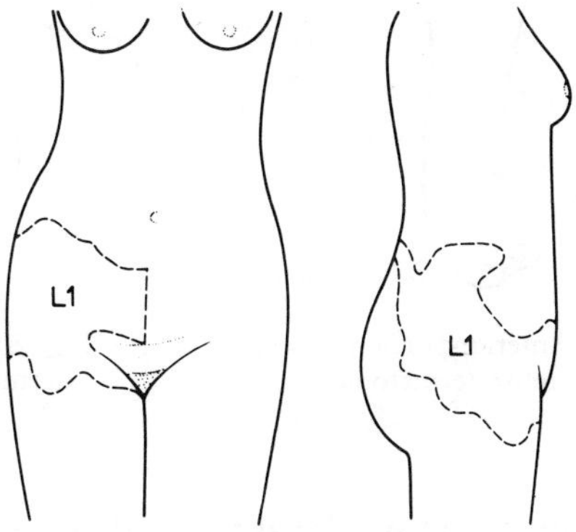


**Fig. 17.** First lumbar dermatome.

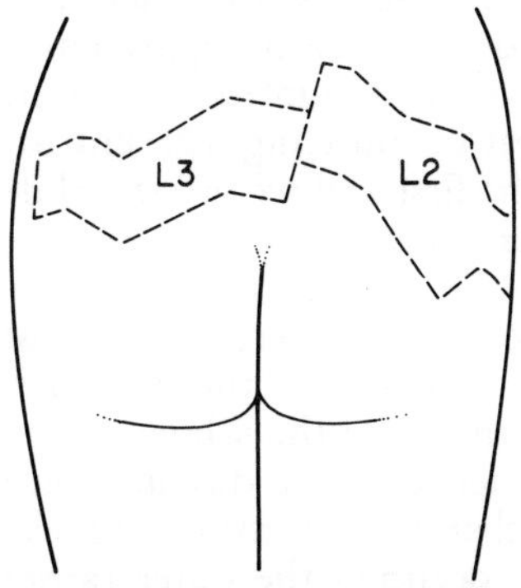


**Fig. 18.** Posterior portion of the second and third lumbar dermatomes.

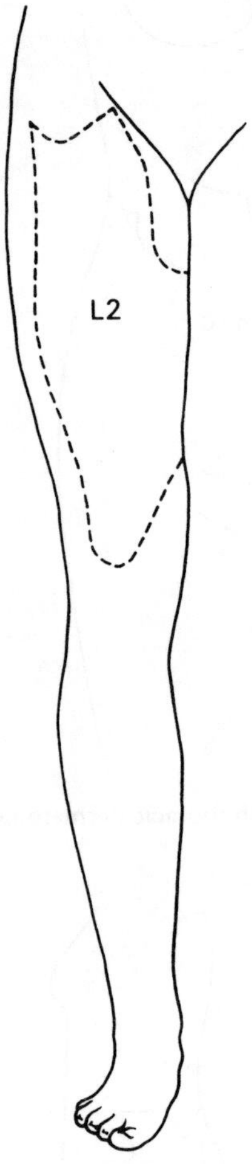


**Fig. 19.** Anterior portion of second lumbar dermatome.

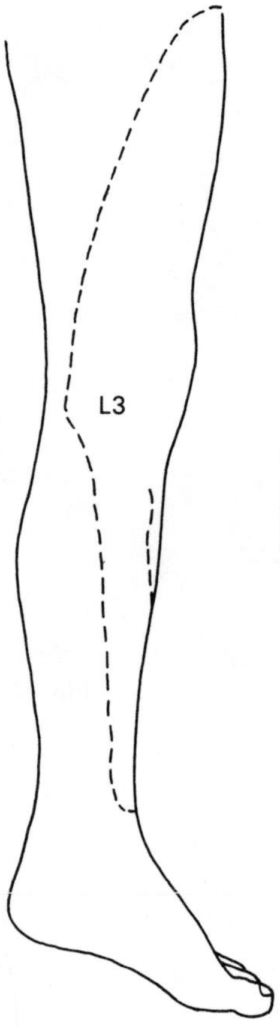


**Fig. 20.** Portion of third lumbar dermatome in the lower limb.

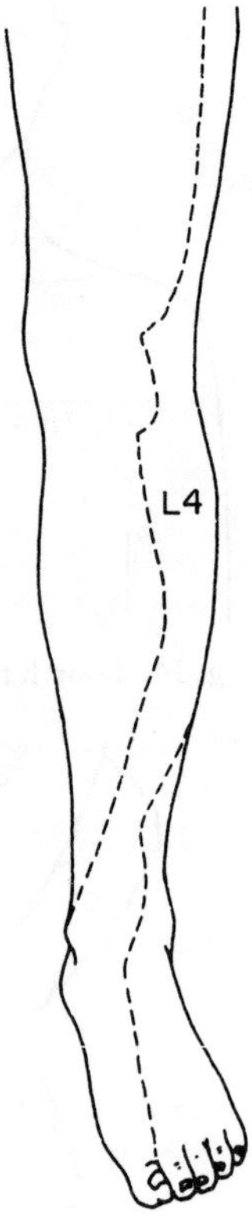


**Fig. 21.** Fourth lumbar dermatome.

of the thigh and leg as far as the medial malleolus (Fig. 20).

It should be noted that cutaneous nerves derived from the first, second and third lumbar roots cross the iliac crest and reach the skin of the upper buttock. No local supply emanates from the fourth and fifth lumbar roots, skin of first to third lumbar origin lying adjacent to the upper extent of the first and second sacral dermatomes at the lower buttock.

*Lumbar 4.* The anterior and medial aspects of the leg according to Foerster; the posteromedial part of the upper calf; the medial side of the dorsum of the foot; the whole hallux (Fig. 21). *N.B.* Experience of the distribution of pain in fourth lumbar root pressure suggests that the dermatome occupies the outer rather than the inner aspect of the thigh and leg, crossing to the inner border of the foot at the ankle.

*Lumbar 5.* The outer aspect of the leg; the dorsum of the whole foot and the first, second and third toes (Fig. 22). The inner half of the sole

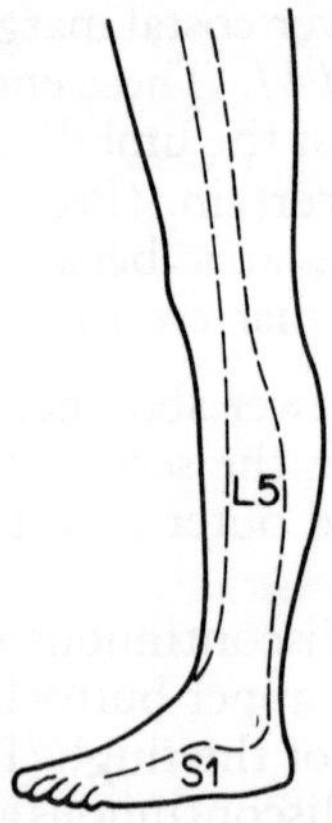


**Fig. 22.** Fifth lumbar dermatome (three inner toes).

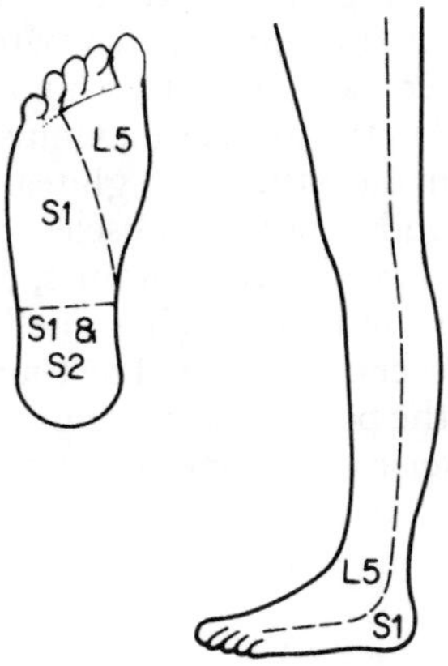


**Fig. 23.** First sacral dermatome (two outer toes).

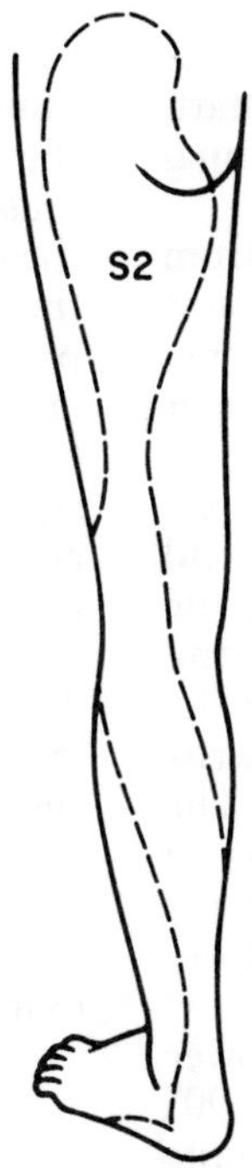

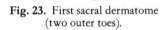

**Fig. 24.** Second sacral dermatome.

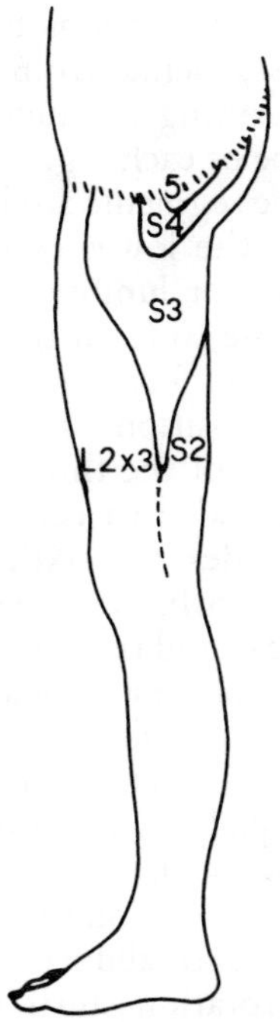


**Fig. 25.** Third sacral dematome. (*After Hansen & Schliack 1962*).

(Fig. 22). *N.B.* The fourth and fifth lumbar dermatomes are all but identical.

*Sacral 1.* The sole of the foot, the two outer toes and the lower half of the posterior aspect of the leg (Fig. 23). *N.B.* During the treatment of chronic sciatica Sicard and Leca (1954) divided the sensory part of the fifth lumbar nerve root in 49 patients and the first sacral root in 83 patients. They found a narrow band of cutaneous analgesia along the posterior aspect of the thigh in each case, and that the first and second toes became numb after section of the fifth lumbar posterior root, and the outer two toes after section at the first sacral level. This fits in extremely accurately with the usual distribution of pain in sciatica and affords the first experimental evidence of a posterior crural extension of these two dermatomes.

*Sacral 2.* The back of the whole thigh, leg, sole and the plantar aspect of the heel (Fig. 24).

The fourth lumbar to second sacral dermatomes were outlined afresh after division of one root by Cole et al. (1968), and the areas described above were confirmed.

*Sacral 3.* A circular area around the anus. A narrow strip following the inguinal ligament and running down the inner side of the thigh to the knee. If this is correct, the analogy with the second thoracic dermatome is close. Fig. 25 shows the third sacral dermatome in the position that clinical considerations had suggested (Hansen & Schliack 1962). Bohn et al. (1956) state that stimulation of the second and third sacral roots sets up pain in the groin; and of the fourth sacral root, pain in the coccyx and rectum. It follows that pain may be referred to the groin in three different ways: (*a*) by ordinary segmental reference along the twelfth thoracic or first lumbar dermatome; (*b*) as part of third sacral reference; or (*c*) as a common site for extrasegmental dural reference, e.g. in lumbago.

*Sacral 4.* Saddle area, anus, perineum, scrotum and penis, labium and vagina, inner uppermost thigh.

*Sacral 5.* The coccyx.

## EMBRYOLOGICAL DERIVATION

The dermatomes do no more than represent the original relationship to the trunk of the limb buds at the earliest stage of development of the embryo. At the end of a month's development the limb buds appear as raised papules at each side of the neck and caudal region. During growth, these projections draw out into themselves the segments from which they start, thereby deforming at these areas the original circular shape of each segment.

Thus, some segments are largely missing from the trunk in the lower cervical upper thoracic and in the lower lumbar upper sacral regions; they have gone to form the limbs. If the upper limb is held out horizontally, thumb upwards, the original position of the bud is recreated. Thus, the base of the thumb represents the end of the elongated fifth cervical dermatome, the thumb and index the sixth, the long and ring fingers the seventh, the ring and little fingers the eighth cervical, and the ulnar border of the wrist and forearm the first thoracic dermatome. The third to twelfth thoracic segments suffer no comparable deformation; the lower merely come to slope obliquely downwards anteriorly to form the abdominal wall.

The original position of the bud for the lower limb is recreated by abduction of the thigh to 90° and lateral rotation until the big toe points vertically. The second and third lumbar segments now lie uppermost, i.e. the adductor and quadriceps muscles covered by the second and third dermatomes, the former extending from groin to patella, the latter covering the same crural area but extending down the front of the leg to just above the ankle. The lower part of the quadriceps muscle and the front of the leg form the fourth lumbar myotome, which is also represented in the buttock by the gluteus medius and minimus muscles. The dermatome occupies the outer leg, the dorsum and inner border of the foot as far as the big toe. Of course, each segment also takes part in the sacrospinalis muscle at the appropriate level. The fifth lumbar segment reaches to the hallux, forming, together with the first sacral segment, the foot and calf. The dermatome ends at the three inner toes. These two myotomes are also represented in the gluteus maximus and take a small share in the other two gluteal muscles. The hamstring and upper calf muscles are formed from the upper two sacral myotomes, except for the biceps femoris muscle which is chiefly derived from the third sacral segment. The fourth sacral segment forms the perineum and anus, where the myotome and dermatome once more correspond exactly.

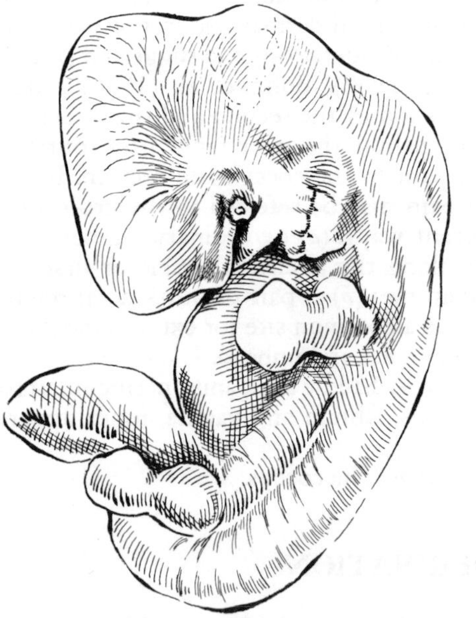

**Fig. 26.** A human embryo five and a half weeks old. (*After Hill*).

## Visceral Embryology

For the convenience of those faced with thoracic or abdominal pain, a list of the approximate segmental derivations of the viscera is appended.

| | |
|---|---|
| Heart | C8–T4 |
| Lungs | T2–5 |
| Oesophagus | T4–5 |
| Stomach and duodenum | T6–8 |
| Liver and gall bladder | T7–8 right |
| Pancreas | T8 left |
| Small intestine | T9–10 |
| Appendix and ascending colon | T10–L1 |
| Epididymis | T10 |
| Ovary, testis and suprarenal | T11–12, L1 |
| Bladder fundus, Kidney, Uterine fundus | T11–L1 |
| Colonic flexure | L2–3 |
| Sigmoid colon and rectum, Cervix*, Neck of bladder, prostate and urethra | S2–5 |

*Theobald et al. (1966) do not agree that the cervix uteri refers pain to the lower sacral dermatomes. They have provoked pain from the cervix by electric stimulation and find that it is felt at first 4 cm above the symphysis pubis. It spreads to the whole hypogastrium, occupying the triangle formed by a horizontal line joining the anterior superior iliac spines and the inguinal ligaments. This corresponds to a reference within the tenth thoracic to first lumbar dermatomes.

## Discrepancies between Dermatomes and Myotomes

There are eight areas where the skin and the structure it covers have different embryological derivations. They are the head, the scapular, pectoral, and intrathoracic regions, and the hand, buttock, thigh and scrotum. Discrepancies also occur within the abdomen but do not appreciably concern the practitioner of orthopaedic medicine.

*Head.* When the embryo is about four weeks old, the projection that will form the head turns twice in the course of growth until it is folded forward on itself like an inverted J. Meanwhile the future mandibular region has appeared as an anterior fold. These two protuberances then fuse about the gap that forms the buccal cavity. In other words, the whole of the head and face as far as the mouth is developed from the back of the neck, and only the lower jaw region develops from the front of the neck. The head and face are formed from the upper two cervical segments.

The nerve that conducts sensory impulses from the skin of the face and scalp as far back as the vertex is the fifth cranial. There is, then, no nerve along which a pain could run from the back of the neck to the forehead. Since such reference of pain is common, it illustrates that a referred pain does not run down a somatic nerve but represents an error in perception. The patient feels a pain somewhere within, or, when the strength of the stimulus is great enough, diffused all over the segment in which it arises.

*Scapular Region.* The growth of the bud that is to become the upper limb draws the lower cervical and uppermost thoracic segments out into itself. The scapula and its muscles (including the latissimus dorsi) are derived from the middle and lower cervical segments, yet the skin overlying them and the ribs beneath them are formed from thoracic segments. Hence, pain in the upper posterior part of the thorax has a cervical or scapular origin if it radiates to the shoulder and upper limb and an upper thoracic origin if it radiates to the front of the chest.

*Pectoral Region.* The interposition is the same as at the scapula. The intercostal muscles, the ribs and the overlying skin form part of the thoracic segments, whereas the pectoral muscles are developed from the lower part of the neck.

*Intrathoracic Region.* The diaphragm is developed largely from the third and fourth cervical segments. The heart forms part of the upper three thoracic segments. Pain from either structure may, therefore, radiate to the shoulder. From the myocardium it may also spread to the arm as far as the ulnar border of the hand, i.e. to the end of the first thoracic dermatome. Hence, pain referred from the diaphragm, heart or the pectoral muscles may have the same quality and may radiate as far as the shoulder; from the heart or the pectoral muscle the pain may spread along the upper limb. Since all three are thoracic structures the local pains to which they may give rise are indistinguishable to the patient.

*Hand.* The skin of the radial side of the hand is developed from the fifth and sixth cervical segments, whereas the thenar and interosseous muscles form part of the eighth cervical and first thoracic myotomes.

*Buttock.* The skin of the outer buttock is derived from the first lumbar dermatome, overlapping the second and third segments at a small area at the upper inner quadrant (see Figs 17, 18). The gluteal muscles, however, are formed within the fourth lumbar to first sacral segments. Hence, at the upper buttock, these muscles extend further proximally than their relevant dermatomes and come to lie beneath skin of first lumbar provenance.

*Thigh.* Patients suffering from fourth and fifth lumbar nerve root pressure repeatedly describe their pain as spreading to the buttock, then to the thigh. Seldom does the patient say that the pain jumps from buttock to calf omitting the thigh. Yet the fourth and fifth dermatomes begin at, or just above, the knee. It is thus theoretically impossible for pain to be felt in the thigh in sciatica; yet that is, in fact, the common site for severe pain. This phenomenon remained unexplained until Sicard and Leca's findings (1954) after posterior radicotomy at the fifth lumbar and first sacral levels. They were able to demonstrate a narrow band of cutaneous analgesia running along the back of the thigh when either posterior root was divided. Hence, a hitherto unsuspected part of the dermatome has been charted, and accounts for the well known crural radiation of the pain in sciatica.

*Scrotum.* The scrotum is derived from the fourth sacral dermatome, yet it encloses the testicles, which are derived from the two lowest thoracic and first lumbar segments. Hence pain felt within the scrotum may have two sources. On the one hand, lesions at the eleventh or twelfth thoracic levels, or at the first lumbar, by pressing on the relevant nerve root, may give rise to pain felt in one or both testicles. On the other hand, when pressure is exerted at a low lumbar level on the intraspinal course of the fourth sacral nerve root, pain or paraesthesia felt in one or both testicles also results. Oddly enough, the patient never mentions the scrotum. There are thus two levels from which testicular pain may be referred, since skin of fourth sacral provenance covers structures of lowest thoracic and first lumbar origin.

## Exception to Segmental Reference

For reasons that remain obscure, the dura mater does not obey the rules of segmental reference at all. For example, patients with cervical root pressure are frequently encountered, the level of whose lesion is clearly indicated by, say, a seventh root palsy. Yet they often complain of pain running up the neck and through to the forehead (C2, 3) and down towards the lower scapular area (T3, 4, 5, 6). The latter is often the first symptom, interscapular pain transferring itself to the whole of one scapular area before the radiation to the upper limb begins. Thus, in the stage first of central, then of lateral dural pressure, the pain is usually felt in areas derived from a segment quite other than that in due course found to contain the lesion. This was recognized by Brown (1828); Teale (1829) described pain radiating from 'the lower cervical portion of the spinal marrow' not only to the upper limbs but also to the upper thorax. Once the protrusion has reached the nerve root, the pain radiates in the expected way; hence it is irritation of the dura only, not its investment of the nerve root, that sets up pain felt at the wrong level. The reverse phenomenon may be experienced during gradual manipulative reduction at the neck; pain and referred tenderness at the lower scapular area can be made gradually to move upwards and proximally as the displaced fragment is shifted bit by bit towards its bed.

Extrasegmental reference is also common in the lumbar region. Backache caused by pressure on the dura mater at a low lumbar level often radiates to the abdomen or up to the back of the chest. Patients may even state that their lumbago is accompanied by a headache that comes and goes with the lumbar symptoms. In acute lumbago due to a lower lumbar protrusion the pain often radiates to one or both groins, or one or both iliac fossae, thus encroaching on lower thoracic segments. Since the possibility of such segmental transgression has never been described and results in pain whose pathway is anatomically inexplicable, suspicion of renal calculus or appendicitis or neurosis may easily arise, and the removal of the appendix for discogenic pain referred extrasegmentally from the dura mater is by no means uncommon.

Other structures in the neighbourhood of the dura mater do not share its independence from segmental reference of pain; hence the mere fact that the patient describes a reference of pain that is theoretically impossible should at once focus attention on the dura mater. Thus the site of

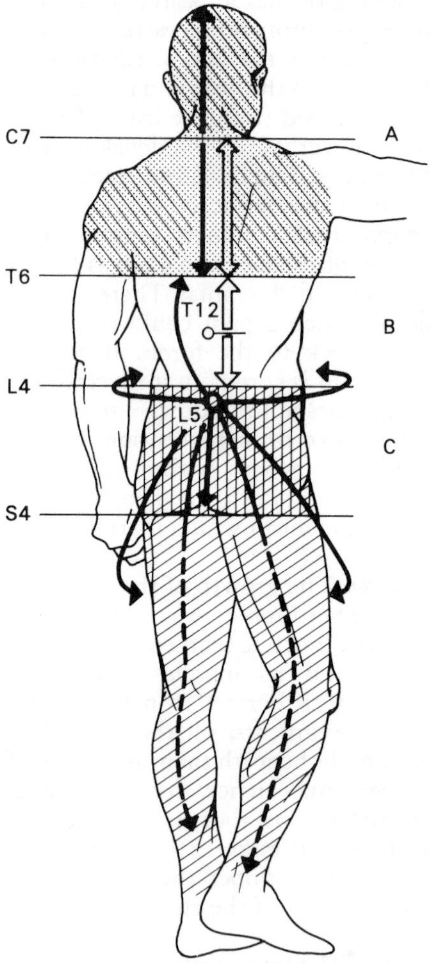


**Fig. 27.** The limits of dural extrasegmental reference. Pain of cervical origin may spread to the head and to the mid-thorax. A middle or lower thoracic lesion may radiate pain to the base of the neck. From a low lumbar level the pain may reach the lower thorax posteriorly, the lower abdomen, the upper buttocks, the sacrum and the coccyx. Dural extrasegmental reference does not extend to the upper limbs or hands, though it often reaches down the lower limbs to the ankles, but not the feet.

pain, taken alone, cannot necessarily differentiate between a cervical or an upper thoracic disc lesion, or a lower thoracic and a lumbar disc lesion.

Extrasegmental reference is also met with in disorders outside the sphere of orthopaedic medicine. For example, in angina the pain is often referred from the myocardium (T1, 2, 3) to the neck and jaw (C3) as well as (properly) to the upper limb.

*Referred Tenderness ('Fibrositis').* The fact that a painful area, though it contains no lesion, is often *diffusely* tender was noted by Lewis in 1942. However, a different type of referred tenderness also exists (Cyriax 1948). When pressure is exerted on the dura mater, usually by a small displaced fragment of disc bulging out the posterior longitudinal ligament, a *localized* tender spot forms within the painful region, and when pressed is instantly identified by the patient as the source of his symptoms. It is a genuine, unilateral, deep tenderness, and not associated with cutaneous hyperalgesia. It is the result of pressure on the dura mater, i.e. a secondary phenomenon, but has been, and still sometimes is, regarded as the primary lesion, the more so since the patient insists that it is the origin of his symptoms. Formerly, 'fibrositis of the trapezius' when it got worse was regarded as leading to 'brachial neuritis', despite the fact that no lesion of this muscle (C2, 3, 4) can refer pain down the upper limb. Today, this localized tender spot in a neck or scapular muscle still leads to concepts such as 'trigger points' and 'myalgic spots' and *cellulite*. These are thought of as primary lesions rather than as a secondary effect of pressure on the dura mater, leading to pain and tenderness felt at a level inconsistent with the segmentation of the body. The formation of metabolites at the muscle has been brought in to explain the tenderness (Weddell et al. 1948) and fatty lobules had a vogue for a time. The simple experiment, whereby the tender spot can be made to shift from place to place in a few seconds, can be confirmed by any physician who manipulates the neck of a sufferer from alleged 'scapular fibrosis'. Moreover, he will find that, when a full and painless range of movement has been restored to the cervical joint, the pain and tenderness in the muscle cease together. Nevertheless, 'fibrositis' has proved a most enduring idea. It was coined by Gowers in 1904 to explain the pathology of lumbago and even now the word remains semi-respectable. The amount of misdirected massage and injections that this secondary tender spot has attracted beggars calculation, and the resulting advantage to lay manipulators has been equally large.

### Referred Pain as a Clue to Segmental Origin

The knowledge that pain is referred segmentally, apart from being employed clinically to estimate the limits within which the source of pain must lie, may also be used experimentally to demonstrate the embryological origin of the tissue concerned. For example, testicular pain is referred along the iliac crest posteriorly, i.e. to the point where the twelfth thoracic and first lumbar dermatomes meet. The capsule of the hip joint provides another good instance. Pain originating in this structure may be felt as a local pain in the groin and buttock referred to the front of the thigh and the knee, and often to the anterior aspect of the leg almost to the ankle. It follows that the capsule of the hip joint is developed within the third lumbar segment. Again the sacroiliac ligaments were regarded by me as developed within the first and second sacral segments. This was confirmed when pain from these ligaments was found to radiate to the posterior thigh and calf. It is a well-established fact that the pain of angina often radiates to the upper neck anteriorly. It seems probable therefore that a small part of the cardiac musculature, presumably of the auricles, is developed from the third cervical segment.

## CONDITIONS FAVOURING REFERENCE OF PAIN

The erroneous perception of the site of a pain depends on four factors: the strength of the stimulus; the position of the painful structure; the depth from the surface, and the nature of the tissue.

### The Strength of the Stimulus

The stronger the stimulus, the less can the patient tell where it originates. For example, arthritis at the shoulder starts as a pain near the shoulder. If it becomes more severe, the pain spreads to the arm and forearm, leaving the shoulder area altogether. When the arthritis regresses the reverse phenomenon takes place. In other words the position of slight pain is often correctly appreciated by the patient; intense pain radiates widely.

The mechanism of this phenomenon remained obscure until 1941. On general grounds it could be assumed that the error lay centrally rather than peripherally, for a larger number of sensory nerve fibres would clearly not be stimulated by an increase in the severity of a lesion unaccompanied by an increase in its extent. The mechanism by which pain is referred was revealed by the experiments of Woolsey et al. (1941) on monkeys. Electroencephalography showed that stimulation of a given area of skin gave rise to an electrical reaction in a fixed and minute area of cortex. Increase in the intensity of the stimulus led to a corresponding increase in the number of cortical cells affected. Such spread to adjacent cells would obviously be interpreted by the patient as an enlargement of the painful area.

The mosaic forming the sensory cortex is arranged dermatome by dermatome, and the extensive reaction resulting from a strong stimulus is confined within the limits of the piece of cortex corresponding to that dermatome. The absence of spread beyond the limit of each piece of cortex is demonstrated most clearly at the two points in the sensory cortex where the arrangement departs from the normal sequence. The region of sensorium corresponding to the fifth cranial nerve adjoins that corresponding to the eighth cervical segment, and the second cervical and first thoracic areas also lie next to each other. Cerebral spread beyond a dermatome would, in these two situations, give rise to bizarre distributions. Clinical experience shows that this type of reference to symptoms (e.g. from the face to the ulnar side of the hand) does not in fact take place. The fact that the diffusion occurs at the cells of the sensory cortex also explains why amputation distal to the lesion does not prevent the radiation of pain to the absent part; for this is still represented—just as before the amputation—in the sensory cortex. The phenomenon that electroencephalography fails to explain is the replacement of an original pain by referred pain, symptoms being no longer experienced at the site of the lesion but distally only.

## The Position of the Painful Structure

Pain will be referred a long way only where elongated segments exist, i.e. in the limbs. The longest segments are the first and second sacral which stretch from mid-buttock to foot.

As a rule, pain is referred only distally, and it is therefore from the proximal ends of the longer segments that diffuse pains usually arise. The structures about the knee and elbow stand almost alone in setting up pain felt to radiate equally in both directions, but the patient seldom fails to realize where his symptoms arise. Pain originating about the wrist or tarsus may also set up an ache in the forearm or leg, but never enough to deceive the patient as to its source. Thus, a diffuse pain may be expected to spring from a structure placed towards the upper end of the painful segment, but by no means necessarily within the area outlined by the patient.

Conversely, the further the lesion lies from the trunk, the more accurate are the patient's sensations. Thus, although there is no theoretical reason why a pain in the foot should not be felt to travel to the buttock, just as a pain arising in the buttock is felt to reach the foot, in fact this does not occur.

## The Depth from the Surface

The more superficially a soft structure lies, the more precise is its localizing ability (Kellgren 1938). One of the most important protective functions of the skin is accurately to localize tactile stimuli. Pains are therefore not referred from its surface; even so, the fingers can localize to within a millimetre, whereas the skin of the back can only do so to within 2 centimetres. It is no part of the ordinary function of deep structures like muscle to localize stimuli accurately. Up to a point, the more deeply a soft structure lies, the greater is its capacity for giving rise to diffuse pains. Lewis (1942) says: 'We assume that a unit area of skin must transmit by its special path, sensory impulses to the sensorum which is able to recognize this unit as the source of the message ... Tissues supplied by deep pain nerves may be regarded as endowed with a similar but simpler form of mechanism, the tissues being represented more in bulk and collectively. The coarsest form of such representation would be that in which tissues in a given segment were represented in such a way that no fine distinctions would be possible in localization.'

While the concept of referred pain as no more than an error in perception on the part of the cerebrum is clear enough, the fact that pain arising from the proximal part of a segment is usually felt diffusely over a much larger area than when its source lies distally gives rise to difficulty. For example, the pain of sacroiliac arthritis may radiate to the calf, but calf pains are very seldom projected as far as the buttock. Further research is required to elucidate the paradox formed by these two conflicting observations—namely, that the buttock and calf possess both common and separate representation in the sensory cortex.

### The Nature of the Structure

When different parts of the nervous system are subjected to pressure, no symptoms whatever need be felt at the point of impact.

Pressure on the spinal cord results in extrasegmental distribution of pins and needles, just as pressure on the dura mater leads to extrasegmental reference of pain. They may be felt in the trunk, all four limbs, the lower limbs or only the feet. Not an uncommon symptom in pressure on the spinal cord in the neck is paraesthesia felt bilaterally from the front of the knee to all the toes, i.e. all the dermatomes from L2 to S1.

Pressure on the dural investment of a nerve root leads to pain, often severe, felt throughout, or in any part of, the relevant dermatome. Pain from neck to hand or from lumbar region to foot is commonplace, but it is equally possible for pain of spinal origin to be felt in, say, the arm or thigh only, or the forearm or leg only. Pins and needles are often, but not invariably, felt distally and occupy the digits appropriate to the dermatome, not to the territory of a nerve trunk.

Pressure on a nerve trunk, by contrast, causes no pain, only distal paraesthesia in an area corresponding to the known cutaneous distribution of that nerve. The symptoms are therefore much the same at whatever point along the main nerve the pressure is exerted. The reason is that a stimulus applied direct to the sensory fibres of a nerve trunk sets up an impulse travelling proximally—an impulse which the sensory cortex interprets as originating from the area of skin supplied by these fibres. Hence no pain is felt at the point of impact. Thus, the spinal cord and nerve trunks refer pain more deceptively than any other structure and much more misleadingly than pressure on a nerve root. This is curious, for the perineurium is not concerned with conduction, and it might have been supposed that pain arising from pressure on a nerve trunk would be felt no more diffusely than those from other fibrous structures in the same neighbourhood.

Pain is apt to be referred from joint capsule, ligament, muscle and bursa in an indistinguishable manner. Bone and periosteum, although the deepest structures of a limb, set up pain that hardly radiates at all. Thus fractures and uncomplicated bony abnormalities due to infection or new growth give rise to pain felt close to their site. There is no obvious reason for this discrepancy between hard and soft structures.

## DIAGNOSIS OF REFERRED PAIN

Referred pain should always be suspected when a patient complains of a deep burning or ache along a limb, from the back of the trunk to its anterior aspect, of 'neuritis', or indeed of any deep pain of large extent and indefinite boundaries. Furthermore, if the painful area presents no physical signs of disorder and there is no disturbance of function of the painful part, the probability is very high that the pain is referred.

Of the structures from which pain is referred, the following concern the orthopaedic physician: joint capsule, tendon, muscle, ligament and bursa, in order of descending importance. To these must be added dura mater and nerve sheath; for it is the orthopaedic physician who is commonly called upon to deal with pressure on dura mater, nerve root or nerve trunk.

There is a great diversity of lesions that can give rise to referred pain and it is essential to consider each case as an isolated problem on the lines described in Chapter 5. Although these pains are often called 'neuritis' by the patient, they are not due to pain arising in, travelling along or even dependent on the integrity of the nerve paths distal to the site of the lesion. They pass upwards from the site of the stimulus by the ordinary sensory paths, but they do not run *down* any structure; their site is merely erroneously localized by the patient's brain, and can be felt in an absent limb, or one deprived of its nerve supply.

### Practical Considerations

Referred pain can be relieved only by treatment to its source. Patients often unwittingly draw attention away from the right spot by insisting that they know from their feelings exactly where the lesion lies, and by rubbing what they maintain is the tender place. Palpation of a tender spot discovered and regarded as relevant by the patient provides a very poor substitute for diagnosis by selective tension. Palpation for tenderness of the structure found to be at fault follows only if the tissue singled out lies within fingers' reach.

It is in difficult cases with referred pain only, without any discomfort felt near the lesion itself, that diagnosis by selective tension is particularly important. Local anaesthesia is then most useful to confirm or disprove the suspected site of the lesion.

Treatment is exactly the same whether a lesion gives rise to referred pain or to local pain only. The diagnostic difficulties are sometimes increased in the former case; but once the right structure has been singled out, it is treated on standard lines. Moreover, since referred pain does not arise from superficial structures, superficial treatment cannot affect its source. Whatever therapeutic measure is employed, it must have a penetrating effect.

CHAPTER 4

# PRESSURE ON NERVES

The layman often uses the word 'neuritis' to designate pain running along a limb. The same pain, when felt at the back of the trunk, is often called 'fibrositis'. The medical profession is apt to use the word 'neuritis' when pain is accompanied by pins and needles. However, paraesthesia, though indicating that some part of the nervous system is at fault, is common to extrinsic and intrinsic disease. External pressure on a normal nerve sets up pins and needles no less than does parenchymatous degeneration. These disorders require radically different treatment and must be distinguished.

Pressure on a nerve from without occupies the territory where the neurologist and the practitioner of orthopaedic medicine meet. The nerves may conduct normally; hence no involvement of the nervous system appears to be present. Examination of the somatic structures may exclude any lesion affecting a moving part of the body. The patient may, therefore, fall between two stools, neither type of examination revealing the existence of a lesion. In fact, the pain results from pressure on a nerve root or nerve trunk insufficient to impair conduction. This possibility has thrown doubt on the view that, for the examination of the peripheral nervous system, estimation of conduction along it suffices (Cyriax 1942).

## PINS AND NEEDLES DUE TO COMPRESSION

This feeling is a most interesting phenomenon, for it appears to provide the only example of a pathognomonic sensation. Lesions of visceral, skeletal or muscular provenance all give rise to identical pains, indistinguishable by the patient. The pains may behave differently (e.g. in colic) but they are identical in quality. Pins and needles, by contrast, arise only from lesions of the nervous, especially the peripheral nervous, system. The different origins of this sensation are set out below.

It is vital to know the exact area where pins and needles are felt. Patients are often very vague, sometimes importantly mistaken, in their recollections. Hence, if paraesthesia is provoked during the clinical examination, this should be interrupted forthwith in order to determine its precise site.

The proximal extent is as important to ascertain as the distal, since the lesion always lies proximal to the upper level of the pins and needles.

### Small Nerve

When pressure is applied to a nerve close to its distal extremity, some pins and needles are felt, but the main symptom is numbness. This occupies the cutaneous area supplied by that nerve; the edge is well defined and towards the centre of the area full anaesthesia is often demonstrable. The analgesic area occupies one aspect of the part. Meralgia paraesthetica is a well-known example of this type of paraesthesia; the numb area lies at the anterolateral aspect of the thigh, the edge is clear, the centre of the region is often anaesthetic, and the numbness more evident to the patient than pins and needles.

### Nerve Trunk—The Release Phenomenon

Minor pressure on the trunk of a nerve sets up pins and needles rather than numbness. They occur as a *release* phenomenon. Faint tingling and numbness appear momentarily when a nerve trunk is first compressed; then nothing is noted until the pressure on the nerve has been released. Painful paraesthesia then comes on some time after the pressure on the nerve trunk ceases. The interval bears a close relationship to the duration of the original pressure. Thus, after five minutes' pressure, the paraesthesia will appear after perhaps 30 seconds; after release from 12 hours' compression, they may not be felt for two to three hours. It is common knowledge that pressure on the sciatic nerve while sitting causes no symptoms; the pins and needles come in when the subject relieves the pressure by standing up. Active movement of the affected digits or stroking the analgesic area of skin usually brings on a shower of pins and needles. This is so wherever along the nerve the point of pressure lies and has no localizing significance. Thus, if moving the fingers provokes pins and needles, it must not be thought that the lesion lies in the forearm or hand. By contrast, if they are elicited by a distant movement, this constitutes the important diagnostic finding. For example, if keeping the shoulders shrugged makes the fingers tingle, it becomes clear that raising the lower trunk of the brachial plexus off the first rib has evoked the release phenomenon.

When a nerve trunk is compressed at the distal part of the upper limb, the release phenomenon ceases to operate. For example, pressure on the ulnar nerve at the elbow causes paraesthesia in the two fingers, which stops a few moments after the pressure is released. Again, when the median nerve is irritated in the carpal tunnel, work involving repeated hand movements is apt to bring on the pins and needles. Curiously enough, this distal change does not occur in the lower limb. If different parts of the sciatic nerve are compressed by, say, sitting on the lower buttock, crossing the knees or applying the outer side of one ankle to the lower thigh, the paraesthesia is felt after the posture has been changed.

The pins and needles are felt only in the distal part of the cutaneous area supplied by that peripheral nerve, no matter at what point in its course the impact occurs; hence *clinical examination must include the full length of the nerve.* The lesion always lies proximal to the upper edge of the paraesthetic area.

Constant pressure on a nerve trunk causes a painless lower motor neurone lesion; there are no pins and needles, but marked numbness.

## Nerve Root—The Compression Phenomenon

The pins and needles are a *pressure phenomenon*, continuing more or less so long as the pressure is sustained. They are abolished instantly by relief from the pressure. Pins and needles in the hand, of however long standing, that result from a cervical disc protrusion, often cease as soon as traction is applied to the neck, and returns when the traction is released. It is very odd that pins and needles should come on with *pressure* on a nerve *root* and with *release of pressure* on a nerve *trunk*. In root pressure, they are felt in the distal extremity of the dermatome, often conspicuously occupying an area not supplied by any one nerve trunk. For example, when a cervical disc protrusion compresses the seventh nerve root, the paraesthesia occupies the index, long and ring fingers—fingers supplied by no one nerve trunk. The paraesthesia has neither edge nor aspect, being felt within the fingers. Stroking the skin may, as in nerve trunk pressure, provoke the pins and needles. However, moving the digits is no longer effective, and this finding may prove helpful when, in a difficult case, distinction must be drawn between pressure on a nerve trunk and a nerve root.

In pressure on a nerve root the pins and needles tend to disappear when the numbness comes on; especially in the lower limb they tend to follow each other rather than coincide—major pressure on the root causing analgesia and minor, pins and needles.

Another major difference exists between pressure on a nerve trunk and on a nerve root. Pressure on a nerve trunk, though it may cause paraesthesia distally, causes no local pain at all. When the pressure is applied to the dural sleeve investing a nerve root, severe pain occupying all or any part of the dermatome results. A nerve is insensitive to pressure along its entire length except at the dural investment of the nerve root (Cyriax 1957*a*). Hence, disc protrusion, since it impinges against the dural sleeve, usually causes severe pain, whereas the same degree of pressure applied a short distance distally along the nerve would have produced no local pain at all. Pain felt in the relevant dermatome has, therefore, a clear significance in distinguishing where along a nerve the impact falls.

At cervical laminectomy, Frykholm (1951*a, b*) showed that stimulation of the anterior division of the nerve root gave rise to deep pain associated with muscle tenderness, thus confirming the views (Cyriax 1948) on the phenomena that had given rise to the idea of 'fibrositis'. He also found that stimulation of the posterior division brought on a more peripheral pain associated with paraesthesia. Since disc protrusions may impinge against one aspect only of a nerve root, they may compress the inferior aspect only and thus affect the motor fibres alone. Or the pressure may come from above, and affect the sensory fibres alone. In consequence, a protruded disc may cause a partial root lesion, sensory or motor, depending on which aspect of the root receives the main impact. Only in the former event are pins and needles brought on.

### Spinal Cord

When the cord is compressed the pins and needles are apt to be bilateral and to ignore the segmentation of the body, occupying areas beyond the cutaneous supply of any one trunk or nerve root. There is no pain and neither moving the digits nor stroking the skin evokes pins and needles. For example, the patient may complain of pins and needles from both patellae to all the toes in each foot, thus spanning five dermatomes. Another interesting complaint is pins and needles in both big toes on neck flexion which ceases after manipulative reduction at the neck.

One cause of pins and needles felt in all limbs or in the upper or the lower limbs only, is a minor degree of pressure on the spinal cord in the neck. When the cord is compressed at its thoracic extent, the paraesthesiae are felt solely in the lower limbs, often only in the feet. Neck flexion is usually the only way to bring the pins and needles on. In central cervical and thoracic disc lesions pins and needles may be felt in the lower limbs, their extrasegmental distribution often providing the diagnostic clue.

## STRETCHING THE NERVE ROOT

Stretching a nerve root whose mobility is impaired may be painful and is sometimes limited in range. The common cause is a disc protrusion and limitation of range occurs only at the lower lumbar levels.

The different ways of stretching the root are given below.

### Straight-leg Raising

When there is impaired mobility of any root between the fourth lumbar and the second sacral, the movement stretching the nerve root is usually painful and restricted in range; moreover, at its extreme, paraesthesia may be evoked at the distal end of the dermatome. Not only is straight-leg raising painful and limited, but neck flexion after the leg has been raised as far as it will go may increase the pain and elicit a shower of pins and needles in the appropriate part of the foot.

### Prone-lying Knee Flexion

This movement stretches the third lumbar nerve root. If a disc protrusion encroaches on the intervertebral foramen, the mobility of this root becomes impaired. In consequence, the movement may be restricted or unilaterally painful at the extreme. Rarely, in addition to the pain, pins and needles are provoked in the anterior tibial area.

### Neck Flexion and Scapular Approximation

When the neck is flexed it is 3 cm longer than in full extension. Hence, when the mobility of the dura mater is impaired at a thoracic or lumbar level, neck flexion often brings on or increases the pain in the lower back or the posterior (seldom the anterior) aspect of the thorax.

Scapular approximation pulls on the eighth cervical and first thoracic nerve roots, thus drawing the dura mater upwards in the same way as does neck flexion. Hence, in thoracic intraspinal lesions the pain at the back or the front of the chest is brought on not only by neck flexion, but also by scapular approximation (Cyriax 1950*a*, *b*). (In lumbar disc lesions, scapular approximation does not alter the pain.) The fact that movement of the scapula has induced posterior thoracic symptoms is apt to be misinterpreted and is thought to incriminate muscles such as the rhomboid and lower trapezius. In fact, the resisted scapular movements do not hurt and, when the active movement already found painful is repeated passively by the examiner, this does hurt. In this way it can be shown that the muscles moving the scapula are not themselves involved.

### Neck Movements

When a cervical nerve root is compressed, one or other of the neck movements may increase the root pain in the upper limb and also provoke pins and needles in the fingers of the appropriate dermatome. In osteophytic root palsy this movement is likely to be side flexion towards the painful side. Sometimes a neck movement evokes pain and paraesthesia only if the upper limb is placed in a special position first, most often held out forwards.

Since neck flexion stretches the dura mater down the whole length of the vertebral column, the fact that this hurts must not be regarded as showing the lesion to lie in the neck.

## PRESSURE ON A NERVE

Pressure on a nerve root causes pain felt in the whole, or any part of the relevant dermatome. Pressure on a nerve trunk is painless; only distal paraesthesia results. Neuritis and neuralgic amyotrophy hurt, although they too affect peripheral nerves. The situation is very confusing, and a most difficult task is to distinguish between painful and painless nerve lesions and their differentiation from the similar pains that arise from disorders of the moving parts.

When the external aspect of a nerve or a nerve root is compressed, none of the classical signs of neurological disease is necessarily detectable. The first paper on affections confined to the external aspect of nerves appeared more than 40 years ago (Cyriax 1942). A book describing the same entities more fully, *Peripheral Entrapment Neuropathy*, appeared in 1963 (Kopell & Thompson).

Pain may originate from pressure on a nerve root, but conduction along it may remain normal. No pins and needles or numbness need be experienced. Stretching the nerve root may leave the pain unaltered and its range full. Nothing in such cases suggests pain arising from any part of the nervous system. However, the possibility arises when the joints, muscles, etc., comprising the same segment as the painful area are entirely normal. This finding draws attention to pressure on a nerve root insufficient in degree to impair either conduction or mobility. Obviously, interference with the external aspect of the root need not be great enough to be transmitted to the conducting element. Secondary parenchymatous change may, of course, develop in due course, if the pressure increases. When these neurological signs appear the label 'neuritis' might seem warranted, but leads in fact to an error in emphasis, focusing attention on the secondary, rather than the primary organic process.

### Rheumatoid Perineuritis

The careful pathological studies of Freund et al. (1942) have shown that long-standing rheumatoid arthritis is often complicated by sharply defined inflammatory nodules in the perineurium. These authors suggest that the paraesthesia and trophic cutaneous changes occurring in chronic cases are due to irritation of the conducting fibres of the nerve by such nodules, since microscopy revealed no abnormality of the nerve parenchyma. Gibson et al. (1946) showed that nodular polymyositis also occurs in advanced rheumatoid arthritis. The nodules in muscle and nerve sheath are absent in ankylosing spondylitis. Arteritis of the vasa nervorum may lead to peripheral nerve palsies, chiefly in patients with severe generalized rheumatoid disease (Weller et al. 1971). The event carries a bad prognosis, a quarter of such patients dying within 12 months.

## SIGNS OF PRESSURE ON A NERVE

The signs fall into seven groups, but all are seldom present in one case. Occasionally no physical signs can be detected, the diagnosis being established on the history, the patient's sincerity, the manner of onset and subsequent migration of the symptoms, the quality of the pain and the absence of signs of any other disorder or of psychogenic pain.

It is noticeable that in almost every case nerve sheaths are affected where they lie in close contact with bone or cartilage or traverse a foramen.

### Pain on Stretching the Nerve

This is the outstanding sign only when the dural sheath of the lower two lumbar and upper two sacral nerve roots is affected; the movement that stretches the nerve, i.e. straight-leg raising, is often limited. The hamstrings go into spasm when traction is exerted via the sciatic nerve trunk on the compressed and therefore immobile root. In third root compression full straight-leg raising is painful only at its extreme, and prone-lying knee flexion may be limited and is nearly always painful at full range. Full extension of the wrist occasionally hurts when the elbow is extended but not when this is kept flexed in cases of compression of the median nerve in the carpal tunnel. Movement of the scapula may painfully stretch the first and second thoracic nerve roots in disc lesions at these levels, and the trapezius may contract to keep the scapula involuntarily elevated to prevent further traction on a recently overstretched axillary nerve.

### Provocation of Pins and Needles

In primary affections of the conducting core of

a nerve, i.e. in neuritis, no movement evokes the pins and needles; they come and go spontaneously. When pressure is applied to a nerve, paraesthesia is provoked in two ways—by active movement of the affected digits and by some distant movement. The mere fact that movement brings the pins and needles on shows the interference to be external. The nature of the distant movement indicates where the pressure is exerted. For example, when elevation of the scapulae brings on a patient's nocturnal pins and needles in the hands, the lower trunk of the brachial plexus has clearly been lifted off the first rib. If neck flexion evokes pins and needles in the lower limbs, pressure is being exerted on the cervical extent of the spinal cord. If straight-leg raising causes a shower of pins and needles in the foot, a low lumbar nerve root is compressed at the intervertebral foramen.

### Tenderness and Swelling of the Nerve Sheath

Both are presumably present in every case and, where practicable, the point should be sought where pressure on the nerve reproduces the distant pain. Swelling occurs at the ulnar nerve in the groove at the elbow and the median nerve in the carpal tunnel. A neuroma, discoverable only at operation, is always found in the later stage of Morton's metatarsalgia.

### Postural Deformity

In severe sciatic and cervical disc lesions, lateral deviation of the spine develops from adopting the posture best calculated to relieve pressure on the nerve root. Cubitus valgus, whether developmental or the result of mal-union of a fracture near the elbow, often results in pressure on the ulnar nerve.

### Evidence of Secondary Parenchymatous Change

Interference with conduction occurs if pressure on the nerve sheath is sufficient also to interfere with the parenchyma of the nerve. At the facial nerve only when palsy supervenes does the condition become apparent at all. If conduction becomes impaired later, a diagnosis of pressure on the external surface of a nerve is clearly correct.

### Cessation of Symptoms for the Duration of Local Anaesthesia

This is the best method of confirming a tentative diagnosis. If this is correct, and the anaesthetic solution reaches the nerve sheath, relief is achieved within a minute or two, and lasts for about an hour and a half. In many cases, a lasting therapeutic effect is also achieved; hence local anaesthesia should always be employed in a doubtful case.

### Relief Following Steroid Infiltration

An injection of triamcinolone into the carpal tunnel is almost always followed by weeks or months of, or even permanent, relief. Hence it provides a good diagnostic test in uncertain cases.

Severe denervation can be prevented in facial palsy by the administration of prednisolone, started during the first two days (Taverner et al. 1971).

## Individual Lesions

These are merely listed, since they are dealt with in the appropriate chapters of this book. They also appear in Kopell and Thompson's book, where my original descriptions have been considerably expanded.

Facial nerve palsy (not dealt with)
Cervical disc lesion
Thoracic outlet syndrome
Axillary nerve palsy
Radial nerve palsy at mid-humerus
Ulnar nerve palsy at the elbow
Carpal tunnel syndromes
Ulnar nerve palsy at the pisiform
Contusion of the radial nerve at the wrist
Pressure on digital nerve in the palm
Thoracic disc lesion
Meralgia paraesthetica
Compression of the anterior cutaneous nerve of the thigh
Compression of the obturator nerve
Lumbar disc lesion
Pressure on the tibial nerve at the knee
Pressure on the long saphenous nerve at the knee
Pressure on the common peroneal nerve at the fibula
Pressure on the superficial peroneal nerve at mid-leg
Tarsal tunnel syndromes
Bruising of the first plantar digital nerve
Morton's metatarsalgia

## TREATMENT

In slight cases, prevention of the causative strain may suffice. Thus, avoidance of prolonged flexion of, or pressure on, the elbow allows irritation of the ulnar nerve at the medial condyle to subside. If mild symptoms of pressure on the lower trunk of the brachial plexus from the first rib appear late in life, prohibition against carrying weights and keeping the scapulae elevated often secure relief.

If simple measures fail, and the symptoms are severe, operation is indicated, thus:

1. Removal of the cause of pressure. When a cervical rib, an osteoma or a protruded intervertebral disc causes pressure on nervous tissue, it may be excised. Intra-articular displacements are often amenable to manipulative reduction. Ganglia can often be aspirated or digitally burst.
2. Elongation of the structure maintaining the position of the skeletal projection. This applies to division of the scalenus anterior muscle in cases of cervical rib. The rib can then sink away from the nerve trunks.
3. Alteration of the course of the nerve. If neuritis is developing, anterior transposition of the ulnar nerve at the elbow is indicated.
4. Enlargement of the foramen by which a nerve pierces a ligament or fascia. This applies especially to meralgia paraesthetica where incision of the foramen of exit of the lateral cutaneous nerve of the thigh may afford relief.
5. Division of the ligament confining the nerve. This applies particularly to division of the transverse carpal ligament in median nerve pressure.
6. Removal of the nerve. This may be required at the sole of the foot and in meralgia paraesthetica.
7. Postherpetic neuralgia. E–5–2 bromovinyl 2 deoxyuridine given in doses of 7 mg per kg of body-weight causes arrest of further vesicles within 24 hours, and disappearance of those already formed in 2 days (Selby et al. 1979). This was confirmed by Clercq et al. in 1980.

CHAPTER 5

# THE DIAGNOSIS OF SOFT TISSUE LESIONS

The clinical work of the orthopaedic physician consists largely in the diagnosis and treatment of soft tissue lesions. Lesions in the moving parts occur frequently, throughout the body, at all ages, and the symptoms may mimic a number of visceral or neurological diseases. In purely orthopaedic and neurological cases diagnosis is exact: there is no doubt about the site of a fracture, the nature of operative intervention, or the type of a nerve lesion. It is therefore mainly in the non-surgical conditions affecting the soft tissues, i.e. the fibrosis in moving parts that follows overuse or injury, the various disorders affecting joints, and pressure on the sheath of nerves, nerve roots and dura mater, that the orthopaedic physician exercises his diagnostic capacity. Radiological criteria are seldom helpful, and may prove misleading; thus the orthopaedic surgeon's standby does not apply.

One of the two main characteristics of deeply seated lesions is the discrepancy between the site of the pain and the site of the lesion. Hence the physician must define the source of the identical diffuse pains that may arise from muscle, tendon, joint capsule, ligament, bursa, dura mater or nerve root. The other outstanding feature of such pains is the paucity of objective physical signs to which they may give rise; hence diagnosis may rest largely on the correlation of a series of subjective data. This elicitation and interpretation of physical signs requires practice. No effort must be spared to localize exactly the source of each pain before treatment can usefully begin. For example massage, unless applied to the exact site of a lesion, can do no good. No less accuracy is essential when local injections are employed, since the solution must be introduced at some definite spot. Likewise, when manipulative measures are contemplated, the site and type of the lesion determine whether they are indicated and what form they shall take. If pain arises in a moving part, some movement or some posture must bring it on. This complex is explored and interpreted in the same way as a simultaneous equation.

This chapter describes the principles of a system of diagnosis that reveals the origin of a pain in a high proportion of cases no matter where the symptoms happen to be perceived. Since pain in lesions of the moving parts is brought on largely by tension, diagnosis depends on applying tension in different ways to different tissues and asking the patient to report the result. (Anoxia and local pressure are the other ways of eliciting or aggravating these pains.) The approach is purely mechanical and leads to full anatomical—though not always pathological—definition of the site of a painful lesion. A complex of painful movements is logically resolved into a number of simple components, each of which is then tested separately. Importance is laid equally on what movements prove painful and/or limited and what movements are of full range and/or painless. This is an approach almost mathematical in its precision and is suited to the mechanical function of the structures under examination.

The patient's cooperation is essential. He is asked to state which activities hurt and which do not, disregarding where the pain is felt and what sort of pain it is. This makes diagnosis more difficult when there is pain in the absence of movement; it is hard for a patient to tell what movement hurts him when he is already in constant pain. In such cases he is apt, unless the nature of the question is explained carefully, to state that all movements hurt, merely meaning that the constant pain continues unabated; he must realize that the examiner is looking for movements that *alter* the symptoms. To get a patient to perform a series of movements at several joints, to say which bring on or increase the pain and which do not, and to let the responses build up a pattern; to perform special tests for certain structures; to search for tenderness of the structure identified, if it is accessible; to induce local anaesthesia at the chosen spot and to await the patient's verdict—all this takes time and patience.

*Positive signs must always be balanced by corroborative negative signs.* If a lesion appears to lie at, or near, one joint, this region must be examined for signs identifying its site. It is equally essential for the adjacent joints and the structures about them to be examined so that, by contrast, their normality can be established. These negative findings then reinforce the positive findings emanating elsewhere; then only can the diagnosis be regarded as established.

At any examination of which the patient's cooperation forms part, the opportunities for deception are many. Since in many cases the only final criterion of a correct diagnosis is the induction of local anaesthesia—the response to which is often also a subjective phenomenon—the physician should be on his guard against feigned illness; for patients have learned that the symptoms least capable of objective evaluation are those with which the orthopaedic physician most often deals. Thus, while it is no substitute for a diagnosis to regard all patients with obscure pains as having a minor or neurotic disability, a balance must be maintained between credulity and excessive scepticism.

### The 'Correct' Pain

It is often not enough to discover that a certain movement evokes pain; care must be taken to make sure that it reproduces the very pain of which the patient complains. For example, a patient with slight backache and a pain in his thigh, or some scapular discomfort and pain in his upper limb, may well have a minor spinal disc lesion responsible for the ache in his trunk but severe arthritis in the hip or shoulder joint causing his important symptoms. In this type of case, the spinal movements do cause some local discomfort, i.e. they set up *a* pain, but inquiry will reveal that it is not the patient's pain. When the hip or shoulder is examined, the movements elicit the symptoms that the patient recognizes, i.e. *the* pain.

When pain in separate areas is evoked in this way, the situation must be clarified by giving greater weight to the movement provoking the recognized symptom. This must appear obvious, but the point is made since lay manipulators take the opposite view. Osteopaths, ever anxious to inculpate the spine as the source of any symptom, regard discomfort on a spinal movement, or even painless limitation of movement at an intervertebral joint, as a good reason for insisting that the distant pain originates from the spine which, by corollary, requires manipulation. Consequently many patients, especially those with arthritis at shoulder or hip, receive endless osteopathy to the unaffected spinal joints, without avail.

## OBJECTS OF DIAGNOSTIC MOVEMENTS

Diagnosis in soft tissue lesions must be approached indirectly. No physician would regard palpation of the chest as the chief method of diagnosis in heart disease; even less would he regard an area of intercostal tenderness as indicating which valve was affected. Palpation of the spine plays little part in assessing the integrity of the spinal cord. Function is tested by remote signs, e.g. feeling the pulse, ascertaining the blood pressure, noting the plantar response, testing urine and so on. For the same reason, immediate palpation of a painful area must be avoided in locomotor disorders. The state of a joint, muscle or nerve is assessed by discovering how well it functions; palpation may or may not follow, and is confined to the tissue identified as at fault, and then only if it lies within reach of the finger.

The object of the diagnostic movements described here is to discover where, i.e. about or at which joint, the symptoms arise. This is not as easy as might be expected; indeed, to tell whether a pain in the buttock has a lumbar, sacroiliac or gluteal origin can prove extremely difficult. This object is best achieved by carrying out a swift review from end to end of the tissues forming the relevant segment. For example, a patient with obscure pain in the arm should receive a preliminary gross examination from neck to fingers in an endeavour to ascertain roughly the relevant area. This part is then examined in detail, in the sure knowledge that the lesion lies within known limits.

## Contractile and Inert

This is a vital distinction. When a voluntary movement is performed, the joint moves and the muscles move it; both are involved. Hence, if an active movement hurts, either tissue may be at fault. Lesions, therefore, in these two types of tissue must be separated on the lines of a simultaneous equation in mathematics.

### Contractile

By *contractile* is meant those structures that form part of a muscle—namely the belly itself, the tendon and their bony insertions. From such structures pain may be elicited both by active contraction and by passive stretching in the opposite direction. But neither of these tests applies much tension to a muscle and both may prove misleadingly negative. The real test for a muscle is contraction against resistance, whereby strong tension is applied to the lesion.

It can be argued academically that neither a tendon nor the bone adjacent to a muscular insertion is a contractile structure; this is true. But in so far as they are attached to the belly of a muscle, they remain contractile clinically, in the sense that contraction of the muscle belly applies tension to them, thus evoking pain. Pain on resisted contraction is caused also when (*a*) a fracture lies close enough to a muscular insertion for the strain to move the broken ends on each other or (*b*) an inflamed lymphatic gland, bursa or abscess lies directly under a muscle.

If the movements show the lesion to lie in a contractile structure, auxiliary tests exist that disclose which one of several possible muscles or tendons is involved, sometimes even which part of it.

### Inert or Non-contractile

This term describes those tissues that possess no inherent capacity to contract and relax. The agency for movement lies outside themselves. Joint capsule and ligaments allow movement to reach a certain point and then arrest it. Many bursae supply synovial surfaces facilitating movement of one tissue on another. The dura mater and nerve roots scarcely move at all. From inert tissues pain can be provoked only by stretching. Confusion arises from the fact that a patient can use his own muscles to stretch an inert tissue painfully, e.g. in arthritis at the shoulder active elevation of the arm hurts when the extreme of the possible range is reached, not because of any fault in the elevator muscles, but because the joint capsule is stretched. Hence pain produced at the extreme of an active movement must not be thought to arise from a contractile tissue. It is only when the stretching is carried out for the patient, i.e. passively, that it has diagnostic significance, since the response to active movement is ambiguous. For this reason active movements are best used in the rough preliminary examination that outlines the region at fault and best avoided in the subsequent detailed examination. For the orthopaedic physician the inert tissues are: joint capsule, ligament, bursa, fascia, dura mater and nerve root.

If the movements show the lesion to lie in an inert structure, it must be decided whether all the structures limiting movement at a joint are involved (i.e. a diffuse capsular lesion), or only a small part of them (e.g. a ligament), or whether an intra-articular block exists (e.g. a displaced part of the meniscus at the knee). If a single inert structure is at fault, its position, whether articular or extra-articular, requires definition.

Finally, correlation of the symptoms and signs determines the stage that the lesion has reached. In some conditions, e.g. internal derangement of a joint or a minor muscular rupture, treatment is the same whether the condition is acute, subacute, or chronic, whereas at other sites treatment on very different lines is required (e.g. arthritis or ligamentous strain).

## HISTORY

Since the orthopaedic physician deals with largely subjective disorders, the patient's account of his symptoms is of great importance. So is his manner of recounting his story. In general, straightforward patients, asked to give a chronological report on their symptoms, do so, and are visibly pleased to talk to an interested physician. They do not digress much and can easily be brought back to the point. Patients with unfounded pains are not sure how their symptoms should have behaved and resent being asked for their exact site, manner of reference and of aggravation. They offer a garbled story with internal contradictions and become restive during questions about the symptom responsible for the disablement described.

### Objects of Listening

Every patient contains a truth. He will proffer the data on which diagnosis rests. The doctor must adopt a conscious humility, not towards the patient, but towards the truth concealed within the patient, if his interpretations are regularly to prove correct.

1. To find out what the symptoms are, in what chronological order they appeared and how

long they have continued, and to compare the patient's account with the examiner's mental map of the dermatomes and his knowledge of the likelihoods. It is well to realize that many patients have given no thought to what their symptoms are before they are actually seated in front of the doctor. Leading questions must be avoided, and all questions must be neutral, e.g. 'What happened after that?' 'Does anything bring the pain on?' Time for reflection and recollection must be given and allowance made for those who do not possess a vocabulary which includes descriptive terms for various sensations or even accurate names for different parts of the body.

2. To discard the irrelevant, and to pursue in detail the pertinent parts of the patient's story, in particular relating to such activity, posture or function as evokes or increases pain. What eases the pain is seldom helpful diagnostically.
3. To piece the symptoms together (some sequences are quite characteristic) and roughly localize the lesion. Such a tentative diagnosis enables relevant questions to be asked in as neutral a way as possible on points that the patient has omitted. Some questions have diagnostic importance; others help to determine treatment or management.
4. To discover the past behaviour of a lesion. For example, whether a fragment of disc is stable or unstable, whether an arthritic shoulder is getting better or worse can be discovered only by listening to the history. Prognosis and treatment may depend almost entirely of the assessment afforded by the progress of symptoms. Is the disorder recurrent; if so, what provokes an attack?
5. To find out what sort of patient sits before the examiner, what is his reaction to pain and how his disorder affects his life and work. Do disablement and symptoms tally? His account of his symptoms suggests the diagnosis, but the patient's digressions and reactions often indicate what sort of person he is.
6. To find out what treatment he has already had, and its results.
7. To decide what sort of examination to conduct and to note pointers suggesting that considerable care or reserve should be exercised.

The history is at its most informative in disorders of the knee and spinal joints, which can be examined only with a clear idea of how the symptoms arose. With the shoulder, by contrast, the history matters little; it is the examination that counts. *The best approach is chronological*, the patient being asked about the events leading up to the onset of the symptoms, what they were then, and then to recount week by week, or year by year, what has happened since.

## Findings Based on History

The patient's age is important, for many diseases affect only certain age groups. Consider hip trouble in childhood, adolescence, early adult life or old age: entirely different diagnoses suggest themselves (pseudocoxalgia, slipped epiphysis, ankylosing spondylitis, osteoarthrosis). Sex is not very relevant in locomotor disorders since both sexes have much the same moving parts; but it may make considerable difference to treatment and management. Occupation has considerable bearing on diagnosis and prevention in industrial hazards, but in orthopaedic medicine it governs chiefly management.

In cases of trauma, the patient should be asked for a description detailed enough to enable the examiner to picture his posture at the moment of the accident and thus to deduce the direction of the strains operating on the injured parts. The events immediately following the accident must be ascertained, especially in patients claiming compensation. The presence of swelling and bruising is considered; blood fills a joint in a few minutes, clear fluid takes hours. The events of that and the succeeding days help to afford ground for giving or withholding credence to the story. Tendinous disorders often follow overuse; hence the activities of the previous few days or the duration and nature of the work done become relevant. A sprained ligament hurts progressively more over several hours; a fracture or an attack of internal derangement is maximal from the first.

Recurrence is to be expected in internal derangement, whether caused by a torn meniscus, a damaged disc or a loose body. The patient is subject to sudden attacks. Since cartilage is avascular, a crack in it cannot unite, and, if it has shifted once, the fragment can shift again. Recurrence is characteristic also of rheumatoid arthritis, gout and ankylosing spondylitis, but now the onset is gradual. If internal derangement is suspected, the question of locking, unlocking, twinges and giving way arises. The position in which the joint locks is material, and whether or not it unlocks suddenly. In dislocation of part of the meniscus at the knee, and in lumbago, the joint is locked in flexion. Sudden twinges, often associated with giving way of the lower limb, occur when a loose body subluxates momentarily, i.e. out–in. Painful twinges occur in three disorders:

1. A loose body in a joint. There are then articular signs on examination.
2. A tendinous lesion. The patient describes attacks of painful momentary loss of power in the part, so that he drops what he is holding or lifting. This is quite common in tennis elbow, less so in tendinitis at the shoulder. In either case the appropriate resisted movement hurts.
3. Neurological twinges. The lightning pains of tabes, the stabbing pains of post-herpetic neuralgia, trigeminal tic or Morton's metatarsalgia provide familiar examples.

A history of trouble arising for no apparent reason is just as important, since it suggests lesions such as gout or rheumatoid arthritis in which trauma plays no part. It is well to realize that many, if not most, disc lesions come on without an obvious causative strain preceding the moment that the symptom appeared.

The length of time that a symptom has been present has diagnostic significance. A constant pain of some years' standing cannot be caused by cancer or tuberculosis, which must in the end make its presence clear. Where the pain is first felt is often close to the lesion; but there are marked exceptions, such as pins and needles (which are felt distally wherever along its length the nerve is compressed) and in disc lesions with primary posterolateral evolution (the pain starting distally in a limb and possibly never reaching the trunk).

There are important differences in significance between (*a*) reference of pain; (*b*) shifting pain; and (*c*) expanding pain.

*Reference of pain* increases in extent as the lesion, though static in position, becomes more severe, and recedes as the trouble abates. Such reference (except in pressure on the dura mater) outlines the dermatome affected and shows in which segment the symptom originates. Hence an important question is always 'Where was the pain originally and where has it spread since?' For example, in minor arthritis at the shoulder or hip, the pain is felt chiefly at upper arm or groin. Should the arthritis become severe, spread to the wrist or ankle is to be expected.

*Shifting pain* results from a shifting lesion. For example, a renal calculus passing down the ureter gives rise to pain felt first in the loin, then in the iliac fossa, finally in the genitals; as the lesion moves, the pain moves. If a patient states that when his sciatica came on, his central backache went away, he describes a lesion projecting centrally that has now moved to one side. Being of constant size, it had to stop pressing centrally when it moved laterally, and the pain followed suit. This account is typical of a disc protrusion altering its position within a central cavity, i.e. the intervertebral joint.

If, on the other hand, he states that, as his backache got worse, it spread down one and later both lower limbs, he is describing the result of an *expanding lesion*, e.g. neoplasm.

The relation to rest, posture, activity and exertion provides much information. In difficult cases, especially suspected thoracic disc lesions of primary posterolateral development (when the pain may remain strictly confined to the anterior trunk for years), it is best also to approach the problem from the other side and inquire into the effect of visceral function on the pain. The rhythmic increase and subsidence of colic, unrelated to any bodily movement, or even making the patient writhe, is characteristic, for trunk pain of spinal origin makes the patient lie still. The effect of eating, hunger and defaecation (which may hurt also in a lumbar disc lesion or in coccygodynia) should be noted, together with any symptoms suggesting a disorder of the urinary tract, or, in women, of the pelvic organs. The fact that a patient declares her backache to be more severe at the time of menstruation does not prove that her pain springs from the uterus, since uterine referred pain may merely superimpose itself indistinguishably on a backache arising from the back. Backache at period times *only* is a different matter. Pain in the trunk on coughing suggests an intraspinal lesion but occurs also in pleurisy. If pain in a limb is induced by breathing or coughing, the lesion almost certainly lies in contact with the dura mater, but a momentary rise in intra-abdominal pressure also distracts the sacroiliac joints. Alleviation of pain during rest is not often significant, but if a certain posture or activity brings it on or increases it, it is highly probable that a lesion of the moving parts is present. (The main exceptions are angina and intermittent claudication.) The nature of the aggravating activity may indicate where to look for the source. Pain at rest may contraindicate active treatment when a joint is at fault.

Whether the symptoms are unilateral or bilateral is sometimes significant. Patients may of course develop osteoarthrosis in both hips and the thoracic outlet syndrome is usually bilateral; however, bilateral symptoms suggest a central origin. Central symptoms do not arise from a unilateral structure—an axiom that is often disregarded. The pain in patients with central backache is so often ascribed to a torn lumbar muscle, sacroiliac strain or lateral facet syndrome that clearly this discrepancy is ignored by those who wish to make a favourite diagnosis.

There is also the question of pins and needles (dealt with in Chapter 4). The most important points are: what brings them on and which part of the skin they occupy: the known cutaneous area of a small nerve, the skin supplied by a nerve trunk, the distal part of a dermatome or extrasegmental distribution. In this way the distinction between a peripheral lesion, affection of a nerve trunk, pressure on a nerve root or on the spinal cord can be made. Vague tingling is also caused by circulatory disturbance, but if this is so the distal part of the limb changes colour.

In joint lesions, inquiry should always be made for involvement, past or present, of other joints. This may bring to light information helpful in arriving at a diagnosis of rheumatoid, spondylitic, gouty or Reiter's arthritis. In gout, the family history may be suggestive.

In spinal nerve root pressure the pain may be constant day and night and is sometimes unrelated to exertion; such movements of the limb as do not stretch the affected root are apt if anything to relieve the symptoms for a short time. Heat diminishes most pains but often aggravates that caused by root pressure or intermittent claudication.

Another virtue of a full history is the warning that it gives to the examiner about when to be careful. Patients with common disorders give an account of their vicissitudes with little variation. The physician recognizes the familiar story, and confirms the diagnosis by examination; but he cannot, especially in an out-patient clinic, always investigate every system in the body. A history noted to differ markedly from the typical arrests the listener's attention and puts him on his guard—partly against psychoneurosis or feigned illness, partly against disorders with which orthopaedic medicine does not deal, and partly against a condition, properly sent to his department, with which the physician is so far unfamiliar.

## INSPECTION

This reveals the attitude in which the part is held; some positions are in themselves characteristic, e.g. the hand supporting the other elbow in fracture of the clavicle. Bony deformity, e.g. genu varum and abnormal postures such as torticollis or scoliosis or a short leg, become evident. The presence of general or local swelling, of muscular wasting and of changes in colour of the skin are noted. Colour changes can be induced by dependence or elevation in claudication and post-traumatic osteoporosis.

Inspection also discloses the type of gait, at times a most important finding especially in internal derangement at the knee, arthritis at the hip, spastic diseases and hysteria.

Inspection of the patient's facies may help to decide how disabling his pain has been; severe pain leading to sleepless nights shows on the patient's face. It provides the most valuable pointer in Parkinsonism. The well-covered individual who, with a bland countenance, describes months of intolerable symptoms is quickly identified.

## PALPATION

### The Joint is Stationary

The dorsum of the examiner's hand detects variations in temperature better than the palm. Localized warmth should be sought, and care taken that the recent removal of a bandage or the application of a rubefacient ointment does not deceive. The detection of heat means that, whatever the lesion, it is in the active stage. Heat is present, therefore, after an operation on a joint, during the stage of active healing of the divided tissues. Heat unaffected by rest is present after a ligamentous sprain, or over a broken bone, if it lies superficially, so long as active healing continues. If adhesions exist, or an impacted loose body lies displaced in a joint subjected to weight-bearing, exertion provokes heat which is quickly abolished by rest. Haemarthrosis is always accompanied by heat, and, if the joint is tense with blood, gross limitation of movement. In all these conditions, there is no synovial thickening. In active Reiter's, gouty, psoriatic, rheumatoid or spondylitic arthritis, heat is present in conjunction with synovial thickening. A superficial malignant deposit eroding bone (e.g. a rib) may feel warm. This has also been detected by thermography in cancer of the breast. Sympathectomy produces a warm foot and arterial thrombosis a cold one.

Palpation reveals the size, behaviour and consistency of any swelling and whether there is fluctuation. Bony enlargement results from callus, osteitis deformans or neoplasm. Oedema may pit. Loose bodies may be made to move about inside a joint cavity or a tendon sheath. Localized swelling of a tendon, osteophytes, a thickened bursa, a cyst, a haematoma or a ganglion are all readily felt. A gap at the point of rupture in a muscle or tendon may be palpable, as is the hard swelling of a muscle belly suffused with blood. Palpation discloses the presence or absence of pulsation in an artery; the extremity of the limb may feel cold to the touch. Any lesion of the lower limb causing muscle weakness in the leg (e.g. sciatica with root palsy) may make the foot cold. In iliac thrombosis the foot becomes colder than its fellow after exertion only; hence there is often no difference if the patient is examined in bed.

Palpation for tenderness provides much misinformation and should therefore be avoided except for good reason. It should be performed only after the tissue at fault has been identified by testing function. It must be confined to that tissue and is practicable only when the tissue lies within fingers' reach. The digital pressure is applied evenly along that tissue and the patient declares where it hurts most.

There is another object of palpation: to ascertain the site of a structure. When this needs precise identification, the finger is moved, feeling for the edges. Palpation starts beyond the edge of the structure and approaches it at right-angles to its long axis. The moving finger feels the ridge, then crosses the substance of the tissue until the dip on the far side is reached. It is, for example, impossible to find the infraspinatus tendon or the intercornual notch of the sacrum except by using this technique.

### The Joint is Moved

Crepitus indicates the state of the gliding surfaces. Fine crepitus at a joint indicates minor roughening of the joint surfaces; coarse crepitus indicates considerable superficial fragmentation of cartilage; the intermittent creaking of bone against bone shows articular cartilage to have been wholly eroded. Tenosynovitis due to overuse may give rise to fine crepitus as the inflamed tendon moves within its close-fitting sheath. In rheumatoid or tuberculous tenosynovitis the crepitus is much coarser. A fracture may crepitate.

A click may be felt as one bone moves suddenly against another. A partly detached intra-articular body may also click to and fro on movement.

At the spinal joints, each may be moved in turn passively, in order to discover at what level the symptoms are best reproduced. A series of extension pressures may demonstrate, for example, that greater discomfort is evoked at the fourth than at the third lumbar levels. Another approach is to ascertain lack of mobility at a spinal joint. This is difficult to be sure of, and in any case there is no certainty that a joint found mobile is not the source of symptoms rather than the joint found too stiff. At the spine feeling for muscle guarding is not very satisfactory either, since this always extends over several joints. For example, in tuberculosis or neoplasm in one lumbar vertebra, gross limitation of movement is visible and palpable at every lumbar joint. Again, in the radiograph of a fourth lumbar disc lesion causing marked lateral deviation (Plate XIII), the reader can see that the correcting deviation in the opposite direction starts only at thoracic levels.

Finally, there is the osteopathic and chiropractic claim that palpation can detect one vertebra to be tilted or rotated on its fellow or on the sacrum. This contention I do not regard as valid; and the experiments of Schiotz (1967) and Cyriax (1973) showed that when this was carried out by separate individuals on the same series of cases, their alleged deviations did not tally at all.

## DIAGNOSIS BY SELECTIVE TENSION

Five different aspects of this examination have to be considered, though not all are necessarily relevant to any one case.

### Active Range of Movement

Active movements indicate a combination of three things: the patient's ability and willingness to perform the movements requested, the range of movement possible and muscular power. Their chief value is to indicate quickly the region whence symptoms originate and which set of tissues to test in detail. They must be carried out first and then compared with the findings on passive and resisted movements. Since passive range and muscle power are assessed separately later, a strong contrast between what the affected part can in fact perform and what the patient is prepared to do shows will-power to be defective, involuntarily (neurosis) or voluntarily (malingering). The way a patient moves informs the examiner how gently to conduct his subsequent examination.

The active range may be normal, limited or excessive. If limited, it may be limited in every direction, in some directions but not in others, or in one direction only. If in only one direction, the limitation may be of the proportionate or disproportionate type (see below).

## Passive Range of Movement

The passive range of movement indicates the state of the inert tissues. The patient relaxes his muscles while the range of movement in each direction is ascertained; thus the effect of conscious control and muscular effort are eliminated. The patient states whether or not pain is provoked. In cases of doubt the examiner may have to push fairly hard to arrive at a true assessment. Five degrees of limitation of movement carries a quite different significance from full range with pain and the exact situation *must* be ascertained. Moreover, it may take some persuasion to get beyond a painful arc and to find out that at full range the pain has ceased. Again, the beginning of pain may not correspond with the extreme range; for example, straight-leg raising may start to hurt at 45° but continue to 90° without increased discomfort. The examiner must note what the resistance is like at the extreme of range, i.e. the end-feel, and if the appearance of pain and the extreme of range are reached together or separately.

Each primary movement of the joint must be tested passively, so as to allow emergence of a pattern, i.e. the relation between the degree of movement obtainable in one and in the other directions. This distinguishes capsular from non-capsular limitation of movement. Any discrepancy between the range of movement obtained actively and passively should be noted. Often accessory movements exist that test single inert structures one at a time.

## Resisted Movements

These provide clear information on the state of each muscle group about a joint. The patient contracts his muscles forcibly against resistance strong enough to prevent all articular movement while the joint is held somewhere near mid-range, so that all the inert structures are equally relaxed. No movement takes place at the joint; the only tension that alters is within the muscle. Indeed, when muscles contract, they squeeze together the opposed cartilaginous surfaces of the joint they span. Cartilage contains no nerves, hence this compression is painless. Moreover, such increased approximation of the bone ends relaxes ligaments and joint capsule. Hence, in arthritis the resisted movements are found painless. This remains so, surprisingly enough, when a tendon blends with the joint capsule, e.g. the supraspinatus.

A resisted movement may provoke pain or demonstrate weakness, occasionally both.

The examiner should pay considerable attention to where he stands and how to apply his hands. When strong muscles are tested, minor weakness cannot be detected unless his hands are well placed for resistance and counterpressure, and his body is properly poised. It is because these simple facts are not appreciated that muscle weakness is so often overlooked.

There are a number of rules.

1. Muscles must be tested in such a way that the examiner's and the patient's strength are fairly evenly matched.
2. The examiner must stand in the right place and use one hand for resistance, the other for counterpressure. For example, when the power of resisted abduction at the shoulder is tested, if the examiner stands facing the patient's side, he is toppled over backwards. If he stands in front of or behind the patient, one hand at his elbow the other on the far side at his waist, a true assessment is arrived at.
3. Muscles other than those being tested must not be included. For example, when the resisted movements at the elbow are tested, the examiner must grasp the lower forearm, not the hand.
4. The joint that the muscles control must not move and should be held near mid-range. This implies the examiner so placing himself and his hands that he is somewhat stronger than the patient.

At the extreme of range at some joints, the lever by which the muscle acts may be so much shorter that power appears impaired. For example, when the foot is held fully plantiflexed and dorsiflexion tested from that position, the examiner is much stronger than the patient. By contrast, when the foot lies at right angles to the leg, and dorsiflexion is tested again, the patient is much stronger than the examiner. When the question of slight weakness arises, this fact can be employed provided that both sides are carefully compared.

5. The patient must be encouraged to try his hardest. Many individuals equate pain with weakness and, if a limb hurts, are convinced that power is lost. Alternatively, the resisted movement may cause a stab of pain, making the patient let go. This event feels quite different to the examiner's hand. It is now no longer a force being gradually overcome until it yields slowly with some continuing resistance, but a sudden cessation of power. Altering the patient's posture, exhortation and repeated trial may show that an apparently weak muscle is perfectly strong. This situation is often encountered in hysteria.
6. There is no way of testing for minor weakness of the calf muscles except asking the patient to stand and rise on tiptoe, first on one leg and then on the other.

### Painful Arc

This means pain felt at the central part of a range of movement, disappearing as this point is passed in either direction. It may or may not reappear at the extreme of range; so long as pain ceases on each side of the arc, it is significant. A painful arc implies that a tender structure is pinched between two bony surfaces.

### Abnormal Sensations

These should be studied both when the joint is stationary and when it is moved (see above).

## Commentary

The information gained by studying the nature, degree and direction of the movements which cause pain or are weak is the basis of diagnosis in soft tissue lesions. The further discovery that many other movements are painless and strong provides the negative half that emphasizes the positive findings. Usually this information is obtainable in no other way, for it may relate to structures inaccessible to the finger and translucent to X-rays, or to places where every structure is sensitive to deep pressure in the normal individual, or to areas too small for differential palpation. *Omission of part of this examination, because the diagnosis seems obvious or to save time, is the common source of error.*

Experience in performing diagnostic movements is required so that the examiner may adopt a routine for each joint. He must be careful to use pure movements that test only one tissue at a time, and pay attention to where he places his hand on the patient's limb, to ensure that he is testing only that particular muscle. For example, if lateral rotation at the shoulder is tested by resistance applied at the dorsum of the patient's hand, instead of at the lowest forearm, resisted extension at the wrist is unwittingly included in the diagnostic movement. Hence, the infraspinatus muscle may receive treatment in a case of tennis elbow. The physician must therefore consider the purity of each diagnostic movement that he uses. Even so, there exist common, but avoidable, misinterpretations, to be mentioned later. Unless all the relevant movements are tried, and the responses noted and correlated, an uncommon condition that happens to give rise to common symptoms may be overlooked. Unless a great number of movements is tested, there are not enough data to enable him to assess the patient's sincerity, since the examiner is largely dependant on the discovery of an incongruous pattern and on inconsistencies in the patient's replies to recognize gross exaggeration or pain devoid of organic basis.

Errors in localization are easy enough to make in soft tissue lesions examined under the best conditions; in hospital practice, where patients may be slow to grasp what is wanted of them or inexplicit in their answers, the temptation to shirk some part of the examination may be great and must be resisted. The patient must not be flustered; for time is lost, not gained, by hurry and an unsympathetic manner. In this field diagnosis depends largely on correlating the history (a subjective statement) with the responses to a series of movements (again subjective). Unless the patient realizes what is required of him, there is little hope of reaching a correct diagnosis in other than simple cases.

*The least reliable way to diagnose in soft tissue lesions is to palpate immediately for tenderness in the area outlined by the patient.* Though this may give occasional success, it is most unsatisfactory, partly on account of misleading referred tenderness, partly because the region outlined by the patient does not necessarily contain the lesion, partly because many spots are normally tender, partly because many lesions lie beyond fingers' reach and therefore no relevant tenderness can exist, and partly because successful deception by allegations of feigned symptoms then becomes inevitable. Hence, it must again be emphasized that indirect examination by assessing function is the most important element in identifying a soft tissue lesion.

The orthopaedic physician must be ready to examine patients repeatedly. If diagnosis is uncertain he can seldom hope for appreciable assistance from a colleague or from ancillary methods such as radiography, blood tests, etc. If an apparently relievable lesion fails to improve, either the diagnosis is wrong or treatment has been imperfectly given. If this is given by the physiotherapist, it is my practice to ask her if she has any reason to offer for the lack of progress and whether she agrees with the diagnosis. If this remains in doubt, local anaesthesia is induced in her presence to settle the matter, and we await the result together. If I have ordered manipulation and, though it has failed so far, it still looks as if it ought to succeed, I carry out the manipulation myself. If I succeed, it provides the physiotherapist with a spur to do better; if I fail, it shows that it was my judgement that was at fault, not her technique.

## SIGNIFICANCE OF DIAGNOSTIC MOVEMENTS

*Active and Passive Movements are each Painful in the Same Direction, and the Pain Appears as the Limit of Range is Approached. The Resisted Movements do not Hurt. An Inert Structure is at Fault*

### Diffuse Capsular Lesion

It has always been standard teaching that arthritis leads to limitation of movement in every direction. This is not always so. If passive movement is limited in every direction in the capsular proportions, then arthritis is present. However, arthritis may cause limitation of movement in some directions only. In early arthritis at the shoulder, only lateral rotation may be restricted; in early arthritis at the hip, only medial rotation. In severe arthritis, the hip joint may fix in full lateral rotation, i.e. one movement is of full range. In early arthritis at the elbow or knee, rotation remains of full range and painless. Then there are joints which fix at the extreme of range, e.g. the talocalcanean at which arthritis causes fixation in full valgus, and the mid-tarsal which fixes in full abduction and lateral rotation. There are also joints not spanned by any muscle and supported by ligaments only. At these, e.g. the sacroiliac and the joints at each end of the clavicle, no way exists of maintaining any limitation; there is pain at the extremes of range only. Yet in each case, arthritis is present. By contrast limitation of movement—albeit not in the capsular proportions—may exist without arthritis, for example in acute subdeltoid bursitis.

If all the passive movements are painful at their extremes—even more, if the range of movement is limited—the whole inert cuff about the joint is shown to be involved. This is the clinical picture of arthritis, and the cause of the signs is diffuse capsular irritation in the early stage and actual contracture later on. Arthritis, capsulitis and synovitis all possess identical meanings: that the entire joint is affected. Periarthritis is a misnomer; for it can logically be used only when a tissue (unnamed) in the vicinity of, but not forming part of, the joint is involved. Since all the periarticular structures have names, the word is meaningless and a label stating which periarticular structure is at fault should be substituted. In fact, periarthritis is usually used when arthritis is present, but the radiograph reveals no bony abnormality, because it is wrongly supposed that such evidence of normality precludes arthritis. Periarthritis, synovitis and capsulitis are all terms best abandoned and arthritis maintained alone. The meaning of 'arthritis' is clear; an affection of the whole joint. In early arthritis the whole synovial membrane and capsule of the joint at first resent stretching; later on the capsule shortens. Hence nearly every movement, since it stretches some part of the capsule, hurts towards its extreme and, in all but the slightest cases, is limited in range. In recent arthritis, muscle spasm protects the irritated synovial membrane; in subacute arthritis the limitation results from muscular spasm coming into play to protect the capsule from being stretched; in osteoarthrosis it is the capsular contracture itself, hardly guarded by muscular spasm, that restricts range; in advanced disorganization of the joint, the bony outcrops engage. Clearly, the day after an injury leading to gross limitation of joint movement, no capsular contracture exists as yet; the limitation of movement is wholly due to muscle spasm protecting the capsule; it can be felt to spring into action on gentle forcing. Capsular contracture has a different end-feel. Purists may argue that all limitation of movement at a joint results from muscular spasm. This is not so clinically; indeed the difference is not only clear but carries diagnostic and therapeutic significance. When abrupt muscle spasm limits movement, stretching is contraindicated, whereas capsular contracture, with its softer stop resembling leather being stretched, invites forced movement in treatment. Whatever the cause of the arthritis, and whether it is acute or chronic makes no difference to the capsular pattern, only to the end-feel. That limitation of movement at the cervical joints is not caused by muscle spasm was proved by Lewit (1967), who examined 10 patients' necks before an operation at which complete muscle relaxation was induced by one of the curare group of drugs. During full muscle relaxation, he re-examined their necks and detected no change in the range of movement. There is thus a series of disorders in which articular contracture is the limiting factor, muscle spasm playing no part; and another in which muscle spasm is the active agent. This fits in very well with the different end-feels that are clinically detectable.

Arthritis, i.e. capsular irritation or contracture, is often spoken of as always causing 'limitation of movement in every direction'. Indeed, this remains the universal belief today, and is standard teaching; but this orthodoxy is not always justified (see Chapter 1). Polley and Hunder (1978) have written a book 286 pages long entitled *Physical Examination of Joints* without mentioning the capsular pattern.

It is well to realize that neither cartilage nor the synovial lining of a joint contain nerve endings; hence if pain is present it must arise from the capsule of the joint or, in severe disorganization, friction between two bony surfaces exposed by erosion of cartilage. For this reason marked crepitus may be present at a painless joint with a full range of movement. This combination implies attrition and roughening of the cartilaginous surfaces without capsular contracture. This is a common finding at shoulder and knee.

## End-feel

When the examiner tests passive movement at a joint, different sensations are imparted to his hand at the extreme of the possible range. They possess great diagnostic importance.

*Bone-to-bone.* This is the abrupt halt to the movement when two hard surfaces meet, e.g. at the extreme of passive extension of the normal elbow. Bone felt to engage against bone in this way is not only diagnostic but affords an important pointer in manipulation; for, once this sensation has emerged, further forcing in that direction is clearly vain.

*Spasm.* Muscle spasm coming actively into play with a vibrant twang indicates acute or subacute arthritis. It can be felt particularly clearly when movement at the wrist is tested in recent carpal fracture or when secondary deposits have invaded a cervical vertebra. Spasm of this order leads to the 'hard' end-feel that accompanies a severe and active lesion and provides a strong contra-indication to manipulation.

*Capsular Feel.* This consists of a hardish arrest of movement, with some give in it, as if two pieces of tough rubber were being squeezed together or a piece of thick leather were being stretched. It is the way the normal shoulder, elbow or hip stops at the extreme of each rotation. This feeling, appearing before normal full range is reached, suggests non-acute (not necessarily minor) arthritis. The arthritis may have been 'chronic' from the onset (if the reader will forgive the word being used in this way), or have become so after a more severe stage.

*Springy Block.* When an intra-articular displacement exists, a rebound is seen and felt at the extreme of the possible range. This is most obvious at the knee when the torn part of the meniscus engages between the bone ends, blocking extension. A springy block indicates internal derangement.

*Tissue Approximation.* This is the normal sensation imparted at full passive flexion of a normal elbow or knee. The joint cannot be pushed farther because of engagement against another part of the body, but would clearly move farther as far as the joint itself is concerned.

*Empty Feel.* If movement causes considerable pain before the extreme of range is reached, and yet the sensation imparted to the examiner's hand is 'empty', i.e. lacking in organic resistance with the patient nevertheless begging the examiner to desist even though he can feel that further movement is in fact possible, important disease is present. Acute bursitis, extra-articular abscess, or neoplasm should be strongly suspected. The cause of an empty feel is the normality of the joint itself. Pain stops the passive movement long before the examiner discerns any articular resistance. For example, when metastases are present at the ilium or upper femoral shaft, the hip joint itself is not involved, and the examiner feels this to be so.

This sensation is also imparted to the examiner's hand when the restriction of range is caused by hysteria or neurogenic hypertonus. In such cases there is initial strong resistance to movement, which yields to sustained pressure, disclosing a full range of movement at the joint. In organic disease of a joint the farther the movement is pushed, the greater the resistance, and full range is unobtainable.

### Sequence of Pain and Limitation

Another important point emerges when a passive movement approaches the extreme of the possible range—whether the pain and the resistance to movement come on together or not. The experienced physiotherapist faced with stretching a painful tissue is guided—often unconsciously—by what she feels the joint will accept.

*Pain before Resistance.* The pain comes on well before the extreme of possible range has been reached. This suggests an active lesion or extra-articular limitation of movement, each unsuitable for stretching.

*Pain Synchronous with Resistance.* Capsular feel: gentle stretching can be cautiously attempted. Hard feel: postpone stretching a little longer.

*Resistance before Pain.* The resistance that signals the approach of the extreme of range is felt, but little pain is elicited at this point. Greater pressure moves the joint a little farther, and discomfort begins. This sequence suggests that quite strong stretching will be well tolerated and is particularly noticeable at those lesions of the shoulder and hip joints that benefit from stretching out.

## The Capsular Pattern

The capsule of a joint is lined by synovial membrane. In a lesion of either of these structures limitation of movement of characteristic proportions results. It does not matter if the irritation is synovial only, as in a recent sprain or haemarthrosis, capsular only as in osteoarthrosis, or both, as in rheumatoid arthritis; the same pattern results. This varies from joint to joint, but scarcely at all in different patients; in other words, all shoulders, say, are alike, but the pattern of restriction at the shoulder is not the same as that at the hip. At every joint, the proportion that the limitation of movement in one direction bears to that in other directions conforms to a standard which indicates whether arthritis is present or not. To arrive at a diagnosis of arthritis it is not essential—it is merely usual—for movement to be limited in every direction. For example, at the shoulder lateral rotation is the movement most restricted, and in early arthritis it may prove the only movement to be limited. Again, in advanced arthritis, the hip joint may fix in full lateral rotation. Should movement prove limited in quite other than the capsular proportions, one of the disorders other than arthritis capable of causing limited movement has to be considered. *For the concept of arthritis as characterized by limitation of movement in every direction must be substituted the concept of limitation conforming with the capsular pattern for that particular joint.* The presence of the capsular pattern does not indicate what type of arthritis is present; for the pattern is the same whatever the cause of the arthritis. Troisier's (1957) accurate goniometric measurements have shown that the capsular proportions of limitation of movement are precisely the same whether arthritis at the shoulder is post-traumatic, degenerative or rheumatoid. Further differentiation rests on extraneous factors: e.g. a history of trauma, the discovery of a raised uric acid level, or of arthritis elsewhere.

### Theoretical Considerations

It is obvious that stretching the joint capsule provides the chief cause of pain in arthritis. For years I considered it the only way to cause pain; for cartilage and synovial membrane are both devoid of nerves. The capsule resents stretching in a selective way, some movements being more painful and limited than others. Clinically, this must derive from more capsular contracture at one aspect of a joint than another. For example, in arthritis at the shoulder, stretching the front of the capsule may well be 80° limited at a time when stretching the back of the capsule is merely 10° limited. In arthritis, movement is seldom restricted equally in each direction, but in the capsular proportions. Thus, except at those joints which no muscle spans, arthritis shows itself clinically as limitation of movement in the capsular pattern. The same proportions emerge whatever the nature of the arthritis and provide evidence of the utmost importance in diagnosis.

Pathologically, this concept is insufficient. For example, a few hours after a severe sprain of a ligament at the knee, traumatic arthritis ensues with grossly limited movement in the capsular pattern. Clearly no contracture can yet have developed. This response to injury has been attributed to synovitis, since the joint has by then filled with fluid, but synovial membrane is insensitive. Arthritis can thus be seen to behave *clinically* as if capsular contracture had supervened, even though it has not. Any strong nociceptor impulse arising from the neighbourhood of a joint provokes involuntary muscle spasm coming into play to restrict mobility in the capsular proportions. It would seem, therefore, that there is a basic awareness on the part of the brain of how the capsule would contract even though in that individual it has never yet done so. Such a mechanism would also account for the limited range of movement occurring in a perfectly normal joint when a lesion exists in adjacent bone, e.g. metastasis or abscess.

Pain is not an essential component of limited movement in arthritis. At the hip, for example, osteoarthrosis (confirmed radiologically) leading to considerable restriction of range in the capsular pattern may coexist with complete absence of pain when the capsule is stretched quite hard. It would seem therefore that the nociceptor system can be called into play subliminally. In arthritis there exist two other phenomena that today defy explanation.

## Pain Without Capsular Stretch

In arthritis, pain may be provoked by means unconnected with increased tension on the joint-capsule. For example, in arthritis at the shoulder or hip, lying on that side often brings on pain arising from the joint. Doing so approximates the cartilaginous bone-ends; no movement takes place; the capsule is fully relaxed. The pain cannot arise from bone pressing against bone since it occurs in joints without erosion of articular cartilage.

## Success of Intra-articular Steroids

In rheumatoid arthritis with limited movement in the capsular pattern, pain often ceases within 24 hours of an intra-articular steroid injection. The drug lies in contact only with the synovial membrane; an insensitive tissue intervening between the suspension and the capsule of the joint. It is not conceivable to me that the particles of the suspension permeate the entire thickness of so extensive and tough a structure as capsule. Arthroscopy has shown (Gil and Katona 1971) that the red inflamed synovial membrane becomes pale after the injection, presumably due to inhibition of prostaglandin formation. Is then the pain in arthritis mediated by the nerves that accompany blood vessels?

In the latter case, actual capsular contracture has taken place. Finally, osteophyte formation and advanced capsuloligamentous contracture has supervened. Where such structural alterations have occurred, the cause of limitation of movement is clear enough yet the injection remains successful.

## Arthritis and Radiography

Since evidence of arthritis is often sought by X-rays, it is easy to think of arthritis as an affection of cartilage and bone, and to adopt the view that, if the radiograph reveals no abnormality, arthritis must be absent. This attitude leads to grievous error. Erosion of cartilage, osteophyte formation and changes in the density of the bones characterize advanced arthritis, but are not of themselves painful. Cartilage is devoid of nerve supply and no lesion in cartilage can of itself give rise to pain. Equally, muscle spasm about a joint, osteophyte formation and rarefaction of bone are not of themselves painful. These are secondary phenomena, and are not vital to the clinical concept of arthritis, which displays itself primarily as a capsular contracture, which can continue for many months or years without giving rise to any radiological evidence of disease.

## The Capsular Pattern Listed

The capsular pattern exists at only those joints that are controlled by muscles. These spring into action to prevent further movement when the tension on the capsule of the joint and on its synovial lining is about to cause pain. There is no capsular pattern, therefore, at joints that rely for their stability purely on their ligaments, e.g. the acromioclavicular or the sacroiliac. Here the degree of arthritis is shown by the severity of the pain brought on when the joint is strained, but no mechanism for involuntary prevention of mobility exists.

*Jaw.* Increasing limitation of opening the mouth.

*Neck.* Side flexion and rotation are equally limited; flexion is usually of full range and painful, extension limited. The common cause of a non-capsular pattern is internal derangement, i.e. subluxation of a fragment of disc.

*Sternoclavicular and Acromioclavicular Joint.* Pain at the extremes of range.

*Shoulder.* So much limitation of abduction, more limitation of lateral rotation, less limitation of medial rotation. The common cause of a non-capsular pattern is acute subdeltoid bursitis.

*Elbow.* Rather more limitation of flexion than of extension. In the early stage of arthritis, rotation remains full and painless. The common cause of a non-capsular pattern is internal derangement, i.e. a loose body.

*Lower Radio-ulnar Joint.* A full range of movement with pain at both extremes of rotation. The common cause of limitation of only supination is mal-union of a Colles's fracture.

*Wrist.* Equal degree of limitation of flexion and extension. The common cause of restriction in the non-capsular pattern is a subluxated capitate bone.

*Trapezio-first–Metacarpal Joint.* Limitation of abduction and of extension; full flexion.

*Thumb and Finger Joints.* Rather more limitation of flexion than of extension.

*Thoracic and Lumbar Joints.* The difficulty is to determine, except in gross arthritis, whether the range is limited or not, taking into account the patient's age and habitus. Comparison between the amounts by which extension and side flexion are limited is scarcely possible. It must be realized that limitation of movement in the capsular pattern at the thoracic and spinal joints occurs symptomlessly in ligamentous contracture and osteophyte formation—objective evidence of osteoarthrosis but not the cause of patients' pain.

By contrast, the non-capsular pattern is very easy to detect, e.g. gross limitation of side flexion one way, full range the other way; or full extension accompanied by markedly limited flexion. Again, at the thorax, a full range of rotation in one direction may be matched by 45° limitation in the other. The cause of this type of non-capsular pattern is internal derangement, i.e. displacement of a fragment of disc.

*Sacroiliac, Symphysis Pubis and Sacrococcygeal Joints.* Pain when stress falls on the joint.

*Hip Joint.* Gross limitation of flexion, abduction and medial rotation. Slight limitation of extension. Little or no limitation of lateral rotation. The common causes of a non-capsular pattern are bursitis or a loose body in the hip joint.

*Knee Joint.* Gross limitation of flexion (e.g. 90°), slight limitation of extension (e.g. 5° or 10°). In the early stages of arthritis rotation remains full and painless. The common cause of a non-capsular pattern is internal derangement (displaced loose body or meniscus).

*Tibiofibular Joints.* Pain when contraction of the biceps muscle stretches the upper tibiofibular ligaments. Pain when the mortice is sprung at the ankle stretching the lower tibiofibular ligament. Normally there is no appreciable movement possible at either joint.

*Ankle Joint.* If the calf muscles are of adequate length, rather more limitation of plantiflexion than of dorsiflexion is present. If these muscles are short, they limit dorsiflexion (soft end-feel) before the arthritic limitation (hard end-feel) can be reached. If so, clinically, limitation of plantiflexion is present alone.

*Talocalcanean Joint.* Limitation of varus range increasing until, in gross arthritis, the joint fixes in full valgus. In early cases, the extreme of such varus movement as is possible is painful.

*Mid-tarsal Joint.* Limitation of dorsiflexion, plantiflexion, adduction and medial rotation. Abduction and lateral rotation of full range.

*First Metatarsophalangeal Joint.* Marked limitation of extension (e.g. 60° to 80°); slight limitation of flexion (10° to 20°).

*Other Four Metatarsophalangeal Joints.* Variable. They tend finally to fix in extension with the interphalangeal joints flexed.

## The Non-capsular or Partial Articular Pattern

When limitation of movement is discovered in proportions not corresponding to the capsular pattern, arthritis is absent and lesions capable of causing restriction of range, but not involving the whole joint, have to be considered. They fall into three categories: ligamentous adhesions, internal derangement and extra-articular lesions.

## Ligamentous Adhesions

Ligaments reinforce the capsule of a joint. When adhesions form about a ligament after an injury, those movements that require a fully mobile ligament for their painless performance resprain the ligament whose mobility is impaired. Hence pain, usually localized, is brought on only by those movements that stretch the adherent structure. Thus some movements are painful, perhaps one movement is slightly limited, and some movements are pain-free in a manner characteristic of the affected ligament, not of the whole capsule of the joint. In ligamentous adhesions movement is restricted in the *proportionate* way, i.e. slight limitation exists in one direction but a full, painless range is present in the other directions.

## Internal Derangement

This need be considered only in joints apt to develop intra-articular loose fragments of cartilage or bone. These are the knee, jaw and spinal joints commonly; the elbow, hip and tarsal joints occasionally.

When a loose fragment becomes displaced within a joint, the onset is sudden. A localized block is formed which occupies only one part of the joint. Hence the pain is localized, often at one aspect only of the joint, and those movements that engage against the block are limited, while those that do not are of full range. Examination thus discloses the partial articular, i.e. non-capsular, pattern characteristic of internal derangement.

In minor cases the restriction of movement is often proportionate, but the sudden onset with limitation coming on immediately shows that ligamentous adhesions cannot be present, for they have not yet had time to form. A major block produces gross *disproportion*; for example, in torticollis or lumbago the spinal joint may possess a full range of side flexion in one direction and no range at all in the other, deformity and pain appearing simultaneously. A large displacement causes the disproportionate type of non-capsular pattern, a small displacement the proportionate type. It is merely a question of the size of the loose body and the degree and site of the displacement. By contrast, in spinal arthritis the degree of limitation of side flexion is equal in the two directions. The disproportion is very obvious at the knee when the torn part of a meniscus shifts, blocking extension but not flexion.

## Extra-articular Limitation

*Disproportionate Limitation.* When, for example, the quadriceps muscle is adherent to the shaft of the mid-femur, 90° of limitation of flexion at the knee joint is associated with a full and painless range of extension. Such gross limitation of movement in one direction only, combined with full painless range in all other directions, indicates that the joint itself is normal, and that an extra-articular contracture will not permit that movement. For example the muscle spasm about the breach in a partly torn gastrocnemius muscle grossly limits dorsiflexion at the ankle joint, whereas passive plantiflexion remains of full range and painless.

The same effect can be produced by a large haematoma or cyst in the popliteal space; again the knee will not bend far though it will extend fully, this time because the swelling cannot be compressed beyond a certain point.

In acute subdeltoid bursitis, limitation of movement at the shoulder joint is obvious, but it is gross towards abduction, slight towards the rotations. This disproportion between the range of abduction and lateral rotation, reversing the capsular pattern at the shoulder joint, shifts attention from the joint to the extra-articular structures.

*The Constant-length Phenomenon.* If the amount of limitation of movement at one joint depends on the position in which another joint is held, the restricting tissue must lie outside any joint. This relationship indicates that the lesion lies in a structure that spans at least two joints, thus clearly excluding any articular tissue. A good example is straight-leg raising. Limitation of hip flexion (when compared with the other side) when the knee is held straight, but not when the knee is allowed to bend, indicates that the structure which will not stretch runs from below the back of the knee to above the posterior aspect of the hip joint. Now, if neck flexion during straight-leg raising further increases the pain in the back or lower limb, it becomes clear that the tissue whose mobility is impaired runs from the neck to the calf; and there is only one such tissue—the dura mater and its continuation as the sciatic nerve.

Volkmann's ischaemic contracture provides another example of the constant-length phenomenon. In this condition, the fingers cannot be extended unless the wrist is flexed first. In other words, the amount of movement of which the fingers are capable depends on the position of the wrist—again, a possibility only if the lesion is extra-articular.

* * *

*Passive Movement is Painful in One Direction and Active Movement is Painful in the Opposite Direction*

This indicates a contractile structure to be at fault, i.e. a muscle belly, a tendon, or the attachment of either to periosteum. Since tension is the cause of pain, passively stretching the muscle hurts; active contraction in the opposite direction also hurts. This finding leads to immediate trial of the resisted movements.

The direction of the painful movement indicates which group of muscles is involved. Accessory movements, picking out the various members of the group individually, define the affected muscle, and may even show which part of it is affected. When a muscle spans two joints, e.g. the muscles of the arm or thigh, special tests can be devised.

*Exception.* In acute tenosynovitis at the wrist, pain is set up when movement occurs between the roughened tendon and its sheath. Hence not only such movements as stretch the tendon, but also those that relax it, set up a painful friction; in the latter case by pushing the tendon down the sheath. The occurrence of pain on those passive movements might suggest a lesion of an inert structure at the wrist joint. The diagnosis becomes clear only when the resisted movements are tried; these cannot set up pain in an articular lesion.

* * *

*Resisted Movement Reveals Pain or Weakness*

## Muscle Lesions

Resisted movement discloses the state of the muscles that perform that movement. Strictly speaking, a resisted movement is not a movement at all, and is a contradiction in terms. It is really a forcible frustrated attempt at movement. Some would prefer to say 'static contraction'. However, this term is not without ambiguity, since static contraction is often used voluntarily to fix a joint and then involves all the muscles controlling the part. 'Resisted movement' is merely short for 'attempted movement against resistance'.

Precautions must be observed to obtain a correct response to this type of testing.

1. The joint must be held near mid-range. In this position all the ligaments and the capsule itself are equally relaxed, no tension falling on them when the muscle contracts. Indeed, muscle contraction approximates the cartilaginous surfaces relaxing the capsule further.
2. The resistance must be so strong that the joint is prevented from moving. Hence, the tension on one muscle group alters as the patient pushes, but the tension on the articular structures does not change.
3. The examiner must apply resistance at a point that ensures that only one group of muscles is being tested. For example, testing resisted lateral rotation of the shoulder by pressing against the dorsum of the patient's hand would elicit pain also if the patient had a tennis elbow, whereas resistance applied to the dorsum of the lower forearm unambiguously singles out the infraspinatus.
4. When the question of muscular weakness arises, the examiner must place his hands suitably. Whether a muscle is found weak or not often depends on his posture. If minor weakness is not to pass undetected, the examiner's resistance and a normal patient's strength must be as evenly matched as possible. For example, if the dorsiflexion muscles of the foot are tested by the examiner standing at the end of the couch and applying one hand to the dorsum of the foot, considerable weakness is unnoticeable, for the examiner is toppled forwards by even minor strength. By contrast, if he stands sideways on to the patient, level with his knee, with one hand on the upper tibia and the other on the dorsum of the foot close to the toes, slight weakness becomes apparent at once. For the same reason, the power of abduction at the shoulder must be tested with resistance applied at the elbow, and counterpressure by the other hand at the far flank. Even gross weakness of a calf muscle is undetectable with the patient on the couch; he must stand alternately on each leg and try to rise on tiptoe.
5. The main muscle groups should be tested one by one and the patient asked each time if his discomfort is evoked or increased. If one resisted movement hurts and the others do not, and a full range of passive movement is present at the relevant joint, it is a virtual certainty that a muscle lesion is present. If the resisted movement found painful involves more than one muscle, accessory movements can usually be devised that identify which one within that set of muscles is at fault. For example, if resisted medial rotation of the shoulder hurts, the trouble might lie in the pectoralis major, latissimus dorsi, teres major

or subcapularis muscles. The first three are also strong adductors of the arm; hence, if this resisted movement proves painless (as is to be expected), the subscapularis muscle is singled out.

If two congruous movements hurt (e.g. resisted flexion and supination at the elbow in a bicipital lesion), a muscle lesion is present in the muscle that combines these two actions, i.e. not the brachialis.

If several resisted movements, or two incompatible movements, hurt, a muscle lesion is improbable.

One occasional finding exists that is difficult to interpret. No pain is elicited by a resisted contraction, but the recognized ache is felt as the patient lets go. If this proves the *only* painful movement, the muscle that contracted and then hurt as it relaxed is probably at fault.

If *all* the resisted movements hurt, the last thing to suspect is a muscle lesion. This finding suggests either the exaggeration that denotes psychogenesis or a severe lesion lying close by proximally, to which any movement transmits stress. For example, every resisted movement of the arm often hurts in acute torticollis, and of the thigh in acute lumbago, since the patient has to brace his spinal muscles before attempting to move the limb.

*In tendinous lesions a full passive range of movement always exists at the relevant joint*, and even a lesion in a muscle belly can limit only that passive movement which stretches the healing breach. Many muscles span more than one joint and tests based on the constant-length phenomenon can then be employed to confirm the presence of such a lesion.

There exist two conditions not directly connected with muscle that nevertheless give rise to pain when muscle is tested against resistance. The first is fracture of bone close to the attachment of belly or tendon. Naturally muscle pull tends to move the fractured ends on each other painfully. For example, anterior fracture of a rib may give rise to pain when the pectoralis major muscle is tested, or fracture of one pubis may hurt on testing resisted adduction of that thigh. The second is compression by the muscle belly of a tender structure. As the muscle hardens and broadens, any adjacent tender structure is squeezed and pain may then be evoked. This phenomenon is met with chiefly in the buttock, where for example a tender gluteal bursa can be compressed by contraction of the gluteus medius muscle.

## Interpretation

When the resisted contraction of muscle groups is tested, the possibilities are:

*Strong and Painful.* This designates a minor lesion of some part of a muscle or tendon. The damage is not gross enough to cause weakness, but a strong contraction hurts, thus indicating that the structural integrity of the muscle–tendon complex is impaired.

Tennis elbow provides a good illustration of a diagnosis that can be made adequately only by examination of resisted movements. In this condition, the passive movements of the elbow or wrist, and the resisted movements at the elbow, cause no pain. However, when the movements at the wrist are tested against resistance, extension causes pain at the elbow. The diagnosis can be further refined by resisting this movement while the patient keeps his fingers flexed. This also hurts, although the extensor digitorum muscle is now out of action. Hence, one of the extensor muscles of the carpus is involved. When ulnar and radial deviation movements of the hand are resisted, only the latter hurts. By this means the lesion at the elbow can be shown to lie at the upper extent of the radial extensor muscles of the carpus. Mere palpation of so small an area could not have demonstrated whether the fault lay in the ulnar, digital or radial extensor muscles.

*Weak and Painless.* There is often constant pain, but making the weak muscle contract against resistance does not alter the symptoms. This finding may indicate a complete rupture of the relevant muscle or tendon, but much more often a disorder of the nervous system. Impaired conduction along a nerve leads to muscle weakness, but, since the structural integrity of the muscle is maintained, no pain arises when whatever contraction is possible takes place. It is important to ensure that a patient in constant pain does not merely allude to this fact, but is clear that what the examiner is asking about is an *increase* in his symptoms during the resisted movement.

*Weak and Painful.* This indicates a gross lesion, i.e. the resisted movement proves weak and the attempt increases pain. In, say, fracture of the patella or olecranon resisted extension at knee or elbow is naturally weak and painful. Secondary deposits at the head of the humerus set up pain and weakness when the resisted movements are tested, together with marked restriction of passive joint range. This finding always suggests serious trouble, even if the first X-ray photograph reveals no abnormality. However, if a resisted movement at the shoulder proves weak and painful but the passive range at the joint is not restricted, the cause is merely partial rupture of the relevant tendon.

*All Painful.* The resisted movements have another quite different virtue. They provide a rough measure of individual variation in sensitiveness to pain since tense patients often equate effort with discomfort. When resisted movements are performed at a joint, the muscles about which are normal, all persons perceive the altered tension on the muscle, but find it in no sense disagreeable. There are patients whose degree of perception is so heightened, usually by fatigue or emotional stress, that they interpret changes in muscular tension as painful. For example, when a patient with backache elicited by lumbar movements also experiences an equal amount of pain at the shoulder—or even in the back!—on resisted arm movements, it is highly probable that he is describing as painful those feelings that do not hurt ordinary individuals. Trial of resisted movements at joints remote from the seat of the patient's pain, helps enormously to indicate whether the symptoms arise from emotional hypersensitivity or pain generated organically.

*All painless. If all the resisted movements prove strong and painless, there is nothing the matter with the muscles.* Were this simple and logical concept accepted, the idea of fibrositis would never have arisen. For example, if patients with 'fibrositis of the trapezius' are examined, elevation of the scapula even against the strongest resistance is painless. This shows the muscle to be normal; hence nothing is to be gained by looking for a tender spot within it. Even if one is found, it cannot be relevant to the referred trapezial symptoms.

*Painful on Repetition.* The resisted movements can also be used to provide a measure of arterial patency. If the movement is strong and painless but is found to hurt after a number of repetitions, intermittent claudication is present.

* * *

*The Elicitation of Pain by Internal Squeezing*

Internal squeezing elicits pain in two ways, one very helpful (a painful arc) and the other misleading (at the extreme range).

## Painful Arc

By this is meant pain appearing near the mid-range of a movement, ceasing as this point is passed. The pain may reappear at the extreme of range, *but it must cease on each side of the arc.* If elevation of the arm begins to hurt when the horizontal is reached, and then continues until full elevation is complete, no painful arc is present. If the pain comes on at the horizontal, ceases above it and then returns (or not) at full elevation, a painful arc has been elicited. This phenomenon is best evoked by active movement, and may appear only on the upward movement of the arm, or only on the downward, or both. In any case, the significance is the same; the lesion lies in a pinchable position. If a tender structure is painfully squeezed when a moving part passes a certain point, anatomical considerations can be used to deduce where the lesion must lie. A painful arc at the shoulder is common and indicates that the tender tissue can be pinched between the acromion and one or other of the humeral tuberosities. This finding therefore incriminates the supraspinatus, infraspinatus or subscapular tendon, or the subdeltoid bursa. Accessory tests then define which is at fault. Once the structure has been singled out, the fact that a painful arc exists indicates which part of it is affected. A painful arc on a spinal movement indicates that the lesion moves suddenly when the tilt on the joint alters from lordosis to kyphosis, i.e. it lies squeezed between the vertebral bodies. A painful arc on straight-leg raising indicates that a small protrusion exists over which the nerve root slides. At the knee, a painful arc suggests a loose body or a transverse crack in the meniscus; at the hip, bursitis.

## Pain at One Extreme of Range

This may prove puzzling; for if pain appears at the extreme of range the examiner is apt to think in terms of stretching and to forget the occasional occurrence of pinching. If he is fortunate, other movements also hurt that identify the structure at fault. For example, when the arm is fully elevated, the greater tuberosity of the humerus engages against the glenoid rim and squeezes the supraspinatus tendon. Hence full passive elevation of the arm may elicit tenderness in supraspinatus tendinitis. This is not the same thing as finding that full *active* elevation of the arm hurts. During the active movement, the supraspinatus muscle is contracting, and pain is therefore to be expected wherever in the tendon the lesion lies. Full passive elevation relaxes the muscle and, in supraspinatus tendinitis, pain can thus result only from squeezing; hence it is a useful localizing sign. Similarly, full passive medial rotation of the arm presses the subscapular tendon against the glenoid rim and full adduction presses the subscapular tendon against the coracoid process. When a lesion lies at the tenoperiosteal junction of the biceps tendon at the radial tuberosity, this point is pressed against the shaft of the ulna at the extreme of full passive pronation of the forearm. Both the psoas bursa and rectus femoris tendon can be squeezed by full flexion with adduction of the hip. The bursa lying in front of the tendo Achillis is squeezed between the tibia and the calcaneus on full passive plantiflexion at the ankle joint.

Great diagnostic difficulties arise when only one movement hurts; for example, if, in a painful shoulder only full passive elevation proves painful, is this a pinch or a stretch? The differentiation between early osteoarthrosis and psoas bursitis or a loose body in the hip joint is obscured by the same ambiguity.

* * *

*The Passive Range of Movement is Full but there is Inability to Perform One or More Movements Actively*

This shows one or more muscles to be out of action, either from intrinsic defect such as a cut tendon or myopathy, or from interference with nervous paths, e.g. peripheral neuritis, anterior poliomyelitis, cerebrovascular accident or psychogenic disorder. In partial palsies or when only one of several muscles that can perform a movement is affected, trial of the resisted movements is needed to disclose the weakness. In both neurogenic hypertonus and hysteria, inability to perform a voluntary movement is associated with considerable resistance when the movement is attempted passively, greatest at the first moment of forcing.

* * *

*An Excessive Range of Movement Exists*

This results from capsuloligamentous laxity at joints whose stability is not under full muscular control. The structures most often concerned are the acromioclavicular, sternoclavicular, sacroiliac and sacrococcygeal joints, the symphysis pubis, the collateral and cruciate ligaments at the knee joint, the inferior tibiofibular and the calcaneofibular ligaments. The liability to subluxation is noted when too much movement is found, sometimes on active movement but always on passive testing. Permanent laxity of any of these ligaments may follow a severe sprain.

* * *

*A Bony Block Limits Movement*

When a joint is felt to come to a dead stop at a point short of its full range of normal movement, a bony block is present. If no pain is elicited on forcing a neuropathic arthropathy is almost certain; if forcing is uncomfortable the cause is probably large osteophytic outcrops of bone, myositis ossificans or a malunited fracture close to the joint.

* * *

*No Movement is Possible*

This may result from the intense muscular spasm set up by bacterial arthritis, or fibrous or bony ankylosis. Absence of movement at the shoulder and hip joints is somewhat masked by scapular and pelvic mobility.

* * *

*A Snap Occurs*

This results when a tendon catches against a bony prominence and then slips over it. Such a sequence of events occurs at the shoulder (long head of biceps) and ankle (peroneal tendons); but if a joint is painful and also snaps, it does not necessarily follow that the pain is the result of a frictional tendinitis. At the hip, the greater trochanter may catch against the edge of the gluteus maximus muscle. An osteoma may first declare itself by catching against a tendon. A small semi-membranous bursa may snap as it jumps from one to the other side of the tendon as the knee is flexed. In trigger finger, a swelling of the digital flexor tendon jams inside the tendon sheath and holds the finger fixed in flexion until the engagement is passively released with a snap.

* * *

*A Crack is Heard*

This is a normal phenomenon, occurring when traction is applied to a joint, especially of the fingers. Roston and Haines (1947) showed that traction up to 6 kg resulted merely in slight separation of the bony surfaces at a man's metacarpophalangeal joint. When the traction reached 7 or 8 kg the bones sprang apart with a loud crack, the distance between them suddenly becoming doubled. Radiography demonstrated that, at that same moment, a bubble of air appeared in the joint. This was doubtless derived from gas dissolved in the intra-articular synovial fluid evaporating as the result of the subatmospheric pressure created by the traction. It was absorbed again in 20 minutes; before this had happened no amount of tension would make the joint crack again. These facts were all confirmed by Unsworth et al. (1971), except that they regarded the crack as caused by the collapse of the bubble, not its appearance. Synovial fluid, so they found, contained 15% gas, four-fifths of which was carbon dioxide. Such a bubble has no effect on subsequent movement at the joint; it is infinitely compressible and thus cannot interfere with mobility. If the crack is followed by any alteration in the physical signs, the formation of a bubble cannot be responsible. Moreover, if a patient bends forward and his lumbar joint is fixed with a crack, and manipulation restores movement with another crack, the mechanism cannot be another bubble forming.

* * *

### *A Click is Palpable*

When a loose body lies inside a joint, it may be felt to move from one position to another by both examiner and patient. This is a commonplace at the knee, and often occurs also at the jaw, spinal and elbow joints. Sometimes it may prove possible digitally to manoeuvre a loose body about inside the knee joint. If the knee joint contains fluid, the patella may be clocked down on to the femur.

Laxity of the ligaments may enable a bone to click as it moves in relation to its fellow. This is common at joints unsupported by muscles, e.g. the acromioclavicular, and after capsular overstretching at the shoulder. Painless clicking of a costal cartilage occurs. The patella often clicks on active extension of a perfectly normal knee. The click that is almost always felt on manipulation of a cervical joint may or may not prove significant. If, after it has occurred, the physical signs are found to have altered, a block to movement has clearly been shifted. At the neck several clicks are to be expected, each heralding an improvement. But normal necks also click. In other cases a fragment of disc must have moved insigificantly, perhaps out and immediately back into place again. At the lumbar spine one or at most two clicks are commonplace. They nearly always indicate improvement.

* * *

### *Crepitus is Felt*

The state of the gliding surfaces of a joint is best assessed by palpation of the moving joint. Fine crepitus means slight roughening of the cartilaginous surfaces; coarse crepitus, considerable surface fragmentation. The intermittent creaking of bone against bone clearly indicates that the articular cartilage has wholly worn through.

In the same way, palpation reveals the state of gliding surfaces in those tendons that possess a close-fitting sheath. Fine crepitus characterizes acute traumatic roughening of the surface; coarse crepitus, chronic rheumatoid or tuberculous tenosynovitis.

There are two situations where muscular crepitus occurs. When the extensor and abductor pollicis tendons are affected in the lower forearm, crepitus is elicited locally. However, it is sometimes felt throughout the muscle bellies, almost as far up as the elbow (Cyriax 1941*b*; Thompson et al. 1951). Again, when the musculotendinous junction of the tibialis anterior suffers strain just above the point where the muscle crosses the tibia, a small area of crepitus is usually palpable.

* * *

### *No Movement Hurts*

When there is full and painless passive movement at a joint and no resisted movement hurts either, the pain felt in that region is clearly referred. If this finding is repeated on examination of all the joints and muscles whence pain might spring, the inference is that a tissue outside the sphere of orthopaedic medicine is at fault, most often part of the nervous system but sometimes a viscus. In this connection it should be remembered that in nerve sheath lesions ordinary neurological examination may disclose no fault, since it estimates only conduction along the nerve. The external surface of nerve roots suffer painful interference, often insufficient in degree to affect the parenchyma. It must also be remembered that bones move at adjacent joints. The bone itself is not a moving structure and sympathetic arthritis occurs only when the extremity of a bone is diseased. When the shaft of a bone contains a small lesion, local pain results unaltered by any activity or on testing movement. This is the situation, for example, in osteoid osteoma at the femur.

Normal function of a tissue precludes its containing a painful lesion. Hence the discovery of tenderness at part of a structure, whose function is normal, suggests referred pain.

## OTHER DIAGNOSTIC PROCEDURES

Four other diagnostic procedures may prove useful, but they do not involve testing movement at a joint.

*Localization of Lesion in two Overlapping Tissues.* When a muscle overlies another muscle or some other structure, it may be important to decide which of the two is at fault. Tenderness is estimated by applying equal degrees of pressure when the superficial muscle is first relaxed, then taut. If the pain is greater in the latter event, the more superficial of the two tissues is affected. This method can be used to demonstrate whether the fault lies, for example, in the pectoralis major, an intercostal muscle or rib. Again, visceral tenderness may be distinguished in this way from tenderness of the actual abdominal wall.

*Test for Distant Pain.* When a lesion lies in a long bone, pressure applied distantly may cause pain at the site of the trauma. Thus, pressure on the sternum may set up pain at the site of injury if a rib is broken, or an intercostal muscle torn, or a costovertebral joint arthritic.

*Diagnostic Traction.* If a structure is painfully squeezed, it may prove possible to abolish the symptoms for the time being by traction. This is a very valuable sign, especially in difficult cases of suspected cervical or thoracic articular derangements. For example, pain and/or paraesthesia due to root pressure caused by a cervical disc lesion may disappear for as long as head suspension or manual traction is maintained. Conversely, compression of a joint may increase symptoms, but is a most unreliable sign.

*Aspiration.* It is often important to ascertain whether the fluid in a joint is clear liquid or blood. Aspiration provides an immediate answer and is a safe diagnostic method suitable for outpatient use. Radiography after air has been injected into a joint occasionally reveals a loose body otherwise invisible. Microscopy of the fluid for cells and crystals does not yield much information helpful in diagnosis. The reader is referred to Scott's (1975) paper which provides an excellent illustrated summary.

### Misleading Phenomena

*Referred Tenderness.* The phenomenon of localized 'referred tenderness' can be extremely deceptive, and has been considered in Chapter 3.

*Associated Tenderness.* This phenomenon is even more misleading; for the tender area is sharply localized and very close to the site of the lesion. The tenderness is undoubtedly connected with the lesion, for both disappear together.

Associated tenderness appears to occur at only two sites: the radial styloid process as the result of tenovaginitis of the abductor longus and extensor brevis muscles at the carpus; and the posterior aspect of the lateral humeral epicondyle just above the radiohumeral joint line in the tenoperiosteal variety of tennis elbow. No explanation can be offered for this curious phenomenon.

*Joint Signs in Root Lesions.* In cervical and lumbar disc protrusion leading to root pressure, a highly misleading phenomenon may be found on examination. In the case of a cervical root, each extreme of movement at the shoulder joint may hurt when tested passively; at times one or more of the resisted movements also prove painful. This distracts attention from the neck, focusing it on the shoulder. As the pain in disc protrusion may be entirely brachial, real confusion easily arises. Limitation of passive movement is not, of course, possible in the absence of a local lesion, but patients with acute torricollis often genuinely cannot actively raise the arm on the painful side. When pressure is exerted on a lower lumbar nerve root, testing the hip joint on the same side may reveal that the extremes of movement are of full range but cause unilateral pain. It might well be supposed that the mechanism is the unavoidable transmission of movement to the lumbar joints when the pelvis moves with the hip joint. This is not so; for movement of the other hip tilts the lumbar spine just as much, and does not hurt. I regard the hip movements as capable at their extreme of altering the tension on the sciatic nerve roots in a minor way, analogous to straight-leg raising.

This phenomenon adds considerably to the diagnostic difficulties in spinal nerve root pressure. It also serves to explain how patients mistakenly thought to be suffering from lesions in the shoulder, hip or sacroiliac joint have been cured by manipulation of the spine.

## THE RADIOGRAPH

In soft tissue lesions the radiograph is uninformative except negatively. It shows fractures, and sooner or later must also show lesions involving bone such as abscess formation, tuberculosis or neoplasm. In fracture work, or in the investigation of pulmonary or abdominal visceral disturbances, it provides the greatest assistance. Contrast media can be introduced into any cavity, a blood vessel, the theca, etc., and produce diagnostic appearances. By contrast, only a few simple lesions within the orthopaedic medical orbit, such as osteoarthrosis of the hip joint, show up regularly on the radiograph. Apart from small areas of calcification, not always relevant, the X-ray picture is uniformly negative. For example, whatever is the matter with the shoulder joint, the radiograph shows no abnormality except in cancer, tuberculosis and such rarities as synovial chondromatosis; diseases which provide between them not more than 1% of all non-traumatic painful shoulders. By contrast, a minor radiographic deviation from the normal is often given diagnostic importance when it bears no relation to the patient's trouble. On the strength of visible osteophytes, osteoarthrosis of the spinal or sacroiliac joints is often mistakenly thought to be the cause of symptoms. Osteoarthrosis of the knee—actually an uncommon disorder—is frequently diagnosed through misinterpretation of radiographic appearances, and any middle-aged patient suffering from monarticular rheumatoid arthritis or persistent subluxation of a cartilaginous loose body at the knee is apt to be given this label merely on the strength of changes, present indeed bilaterally, to be expected at that age.

Attempted diagnosis by radiography is proceeding apace nowadays. An elderly patient with, say, tendinitis, bursitis or arthritis at the shoulder (none of which shows on the X-ray photograph), or even with a tennis elbow, is very apt to have a radiograph taken at the site of pain and at the neck. Since the lesion lies in the soft tissues the local photographs reveal no abnormality, but at that age marked trouble is seen at the neck—osteophytosis, one or more diminished joint spaces, etc. If patients old enough to have angina had their necks X-rayed, it could equally unreasonably be alleged that cervical spondylosis caused coronary disease. No doctor would fall for such a facile lack of logic; yet, it is very common to find that patients with disease in an upper limb have received months of treatment to the neck, because the radiographs were inspected without previous clinical examination.

The locomotor disorders that do show up radiologically are usually gross and therefore easy to detect clinically. Surprises are a rarity. But osteitis deformans with involvement of one shoulder or hip might well be mistaken for ordinary osteoarthrosis without X-ray help. When, say, neoplasm of the ilium, sacroiliac arthritis or secondary deposit at a vertebral body is suspected, radiography, if necessary repeated, is essential. Nevertheless, the radiograph need not reveal early disease and must not be taken as excluding such diseases, if the symptoms are of recent date. In my experience, it can take five years for the sclerosis at a spondylitic sacroiliac joint to begin to show. On two occasions, a tuberculous lumbar joint had lasted eighteen months before the invasion of bone became visible. Two years may well elapse before a vertebral myeloma shows up. Cervical chordoma usually takes two years; the first few radiographs are always negative.

On the whole, in orthopaedic medical disorders, irrelevant radiographic appearances must be resolutely ignored. I regard it (but am probably alone in doing so) as far more dangerous to the patient—not to the physician—to omit a proper clinical examination and to rely on radiography, than to do the reverse. Negligence in clinical examination is scarcely capable of proof, whereas failure to X-ray is a simple fact; hence, undue prominence has been given by the Courts to this omission. Hindsight makes it clear that in this particular case an X-ray photograph would have helped, but the Courts ought to take into account the thousand other useless radiographs that would have had to be ordered to prevent the one error. In consequence, doctors nowadays fear not to have a patient X-rayed, since large sums are awarded in damages. But many mistakes, some quite ludicrous and just as culpable medicolegally, were proof to hand, result from attempts at diagnosis in soft tissue lesions mainly by radiography. Moreover, the lulling effect of a normal X-ray picture in early serious disease may prove disastrous. The strength to ignore both a positively and a negatively misleading radiograph comes only from proper clinical examination.

Welcome support for revolt against excessive routine radiography has stemmed from the National Hospital, Queen Square. There Bull and Zilkha (1968) carried out a retrospective survey of 410 patients and a prospective study of 200 more. Their conclusion was that radiography in 'migraine or headache, pain in the neck, vertigo or Ménière's disease, and epilepsy, in the absence of physical signs, does not contribute materially to the diagnosis'.

## EXAMINATION OF THE NERVOUS AND ARTERIAL SYSTEM

This should never be neglected in cases of obscure pain. The search is not for the gross signs that characterize advanced neurological disease, but for minor deviations from the normal. In nerve sheath lesions the patient may complain of pins and needles and numbness; yet examination reveals that cutaneous sensibility at the area felt to be numb is either normal or so little impaired as to leave the issue in doubt. Alternatively, a small degree of muscular weakness or an area of analgesia rather than of anaesthesia are the most that can be expected in the lesions primarily affecting a nerve sheath that so often find their way to the orthopaedic physician.

When a neurological symptom identifies one cutaneous area, *the whole length of the corresponding nerve must be examined*; for the symptoms are felt distally no matter where the nerve trunk suffers compression. For example, ulnar paraesthesia may result from pressure on the eighth cervical root, on the lower trunk of the brachial plexus where it crosses the rib, on the ulnar nerve at the back of the elbow, or at the wrist. Signs of a relevant somatic disorder must be sought at each of these four levels, and the whole attainable stretch of nerve should be palpated as well. Again, paraesthesia of median distribution can arise from fifth cervical disc lesions, the thoracic outlet syndrome, and compression in the carpal tunnel; search from neck to wrist is required. When the paraesthesia occupies, say, every digit of the hand, it is clear that the lesion lies above the differentiation of the brachial plexus, and a much shorter stretch of nerve need be examined, i.e. from the spinal cord to the first rib.

Pins and needles felt in the feet are often an early symptom of pressure on the spinal cord, and may be experienced many years before the plantar response becomes extensor.

## PALPATION

Interpretation of the pattern that emerges when the patient is examined in the manner set out in this chapter nearly always enables the tissue at fault to be singled out. Accessory signs may then disclose at what point in its extent it is affected; if so, palpation is unnecessary. Alternatively, if the structure containing the lesion lies within fingers' reach, palpation for tenderness is most helpful. Such palpation is not indiscriminate; it is confined to the tissue at fault. It must never be undertaken until every movement bearing on the functional assessment has been studied. Palpation too early on in the examination of a patient has been practised on a large scale, and until recently was probably the commonest cause of mistaken diagnosis in the whole of medicine. One has only to consider the former universality of 'fibrositis' to realize how widespread was the adoption of this approach.

The farther down the limb a lesion lies, the more precision in diagnosis palpation affords. At the trunk, shoulder and hip areas, it is seldom of value and often misleading. At the knee and elbow, palpation is helpful, and at the wrist and hand, ankle and foot, it has great importance. Sometimes there is no tenderness over the site of a proximal lesion. The examiner must not let himself be dismayed in such a case since, for example, in supraspinatus tendinitis the tendon is no more tender than its fellow on the other side; and in subdeltoid bursitis the part of the bursa involved may lie under the acromion, inaccessible to the investigating finger. Only when the decision has been reached that the lesion lies quite superficially can absence of tenderness be regarded as showing the diagnosis to be wrong. By contrast, he must be on his guard against the phenomenon of referred and associated tenderness already discussed.

The presence or not of pulsation in the arteries is often important diagnostically. In intermittent claudication the popliteal pulse can seldom be felt. In arterial thrombosis or in coarctation of the aorta, of which an early sign may be vague pains in the lower limbs on walking, the femoral pulses are absent. Thrombosis of the external iliac artery leads to claudication and a cold foot after walking; again the femoral pulse is absent. Sometimes in the thoracic outlet syndrome, and in many normal people, approximation of the scapulae abolishes the radial pulse.

Palpation may also reveal the presence of

deformity, e.g. a Paget tibia, warmth, swelling, fluid or crepitus. Fluctuation may identify a haematoma or fluid in a joint or bursa. (Any muscle appears to fluctuate when tested transversely; hence the examiner's fingers must lie at different levels along the length of the belly.) Bony tenderness may provide the sign suggesting a fracture. In rupture of a muscle or tendon the gap may prove palpable.

Palpation can detect a difference in mobility at one spinal joint as compared with its fellows; lay manipulators lay great stress on this examination. But the question arises whether it is the hypomobile or the hypermobile joint that should be considered pathological. In fact, laymen often find lesions at the upper two lumbar joints by palpation, whereas these are the very levels where trouble is so rare; hence I am not convinced of its diagnostic value. Laymen also allege that they can single out subluxations of one vertebra on another by this means; however, different exponents' findings show marked discrepancy.

In my view, the best criterion is to move each spinal joint in turn and find out at which level symptoms are most strongly evoked.

## LOCAL ANAESTHESIA

When an anatomical localization has been arrived at by correlation of the patient's symptoms with the deductions based on a series of responses to many diagnostic movements, followed or not by palpation, there is still room for error. Whenever possible, therefore, confirmation or disproof should be sought from the induction of local anaesthesia, at any rate for the first few years of the clinical work of the future orthopaedic physician. Otherwise he may erroneously ascribe some particular pattern to a certain disorder and never find out his mistake. If 2–10 ml (depending on the size of the lesion) of a 1 : 200 solution of procaine in saline is injected into the point of origin of the pain, the symptoms disappear for the duration of anaesthesia—about 90 minutes. A stronger solution affords no better anaesthesia and the after-pain is more severe.

In the limbs, if the wrong spot is chosen, the pain, being merely referred thither, fortunately does not cease. Hence, the criterion in these parts of the body is good. Unhappily, the same does not apply to the trunk, especially its posterior aspect. *Pain due to unilateral disc protrusion in the neck, thorax or lumbar region can sometimes be abolished for the time being by a local anaesthetic injection into the tender paraspinal areas.* This phenomenon is difficult to account for, but a possible explanation has been put forward by Whitty and Willison (1958). They suggest that *any* reduction in the impulses which pass to the centre of summation may modify the referred sensation by diminishing the total sensory inflow.

Five minutes after the infiltration, the patient is requested to repeat whichever movement was found on examination to be the most painful, and is asked if it still hurts. It is by no means enough to ask the patient as he lies on the couch if his pain has gone. In addition, if limitation of some movement existed, its range should be estimated again, e.g. straight-leg raising in sciatic root pressure after epidural infiltration or active elevation of the arm in patients with a painful arc. If the pain has nearly or quite disappeared, the right spot has clearly been chosen. If it remains, and the solution has been injected into the intended spot, the diagnosis has been shown to be mistaken; hence the patient must be examined again to see where the error in deduction lies. If he says that the pain is only slightly eased, no attention should be paid, since many patients like to avoid discomfiting the doctor, especially if students are present.

Local anaesthesia is a most valuable method of confirming localizations arrived at in soft tissue lesions. There is no other criterion comparably effective. By using it in every suitable case, the physician makes the patient the judge of the correctness of the diagnosis. It is very easy to fall into the habit of assuming that a certain set of symptoms and signs designate some lesion, and it is only when local anaesthesia has conspicuously failed in several consecutive cases that the physician is brought to realize that he has misconceptions on this particular point. In those numerous soft tissue lesions which lie deeply and in which the radiograph cannot help, it is the patient who, with the help of local anaesthesia, assists the physician to confirm where the lesion lies.

## FAILURE TO ARRIVE AT A DIAGNOSIS

Patients in whom a thorough examination on the lines suggested in this chapter fails to disclose the source of the pain fall into five main categories.

### Slight Pains

When the degree of pain is small, the diagnostic movements may not elicit it in the expected way. If such patients are examined again a week or two later, some of them will be found to have recovered spontaneously. Others will have got worse, and the lesion becomes clearly definable. This applies particularly to some cases of neuritis or of herpes zoster in which the first symptom may be severe pain unaccompanied by any physical signs. The characteristic signs may not appear for several days; until then no certain diagnosis is possible.

### Very Severe Pain

During the first day or two after an injury of any severity, the pain may be such that the patient cannot state accurately which movements hurt and which do not. Moreover, especially at the shoulder and ankle, every passive and resisted movement may be found to cause pain, no clear pattern emerging at all. When localized tenderness is sought, widespread swelling may obscure it by making all spots painful on pressure. When real doubt exists, re-examination at the end of a few days suffices.

In the presence of severe pain, clinical examination may prove extremely difficult on account of an excess of physical signs. For example, in severe lumbago or sciatica the patient may be found lying very still, the smallest movement of any part of his trunk or lower limbs causing intense exacerbation. In such a degree of pain, the patient cannot allow the range of movement at unaffected joints (e.g. the hip) to be tested, nor can he cooperate when the power in his muscles is to be ascertained. Justifiable fear of pain rightly prevents him from moving.

In these cases the history must be given its full weight; gross signs such as muscle wasting or absence of tendon reflexes must be noted and considered in the light of the fact that only a limited number of lesions cause agonizing pain. A radiograph may not be obtainable at first because of the difficulties of moving the patient. One must not forget to take such a patient's temperature; for a septic process of slow onset may give rise to pain starting in much the same way as disc lesions or secondary malignant deposits.

### Lesions Outside the Sphere of Orthopaedic Medicine

The diffuse pains that characterize some diseases of the nervous system and viscera may be difficult to distinguish from the equally diffuse pains so often set up by lesions of the moving parts. Thus the absence of signs of disease of the bones, joints, muscles, etc., of a limb should lead to a neurological and arterial examination. X-ray of the lungs should be included. Inquiry about general health and visceral function must be made and, if necessary, followed up.

### Genuinely Difficult Cases

Most of these are patients with obscure pain in the trunk, especially when the symptoms are felt anteriorly only. The distinction between visceral pain and that caused by lesions of the vertebral column may be most difficult. Moreover, not only may thoracic disc lesions give rise to purely anterior thoracic or abdominal pain, but both cervical and lumbar disc lesions may set up dural pain felt in the trunk far beyond the relevant dermatome. Hence the search must be wide and areas examined from which, in theory, symptoms of such distribution cannot arise.

Another source of difficulty is a minor lesion obscured by psychogenic overlay, the patient putting forward a reasonable story but alleging a number of inconsistent responses on examination. It is then often advisable to have the patient treated for a week or two by the physiotherapist, even without a definite diagnosis, and to ask the hospital social worker for a domestic inquiry. The handling to which the patient becomes accustomed, together with contact with two sensible and dispassionate persons, improves his capacity as a witness when he is next seen. Such treatment is less an evasion of responsibility than preparation for further examination after a clear picture has developed.

Yet another difficulty is a double lesion. When two lesions lie close together, especially when a major lesion overshadows a minor one in its vicinity, or two adjacent tissues appear both affected, a decision on what action to take is not easy. For example, both the supraspinatus and the infraspinatus tendons may appear at fault, or a neck and a shoulder lesion to coexist. In determining the best approach, the following criteria are useful:

*The Most Tractable.* If, say, a patient has a minor cervical disc displacement causing scapular pain and appears to have some disorder at the shoulder too, it is a matter of only a few minutes to carry out manipulative reduction at the neck and, when the pain derived from the neck has ceased, re-examine the shoulder.

*The Commoner.* Since supraspinatus tendinitis is twice as frequent as infraspinatus tendinitis, the statistical approach is reasonable in such cases.

*The Most Obvious.* If one disorder is identified with certainty, it is either anaesthetized or treated until it no longer causes symptoms. This allows the second lesion to stand out during clinical examination later.

*The Most Painful.* Severe pain from one lesion overshadows discomfort emanating from a lesser disorder. This will declare itself only after cure of, or anaesthesia induced at, the greater trouble.

*The Articular.* Vague aches apparently arising from extra-articular sources may be elicited when in fact only the joint is affected. The joint should be treated first and, when it has recovered, the patient is examined again.

## Pain Devoid of Organic Basis

Patients with assumed or purely psychogenic symptoms constitute a real problem in orthopaedic medical clinics, to which are properly sent all cases of obscure pain for which an adequate physical explanation seems lacking. For the sake of the practitioner of orthopaedic medicine himself, no less than that of the staff of the department, such cases *must* be sorted out. Otherwise he may be led to adopt unwarranted opinions on the efficacy of some form of treatment, since dramatic (though usually ephemeral) cure may follow any therapeutic measure, merely as a result of suggestion. Moreover, it is most disheartening to the staff of a department to have to give treatment endlessly to patients who have no organic lesion.

Detection is seldom difficult. The patient's story may arouse suspicion when a most uncommon sequence of events is described, transgressing the rule of 'inherent likelihoods'. The pain is found to spread more and more distantly as the narrative continues. The circumstances attending the onset of pain may be curious and tendentiously put forward and the patient emphasizes suffering rather than symptoms throughout. There may be reference that ignores the segmental boundaries. The pain may come and go in a most unlikely manner and may not obey the generalization that referred pains do not cross the midline. The degree of disablement may vary from day to day, and be much in excess of the patient's complaints and of what examination reveals later.

A great number of active, passive and resisted movements should be performed, the examination beginning at joints as distant as possible from the site of alleged pain. Thus, if the upper limb is stated to hurt, the trunk movements may well be tried first. The examiner may find that the painfulness or not of a movement depends on variations in his tone of voice when asking if pain is elicited, or on the care and expectant attitude with which he attempts some passive movement. The same movement tested in different ways may elicit different answers, as may even the identical movement repeated a few minutes later.

The most striking finding in patients with pain devoid of organic basis is that no coherent pattern emerges, the patient appearing to answer at random and often contradicting himself. Alternatively, every movement at every joint may be stated to cause pain. Again, movements may be said to hurt in areas that they cannot affect. No patient, not even a doctor, when asked to perform a series of movements at several joints, can work out quickly in his mind which should and which should not cause pain. Diffuse tenderness is to be expected, and has led to the erroneous idea of 'diffuse fibrositis', 'generalized muscular rheumatism', and 'polymyalgia'.

It is less, however, on the failure to make a pattern out of the patient's responses than in the discovery of clear inconsistencies that a diagnosis of psychogenic pain may be confidently made. The response to the same movements may alter when performed with the patient standing and lying or on lying prone and lying supine. The range of movement at a joint may be found much limited in one direction and full in all the others in a manner that does not occur at that joint. Or the patient may be unable voluntarily to move a joint at which the passive range is full and muscle power, as tested by resisted movement, normal. If real doubt still exists, the patient may be put on to some indifferent treatment for a fortnight and then examined again. The examiner has recorded the findings, but the patient cannot remember his previous responses (unless they were all positive or all negative) and differences found on the two occasions afford a clear pointer.

The examiner should be on his guard against considering the symptoms of hypersensitive patients as psychogenic. Mere exaggeration does not prove that there is no lesion, for many patients endeavour to impress the examiner by too great a show of pain. In such cases there are no errors of quality but only of quantity. It is both unfair to patients and a hindrance to advancement in diagnosis to label every obscure pain as psychogenic or of little account. On the contrary, if difficult cases are examined repeatedly, some patients will be found ultimately to be suffering from a condition with which the examiner was previously unfamiliar. In others, the increasing disparity between the findings at different times confirms the lack of organic basis for the complaint.

Unfortunately, no test has yet been devised to distinguish between pain deliberately assumed (e.g. for financial purposes or to evoke domestic sympathy) and psychoneurosis, in which the disorder is unconsciously motivated.

*Note:* The matter set out in this chapter in successive editions of this book over the last 40 years has been in part repeated and confirmed by Beetham et al. (1965), to whose work the interested reader is referred.

CHAPTER 6

# THE HEAD, NECK AND SCAPULAR AREA

The chief difficulties when investigating pain in the head, neck and scapular area are the misleading way in which pain and tenderness are referred, belief in cervical spondylosis as a cause of pain and as a contraindication to manipulation, and uncertainty about 'fibrositis'.

## THEORETICAL CONSIDERATIONS

Pain of ligamentous origin appears to occur at the joints between occiput and atlas, and atlas and axis; it results in the old man's matutinal headache. This arises spontaneously in the elderly and is connected with the degeneration and limited movement that designate osteoarthrosis, although equal degrees of osteophytosis can exist radiographically in those who do, and do not, have headache. This concept was put forward by Harrison in 1821 who, referring to the spinal ligaments, stated that 'these get relaxed and suffer a single vertebra to become slightly displaced'. At the remainder of the cervical joints osteoarthrosis of itself causes no symptoms; there is no discomfort, merely a painless limitation of movement that makes the patient complain of stiffness and inability to turn the head properly when backing a car. An intra-articular displacement, i.e. pressure from a protruded fragment of disc, causes pain at a cervical joint no less than at a thoracic or lumbar level, whether or not osteoarthrosis is present. The fact that attrition of the disc and osteophyte formation are symptomless becomes clear after manipulative reduction has been carried out on an allegedly 'osteoarthrotic' neck. Moreover, in most cases the history—even taken by itself—rules out 'osteoarthrosis', for patients complain of intermittent pain, unilateral pain, pain on coughing, sudden twinges on some movements. In such cases examination reveals the partial articular pattern of internal derangement. During manipulation the end-feel is not the bone-to-bone of osteophytes engaging but the softer resistance that is overcome with the production of the small click that heralds cessation of symptoms. Understanding of disc lesions in middle aged and elderly patients will remain clouded until the idea of osteoarthrosis or osteophyte formation as a cause of pain at any level between the third cervical and the fifth lumbar is laid at rest. Osteophytosis is the result, not the cause, of the disc lesions, and it is the latter which cause all the intermittent pain.

Osteophytes do at least exist. By contrast, cervical, scapular or pectoral 'fibrositis' is a purely imaginary concept based on palpation without previous assessment of the function of the relevant tissues. The secondary nature of what used to be called 'fibrositis' can be shown by clinical examination. This discloses that some of the active and passive neck movements evoke or increase the scapular pain, whereas the resisted neck, scapular and arm movements do not. The lesion ascribed to 'fibrositis' is thus shown to have a cervical articular origin, devoid of muscular component. An even more convincing proof lies in manipulation. Before this begins, the patient and examiner identify the very spot. As manipulative reduction at the neck progresses, the spot shifts from, let us say, the infraspinatus muscle to the supraspinatus, then to the rhomboid, then to the trapezius and, finally, when a full range of painless movement has been restored to the affected cervical joint, it has disappeared. In no circumstances could an area of real inflammation in a muscle be made to shift to another muscle and then to yet another in the course of seconds by manipulating a near-by joint.

### Cervical Spondylosis

Spondylosis is a general term for the many different results of degeneration of the intervertebral discs. *It is not a diagnosis,* since the results of degeneration are so varied. A blunderbuss name of this sort is useful as an indication of aetiology, but is not exact enough a description for any decision on treatment; for no indication is afforded whether the pressure is due to an osteophyte or a protruded disc.

Since clinical differentiation is not difficult if the instructions in this chapter are followed, the word should be dropped and replaced by the appropriate diagnosis.

Spondylosis is in part a beneficent phenomenon. The osteophytes that form limit movement and ultimately serve to stabilize a joint containing a fragmented disc. They also increase the size of the weight-bearing surfaces, thus distributing the load over a larger area. Indeed, Adams and Logue (1971) found that, after laminectomy, the less the range of movement, the better the prognosis.

'Spondylosis' at the neck includes:

1. Symptomless osteophyte formation, seen radiologically, at vertebral body or foramen.
2. Symptomless narrowing of one or more joint spaces, indicating erosion of the disc.
3. Osteoarthrosis causing upper cervical pain or headache.
4. Osteophytic compression of one or more nerve roots.
5. Osteophytic compression of the spinal cord, causing paraesthesia in hands and feet.
6. Osteophytic compression of the anterior spinal artery, causing paraplegia.
7. Osteophytic kinking of the vertebral artery by an outcrop on the superior articular process, affecting the basilar circulation.
8. Cervical disc lesion with unilateral or alternating scapular pain.
9. Cervical disc lesion with bilateral pain in the neck.
10. Cervical disc lesion causing headache by extrasegmental dural reference.
11. Cervical disc lesion with unilateral scapulobrachial pain without root palsy.
12. Cervical disc lesion with unilateral scapulobrachial pain with root palsy.
13. Cervical disc lesion with bilateral aching in the upper limbs and paraesthetic hands as the result of bilateral protrusion.
14. Cervical disc lesion causing paraesthesis in hands and feet, as the result of central protrusion.
15. Cervical disc lesion compressing the spinal cord with one or more root palsies in one or both upper limbs and spastic paresis in the lower limbs.
16. Cervical disc protrusion compressing the anterior spinal artery.
17. Adherence of the dura mater to the posterior longitudinal ligament.
18. The mushroom phenomenon at a cervical level.

Clearly, many of the conditions that are lumped together as 'cervical spondylosis' cannot be anything of the sort, since they get well after a time. Any disorder that was genuinely caused by a narrowed disc and osteophyte formation could never improve, since cartilage is avascular and cannot regenerate and osteophytes cannot become smaller.

## REFERRED PAIN

### Headache

Riadore (1843) stated that in cervical spinal disorders the pain may spread from the occiput to the forehead but much doubt exists concerning the circumstances in which pain in the head can spring from the neck. Some disbelieve in the possibility altogether, ignoring the way pain may be made to radiate experimentally from the neck to the head (Cyriax 1938). This was confirmed by Campbell and Parsons (1944) and by Brain (1963) who supported the concept of what he termed 'spondylotic' headache. Others point out that no nerve runs from the occiput to the forehead; but this anatomical objection is invalid, since referred pain does not travel down any nerve, being an error in cortical perception. In fact, reference of pain from neck to head is a commonplace, and has been described in succeeding editions of this book since 1947 but, as the symptoms do not correspond with the known headaches and may go on for years without altering or giving rise to signs of overt disease, these are often mistakenly dismissed as due to neurosis or, at best, as possibly organic but incurable. At times, differentiation is indeed difficult, but the distinction is important; for headache arising from the neck is among those most easily and lastingly relievable. It is therefore a great pity when the diagnosis is missed, since a situation arises in which lay manipulators receive a gratuitous advertisement from medical men. A not uncommon sequence is that an elderly man is told that his headaches are caused by high blood pressure whereas they are in fact unconnected and result from upper cervical osteoarthrosis so apt to occur coincidentally at this age. He goes to a bonesetter; his neck is manipulated; his headache ceases. The patient, and doubtless the layman too, is misled into supposing that manipulation of the neck alters autonomic tone and is the cure for hyperpiesis. Since these laymen assert their ability to cure a number of disorders that manipulation does not in fact alter, unhappy verisimilitude is given to these claims, and patients who really do suffer from arteriosclerosis are induced to waste time and money on fruitless visits. It is well to realize in this connection that several recent surveys have shown that hyperpiesis seldom causes headache. Only when the diastolic pressure reaches 130 mm is there any enhanced liability (Waters 1971).

There are two ways in which headache arises from the neck: by segmental or extrasegmental reference (Cyriax 1938, 1962). Headache, especially migraine, can be triggered off by impulses arising from the neck—perhaps a vascular effect.

*Segmental Reference.* The head is formed from the first and second cervical segments (the mandible from the third). The first and second cervical vertebrae are also derived from these two segments. Hence, on anatomical grounds, lesions of the occipito-atlantoid-axial joints may set up pain felt to spread to any part of the head. Painful capsular contracture occurs some time after an injury—traumatic osteoarthrosis leading to post-traumatic headache—or as age advances. The pain is usually felt to start at the centre of the upper neck, spreading to the occiput, to the vertex (C1) and/or to the temples and forehead (C2). As happens elsewhere, local pain may be wholly absent, the patient then complaining only of the referred headache.

In matutinal headache, the cardinal symptom is pain on waking every morning, felt in the occiput and head, or head only. This begins to ease after some hours, and it has gone by midday. The patient is then free till the next morning. There is nothing periodic about this headache; it appears on waking every day without fail, tending to last longer into the day as the years go by. Analgesics like aspirin have no effect on it. Yet it can be lastingly abolished by one session of manipulation.

*Extrasegmental Reference.* As has already been stated, the dura mater is the only tissue related to the locomotor system from which pain is referred extrasegmentally. Patients often describe pain felt to radiate from the mid-neck down to the scapular area and up to the temple, the forehead and behind one or both eyes, rarely to the bridge of the nose. This description of a pain occupying the territory of the upper thoracic to the second cervical dermatomes (i.e. traversing 12 segments) naturally directs attention to the dura mater, and therefore to the common cause for pressure on it: a disc protrusion.

A central disc lesion at a mid or lower cervical level may give rise to bilateral pain extending from the scapular to the occipital area. Such widespread symptoms may suggest a multiple origin, and the cause is often thought to be cervical osteoarthrosis at several levels, a notion to which the radiographic appearances in any elderly patient will lend spurious colour. An important diagnostic feature in these cases is provocation of dural pain by coughing, a symptom that is, of course, absent in pain of articular origin. Realization that osteoarthrosis at the cervical joints other than the two uppermost of itself causes no discomfort should prevent this misdiagnosis. It is an important error; for such patients can often be fully relieved of their symptoms, but the manipulative technique required is different from that suited to matutinal headaches resulting from segmental reference. It is also different from osteopaths' and chiropractors' manoeuvres.

## Pain in the Face

*Local.* There are a number of well recognized local lesions that cause pain in the face. This may stem from an infected tooth or sinus, from the temporomandibular joint or from the facial bones themselves as the result of fracture, neoplasm, abscess or osteitis deformans. Then there is post-herpetic neuralgia, trigeminal neuralgia (sometimes bilateral in disseminated sclerosis) and arteritis, which may set up intermittent claudication in the tongue or masseter muscles. Just as intracranial arterial dilatation gives rise to migraine, so may a similar affection of the arteries of the face give rise to periodic attacks of pain in one cheek, with a hot ear.

*Referred.* It must be remembered that the face forms part of the second cervical segment; hence pain in the face may originate from the neck. There are two mechanisms: (*a*) segmental reference from a disc lesion at the axial–third cervical joint; (*b*) extrasegmental reference from pressure on the dura mater exerted at any part of its cervical course. It is important, therefore, to examine the joints of the neck in any patient with obscure or long-lasting pain in the face. This also applies to patients with vertigo, tinnitus and positional nystagmus (Cope & Ryan 1959), when no aural cause can be found.

## Thoracic Reference

Pain can be referred extrasegmentally upwards to the head from a lesion causing pressure on the dura mater at an upper thoracic or any cervical level. Pain at one or both aspects of the upper posterior thorax may originate locally, but it is far more often referred from the lower cervical extent of the dura mater. Indeed, the probable cause of scapular pain is a cervical disc protrusion in the early (reducible) stage. Uncommonly, the pain may be pectoral, but felt within the body, less superficially than the scapular aching which appears to the patient to lie close under the surface. Anterior extrasegmental referred pain is no more a transgression of the boundaries of the dermatomes than posterior pain, but is rare, and may well be misdiagnosed as angina. Equally unanatomical is the interscapular pain, without any neckache, that may result from a cervical disc lesion protruding centrally and compressing the dura mater. Since it is accompanied by the same referred tenderness, this time centrally, as occurs unilaterally with scapular pain, the central thoracic pain and tenderness may well be ascribed to an upper thoracic spinal lesion. Compression of the eighth cervical or first or second thoracic nerve roots by a disc protrusion causes lower scapular pain, often felt at the fifth to seventh thoracic dermatome area. Diagnosis may prove difficult before the pain in the upper limb appears and outlines the relevant dermatome there (Brown 1828). When the root pain is absent, it can be extremely difficult to know whether such thoracic pains start from the neck or the upper thoracic part of the spine.

This diagnostic difficulty is enhanced by the fact that neck flexion stretches the dura mater in both the cervical and the thoracic regions; pain elicited by this movement is therefore ambiguous. If the other cervical and not the thoracic, or the other thoracic and not the cervical, movements hurt, the diagnosis is established, but there are cases with rather mixed signs which are anything but clear. Pain on scapular approximation strongly suggests a thoracic lesion, but is not a certainty. Yet, one must at least know beforehand whether manipulative reduction is to be attempted at a cervical or an upper thoracic joint.

## Paraesthesia

Which fingers are involved and how far proximally the pins and needles extend should always be ascertained. If the inner one and a half, or one aspect of the outer three and a half digits, are involved, the relevant nerve trunk must be examined from the base of the neck as far as the hand; no indication of the level of the impingement is afforded, except that it is not at the intervertebral foramen itself. If pins and needles are felt running from the hand to, say, the forearm, the source of pressure cannot lie at the wrist, since the lesion is always proximal to the upper level of the paraesthesia. If, by contrast, all the digits are affected, or any combination other than those mentioned, the level of pressure must lie above the final differentiation of the nerves forming the brachial plexus. Hence a complaint of pins and needles in fingers not supplied by *one* peripheral nerve affords a good indication that the pressure is exerted above the level of the shoulder. In such cases, a dermatomic distribution is to be expected and affords great diagnostic help. If pins and needles are felt in the feet as well, a cervical disc or osteophyte may be projecting centrally and transfixing the spinal cord, but diseases like a spinal neuroma, pernicious anaemia, diabetes and peripheral neuritis must then be excluded.

## Misleading Tenderness

When the dura mater is compressed, tenderness of the muscles at the site of the pain thus caused is a constant and most misleading phenomenon. This is a genuine, deep, localized muscular tenderness, and digital pressure here is stated by the patient not only to have established the exact site of his trouble, but also may evoke the pain referred to the limb. Palpation without previous examination of function in such cases has led to the ascription of such pains to a disorder—regarded as imaginary (Cyriax 1948)—called 'fibrositis', and various authorities have described myalgic spots and trigger areas. These exist; but they are the result, not the cause, of the lesion, as reasoned evaluation of the physical signs present will quickly demonstrate.

The suggestion has been made that such tender areas are the result of small areas of fasciculation, secondary to the lower motor neurone lesion. This is not so; for the tender areas are commonly found at the trapezius, rhomboid or spinatus muscle in, for example, seventh cervical root palsies: muscles belonging to quite other segments, at which the electromyograph can in any case be employed to prove that fibrillation is absent. This phenomenon must be recognized, otherwise minor subluxations in the cervical joints will continue to be misdiagnosed as muscle lesions until root pain supervenes ('fibrositis of the trapezius leading to neuritis'), and the best moment lost for performing manipulative reduction. Palpation for tenderness must be avoided in cervical disc lesions, for it is positively fallacious. It is only in the rare event of the pattern for a muscle lesion appearing when the diagnostic movements are interpreted that the muscles at the base of the neck and scapula should be palpated.

## TEMPORAL ARTERITIS

Giant-cell arteritis scarcely occurs before the age of 60 and the main incidence is over 70. It is a self-limiting disorder, seldom lasting longer than a year. As elderly patients usually have evidence of osteoarthrosis in X-rays of the neck, the pain of arteritis is often mistaken for 'cervical spondylosis'. In these cases the name 'polymyalgia arteritica' is more appropriate. Years of matutinal headache should not be confused with the short history of increasing pain in scalp, face and neck of arteritis. The scalp may become so tender that the pressure of the pillow at night hurts. The ESR is greatly raised, usually to between 50 and 100 mm.

Examination shows the temporal arteries not to pulsate, to be tender and often nodular. The pterygoid muscles may claudicate, and if the lingual arteries are affected the tongue cannot be protruded fully.

Energetic treatment with high doses of cortisone is an urgent necessity; for thrombosis of the ophthalmic artery with irretrievable blindness may otherwise come on without warning.

## THE BASILAR SYNDROME

Vertigo may be dependent on the position of the neck. It is very apt to follow prolonged maintenance of neck extension, e.g. going round an art gallery or painting a ceiling—postures to be avoided by the elderly.

The basilar artery is formed by the junction of the two vertebral arteries. Blood is supplied to the temporal lobes and visual cortex by the two posterior cerebral arteries that spring from the basilar artery. If the circle of Willis is atheromatous and cannot quickly supply extra blood, temporary ischaemia (without thrombosis) of these areas of the brain can be caused by pressure on the vertebral arteries. Vertigo on neck extension is the common complaint; or the patient may have to change from sitting to lying very slowly for fear of severe giddiness. Vision may be momentarily blurred as posture alters.

Rotation about the odontoid process accounts for at least 60°, the remaining movement up to 90° being distributed between the other cervical joints. Gerlach (1884) and later de Kleyn and Nieuwenhuyse (1972) showed that rotation and extension of the neck to one side could obstruct the vertebral artery on the stretched side at the level of the atlas, vertigo and nystagmus resulting. Tatlow and Bammer (1957) showed by angiography that the vertebral artery is also compressed at the second to sixth levels by rotation towards that side. Hence the vertebral artery may be menaced by osteophytes: both those projecting anteriorly from a facet joint and those projecting laterally from the intervertebral joint. It is also endangered by each inferior articular facet if the vertebra moves backwards during movement towards extension. Since marked asymmetry is present in the vertebral arteries in nine-tenths of normal individuals, it is clear that occlusion of only one artery, if it happens to be the major one, can exert a profound influence on the amount of blood reaching the brain. When, therefore, an elderly patient complains of non-progressive symptoms of this kind related to posture and neck movement without deafness, tinnitus or evidence of neurological disease, it is highly probable that osteophytes are compressing the vertebral arteries, thus reducing the basilar flow momentarily. Pins and needles in the face, especially round the lips, are an occasional symptom in basilar ischaemia.

A test has been devised to detect deficient circulation through the vertebral artery. The patient stands with his eyes closed and his arms stretched out horizontally in front of him, keeping quite still. He is then asked to rotate his head fully to one side and stay so for a minute, then to turn his head the other way. His outstretched arms are observed and any straying of the arm away from the parallel suggests cerebral ischaemia caused by the cervical rotation. If the test is positive and careful manipulation during strong traction has no effect, decompression of the vertebral artery at the point of impact as demonstrated by arteriography may be indicated.

## MIGRAINE

The vascular origin of migraine is not in doubt, for angiography has demonstrated the vascular spasm in the cerebral arteries. By contrast, the extracranial blood vessels dilate, and may be felt throbbing not only by the patient but by the examiner. The factors that trigger off an attack in susceptible subjects are unknown, nor do we know whether, in different individuals, the attacks are provoked by a common mechanism.

The history is particularly valuable in distinguishing migraine. In clear cases, a long history—often starting in adolescence—of sudden onset of unilateral throbbing headache is characteristic. It may change sides; it spreads to the whole neck; photophobia, visual hallucinations, tunnel vision and prostration occur; vomiting brings relief. Sometimes, however, the headache is bilateral and not accompanied by typical symptoms; then the diagnostic feature is recurrent severe headache of unprovoked onset, without stiffness of the neck, followed by sudden complete subsidence of all pain until the next attack. Occipital migrainous neuralgia also behaves in this way.

An attack of migraine can sometimes be instantly aborted by strong traction on the neck. Half a minute's traction in some cases is regularly successful, in others not. The mechanism is obscure (it may be connected with stretching the carotid artery) and the phenomenon would clearly repay further study, since it affords one criterion whereby two different types of migraine can be differentiated.

For many years, I supposed, on what appeared to me logical grounds, that manipulation of the neck could have no preventive effect on migraine, but only on those headaches mistaken for migraine. But a minority of patients reported, some years after the reduction by manipulation of a cervical disc replacement, that ever since then attacks of obvious migraine had ceased. Since this happy result is obtained only in the middle-aged or elderly, it may well be that an occasional factor in periodic headache is that described by Kovass (1955). His careful radiological studies showed that the superior articular process of a cervical vertebra can develop an osteophyte that presses on the vertebral artery and the sympathetic fibres running with it. Were pressure at this point exerted by a small displaced fragment of exfoliated articular cartilage within the lateral joint, manipulative reduction couid prove lastingly successful. Be that as it may, it is always worth while manipulating the cervical spine in patients over 40 who suffer from migraine. Curiously enough, migraine dating from adolescence, and therefore most unlikely to be triggered off by trouble in the neck, may respond well in middle age. One session suffices for those whose neck movements are found painless. This negative finding does not preclude a good result. If the neck movements hurt, treatment may have to be repeated two or three times, until all discomfort at the extreme of each range has ceased.

### Cluster Headaches

These are not identical to migraine. They are really severe, much commoner in men and come on at the same hour each day. This goes on for one to three months; then they cease, only to return six months to two years later. They are apt to come on at night, lasting thirty minutes to two hours, always on the same side from occiput to forehead. The eye waters and goes red; the cheek may flush. If the attacks are predominantly nocturnal an ergotamine suppository at bedtime usually suffices. By day, a tablet taken shortly before the attack is due is effective. Peatfield (1981) reports good results with lithium 0.8 g to 1.6 g taken at bedtime.

## TINNITUS AND VERTIGO

That vertigo can originate from the neck has been known for many years. Mayoux et al. (1951) and Ryan and Cope (1955) report instances brought on by traction for cervical spondylosis, accompanied by severe nystagmus in the formers' patient. Ford (1952) drew attention to the syndrome of syncope, vertigo and disturbed vision resulting from obstruction of the vertebral arteries secondary to a defect in the odontoid process. Powers et al. (1961) pointed out that a congenital abnormality of the origin of the vertebral artery from the subclavian artery, whereby it emerged posteriorly and level with the thyrocervical trunk instead of 2 cm medial, resulted in compression against the medial border of the scalene muscle, with consequent vertigo and tinnitus. Division of the scalene and of the branches of the thyrocervical artery, combined with stripping the vertebral artery of its sympathetic supply afforded full relief in 63% of their cases. There is thus no doubt that interference with the vertebral artery can cause vertigo and tinnitus. Indeed, Riadore (1843) had already drawn attention to 'noise in the ears' in cervical spinal trouble.

It is my experience that, when no aural cause has been discovered, tinnitus can sometimes be abolished by cervical manipulation. In one case of 10 years' standing, manipulative relief lasted another 10 years. One such case has been recorded (Broderick 1972). Gurdjian and Thomas (1970) studied 137 cases of whiplash injury and found tinnitus to have resulted in three cases. Many patients feel giddy during an attack of acute torticollis, the vertigo ceasing as soon as manipulative reduction becomes complete. This is not so surprising as it seems at first sight since Wyke (1973) has pointed out that the adoption of the upright posture had the effect of diminishing the importance of the vestibular system and increasing reliance on impulses from the cervical facet joints. Understandably, therefore, asymmetrical impulses from these joints may well cause vertigo. Postural vertigo occurs also in basilar ischaemia.

Important new facts were supplied by Wing and Hargrave-Wilson (1973). They collected 80 cases of cervical vertigo, three-quarters of them women. Half of all patients were aged 40 to 60, and five-sixths had associated occipital or upper cervical pain. Half had had an injury to the neck in the past. One-fifth complained of tinnitus as well. Aural examination had revealed no cause for these symptoms, but encephalograms taken in flexion, extension and rotation of the neck all showed abnormality, especially on rightward rotation. After manipulation of the neck in the osteopathic manner by Hargrave-Wilson half of all cases were fully relieved, and a further third were much better. In three-quarters, the encephalogram revealed significant improvement. Toglia (1976) submitted to electrical testing 309 patients whose chief complaint after a whiplash injury was dizziness. He found more than half with objective signs of a vestibular lesion, in spite of neurological examination having revealed no abnormality. In patients with symptoms of tinnitus or vertigo persisting six months to two years after the accident (three-quarters) the incidence was the same whether litigation was pending or not. He attributes these two symptoms to reduced vertebrobasilar blood flow.

The technique that I employ for this type of case is very strong traction with a minimum of articular movement.

## AURICULAR NEURALGIA

One instance of this rare disorder has come my way. Seventeen years previously the patient had bent his head sharply backwards and had felt an electric shock at his left ear. He had suffered with increasing frequency from agonizing bouts of pain, lasting a minute or two each, up to 30 times a day. Swallowing or a sour drink was apt to precipitate an access of pain.

Two sessions of manipulation proved curative.

## LINGUAL PARAESTHESIA

On one occasion manipulation of the neck served to abolish pins and needles felt at the inferior surface of the tongue as well as in both feet.

## HISTORY IN NECKACHE

In the case of cervical disc protrusion the history is usually characteristic. There are eight recognizable stages. *First*, the young patient is apt to suffer attacks, once a year perhaps, of waking with severe unilateral pain in the neck, which is fixed in visible deformity: acute torticollis. The pain is constant and severe for two or three days, spontaneous recovery taking seven to ten days. Recurrence is to be expected. Acute torticollis is the analogue of lumbago: a large nuclear protrusion appearing during sleep. *Secondly*, attacks of intermittent scapular aching begin during the patient's late twenties or thirties. They last several weeks and again are unilateral, but not always on the same side of the neck. *Thirdly*, during the fifties or later the ache becomes constant, the loose fragment of disc no longer spontaneously returning to its bed. *Fourthly*, at any time after the age of 35, the scapular ache may become much worse and progress to unilateral severe root pain, increased at night with or without pins and needles in the hand. The brachial pain gets worse for a fortnight, remains severe for four to eight weeks and then subsides gradually. Patients with a root paresis usually lose their pain in three months; those without, in four months. *Fifthly*, a bilateral protrusion may set up discomfort in both upper limbs with pins and needles in all the digits of both hands. *Sixthly*, a central protrusion may bulge out the posterior ligament and compress the dura mater, which becomes adherent. At this stage, constant bilateral aching from occiput to scapulae is to be expected in a patient aged 60 or more. *Seventhly*, the spinal cord becomes compressed and pins and needles appear in hands and/or feet, with bilateral aching in the upper limbs. *Lastly*, an osteophyte obliterates the anterior spinal artery and paraplegia results.

The common site for pain arising from a cervical disc lesion is the scapular area, often with upward reference towards the ear. Rarely the pain is pectoral or felt in one axilla only. Naturally pectoral pain in fact of cervical origin radiating down the arm suggests heart disease (Nachlas 1934; Semmes & Murphy 1943). Cough seldom hurts, whereas in a thoracic disc lesion both cough and a deep breath usually increase the pain. Swallowing may be uncomfortable in cervical disc protrusion. Scapular pain occurs in neuralgic amyotrophy and spinal accessory, suprascapular and long thoracic neuritis. Rarely, pain may be referred from the shoulder joint or the sternoclavicular joint to the base of the neck. There is nothing very characteristic about the head- and neckache of temporo-occipital arteritis. It should be suspected if the headache is severe and comes on without previous attacks of neckache in an elderly patient, whose neck on examination reveals no articular signs sufficient to cause more than minor discomfort.

In elderly patients, headache or bilateral occipitocervical pain can arise from the ligaments of the upper two cervical joints. This is the elderly patient's matutinal headache, easing after some hours. Though the pain is not severe, it is very trying since the ordinary analgesics have little or no effect on it. Unilateral cervical pain in the elderly is usually caused by a disc lesion with displacement of a fragment of cartilage within the osteoarthrotic joint; it is *not* due to osteoarthrosis as such. It is the displacement that hurts, whether or not osteoarthrosis is present, as manipulative reduction quickly demonstrates. In younger patients, ankylosing spondylitis gives rise, of course, to stiffness and pain at the neck radiating to the head. As a rule the history of lumbosacral pain finally reaching the neck gives the clue; but the lumbothoracic ankylosis may evolve painlessly, and difficulty in turning the neck be noticed as the first symptom.

Drop attacks may result from congenital laxity of the occipito-atlantoid ligaments or from a deformed odontoid process. Brust's (1979) post mortem findings showed transient ischaemia in the corticospinal tracts in one such case. Again, spondylolisthesis with vertebral fission may lead to similar instability. In each case, both vertebral arteries may suddenly become occluded, the patient falling to the ground without warning and without losing consciousness.

Metastatic deposits give rise to central pain and marked limitation of movement coming on much more quickly than the slow onset of osteoarthrotic stiffness. This speed of onset is characteristic. Movement becomes rapidly limited and the pain more severe week by week rather than year by year.

# INSPECTION

## Inspection of the Neck

The neck may be held in an asymmetrical posture; if so, note should be taken whether the deformity is a pure lateral list or contains an element of rotation as well; if there is pain, the deviation may be towards or away from the painful side. The existence of a compensating thoracic curve is determined. If this is present, the probable cause is adolescent scoliosis, unilateral cervical rib, Klippel-Feil deformity or a past thoracoplasty.

### Congenital Torticollis

Painless congenital contracture of one sternomastoid muscle results in the neck being fixed in side flexion towards the affected side and rotation away from it. In babies there may be a swelling on the muscle, but usually there is not.

Neglected cases are seen in which the contracture has resulted in permanent postural deformity of the neck and facial asymmetry. Treatment should have been instituted by stretching out the sternomastoid muscle and subsequent maintenance of the overcorrected position as soon as the baby was born. If this was not done, division of the muscle is required in adolescence, followed by vigorous after-treatment.

### Acute Torticollis in Children

This is an interesting condition. Children between the ages of 5 and 10, usually after a sore throat, suddenly develop a stiff neck, with little or no pain. Inspection shows the neck to be held in flexion towards one side and rotation in the opposite direction. The resisted neck movements are not weak but may be slightly painful. There may be glands in the neck, particularly on the contracted side, suggesting recent tonsillitis. The radiograph reveals the postural deformity, of course, but no other lesion.

I feel sure that this condition is not caused by a cervical intervertebral disc lesion, nor by acute myositis or anterior poliomyelitis. It resolves spontaneously in about a fortnight, and probably results from a swollen gland lying under and irritating the sternomastoid muscle, thereby causing reflex spasm. This seems to be a minor form of the well-known fixation of the neck from glandular enlargement that characterizes the anginal variety of glandular fever. Manipulation and exercises are useless.

In children occasional cases of afebrile otitis media occur. The presenting symptom may then be merely pain in the neck, and the only sign, for the first week or two, asymmetrical fixation. The neck is held immobile by muscle spasm and the slightest attempt at any passive movement provokes pain and is resented and strongly resisted. This is a greater degree of limitation of movement than occurs in the transient torticollis described above, moreover, movement is limited in every direction. Such signs, in the absence of X-ray evidence of disease of the cervical spine, should lead to aural examination. Retropharyngeal abscess may also start in this way. A child with a rectus palsy cannot look sideways with the affected eye. He therefore turns his head instead. In such ocular torticollis the limitation of movement lies at the eye, not the neck.

### Acute Torticollis in Adults and Adolescents

Acute torticollis is rare before the age of 12 but begins to be quite common at about 15. Whereas disc lesions at thoracic and lumbar levels causing root pain are not infrequent in adolescence, cervical disc lesions, though a common cause of scapular aching, appear not to cause other than ephemeral brachial pain before the age of 35. Exceptionally, patients who have suffered a severe accident to the neck may develop root pain some years younger, but in my experience never before the age of 30.

The patient, usually aged 15 to 30, wakes with a 'crick in his neck', i.e. the neck fixed in side flexion sometimes towards, sometimes away from, the painful side, but without rotation deformity. Marked limitation of only one lateral and only one rotation movement is found on examination, and the pain is unilateral. In other words, part of the joint is blocked by an intra-articular displacement. The nucleus has oozed out slowly during the night, while the patient has lain with the neck held sideways and rotated for hours (Fig. 28). The constant angulation of the joint has led to a progressive bulging. This becomes suddenly and very painfully apparent when the patient sits up and applies weight-bearing to the joint at the same moment as he tries to move it to the neutral position. The pain is constant and severe for a few days and then

**Fig. 28.** Acute torticollis. *Left*, the patient lies with his neck sideways all night. *Right*, prevention.

eases; all symptoms have gone by seven to ten days after the onset.

Lumbago may cause lateral deviation of the lumbar spine, but more often fixation in flexion. In acute torticollis, the frequency is reversed and a list to one side is common, but a neck fixed in flexion is rare, except after a whiplash injury. But it does occur in early posterocentral displacement in youngish persons, and such cases must be treated with great care to avoid further retropulsion towards the spinal cord or stretching of the posterior longitudinal ligament.

During the earliest stage of glandular fever, before the patient has begun to feel unwell, a stiff and aching neck may be the first symptom. The discomfort is diffuse, and every active movement of the neck is uncomfortable in a manner quite unlike a blocked joint. Even if one active movement is limited, the end-feel on passive movement is normal. The resisted movements often hurt, since they press on the tender glands on contracting. These findings lead to search for glandular enlargement and pyrexia.

## Spasmodic Torticollis

The diagnosis is made on inspection. The patient is seen suddenly to twist his head, always in the same direction, by an apparently irresistible active movement. The complaint is of social inconvenience, not pain. The movement can be prevented by the patient's or the examiner's manual pressure, which can also be used to overcome the muscles and rotate the head back into the neutral position. The muscles give way in the manner suggesting neurological hypertonus; there is strong resistance at first, but once the muscles begin to give, resistance ceases. Apart from the repeated movement, nothing abnormal is found when the neck is examined. In severe disease, associated movements may relax the spasm. For example, the patient's head may be fixed in extreme rotation from which position he cannot move it except by bringing his hand to his mouth, whereupon the head automatically turns forward.

Spasmodic torticollis had always been regarded as a tic, hysterically produced. Critchley (1938), however, distinguishes four types: (*a*) purely psychogenic; (*b*) following epidemic encephalitis (often transitory); (*c*) forming part of a more widespread extrapyramidal lesion; and (*d*) a gradually progressive tonic–clonic spasm not confined to the neck muscles. By performing an intracerebral injection, Russell (1938) produced spasmodic torticollis accidentally in a monkey. Post-mortem examination showed a subthalamic infarct.

In early mild cases, it is worth while trying to teach a cooperative patient to move the head in the opposite direction at the moment when he feels the involuntary movement about to begin; this may keep the head still. Other physiotherapy is useless; hypnotism has an occasional success. If the symptoms warrant, assessment of which muscles are causing the movement should be attempted; denervation by means of root section and/or division of the spinal accessory nerve may then bring about marked improvement. Sorensen and Hamby (1965) describe excellent results in half of all cases. Since sterotactic surgery has proved a success in dealing with the torsion spasm of muscular dystonia deformans, Cooper (1965) has reported on this approach in spasmodic torticollis. He has no doubt about the organic nature of most cases; neither has Meares (1973). Indeed, spasmodic torticollis was produced artificially in cats by Jung and Hassler in 1960. They place the lesion at the cerebellothalamic connections and report on 90 cases treated surgically. Meares (1971) states that the late result is often unsatisfactory; only four out of eight cases benefited lastingly from thalamotomy.

## Spastic Torticollis

This is a rare disorder, not always the late result of spasmodic torticollis, for there may be fixation from the first. Instead of the neck rotating involuntarily to one side again and again, it becomes fixed and stays so in rotation and side flexion in the same direction. It takes the patient a strong voluntary effort to bring the head back to the neutral position. As soon as this is relaxed,

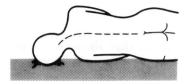

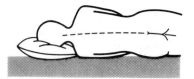

the head turns again and stays so. When the patient lies down and the weight of the head is no longer borne by the neck, the spasm abates and effortless voluntary movement in every direction is restored. The disorder is clearly a perversion of postural tone; when this ceases, the added spasm is simultaneously abolished.

If spontaneous remission has not taken place within five years, the upper three cervical nerve roots are divided at laminectomy together with section of the spinal accessory nerve.

### Associated Movement

In 1978 I saw as a patient a professional tennis player who, for the past five years, had found that when he threw the ball up with his left hand, his head turned involuntarily to the right; thus he could not see the ball to serve. He had had minor backache in the past.

This seemed to me an avoidance reaction, mediated cerebrally, akin to writer's cramp, since it came on only at tennis. I sent him on to Mrs Bobath, MCSP, hoping that she could break him of this habit. He was seen at her clinic by Mrs Bryce, MCSP, who decided that the rotation of the head was brought on by extension at the lumbar spine, though this set up no discomfort. I found this hard to believe, but gave him an epidural injection, whereupon he played tennis during the period of anaesthesia. His head no longer turned, and he has been much better ever since.

### Hysterical Torticollis

These cases are easy to detect; for the patient contracts his vertebroscapular muscles, thus keeping the scapula hunched, as well as flexing the neck towards that side. Elevation of the scapula can play no part in an organic lesion resulting in the head being held fixed in side flexion. No disorder exists in which an adult's neck becomes suddenly so painfully fixed that no movement is possible in any direction. This is also an hysterical manifestation, the muscle contraction being easily overcome by sustained passive pressure during persuasion.

In Parkinsonism, the neck may become gradually stiff and painful, owing to muscle rigidity, and in such elderly patients the radiograph is sure to show 'osteoarthrosis', thus obscuring the true diagnosis. Discovery that the passive range is much larger than the active range affords the clue, and inspection of the facies is confirmatory.

## Inspection of the Scapular Area

The level at which the scapulae lie is noted; unilateral downward and outward displacement suggests trapezial weakness secondary to accidental division of the spinal accessory nerve during an operation for glands in the neck or, less often, localized neuritis of this nerve. Prominence of the vertebral border of one scapula suggests a long thoracic neuritis with paralysis of one serratus anterior muscle: this may be called 'winged scapula' but should not; for it draws attention to the result and not the cause. If both scapulae are affected thus, and both muscles found weak, myopathy is highly probable. A thoracic kyphosis in children and thin adults makes the lower angles of the scapulae stand out prominently. The appearance results from a flat bone being held against a convex surface. As the scapula is applied to the thorax superiorly by muscular tension, it is the lower part of the bone that projects. (Such patients should be treated for the causative kyphosis; exercises to strengthen the thoracoscapular muscles naturally have no good effect.) Occasionally inspection of the scapula reveals isolated wasting of the infraspinatus muscle; rupture, myopathy, traumatic or suprascapular neuritis or severe arthritis of the shoulder then have to be considered. The contour of the thorax itself and of the arm is also noted.

Fixation of one scapula at a higher level than the other characterizes congenital elevation of the scapula (Sprengel's shoulder). The levator scalupae muscle is then replaced by abnormal bone—the suprascapula.

Enlargement of the clavicle provides an occasional manifestation of osteitis deformans; subluxation at the sternoclavicular joint gives rise to false appearance of enlargement by making the bone prominent. Congenital absence of the clavicle, nearly always bilateral, and with such undue mobility of the scapulae that the shoulders can be made to meet in the front of the sternum, characterizes cleidocranial dysostosis.

# EXAMINATION

## Neck Movements

For examination of the active, resisted and passive movements of the neck, the patient sits on a couch or stands. The former is preferred as he is then prevented from moving his trunk as well when asked to move his neck, and the examiner is well placed for resisting the neck and scapular movements. Neck movements are: flexion, extension, flexion to each side, rotation to each side. Their range is noted, whether or not each sets up pain, and if a movement hurts, where the pain is felt. The painfulness of the resisted movements is assessed; weakness is a rarity. If any neck movement hurts in the cervicoscapular area, the lesion clearly lies at the neck. If, as is to be expected, some of the passive movements hurt in the same pattern, but the resisted movements do not, the lesion must be articular.

It is well to realize that restriction of range at the cervical joints is seldom caused by muscle spasm; hence the diagnostic importance of different end-feels. At the neck these are best elicited at the extremes of passive rotation. The normal joint stops with a leathery sensation indicating the end of ligamentous stretching. In osteoarthrosis bone is felt to hit bone. In vertebral metastasis, the twang of muscle spasm is felt coming into play abruptly. Lewitt (1967) reached the same conclusion by another route. In order to ascertain whether restricted movement at the cervical joints was structural or due to muscle spasm, he selected ten patients about to undergo an operation under the full muscular paralysis induced by succinylcholine. Range was assessed just before and during the operation, and was found to be the same.

The passive movements show whether or not a full range at the cervical joints exists and provide useful data for correlation with the findings on active movement. If the passive movements are tested with the patient lying supine, it must be remembered that a greater range exists in this position than when the patient sits up, on account of the postural tone present in the muscles during the erect position. Hence, minor discrepancies in the range of movement have no significance and provide no evidence that a psychogenic disorder is present.

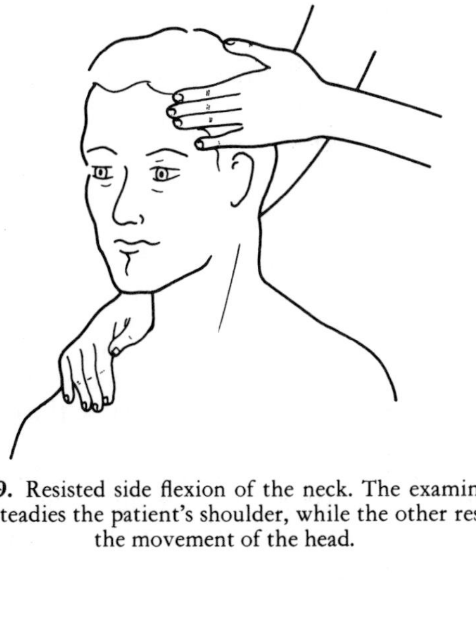

**Fig. 29.** Resisted side flexion of the neck. The examiner's hand steadies the patient's shoulder, while the other resists the movement of the head.

Since testing the resisted movements so seldom causes pain (except in fracture of the first rib, anginal glandular fever, acute adult torticollis, vertebral metastasis or neurosis), it becomes clear that at the neck articular lesions predominate and muscle lesions hardly occur. Therefore, the chief virtue in examination of the muscles against resistance is the information afforded in cases of suspected psychogenic disorder.

Gross wasting of both trapezius muscles and of the erector muscles of the neck occurs in myopathy. The patient has difficulty in holding the head up for long, and the muscle wasting on each side results in great prominence of the spinous processes of the cervical vertebrae. Scleroderma of face and hands may coexist in these cases. On account of the flexion deformity and muscle wasting, these signs may be mistaken for arthrosis at the cervical joints, an error that the radiograph, if the patient is middle aged, appears to confirm. Myasthenia gravis occasionally first shows itself as an inability to hold the head up for long, e.g. at the theatre. In paralysis agitans, pain and limitation of active neck movements are sometimes the presenting symptoms, but the passive range is not limited. This discrepancy leads to immediate realization that voluntary control is at fault. A sudden extension strain to the neck muscles may overstretch the longus colli muscles; if so, the patient cannot lift his head from the pillow in bed and resisted flexion remains weak for about a fortnight.

## Scapular Movements

The patient is asked to shrug his shoulders; this demonstrates whether or not the scapula possesses normal mobility in relation to the thorax. Crepitus on this movement is noted. Pulmonary neoplasm, contracture of the costocoracoid fascia and secondary malignant deposits in the scapula limit passive mobility. In advanced spondylitis ankylopoetica the acromioclavicular joint may suffer ankylosis; scapular movement is then grossly limited and the arm cannot be raised beyond the horizontal. If paraesthesia appears in the hands after the scapulae have been kept elevated for a minute or so, the thoracic outlet syndrome is present. Bringing the scapulae strongly backwards may abolish the radial pulse when the space between the clavicle and the first rib is unduly small. This occurs in some normal persons, but suggests the thoracic outlet syndrome.

The resisted scapular movements are tested next: elevation (trapezius and levator scapulae muscles), forward movement (pectoralis minor and serratus anterior), backward movement (rhomboids and lower trapezius) and pressing against a wall with the arms held forward horizontally (serratus anterior). It must be remembered that the active scapular movements also affect the joints at each end of the clavicle. Scapular approximation stretches the dura mater via the first thoracic nerve root, causing interscapular pain in thoracic disc lesions.

Although the neck, thorax and scapulae have now been tested, it is quite unsafe to stop the examination at this point, even if the patient has purely scapular or cervical pain. The upper limb must be examined next for evidence of a neurological lesion. Unless muscular weakness is carefully sought, a lesion of a nerve root or a nerve trunk may escape detection. Moreover, pulmonary sulcus tumour or neoplasm in the cervical spine cannot be excluded in the earliest stage merely by relying on the radiograph. This may reveal nothing at a time when examination of the forearm and hand reveals marked muscle weakness. Finally, evidence of an upper motor neurone lesion should be sought; for a central posterior protrusion at a cervical or thoracic joint may compress the spinal cord.

### Summary

Full examination for scapular pain of somatic origin thus consists of:

1. Inspection.
2. Testing the joints of the neck, scapula and thorax by active and passive movements.
3. Testing the muscles of the neck, scapula and arm for pain on resisted movements.
4. Neurological examination of the upper limb for lower motor neurone lesion.
5. Neurological examination of the lower limb for upper motor neurone lesion.
6. Radiography (often misleading).
7. Myelography (useful in the later stages).
8. Discography (often misleading).

## INTERPRETATION

### Neck Movements

Neck flexion stretches both the cervical and the thoracic extent of the dura mater; hence this movement will elicit the pain in both a cervical and a thoracic disc lesion; from either region central or unilateral pain at any scapular level may result. The diagnosis rests on which *other* movements prove painful—cervical or thoracic. Pain on scapular approximation nearly always indicates that the thoracic spine is affected, since this movement draws up the thoracic but not the cervical extent of the dura mater.

The *capsular pattern* at the cervical joints is: no limitation of flexion, equal degree of limitation of side flexion and rotation, some or great limitation of extension. Painless restriction in an elderly patient signifies osteoarthrosis, i.e. painless stiffness. If any passive movement other than flexion causes pain, and especially if this is unilateral, a disc lesion is present at the symptomless osteoarthrotic joint. Gross limitation of passive movement in a young person, coming on slowly, characterizes ankylosing spondylitis. If so the lumbothoracic spine is already fixed and the sensation of bone-to-bone is evoked early at the extremes of passive rotation and side flexion at the neck. Marked limitation of movement in the capsular pattern, coming on quickly (i.e. in the course of weeks or at most a few months), accompanied by pain steadily increasing in severity, strongly suggests secondary neoplasm. Invasion at the fourth to seventh levels is easily identified by the neurological signs when the upper limbs are examined, even though no particular discomfort has yet reached the arm. But at the upper three levels no neurological muscle weakness is to be expected; hence detection is more difficult. However, in secondary neoplasm the muscles are affected too, with the result that resisted rotation proves painful, so painful sometimes that the patient is unwilling to press hard. If doubt still exists, and the radiograph is uninformative, gentle passive movements are carried out with the patient supine. The twang of muscle spasm identifies metastasis. If this sensation is elicited a radiograph taken a few weeks later will disclose the osseous rarefaction.

Upper cervical myeloma is indistinguishable from chordoma at first—gradually increasing central pain with marked limitation of movement and the end-feel of muscle spasm. It is only after perhaps two years that the radiograph proves diagnostic. In lower cervical myeloma a root palsy that is too extreme, has lasted too long, or is bilateral arouses suspicion.

## Arthritis

Limited movement in the capsular pattern at the cervical joints may be caused by osteoarthrosis, spondylitic arthritis, rheumatoid arthritis, recent fracture, post-concussional adhesions and disease of bone.

Osteoarthrosis at the upper two cervical joints leads to ligamentous contracture sometimes causing pain in the occiput and forehead, worst in the morning. The patient also finds, for example, that he is embarrassed in trying to reverse a car by inability to turn his head fully. Osteoarthrosis at the lower cervical joints causes no symptoms, merely painless stiffness. If a disc lesion occurs at an osteoarthrotic joint, pain results identical with pain caused by a displacement at a joint devoid of osteoarthrosis.

Since osteophyte formation is the result of degeneration of the disc leading to ligamentous pull and consequent raising up of periosteum at the articular margins, disc lesions are particularly common at osteoarthrotic joints, not as the result but as the cause of the osteophytes visible on the radiograph. This has led to the idea that osteoarthrosis at the neck is painful. This is an important theoretical error for, if osteoarthrosis were the cause of patients' symptoms, no treatment could avail. In fact, if the displacement can be corrected, the allegedly osteoarthrotic pain ceases. The demonstration of osteophytes and diminished joint spaces by radiography in no way contraindicates manipulation by the methods employed by the orthopaedic physician, whereas forcing movement by the methods of osteopathy or chiropraxy is apt to aggravate the condition, as does manipulation under anaesthesia. The elderly patient's tolerance of discomfort is diminished and the amount of distraction possible at his joint is reduced by osteophytes and ligamentous contracture. Hence, the orthopaedic physician's technique involving strong traction is the only safe method in such cases.

Ankylosing spondylitis results in increasing fixation and finally ankylosis in flexion; stiffness in the joints in this disorder precedes local radiographic evidence of the disease by many years. If lumbothoracic involvement has progressed painlessly—as may happen—the diagnosis may remain obscure unless the whole back is inspected. The radiographic appearance, not of the cervical spine, but of the sacroiliac joints, is diagnostic.

Wedge fracture of a cervical vertebral body, left untreated, usually becomes symptomless after a month. It is often first discovered years later when the neck is X-rayed on account of a disc lesion. Radiographic signs of osteophyte formation at the cervical spinal joints is compatible with full painless function; by contrast, in some elderly patients with capsular contracture causing marked limitation of each cervical movement, the radiograph does not show a single osteophyte.

Rheumatoid arthritis may affect the spinal joints, usually after many years of chronic disease, causing bone atrophy and even such inflammatory destruction of ligament that the bones subluxate. Conlon et al. (1966) studied 658 patients' necks, half with osteo- and half with rheumatoid arthritis. They found disc degeneration equally in both groups most often at the fifth–sixth joint, but multiple disc narrowing without osteophytosis and atlanto-axial subluxation were confined to the rheumatoid cases. Cervical subluxation seldom begins less than ten years after the onset of the disease. Different investigators have, in long-standing cases, found radiological evidence of forward displacement of atlas on axis in 10–20% of such patients, of whom only 10–20% had neurological complications.

Rheumatoid arthritis of the cervical joints occurring in the early stage of the disease or as an isolated phenomenon is rare. The diagnosis is made when the patient lies down and the feel of the joint on passive movement is ascertained. In spondylitis the end is reached abruptly by bony block; in osteoarthrosis the movement comes to a fairly hard stop, but in early rheumatoid arthritis the joint has the characteristic 'empty' feeling, i.e. the movement ends without any contact of bone, ceasing at a point which the examiner can tell is far short of how far the joint will go structurally. Manipulation is strongly contraindicated.

There is one disorder that may give rise to combined articular and muscular pain: post-concussional syndrome. The patient lies in bed for some months after a head injury, often fracture of the skull. During this time it is not feasible to give neck exercises. Hence healing in the absence of adequate movements occurs both at the damaged upper cervical joints and at the muscular attachments at the occiput. Such patients are often suspected of psychoneurotic pain; yet massage to the muscle origin together with manipulation of the joints often affords lasting relief.

## Disc Lesions

In disc lesions the partial articular pattern is found. In acute torticollis, the pain is unilateral and though the extremes of five, rarely all six, passive and active movements provoke considerable pain, the pattern of limitation is diagnostic. Gross limitation is present of one side flexion movement, and of the rotation movement towards the same side; often no movement at all in either of these directions is possible. By contrast the other four movements are of full range. In minor more chronic displacement, four, three or two movements prove painful at the extreme, and two, three or four do not. The examiner should beware if only one passive movement hurts, the other five do not, especially if the painful movement is side flexion away from the painful side. Any costoscapuloclavicular lesion, or one at the apex of the lung, may cause pain when it is passively stretched. If resisted side flexion towards the painful side also hurts, a lesion at the first rib, e.g. stress fracture, is the probability. A painful arc, usually on extension or on rotation is pathognomonic of a disc lesion. When root pain is present, some of the neck movements increase the scapular pain in exactly the same way as if root pain were not present. Occasionally, one, two or three of the six movements provoke brachial pain, or paraesthesia in the hand, or both. If so, the likelihood of reduction proving possible is very small. When a patient has nearly recovered from an attack of root pain, the neck movements may no longer hurt in the scapular area, the diagnostic clue (apart from the history) being the characteristic pattern of root weakness on examination of the upper limb. In chronic central posterior disc protrusion, the neck movements, surprisingly enough, may be merely uncomfortable in a vague general sort of way; alternatively a full (for his age) and painless range may be present. Sometimes the extreme of neck flexion may elicit the pins and needles in hands or feet or both—a sign that is shared with disseminated sclerosis, when an active plaque is present at a lower cervical or upper thoracic level of the cord.

## Subacute Arthritis of the Atlanto-axial Joint

This is a rare condition, encountered in my experience only in men aged 25–40 years old. The patient complains of several weeks' increasing stiffness and discomfort in the centre of the upper neck. There has been no previous neck trouble, and, if the patient has had osteopathy, it has merely caused some hours' added pain.

Examination shows a full range of flexion, extension and side flexion at the joints of the neck, but gross limitation of rotation, which may be restricted to 10 or 20° in both directions. This unusual finding naturally engenders caution, but fever is absent, the X-ray picture and the ESR are normal; there has been no sore throat; no glands or mastoid tenderness is present, and examination of the lumbothoracic spine shows no evidence of ankylosing spondylitis.

The patient is asked to lie down and the end-feel of rotation is assessed. The movement comes to a soft stop, quite unlike the bone-hard end-feel of spondylitis or advanced osteoarthrosis (neither of which could come on in a few weeks), the crisp end-feel of a disc lesion, or the twang of the muscle spasm that characterizes secondary malignant deposits.

The cause of this condition is not clear, but it is presumably caused by non-specific inflammation since a few days' indomethacin (25 mg three times a day) restores full painless range. The fact that this disorder is often treated in vain by lay manipulators makes me very sceptical of the alleged sensitivity of their hands, since I should have thought that anyone could perceive the unsuitability of the end-feel.

## Retropharyngeal Tendinitis

Pain in the head and neck of sudden onset and such severity that retropharyngeal abscess may be suspected occurs in tendinitis of the longus colli muscle at its upper extent. Differential diagnosis is made more difficult by the fact that some of the patients have a slight fever. The disorder was first described by Fahlgren et al. in 1966; they had collected 12 patients aged 26–81. Biopsy material from one revealed amorphous chalky material. I have recognized only one case, but can recollect a few others undiagnosed before I became aware of this syndrome.

The onset is sudden and severe, bilateral pain occupying the whole head and neck. Swallowing hurts and a cough is so painful that it makes the patient support his head in his cupped hands. The symptoms ease after two days and cease in about ten days.

The range of active neck movements is markedly restricted in a symmetrical way. Passive flexion and side flexion can be coaxed to full range, but rotation and extension remain obstinately limited. Resisted rotation and flexion are painful.

The diagnosis is established when the lateral X-ray photograph shows a calcified deposit lying in front of the body of the axis and thickening of the shadow thrown by the longus colli muscles, such that it increases from the usual 3 mm to 10 or 15 mm.

### Other Disorders

Limitation of movement in the capsular pattern appearing at once after injury suggests fracture. The same limitation of movement coming on gradually after a severe injury suggests 'traumatic osteoarthrosis'. This lesion, if organic lesion it is, appears confined to patients who are claiming compensation for an injury, and though the limitation of passive range is perfectly genuine, and can be felt to be so when the joint is moved during manipulation, I am in two minds whether it really causes symptoms. Limitation of active, but not passive movement at the neck occurs in paralysis agitans. Annoyingly enough, in the early stage of neuralgic amyotrophy, although there is no articular lesion, the neck movements often hurt in the cervicoscapular area in an uncharacteristic manner. The nature of the disorder is ascertained when the upper limbs are examined and muscles found paralysed at random, not according to the pattern of one root.

Pain on resisted movement occurs in neoplasm and occipital arteritis, when resisted extension and side flexion compress the tender artery. After concussion, a patient may have lain unconscious or uncooperative for days after the accident and adhesions may have formed both about his cervical joints and at the muscle insertions at the occiput.

No lesion, except retropharyngeal tendinitis, exists that causes sudden complete inability to move the head in an otherwise healthy patient. This event characterizes hysteria, when active movement may suddenly become impossible in all directions. Examination shows the exaggeration, and when passive movement is attempted, much resistance is encountered at first. It gradually gives, and finally a full range of passive movements is disclosed, with no pain at extremes but a gush of tears instead.

## Scapular Movements

If scapular pain is brought on by the scapular movements, the following seven patterns exist.

1. The active and passive scapular movements all hurt; the resisted do not. A first or second thoracic root lesion. Some radiation will soon appear to the ulnar border of the forearm and palm (T1) or along the medial aspect of the arm to the inner side of the elbow (T2).
2. Active, and full passive, elevation of the scapula hurts; the forward and backward movements do not. The resisted movements are painless. (*a*) Arthritis at the sternoclavicular joint. When its posterior ligaments are affected, the pain may be felt only at the back of one side of the neck. (*b*) Strain or neoplastic invasion of the costocoracoid fascia. If so, full elevation of the arm also hurts at the pectoroscapular area. (*c*) Healed apical phthisis. Dense scarring here also limits the mobility of the costocoracoid fascia.
3. Active and passive elevation of the scapula are painful and limited but the resisted movements painless. History of trauma and no damage to bone: haematoma lying in contact with the costocoracoid fascia. No history of trauma: apical pulmonary neoplasm should be suspected and the small muscles of the hand examined. The radiograph soon becomes diagnostic.
4. Weakness of adduction of one scapula coupled with 5° limitation of active but not passive elevation of the arm characterizes spinal accessory neuritis.
5. Active and passive approximation of the scapulae hurt; the resisted movement does not. An upper thoracic intraspinal lesion is compressing the dura mater: almost certainly a thoracic disc protrusion.
6. Moving the scapula up and down may elicit discomfort and crepitus, sometimes marked enough to be audible across the room.
7. If active and passive elevation of the scapulae hurt at the pectoral area, in combination with pain elicited also by resisted depression of the bone, the subclavius muscle is at fault.

Unilateral scapular pain unaffected by neck or thoracic movements, taken together with normal X-ray appearances of the lungs and ribs, suggests herpes zoster or infectious neuritis. The vesicles appear after four days, and the pain of infectious neuritis lasts only three weeks. In neuralgic amyotrophy the brachial pain comes on within a few days. Hence pain that has continued for more than a month without radiating suggests visceral disease such as atypical angina.

### First Costotransverse Joint

The pain is felt at one side of the base of the neck. It is evoked by stretching, i.e. neck flexion and side flexion towards the painless side, and by resisted side flexion towards the painful side which pulls the rib upwards when the scalene muscles contract. Active and passive elevation of the scapula also hurt, as does full elevation of the arm. This pattern indicates a lesion lying half-way between neck and scapula, and thus suggests the uppermost costotransverse joint.

## X-RAY EXAMINATION

This yields mostly negative information, showing the absence of tuberculous disease, fracture or neoplastic erosion. But secondary deposits can be detected clinically before enough erosion takes place to show by X-rays. Minor wedge fracture of the body of a vertebra does not set up symptoms after the first few weeks unless the disc was damaged at the same time. When radiographs are taken in full flexion and full extension, it will be noted that, especially in young people, each vertebra slips a little forwards on the one below. This is normal and due to forward sliding on the curve of the lower facet.

Diminution of one or more joint spaces is a commonplace in painless necks. Some osteophyte formation is all but universal in other than young patients, and is compatible with a full and painless range of movement. Gross osteoarthrosis leads to limitation of movement, not necessarily to any discomfort. Ossification in the anterior longitudinal ligament leads to painless stiffness at the affected joint. Congenital fusion of two vertebrae limits movement slightly and is symptomless in itself but leads to overuse of the joints above and below. Disc lesions occur at joints whose space is not visibly diminished; and a narrowed joint space, though it shows the disc to be thin, cannot be taken as evidence of protrusion. If a disc lesion is known to be present, the fact of narrowing does not prove that that joint contains the lesion. Treanor stated at a conference in San Francisco in 1970 that he had found correspondence between the radiological and operative findings in only 34% of cases. A diminished space at the fifth cervical level is often found in cases of seventh or eighth cervical root palsy, i.e. a sixth or seventh cervical disc lesion. Decker (1975), whenever he carried out a myelogram for lumbar trouble, let the contrast medium flow up to the neck and found that 25% of these patients had large asymptomatic defects there. Lateral angulation at one joint only (as is occasionally seen at the lumbar spine) can never be detected, even when the neck is recently fixed in gross deformity. In normal individuals spondylolisthesis may be seen at the third or fourth cervical joint; this has no pathological import and is no bar to manipulation, but the secondary spondylolisthesis of advanced rheumatoid disease is of course significant, and would provide a contraindication to manipulation except for the fact that manipulation is already contraindicated in rheumatoid arthritis without spondylolisthesis. Spondylolisthesis with body defect leading to marked instability leads to drop attacks; this finding provides an absolute bar to manipulation. The radiograph serves merely to exclude unsuspected disease of other kinds, but in early cases of vertebral malignant invasion, it cannot even be relied upon always to do that. It is, of course, patients with secondary deposits not yet visible by X-rays who reach the orthopaedic physician.

A common source of error today is attempted diagnosis by radiography. A patient aged, say, 50 develops an arthritis in his shoulder, or supraspinatus tendinitis or a tennis elbow. The radiograph at that age is sure to show some narrowing of a disc or two with osteophytosis. The radiographic appearances of the shoulder and elbow are normal, since the capsule of a joint and a tendon are both radiotranslucent structures. The patient's pain is now attributed to his neck on radiographic grounds. Things have gone so far that articles have even been published stating that cervical spondylosis *causes* tennis elbow. It would be equally easy to prove, since both occur at the same age, that it causes angina or intermittent claudication.

The posterior osteophyte that compresses the spinal cord is not visible on a plain radiograph, though it is disclosed by myelography. When the anterior spinal artery is, or is in danger of becoming, compressed, radiography with contrast medium is indicated, since decompression or removal of the osteophyte offers the patient the only hope of arrest. Such osteophytes are often multiple. Naturally, a suspected neuroma requires myelography at once.

Osteophytes encroaching on the intervertebral foramen show up well on an oblique view. Even when quite large they may not cause root pressure, since the aperture is four times the size of the root (Wolf et al. 1956). By contrast, if a monoradicular palsy has come on slowly and painlessly in an elderly person, the finding is clearly relevant.

## SECONDARY MALIGNANT DISEASE

### Upper Three Cervical Vertebrae

Malignant deposits at the upper three cervical levels are difficult to detect, for the nervous involvement that makes the situation so clear at lower cervical levels is absent. The patient complains of rapidly increasing stiffness and pain in the neck coming on in the course of one or two months. Examination shows gross limitation of active movement in every direction, and when the passive movements are tested, muscle spasm is felt to spring into action to prevent movement; the bone-to-bone feel at the extreme of range of an osteophytic joint is noticeably absent. The resisted movements are then found also to hurt so much as to be weak—evidence of a gross lesion. Since the patient is usually elderly, and the radiograph may at first show just osteophytes, a mistaken diagnosis of osteoarthrosis is often made. Any patient whose 'osteoarthrosis' has caused grossly restricted movement and increasingly severe pain at the neck in the course of weeks or a very few months should be regarded as suffering from malignant invasion, and X-rayed at intervals until the deposit shows or time proves the ascription to be incorrect.

### Lower Four Cervical Vertebrae

Diagnosis is easy. Suspicion is aroused when marked articular signs (as above) are found in conjunction with a short history. But, when the upper limbs are examined, neurological signs are detected far in excess of anything a disc lesion can produce. In disc lesions there is severe pain and some muscle paresis; in malignant disease the root pain is far less severe, but the paresis much more complete and extensive. Discrepancies are of several sorts. In disc lesions, one root only is affected; in cancer often two or three. Disc lesions set up unilateral weakness; in cancer the paresis is often bilateral, and perhaps at different levels. Discovering that too many muscles are weak puts the examiner on his guard.

### Upper Thoracic Vertebrae

At first thoracic root palsy is, in my experience, never the result of a disc lesion. This causes lower scapular pain with radiation of root pain to the ulnar aspect of the hand, but I have never yet detected any root weakness. If the small muscles of the hand are weak, Horner's syndrome is often present as well; if so, a pulmonary sulcus neoplasm must be sought radiologically. If the apex of the lung is clear, the vertebrae must be X-rayed at intervals.

Difficulty arises with the upper thoracic vertebrae below the first. Malignant invasion, as happens also at the upper three cervical vertebrae, causes no detectable root palsy. But at the upper cervical joints marked limitation of movement is obvious, whereas at upper thoracic levels limitation of movement, however gross, cannot be detected. Unless the root pain is bilateral, only a past history of operation for cancer puts the physician on his guard. In difficult cases (as they all are) one can manipulate if patient, family doctor and previous surgeon agree; or wait several months and only then, if the radiograph remains clear, manipulate.

## FRACTURE

A recent fracture of a vertebral body leads to marked limitation of movement in each direction, especially of extension. The pain is bilateral or central, and the patient has had to hold his neck quite stiff ever since the accident. The patient is not often of the age for malignant deposits, although a pathological fracture occurring, e.g. at tennis, may afford a misleading history. The radiograph is confirmatory, but the appearances are often difficult to interpret.

## CERVICAL NEUROFIBROMAS

These are rare and diagnosis may be anything from very easy to impossible. Any patient who appears to have a cervical disc lesion causing root pain in the upper limb for more than six months should be suspected of a neurofibroma and the case reviewed with this possibility in mind. Naturally enough, articular signs are absent, for there is nothing wrong with the joint. Unhappily, when a cervical disc lesion with brachial pain has been present for some months and spontaneous cure is well advanced, the articular signs often disappear; however, this coincides with relief from pain, whereas the pain of a neuroma goes on increasing.

Neurofibromas have lately appeared in my department at the rate of three or four a year and the possibility must always be considered. Warning points are:

1. The patient's age. A cervical disc lesion causing considerable root pain does not occur under the age of 35; even after a severe accident to the neck it does not appear before 30. Any patient, therefore, in his twenties suffering from what might otherwise be thought to be persistent root pain caused by disc protrusion should be regarded as suffering from a neuroma.
2. Cough hurts the arm. The pain of a cervical disc lesion is seldom aggravated by coughing, and if it is, it is nearly always felt in the scapular area, not down the arm.
3. Primary posterolateral onset. Though it is true that a disc lesion in the neck may start in the reverse fashion (i.e. paraesthetic hand, aching forearm then arm, finally scapular pain), this is uncommon. By contrast neuromas usually start this way.
4. Length of history. Unilateral root pain, especially if a root palsy supervenes, very rarely lasts more than three or four months, and does not get worse after the first month. A neuroma causes pain increasing indefinitely.
5. Extent of weakness. The experienced clinician knows what is the maximum amount of root palsy that a disc protrusion will cause. Weakness too great in degree, or affecting muscles that are not usually involved, is strongly suspicious. Since the cervical nerve roots emerge horizontally, one disc protrusion can squeeze only one nerve root. Hence weakness in muscles derived from more than one segment is almost certainly caused by a tumour.
6. Bilateral development. If a disc protrusion shifts to one side, it moves away from the other side; hence the pain is strictly unilateral. Elderly patients, it is true, may suffer minor bilateral protrusion, and thus get pins and needles in both hands, but they have scarcely any root pain. Hence any young or middle-aged patient, whose unilateral root pain becomes bilateral, probably has a neuroma.
7. Cord symptoms. Pins and needles felt all over the body and evoked by neck flexion are characteristic of a neuroma. Elderly patients with cord pressure from a disc or an osteophyte may have intermittent paraesthesia in one or both hands and feet, but scarcely ever in the entire trunk as well. Moreover, in neuroma the pins and needles often come and go causelessly, and are only seldom brought on by neck flexion.
8. Cord signs. If pressure on the pyramidal tracts is displayed by a spastic gait, incoordination or an extensor plantar response, myelography will be considered whatever the lesion is thought to be.

In neuroma, the straight radiograph reveals nothing relevant at first, but may show misleading narrowing of one or more joint spaces if the patient is no longer young.

If suspicion arises but no convincing signs are detectable, the patient should be kept under observation for as long as is necessary—not less than a year. He should not be referred to a neurological department. Here, when nothing much is found, a patient may be discharged. I have had to wait as long as 18 months for acceptable neurological signs to appear; hence the patient should be encouraged to continue attending.

## CHORDOMA

This tumour is apt to attack middle-aged people. A central ache starts at the upper neck and gets slowly worse. Movement becomes increasingly limited in the course of months, especially rotation. The radiograph shows no lesion for the first 18 months. But the limitation progresses much faster than say that caused by osteoarthrosis, and the end-feel is a soggy stop, neither the hard feel of bone to bone nor the sudden twang of muscle spasm. Forcing movement has usually already been performed by a lay-manipulator, and results in merely a few days' increased pain.

As soon as the radiograph or the myelogram shows the invasion, the surgeon attempts removal, but this is seldom possible fully. Hence the prognosis is bad.

## THE FACET JOINTS

### Osteoarthrosis

Many patients with marked osteoarthrosis of the facet joints, as seen on the radiograph, have no symptoms except restricted movement without discomfort. In what circumstances pain arises is unclear.

The patient is elderly and complains of the gradual onset of an ache at each side of the mid-neck and marked restriction of movement. The ache is never severe and does not radiate, since the dura mater cannot be compressed by a structure lying away from the midline. The pain does not come and go in the manner characteristic of recurrent internal derangement. The ache is never central, nor suboccipital, nor felt at the base of the neck; it would seem that facet osteoarthrosis causes symptoms only at the third and fourth cervical levels.

There is no discomfort when the neck is held motionless, but a!' che neck movements hurt at one or other siae, sometimes on both sides at once. The passive movements hurt more, the resisted do not, and there is no possibility of a neurological deficit.

### Primary Rheumatoid Arthritis

It is rare for rheumatoid arthritis to attack only the cervical facets, without further spread. Nothing suggests the diagnosis at first except the uncommon complaint of years of unremitting discomfort at the sides but not the centre of the mid-neck in a patient perhaps in his thirties or forties. By contrast, disc symptoms come and go and radiate to the scapular area. The nature of the disorder becomes clear only when the neck is given its first tentative manipulation. The operator immediately detects a soggy end-feel and abandons the attempt forthwith. Even so slight a manoeuvre increases the pain for several days. This combination of two unlikely findings brings rheumatoid arthritis of the facet joints to mind.

Recognition is important for one or two intra-articular injections afford several years' relief. My best example was a woman of 40 who was rendered pain-free for the first time for 16 years.

### 'Facet Syndrome'

Many doctors have accepted laymen's idea of symptoms arising from the facet joints in the neck, though the advocates of this theory have put forward no evidence to support this view.

For myself, I have not been able to devise a system of clinical examination that would distinguish a unilateral pain arising from an intervertebral joint from one arising from a facet joint. Certainly, symptoms do arise from the ligaments of the upper two cervical joints and osteoarthrosis at the third and fourth cervical facet joints occasionally causes aching.

Such a condition may exist and cause symptoms; we must await evidence from those who put this idea forward. In the meanwhile, criteria are far easier to intepret at lumbar levels where the burden of clinical findings is strongly against any such ascription (see p. 239). Meanwhile, Crelin (1973), professor of anatomy at Yale University, subjected spines excised within six hours of death to increasing pressures up to the cracking point of the bones. He discovered that subluxation of a vertebra as propounded by chiropractors did not occur.

## OSTEOPHYTIC ROOT PALSY

The symptoms and signs are quite different from those of a cervical disc lesion. The bony outcrop enlarges very slowly, thus causing very little aching, as it gradually grows to transfix the nerve root in the course of years. There is not much neckache; the upper limb may not hurt at all, the patient complaining merely that it is weak. Alternatively, some root pain may be present, changing little in the course of months. Scapular pain is often slight or absent.

Naturally the patient is elderly, 50 or over. Examination shows a neck stiff from osteoarthrosis but often the movements of the neck do not alter such symptoms as are present. Occasionally, side flexion of the neck towards the affected side engages the osteophyte further against the root and sends a pang down the arm. When the upper limb is examined, a severe root palsy at one level only is discovered, most often at the fourth level, since inability to abduct the arm draws attention to itself much more forcibly than a sixth or seventh paresis.

An oblique radiograph of the relevant foramen shows the projection, but the converse does not hold, for many patients with such intraforaminal osteophytosis have no symptoms and no weakness.

If the palsy is severe, the foramen should be explored and the osteophyte drilled away with a dental burr. If it is not severe, the patient should be reviewed at three-monthly intervals for assessment of the degree of root weakness. If it increases, as is to be expected, operation should not be deferred, especially if the abductor muscles of the shoulder are wasting, since inability to raise the arm from the side is a severe disability. If the paresis remains stationary, it is safe to wait. Only once have I encountered a patient whose palsy recovered spontaneously in the course of a year, and it is scarcely worth waiting for this slim chance. Lay manipulation has often been carried out on these patients, and as far as I can see no real harm has resulted. Nevertheless, it can only drive the osteophyte harder against the nerve, and I regard manipulation as contraindicated in these cases.

## NEURALGIC AMYOTROPHY

This is an uncommon disorder, often mistaken for a cervical disc lesion with root pain. However, the history is different and examination shows the disorder to have picked out muscles regardless of root derivation, or all the muscles of several roots.

Violent pain starts suddenly at the centre or both sides of the neck. There is no trauma nor causative strain and the patient remembers that, despite the pain, he could move his head quite well, thus contrasting strongly with the marked restriction of movement that accompanies the early stages of internal derangement. Moreover, the pain is central, whereas in a non-traumatic stiff neck the symptoms are nearly always unilateral. After a few days, the pain spreads down both arms often to the hands, but there are rarely pins and needles. It then leaves one upper limb, but remains in the other, which aches very severely for about two months, and it takes another two or three months for the pain gradually to subside completely.

Examination reveals a full range of movement at the neck, but some of the cervical movements may provoke local discomfort, which may also be aggravated by a cough or a deep breath. Examination of the painless upper limb occasionally reveals that one muscle, usually the infraspinatus, is paralysed, all the other muscles being of full strength. Examination of the painful limb shows that several muscles are paralysed, the others belonging to the same segment retaining full power. A common pattern is paralysis of the infraspinatus with the triceps, or with the extensors of the fingers, or with the extensors of the thumb. It is rare, whatever other muscles are affected, for the infraspinatus muscle on the painful side to escape. The affected muscles are paralysed, not just weak, as in a disc lesion.

Severe cases occur, but do not reach the orthopaedic physician. When a complete palsy of most of the muscles in both upper limbs results from a sudden attack of neuralgic amyotrophy, the patient is bedridden and requires strong analgesics for several months.

The pain in the upper limb remains severe for about two months and then slowly abates. By four months from the onset the patient is comfortable. In the course of the next three or four months muscle power returns spontaneously.

## POST-CONCUSSION HEADACHE

Much confusion exists about this syndrome. Sympathetic doctors regard it as organically determined; the more objectively inclined, as due to neurosis. There being no objective criteria for evaluating headache, the diagnosis is apt to reflect individual doctors' attitude to disorders that do not set up detectable physical signs. Headache—an undisprovable symptom—is, of course, often alleged by patients wishing to strengthen their claim for compensation after injury to the head and neck.

Clearly organic headache complicates concussion; so does neurotic headache; so does assumed headache. But the only rapidly relievable headache of these three is that arising from the neck. Naturally, any force severe enough to cause concussion must expend some of its impact on the neck as well. The joints, less often the muscles, are damaged at the moment of the blow, and the immobility imposed by the damage to the brain prevents early movement. Adhesions form about the occipito-atlanto-axial ligaments, and scars may also form at the occipital insertion of the semispinalis muscles. The former are easily rupturable by manipulation, and the latter by deep friction.

The only difficulty is diagnosis. The headache caused by cerebral commotion is not, of course, alterable by manipulating the neck. Nor will the traumatic neurasthenic be persuaded thus to drop his lawsuit. In either case, the neck is not at fault, and treating it is fruitless. In any case, Pearce established (1974) that in 80% of patients the headache ceased after the lawsuit was settled.

Diagnosis is made first by careful assessment of the history—the lack of tendentious statements, the correspondence between symptoms and disablement, the absence of additional symptoms such as giddiness and inability to concentrate. A straightforward account given in an objective manner inspires confidence. When this is supported by an examination devoid of inconsistencies or exaggeration, the patient must be regarded as sincere. Such patients should receive manipulation of the upper two cervical joints and deep friction to the occipital insertion of the muscles. Success results even in cases where the neck signs are so slight that little benefit is anticipated. Hence one treatment should be given as soon as the patient is seen, and repeated if necessary. Only two or three treatments are required; if the patient is not well by then, it is useless to go on.

Bechgaard (1966), in a review of over 300 cases of injury to the cervical spine, found that in 64% there was a dramatic initial improvement in symptoms after manipulation. Of these, 23 were patients with late post-traumatic headache. Three-quarters of these patients improved after one to three manipulations. Follow-up showed that two patients relapsed after a fortnight, six experienced partial relief only, two remained symptom-free six months later and eight were still well after a year. Since it is in this type of case that orthopaedic medical manipulation during traction is considerably more successful than manipulation by other techniques, these results represent a minimum.

## CRICO-ARYTENOID ARTHRITIS

The crico-arytenoid joints can be affected in severe rheumatoid arthritis (Montgomery et al. 1955) and in long-standing ankylosing spondylitis (Wojtulewski et al. 1973). Their article illustrates the histological appearance of rheumatoid pannus invading the surface of the joint.

Dyspnoea, a hoarse voice and a feeling that the throat is obstructed should lead to laryngoscopy which shows fixation of the arytenoid cartilages and no abduction of the cords on inspiration.

CHAPTER 7

# CERVICAL INTERVERTEBRAL DISC LESIONS

From the clinical point of view the cervical spine includes the upper two thoracic vertebrae, which are examined with the other segments forming the upper limb. Hence the two uppermost thoracic joints are tested with the neck, the thoracic type of examination becoming relevant from the third to the twelfth thoracic levels.

## ANATOMY

The range of movement at the cervical joints was worked out by Bearn and is set out in MacConaill and Basmajian's book (1959). It will be noted that the upper two cervical joints work together as a gimbal, flexion–extension taking place at the atlanto-occipital joint and rotation at the atlanto-axial.

*Atlanto-occipital joint*

| | |
|---|---|
| Flexion–extension | 30° |
| Rotation | 0° |
| Side flexion | 10°–20° |

*Atlanto-axial*

| | |
|---|---|
| Flexion–extension | 5° |
| Rotation | 60°–80° |
| Side flexion | 5° |

*Remaining cervical joints*

| | |
|---|---|
| Flexion–extension | 100° |
| Rotation | 60° |
| Side flexion | 60° |

These anatomical facts do not correspond with clinical findings; for at the spine muscle guarding spans several joints. Just as side flexion in one direction may be wholly barred at all five lumbar joints by a disc protrusion only at the fourth level, so is limitation of movement at distant joints a commonplace at the neck, particularly in acute torticollis. Then rotation in one direction may prove 90° limited as the result of a lower cervical disc protrusion, though the main level at which rotation occurs is the unaffected atlanto-axial joint.

The intervertebral discs lie between the opposing surfaces of the bodies of the vertebrae, except at the joints between occiput and atlas, and atlas and axis. Here no discs exist; hence the first disc lies between the axis and the third cervical vertebra. The first and second roots are very seldom pinched. The disc compresses the nerve root one greater in number than itself; i.e. a protrusion at the fourth level compresses the fifth root and so on. The discs are adherent to the cartilaginous end-plates that cover the articular surface of the adjacent vertebral bodies and blend with the anterior and posterior longitudinal ligaments. They are somewhat thicker anteriorly, thus contributing to the cervical lordosis. As elsewhere, the disc consists of annulus fibrosus and nucleus pulposus, but from the clinical point of view nuclear protrusions form only a small minority of cervical disc displacements. Wolf et al. (1956) found the average anteroposterior diameter of the neural canal to be 1.7 cm, and consider that a protrusion that diminishes the canal to less than 1 cm will compress the spinal cord, but before this has happened adherence of the dura mater to the posterior longitudinal ligament may lead to damage to the cord on neck flexion. In the normal adult, the root foramen is four times the size of the nerve root; hence encroachment must be considerable before conduction is interfered with and in fact quite large foraminal osteophytes may be visible radiographically that cause no pain and no interference with root conduction. Each nerve root possesses a dural sleeve, pressure on which sets up pain felt in any part, or the whole of the relevant dermatome. Pressure on the nerve trunk just beyond its exit from the foramen is painless, distal paraesthesia and a lower motor neurone lesion resulting.

Wilkinson (1964) points out that pressure from disc material may compress the nerve root in two ways:

1. Posterolateral protrusion that does not invade the foramen, but compresses the root against the lamina.
2. Posterolateral protrusion lying a little farther laterally which compresses the nerve root against the articular process.

In her series of 17 patients, all of whom came to autopsy (most of them with multiple protrusions), the frequency was:

| | |
|---|---|
| C2 | 4 |
| C3 | 11 |
| C4 | 12 |
| C5 | 16 |
| C6 | 9 |
| C7 | 2 |

This is quite different from the frequency in the cases of less advanced disease seen by the orthopaedic physician. The root signs indicate that protrusion is very rare at C2 and 3, uncommon at C4 and 5 and 7, and very common at C6. In nine patients out of ten with a root palsy, it lies at the seventh level, i.e. a C6 disc lesion. These root syndromes were worked out clinically and appeared in the 1954 edition of this book. They were confirmed in surgically corroborated cases in considerably greater detail by Yoss et al. (1957). Their findings tally with clinical experience:

| | |
|---|---|
| C5 root | 2% |
| C6 root | 19% |
| C7 root | 69% |
| C8 root | 10% |

80% of their patients were male.

Todd and Pyle (1928) measured the thickness of adults' cervical discs and found the spaces: C2, 3.7 mm; C3, 4 mm; C4, 4.4 mm; C5, 4.8 mm; C6, 5.6 mm; C7, 4.4 mm. Clearly the instability is likely to be greatest where the intervetebral ligaments are longest, and this may well be the cause for the great preponderance of seventh cervical root palsies.

The following operative figures have been reported from Switzerland (Brügger 1960):

| *Joint* | *No. of protrusions* |
|---|---|
| C4 | 1 |
| C5 | 8 |
| C6 | 12 |
| C7 | 0 |

Naturally, a bulging disc exercises ligamentous traction and lifts up periosteum; bone grows to reach its lining membrane and an osteophyte forms. Spondylotic myelopathy is 'one of the commonest diseases of the spinal cord found in middle aged and elderly people' (Wilkinson 1964) and 'it has become increasingly apparent in recent years that cervical spondylosis is the commonest cause of disease of the spinal cord over the age of 50' (Leading article in *British Medical Journal*, 1963).

These two quotations are cited to emphasize that many neurologists now regard cervical protrusions (of disc material and of bone) as the main cause of disease at the cervical extent of the spinal cord. Once gross osteophyte formation or adherence of the dura mater to a bulging posterior ligament has taken place, obviously nothing can be done by conservative treatment to remedy, let alone reverse, this process. But it stresses the importance of the view that I have expressed for so many years, that reduction at a time when this is still possible is the only effective prophylaxis against irremediable damage to the spinal cord years later. This is contrary to current treatment of a protruding disc, which is to leave it where it is, apply a collar and hope for the best. Judging by the neurological opinion recorded above, this attitude does not get the spinal cord very far in the long run.

During full flexion, the neck is 3 cm longer than in full extension. Patients with dural adhesion to the posterior ligament may well damage the cord when they stretch it by neck flexion; now wearing a collar is a rational precaution. This increase in length provides the reason why neck flexion so often aggravates the pain of a thoracic or lumbar disc protrusion: the dura is pulled upwards along its whole extent, engaging or tautening the relevant nerve root against the intraspinal projection. Though the cervical nerve roots also angulate as the dura mater is drawn upwards during neck flexion, it is remarkable how seldom this movement sets up increase of the brachial pain in root compression whether from an osteophyte or a disc protrusion.

## Anterior Spinal Artery

Direct pressure on the dura mater from the bars that project backwards at each interspace, like the rungs on a ladder, leads to cervicoscapular pain, sometimes referred to the occiput and forehead. Further bulging reaches the spinal cord and pins and needles in hands and feet are experienced. Still further protrusion from disc material or from osteophytes reaches the anterior spinal artery and causes ischaemia of the spinal cord. Finally thrombosis of the artery develops leading to quadriplegia.

Anatomists no longer regard the anterior spinal artery as an artery, but as a channel for upward and downward distribution of blood derived from the radicular arteries emanating from the vertebral arteries. Since the vertebral arteries are so seldom symmetrical in calibre (less than one in ten) compression of the radicular branches on the dominant side only as the result of root fibrosis or foraminal stenosis can deprive the anterior spinal artery of much of its blood supply. Then ischaemia of the spinal cord follows without direct pressure on it.

## EXAMINATION

The objects of the examination are four. *First*, examination of neck, by active, resisted and passive movements to decide if an articular lesion is present. *Secondly*, examination of the upper limb for root paresis. *Thirdly*, examination of conduction along the spinal cord. *Fourthly*, if complaint is made suggesting root pain, examination of the upper limb for an alternative cause for the pain in the arm. Cervical disc lesions are so common that patients often develop a painful disorder of the upper limb at a time when they happen to have scapular pain caused by a cervical disc lesion, and the brachial pain is then apt to be mistakenly attributed to root pressure: an error to which the radiographic appearances of a middle-aged patient's neck misleadingly afford apparent confirmation. It will be noted that the expected fifth component of clinical examination does not apply—estimating the mobility of the nerve roots. The fourth to eighth cervical roots are already fully stretched when the patient's arm hangs by his side. Tension on the fifth, sixth and seventh roots is prevented by their being tethered at the lateral border of each foramen. Though they shift within the spine on neck movements, they do not do so extraspinally (Adams & Logue 1971). Hence the nerve fibres of the brachial plexus follow a zig-zag course, which allows for elongation (Fontana 1781). Clark and Bearn (1972) showed that the brachial nerves had spiral bands which enabled them to stretch a further 16% without damage. This elasticity was absent at the lumbosacral nerve roots: hence the phenomenon of limited straight-leg raising.

### Articular Signs

The patient performs six active movements: flexion, extension, side flexion each way, rotation each way. He states whether or not each movement hurts, and if so where; the examiner notes the range of movement. The same six movements may then be tested again passively and against resistance, the patient reporting each result. These findings are then collated.

Since cervical disc lesions often give rise to upper posterior thoracic pain, as may also upper thoracic disc lesions, it is important to realize that neck flexion is an articular movement as regards the cervical joints, but pulls the dura mater upwards at its thoracic extent. Adams and Logue (1971) have shown that neck flexion causes unfolding of creases in the dural tube to the extent of one-third. The remaining two-thirds involve actual upward movement of the theca. Hence upper thoracic pain provoked by neck flexion is an ambiguous finding; diagnosis depends on what other movements of the neck, scapula and thorax do, or do not, reproduce the symptoms.

The articular signs are the same whatever the level of the lesion; this can be deduced with certainty only if root signs appear. In recent cases, an oscillatory technique can be used to detect the joint that resents passive movement. The examiner applies his thumbs at each side of a cervical spinous process, and can feel the muscles contract to protect the affected joint. Alternatively, the patient can lie supine with the examiner's fingers under his neck. An anteroposterior gliding movement can be imparted to each joint in turn, the patient stating at which level his symptoms are reproduced best. These tests are useful if manipulation in the osteopathic or chiropractic way is contemplated, but unnecessary if orthopaedic medical methods are employed.

In internal derangement, the pain is usually unilateral and felt all over or anywhere in the neck and scapular area. The symptoms are provoked in the manner of a blocked joint, some active movements hurting unilaterally, others not. Common patterns are two, three or four movements out of the six hurting and four, three or two proving painless. A painful arc is not uncommon on rotation in unilateral pain, or on extension if the pain is central. Active rotation towards the painful side nearly always hurts at the extreme; this movement is sometimes unilaterally limited. The passive movements reproduce the same pattern, and hurt more than the active. The resisted movements prove painless, except that resisted flexion may be uncomfortable, presumably as a result of the consequent compression strain on the affected joint.

In acute torticollis in young people (15–30), the articular signs are gross and obvious: the onset is sudden, usually on waking; the neck deviates, often away from the painful side; side flexion and rotation in one direction cannot be performed actively or passively; yet movement in the other directions remains little affected.

When a patient is recovering from severe root pain, there is often a moment when the neck movements reach full painless range but the upper limb still hurts considerably. The history, the presence of the root palsy and the fact that he states that his neck was very stiff originally provide the clue.

The articular signs in central posterior protrusion vary a great deal. In a recent case in a young or middle-aged patient the neck may be fixed in flexion; the analogue of lumbago. Long-standing gradual protrusion in the elderly may leave the neck movements entirely painless even in the presence of a large projection squeezing the spinal cord, and the limitation of movement may be no more than is usual at that age in trouble-free patients.

Bilateral posterolateral protrusion also sets up little in the way of articular signs. The patient is elderly, complains of an ache in both upper limbs and paraesthetic hands. Examination shows some discomfort at each side of the neck on the cervical movements; there is often considerable limitation, but often not more than can exist in patients without symptoms.

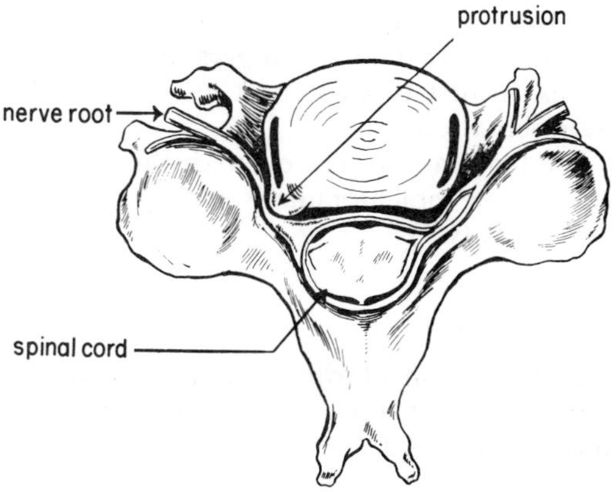


**Fig. 30.** Protrusion of the disc substance at a lower cervical joint causing root pressure.

## Root Signs

Root-pain and signs due to disc protrusion occur between the ages of 35 and 60. In younger patients, neuroma should be suspected; in older patients, osteophytosis or metastasis.

The symptoms are three-fold; scapular pain caused by unilateral compression of the dura mater; root pain due to pressure on the dural sleeve of the nerve root; weakness and tingling due to parenchymatous involvement. The signs are threefold; for there is no way of testing the mobility of a cervical nerve root at the intervertebral foramen in a manner analogous to stretching the lower three lumbar nerve roots. Adams and Logue (1971) showed that the lower cervical nerve roots are tethered at their exit from the foramen. Thus they move within the spine on neck movements but not at their extraspinal extent. They are thus: (*a*) articular signs; (*b*) ascertaining if a cervical movement increases the pain in the arm or brings on the pins and needles in the hand; (*c*) estimating conduction along the root. However, the examiner must not expect the neck movements to hurt down the arm; this is uncommon. Nor must he await the appearance of a clear root palsy before diagnosing cervical disc lesion; this must be done on the articular signs alone. By the time a root paresis makes the diagnosis obvious, the time for effective treatment has passed. If this were realized, root pain would become a rarity, manipulative reduction having been carried out at the stage of scapular pain only.

The upper limb is examined for root paresis; if present, this indicates the level of the protrusion. The following movements are tested against resistance:

| | |
|---|---|
| Rotation of neck | C1 |
| Shrugging shoulders | C2, 3, 4 |
| Abduction and lateral rotation at shoulder | C5 |
| Adduction of arm | C7 |
| Flexion at elbow | C5, 6 |
| Extension at wrist | C6 |
| Extension at elbow | C7 |
| Flexion at wrist | C7 |
| Ulnar deviation at wrist | C8 |
| Extension and adduction of thumb | C8 |
| Approximation of fourth and fifth fingers | T1 |

Cutaneous analgesia is sought at the fingers: it is absent in fifth root lesions, often present at the thumb and index in sixth root lesions, the index, long and ring fingers in seventh root lesions; the middle and two ulnar fingers in eighth root lesions. In first thoracic root lesions the fingers retain sensation.

The tendon jerks are elicited, the biceps jerk (C5, 6), the brachioradialis jerk (C5) and the triceps jerk (C7).

### Cord Signs

A spastic gait, incoordination of the lower limbs and an extensor plantar response indicate pressure on the spinal cord.

### Upper Limb Signs

An alternative cause for the ache in the arm becomes apparent during examination of the upper limb for root paresis. If limitation of passive movement at the shoulder or, say, a tennis elbow is found, the patient with articular signs at his neck as well must have two lesions. Difficulty arises when a patient has a cervical disc lesion and also presents rather vague signs at the shoulder joint—a full range of movement but a suggestion perhaps of subdeltoid bursitis or a tendinitis as well. These secondary signs may prove false. The situation is clarified when manipulative reduction is carried out at the neck. The shoulder is then examined again. In at least half the cases, the shoulder 'signs' will be found to have disappeared.

## Pressure on Individual Roots

The first intervertebral disc lies between the second and third cervical vertebrae. The first cervical root emerges between the occiput and the atlas, and the eighth cervical root between the seventh cervical and the first thoracic vertebrae. It follows that a cervical intervertebral disc, when it protrudes, compresses the root one great in number: e.g. the disc at the sixth joint affects the seventh root. In the list appended here, the maximum root signs are set out, but partial palsies do occur, though not so often as in the lower limb.

### First and Second Cervical Roots

*False Reference.* Cases are not infrequently encountered of pain in the neck spreading to the vertex of the skull (C1) or to one temple, the forehead and behind one or both eyes (C2). Examination shows the pain to originate in the joints of the neck. In young patients there is no question yet of occipito-atlanto-axial osteoarthrosis leading to bilateral capsular pain felt in the head; moreover, the pain may be unilateral. The cause cannot be a disc lesion at the upper two joints, since they do not contain a disc. Pain in the head associated with a cervical disc lesion is only another example of extrasegmental reference from the dura mater; it has nothing to do with the first and second cervical nerve roots. In fact it is no more unreasonable for a disc lesion at the sixth or seventh level to set up pain in the upper neck (C3) and occiput (C2) than in the forehead, which is also part of the second cervical segment. The degree of extrasegmental reference is the same.

*Root Pressure.* Unilateral pain felt at the upper neck accompanied by *tingling* in the occipitoparietal region on the same side is a rare complaint in elderly patients; this appears to be a true localizing sign. Examination of movements shows the articular pattern accompanied by marked limitation of movement in every direction. Rotation may be reduced to 10° range. Gross osteoarthrosis at one side of the atlanto-axial joint is presumably responsible, with an osteophyte engaging against the second cervical root.

### Third Cervical Root

This is rarely affected. Possible symptoms in addition to the unilateral pain in the neck are pins and needles and numbness felt at the lower pinna, the posterior part of the cheek, the temporal area and any part of the lateral aspect of the neck with a forward projection along the chin. I have met with two cases in which the paraesthesia extended to half the tongue. Clinically I have never detected muscular weakness. Occasionally unilateral analgesia of the skin of some part of the neck is present. Rarely, paraesthesia in one cheek is the only symptom; naturally this draws immediate attention to the trigeminal nerve. When repeated expert neurological examination reveals no lesion of this nerve, and time shows that the trouble is not progressive, the patient is usually regarded as imaginative or, at best, as suffering from an undiagnosable disorder.

### Fourth Cervical Root

These cases are rare. The pain spreads outwards from the mid-neck and is concentrated at the shoulder. This distribution is slightly different from that caused by pressure on the side of the dura mater at any cervical level; for in the latter event scapular pain is felt posteriorly, seldom at the point of the shoulder, and it does not end abruptly at the deltoid area. Pins and needles are absent, but a horizontal band of cutaneous analgesia, 2–4 cm wide, may be found along the spine of the scapula, the mid-deltoid area and the clavicle, like a half-hoop. No muscle weakness is detectable.

## Fifth Cervical Root

The pain extends from the scapular area to the front of the arm and forearm as far as the radial side of the hand; it does not extend to the thumb; pins and needles are, in my experience, absent. Yoss et al. (1957) also comment on the absence of paraesthesia in fifth cervical root pressure. *The weak muscles are* the two spinati, the deltoid and the biceps. The biceps jerk may be sluggish or absent; the brachioradialis jerk sluggish, absent or inverted.

*Differential Diagnosis.* The most difficult finding, leading to frequent errors, especially in elderly patients, is a combination of cervical disc lesion causing scapular pain, and some other lesion (e.g. supraspinatus tendinitis or arthritis of the shoulder) giving rise to pain felt in the arm. Since at this age, radiological alterations are always visible at the cervical vertebrae, and the radiograph in most painful shoulders reveals no local abnormality, X-ray examination can be most misleading.

The other conditions to be kept in mind are enumerated below:

1. Traction palsy of the fifth cervical root.
2. Palsy of the axillary nerve after dislocation at the shoulder.
3. Neuritis of the spinal accessory, long thoracic or suprascapular nerve.
4. Traumatic palsy of the suprascapular nerve.
5. Herpes zoster.
6. Myopathy affecting the deltoid and spinatus muscles, complicated by capsular pain (due to disuse contracture) emanating from the shoulder joint.
7. Rupture of the supraspinatus tendon.
8. Rupture of the infraspinatus tendon.
9. Secondary malignant deposits at the scapula.
10. Diaphragmatic pleurisy.

## Sixth Cervical Root

The pain spreads down the front of the arm and forearm to the radial side of the hand, and pins and needles felt in the thumb and index finger are often a conspicuous feature; cutaneous analgesia may be detectable at the tips of these digits. *The weak muscles are* biceps, brachialis, supinator brevis and the extensores carpi radialis. Wasting of the brachioradialis muscle may be visible. Occasionally the subscapularis muscle is weak too. The biceps jerk is sluggish or absent, sometimes as an isolated finding.

*Differential Diagnosis.* At this level, the difficulty lies in the fact that the muscular weakness is often slight. Electromyography may assist, but paresis detectable clinically often appears before electrical testing reveals any abnormality. The conditions that give rise to similar symptoms are:

1. Pressure on the median nerve in the carpal tunnel.
2. Pressure of the first rib or of a cervical rib on the lower trunk of the brachial plexus.
3. Tendinitis or partial rupture of the biceps muscle.
4. Radial pressure palsy at mid-humerus. Extension of the wrist is not just weak, as in a disc lesion, but completely paralysed, together with extension of the fingers at the metacarpophalangeal joints. Extension of the thumb and supination at the elbow are weak. The cutaneous analgesia extends from the outer aspect of the elbow, along the radial side of the forearm, to the dorsum of the whole thumb and of the proximal phalanges of the index and long fingers.

   As a rule, the patient wakes with painless drop-wrist, having fallen asleep with his arm over the edge of a chair. Nowadays, 'Saturday night paralysis' is more apt to occur in drug addicts than in heavy drinkers. Other causes are: lying all night with the arm resting against the hard edge of a bunk, using the old-fashioned axillary crutch or fracture of the humerus.
5. Rheumatoid perineuritis, especially if it complicates monarticular rheumatoid arthritis of the shoulder joint.
6. Tennis elbow.

## Seventh Cervical Root

This is by far the commonest root affected; at least nine out of ten cervical disc lesions causing a root palsy occur at this level. The pain extends from the scapular area down the back of the arm, via the outer forearm, to the fingertips; pins and needles are usually felt in the index, long and ring fingers. Rarely the pain is pectoral instead of scapular; indeed, a few patients with weakness due to a seventh root palsy never develop any brachial discomfort at all, but only unilateral anterior upper thoracic pain. Some of the neck movements provoke the pectoral pain; the thoracic movements and resisted adduction of the arm do not, and it is examination of the symptom-free upper limb that clarifies the diagnosis. *The outstandingly weak muscle* is the triceps; the radial flexor, much less often the extensors (or both), of the wrist may be weakened too. The triceps jerk is seldom affected even when the triceps muscle is extremely weak. Cutaneous analgesia is often found at the dorsum of the long and index fingers. After severe and prolonged pressure, complete wasting of the mid-fibres of the pectoralis major muscle may appear as a triangular depression lying between the parts of the muscle developed from the sixth and eighth myotomes. Rarely, a larger part than usual of the serratus anterior is developed from the seventh myotome and partial winging of the scapula results. Adduction of the arm becomes weak because the latissimus dorsi muscle is largely derived from the seventh cervical segment. Though the seventh root cannot be painfully stretched, the patient finds relief from putting his hand on his head: a posture that relieves tension on the root. Patients should be told to adopt this position when trying to fall asleep.

*Differential Diagnosis*

1. Lead poisoning (always bilateral).
2. Carcinoma of the bronchus.
3. Tennis elbow; golfer's elbow.
4. Tricipital tendinitis.
5. Fracture of the olecranon.

## Eighth Cervical Root

The pain occupies the *lower* scapular area, the back or inner side of the arm and the inner forearm; pins and needles are usually felt at the third, fourth, and fifth fingers. *The weak muscles* are the ulnar deviators of the wrist, the extensor and adductor muscles of the thumb, the extensor muscles of the fingers and the abductor indicis. The triceps muscle is sometimes a little weak too. Cutaneous analgesia may be detected at the fifth finger.

*Differential Diagnosis*

1. Cervical rib. The muscles derived from the first thoracic myotome are affected.
2. Pressure on the lower trunk of the brachial plexus by the first rib.
3. Malignant deposits at the seventh cervical or first thoracic vertebra. This is their usual site at the cervical spine and the condition is easy to detect; for the pain is not severe in proportion to the weakness, which is extreme. Moreover, the seventh and eighth, alternatively the eighth cervical and first thoracic, roots are *both* involved, with the result that the whole hand and forearm are virtually paralysed. Disc lesions in the neck do not give rise to multiple palsies; hence evidence of involvement of two roots immediately suggests secondary neoplasm, whether or not the radiograph shows bone erosion as yet.
4. Pancoast's tumour. The neck movements are usually of full range and painless, although side flexion away from the painful side may prove uncomfortable. Elevation of the scapula is usually painful and may be limited; if so, full passive elevation of the arm hurts too. Horner's syndrome and a first thoracic palsy are present; X-ray examination of the apex of the lung reveals an opacity.
5. Angina. Although cervical disc lesions usually give rise to scapular pain spreading to the upper limb, cases are occasionally encountered of unilateral reference to the front of the chest. Pain in the neck and the left pectoral area spreading down the upper limb to the ulnar aspect of the hand naturally suggest a myocardial disorder, especially if the patient is no longer young.
6. Traction palsy of the lower two roots of the brachial plexus.
7. Frictional ulnar neuritis at the elbow.
8. Pressure on the ulnar nerve at the wrist. Occupational; or a ganglion connected with the flexor carpi ulnaris tendon.
9. Thrombosis of the subclavian artery. The upper-limb pain is claudicational and the radial pulse is lost.

## First Thoracic Root

Disc lesions at the first thoracic level are very rare. One case has been reported by Gelch (1978). The patient was a man of 40 with five weeks' pain in the neck and pectoroscapular area radiating down the inner side of his arm. The small muscles of his hand were weak together with Horner's syndrome. Myelography revealed a defect at the first thoracic level, and removal of the disc protrusion brought about recovery. Most patients with symptoms attributable to this root are, in fact, suffering from some other disorder, e.g. cervical rib, pulmonary sulcus tumour, secondary vertebral neoplasm, or pressure on the median or ulnar nerve trunk.

The pain is felt diffusely in the lower pectoroscapular area and spreads down the inner aspect of the arm to the ulnar border of the hand, where pins and needles and slight numbness may be noted. The fingers are unaffected. In first thoracic disc lesions, *there is no weakness of the hand*; if this is found, neoplasm or a cervical rib is the likely cause.

The first thoracic root can be painfully stretched by forward movement of the scapula and also by abduction of the arm to the horizontal and then stretching the ulnar nerve by flexing the elbow. Both these movements should aggravate the thoracic pain, as do coughing and neck flexion. Reduction by manipulation is difficult; if it fails, spontaneous recovery is not to be expected in less than six to twelve months.

### Second Thoracic Root

I have met with four cases. A man of 40 lifted a heavy weight while crouching and felt a click in one scapular area. Within some hours he had unilateral pain in the pectoroscapular region, spreading to the inner side of the elbow. He had had constant pain for six weeks, aggravated by a deep breath or cough. The movements found to increase the brachial pain were neck flexion during full elevation of the painful limb, neck flexion during scapular approximation and elbow flexion with the arm horizontal, i.e. touching the back of his neck. In one case a fortnight's treatment by daily head suspension, and in the other two sessions of manipulation, afforded full relief. The third patient started with pain felt only at the manubrium sterni, spreading to the scapular areas and inner arms after a fortnight. Manipulation did not help but a series of strong manual tractions on five occasions afforded reduction. The fourth patient was only 16 years old and the pain along the inner aspect of his arm ceased after side flexion away from the painful side had been maintained for minutes on end. Two sessions sufficed.

## Cervical Disc Lesions Causing Pressure on the Spinal Cord

Nowadays it is generally agreed that the commonest cause of upper motor neurone disease in elderly patients is central posterior protrusion of disc substance, or the development of an osteophyte in this situation. In either case the spinal cord suffers compression and/or ischaemia.

### Sudden Onset with Pain in the Neck

These cases used to be called transverse myelitis if the onset was unprovoked, and contusion of the spinal cord if the cause was severe trauma to the neck. Severe pain in the neck is followed by pain, weakness and tingling in both upper limbs, or in all four limbs. A central posterior protrusion or a fold of ligament has squeezed the spinal cord.

### Pain in Both Upper Limbs

The patient develops pain in both scapular areas, soon radiating to the arms and forearms. The hands tingle, rarely the pain in the arms alternates; if it is more severe on one side, it is correspondingly less on the other. Then pins and needles appear at the soles of the feet, often increased or brought on by neck flexion.

In these cases, since the displacement is central and interferes little with the joint from which it protrudes, the articular signs at the neck may be quite inconspicuous, the commonest being considerable limitation of extension. The symptoms often suggest the thoracic outlet syndrome or, less often, a sensory stroke, and differential diagnosis is not easy. The protrusion being central, there is no tendency to spontaneous cure such as characterizes unilateral pain caused by a posterolateral protrusion. The brachial pain may thus last for years; by corollary, manipulative reduction may prove possible also after years of pain and paraesthesia.

### Painless Slow Onset

The patient finds difficulty in walking and on examination is found to have an upper motor neurone lesion affecting both legs. Hands and feet tingle; a common complaint is pins and needles from the front of both knees to all the toes. Contrast radiography shows the protrusions, which are often multiple. They may be the result of osteophyte formation or of disc herniation; the two are distinguishable only at laminectomy. Later on, pressure may be exerted on the radicular arteries or the anterior spinal vascular channel causing widespread local degeneration of the cord with paraplegia. The posterior longitudinal ligament forms adhesions to the dura mater, which becomes thickened. Neck flexion may then overstretch and damage the spinal cord further; hence wearing a collar may well prevent aggravation and even bring about some improvement in the course of months.

In patients who have had, say, a severe car accident, considerable damage without fracture at the neck is a commonplace. These younger patients may develop central disc protrusion at any time during middle age; the resemblance to disseminated sclerosis is then considerable. The patient starts limping and drags one leg; there is not necessarily any neckache. Examination shows the upper motor neurone disturbance. Myelography is always called for.

### Paraesthetic Digits: Acroparaesthesia

In elderly patients, pins and needles in the hands can arise from the cervical spine in two ways. Bilateral protrusion of disc substance and bilateral foraminal stenosis both cause paraesthetic hands. All five digits are affected and there is a certain amount of root pain in arms and forearms. A central protrusion or a central osteophyte may compress the spinal cord slightly. Pins and needles in the hands result, sooner or later spreading to the feet. Root pain is absent.

Even myelography does not always help in differential diagnosis but, if manipulation abolishes the symptoms, the lesion was clearly a disc protrusion, not an osteophyte. In patients without signs of cord compression, manipulation by the methods of orthopaedic medicine is safe, whereas osteopathy and chiropractice are dangerous.

## The Mushroom Phenomenon

This is a rarity at the neck. The patient is elderly and states that, lying down, he is perfectly

| Disorder (traditional name) | History | Articular signs | Root signs | Cord signs | X-ray signs | Differential diagnosis | Treatment |
|---|---|---|---|---|---|---|---|
| Acute 'rheumatic' torticollis | Young; wakes with neck fixed by unilateral pain. Whiplash | +++ Partial articular pattern of internal derangement | − | − | − | Glandular fever. Hysteria | Reduce. Method different in patients under and over 30 years old |
| 'Scapular fibrositis' | Any age after childhood. Intermittent scapulocervical pain | + Partial articular pattern | − | − | Irrelevant | Neuritis. Pancoast tumour. Pleurisy | Reduce |
| 'Brachial neuritis' | Between 35 and 60. Unilateral scapular pain spreading to upper limb. Often pins and needles in hand | + Neck movements hurt in scapular area, seldom down limb | −<br>+ (uniradicular) | − | Irrelevant | Neuroma. Cervical metastases. Neuralgic amyotrophy. Angina. | No root palsy and brachial pain for less than 2 months: attempt reduction. Root palsy: wait 3 to 4 months from onset of root pain |
| Acro-paraesthesia (bilateral posterolateral protrusion) | Elderly. Pins and needles in both hands. Vague armache | Elderly stiffness | − | − | Elderly changes | Thoracic outlet syndrome. Bilateral carpal tunnel | Attempted reduction often fails, if so, collar required; often intractable |
| Osteophytic root palsy | Elderly. Slowly increasing weakness of arm, little ache | Elderly stiffness | ++ | − | Oblique view shows foraminal osteophyte | − | Grind osteophyte away |
| Posterolateral sclerosis | Elderly. Weak legs, perhaps upper limbs also. Pins and needles | Elderly stiffness | ±<br>− | +<br>+ | Filling defect on myelogram | Other cord disease | Laminectomy |

comfortable and with his head supported on a pillow he can move it painlessly. After sitting or standing for some time, he feels neckache, i.e., after the affected joint has borne the weight of the head. If this compression is maintained for long, discomfort in both arms and pins and needles in the hands begin. The patient has found that lifting his head upwards with his hands stops all symptoms.

Examination reveals an osteoarthrotic neck with limited movement, not necessarily with much aching at the extremes of the possible range. Neurological signs attributable to the root pressure are absent and conduction along the spinal cord is unaffected.

The diagnosis rests on the typical history and the negative examination. A weight-relieving collar or arthrodesis provide the only effective alternatives.

## Whiplash Injury

There exists a tendency to regard this accident as causing a disease *sui generis* and to suppose that the use of the term 'whiplash' indicates that a diagnosis has been made. This is not so; 'whiplash' is merely a statement on how the injury was caused. In severe cases, the anterior longitudinal ligament may rupture; the upper facets then slide downwards on the lower facets. This causes marked anterior folding of the now relaxed ligamentum flavum. This fold compresses and damages the spinal cord, even causing death. In such cases the radiograph shows neither fracture nor dislocation and post-mortem examination reveals no disc protrusion.

More often an ordinary cervical disc lesion results, no different from that acquired without a memorable accident. In an analysis of 41 cases of fatal whiplash injury, Hinz (1968) found that the commonest lesion was rupture of a disc, more often at the third than the second or fifth levels. Muscular ruptures occurred only in complete avulsion of occiput from atlas. Quite occasionally, however, the disc takes the brunt and suffers severe damage, sometimes on one side only. If so, the head is held permanently to one side, marked limitation of movement persisting indefinitely. Root pain supervenes, not particularly severe, but going on for many months accompanied by paraesthesia in the fingers. In this type of case manipulation is only partly successful. If the end-feel is found to be bone-to-bone at the first attempt, no treatment is likely to help.

Typically, the patient is seated in a stationary car which is run into from behind. He has no warning and cannot brace his muscles as he would when seeing a car about to collide with him head on. His body is shot forwards, leaving the head behind and the cervical joints are forcibly hyperextended. The head recoils now into excessive flexion, unless the forehead hits the windscreen, which is just as damaging, owing to the severe articular jarring. The patient is stunned for a moment and taken to hospital complaining more of his head injury than of his neck. The X-rays taken there prove negative and he is sent home perhaps with a stitched scalp. It is not till next day that he wakes with a neck so stiff and painful that he can scarcely move it at all. The ache is central and bilateral, and fixes the head in flexion; the cause is clearly a posterocentral disc protrusion akin to lumbago. Indeed, a cough often hurts the neck. After some days in bed the patient starts getting up little by little, usually remaining housebound for two or three weeks. The neck aches badly for one or two months, then slowly recovers in about a year. Movement returns equally slowly, and may never become fully restored, unless manipulative reduction is carried out within the first six months or so—exactly what medicolegal considerations usually prevent. These posterocentral protrusions draw out osteophytes fairly quickly and extension, or rotation to one side, may become permanently blocked.

'Treatment' usually involves repeated radiography, physiotherapy, traction or a collar—all to no avail. Refractoriness to such vain measures unjustly raises the question of exaggeration or of hysterical prolongation. These attitudes exist, of course, but many cases are genuine and the result of failure to carry out manipulative reduction.

### Legal Problems

Some doctors are incurably sanguine in their prognoses in whiplash injury. They find evidence merely of muscle and ligamentous strain from which they predict a rapid recovery. Alternatively, they detect radiographic evidence of osteophytosis or of attrition of the disc, and allege that this finding indicates that the patient would soon have developed pain anyhow. This ignores the fact that cervical osteophytosis usually causes merely painless stiffness. Naturally, lawyers protecting firms that may have to pay out compensation do not relish the idea of damage to the cartilaginous disc: an avascular tissue that can never repair itself.

Then the question of compensation (or traumatic) neurasthenia arises. Is the patient exaggerating his symptoms or not? Differentiation is difficult, since the history often includes symptoms whose factual basis cannot be assessed, e.g. headache, inability to concentrate, loss of memory, and so on. However when the 18 movements of the neck are tested, insincerity is quickly revealed. The neurasthenic is apt to equate effort with pain; it is best therefore to test the resisted movements first. He often alleges that they hurt, and the examiner finds that they are weak (particularly flexion) or jerkily performed. The active and passive neck movements may now elicit a self-contradictory pattern, and when the scapular movements are tested, elevation is often found limited or weak. When the upper limb is tested further evidence of inconsistency emerges. By contrast, the plaintiff in a compensation case must not be regarded merely on that account as exaggerating; hence the sincere patient must have his claim warmly supported when the defendants belittle his symptoms.

Unfair attitudes abound on both sides. Considerable damage to a disc without concomitant fracture may cause genuine severe symptoms which are apt to be disbelieved; by contrast, a fracture without concomitant injury to the disc unites and usually causes no further trouble. But the deformity is visible radiologically and a 'fractured spine' is very acceptable legally. The patient is in a cleft stick; if he is sincere and alleges only the actual amount of aching, he gets little compensation; if he exaggerates his symptoms considerably, he is apt to receive a larger sum, even if the traumatic neurasthenia is recognized. If he overdoes his symptoms blatantly he may be regarded as a malingerer and lose his case. A properly designed clinical examination alone can decide what is the true position, and ensure a report based on observed facts and not on opinion.

### Treatment

It is my habit to explain the position to those patients who are sincere. I offer them an immediate attempt at manipulative reduction, if their main interest is relief from symptoms; but point out that, if this proves successful, the amount of compensation will be much reduced. If they are uncertain, I advise them to consult their solicitor before receiving treatment, and emphasize that, although the lesion is most probably reducible today, there is no certainty that this situation will continue until the suit has been concluded several years hence. Patients with responsible work to do seldom hesitate; they merely wish their pain relieved so that they become effective again. Those with an uninteresting job are naturally more concerned with the benefits of compensation; they often decide to take their chance that reduction will still be feasible after the case has been settled.

## TREATMENT OF CERVICAL DISC LESIONS

### Prophylaxis

Young patients wake up with a stiff neck, having gone to bed comfortable the night before, obviously as the result of lying for many hours on end with their head twisted on their shoulders. Intra-articular displacement comes on gradually during this time and, on waking, they think they 'have been sleeping in a draught'. Hence posture at night is an important point in prophylaxis. The patient, if he sleeps supine, should have one thin pillow; if he lies on his side, the thickness of the pillow should be so adjusted that his cervical and thoracic vertebrae form a horizontal line. The habit of lying prone in bed, so useful for patients with lumbar disc lesions, results in the head being kept fully rotated for hours during sleep. Patients should be warned that this otherwise beneficial position must be avoided once stiff neck has begun to show itself. A bath towel twisted into a rope 10–15 cm in diameter and wound round the neck provides an effective stabilizer at night for those who keep getting attacks.

A head rest on the car seat prevents the sudden extension movement of the neck on impact from behind, but a safety belt increases the force of the flexion rebound by limiting it to the cervical spinal joints.

By day, the cervical lordosis should be maintained. Patients liable to stiff necks, or who have just had a displacement reduced, must avoid keeping the neck bent for a long period: they should extend the neck every so often for a second or two when reading, writing, sewing, knitting, etc. Alternatively, during reading they should raise a book to the level of their eyes. Yoga exercises in which the weight of the whole body is borne on the flexed neck should never be attempted. At night, those who sleep supine should use a thin pillow; those who lie on their side should use one thick enough to occupy the

**Fig. 31.** Pillow for those who turn from supine to side-lying.

full distance between ear and mattress. For those who do both a pillow must be made in three parts. When lying on his back the thinner part lets his head come lower, but if he turns on to his side the thicker side-pieces keep the neck straight (Fig. 31).

## Root and Cord Pressure

If a damaged cervical disc protrudes repeatedly, sooner or later the displacement, instead of undergoing spontaneous reduction again, will increase in size, and any time after the age of 35 an attack of severe root pain may incapacitate the patient for several months. Alternatively, a posterior central bulge may form and increase slowly in size; it may draw out an osteophyte by ligamentous traction lifting up the periosteum. Both these processes are encouraged by today's normal attitude towards even an obvious disc displacement—passive resignation. There are various ways of doing nothing that do not make this negative attitude obvious to the patient: e.g. the prescription of analgesic drugs, or heat, or massage, or exercises, or the provision of a collar. If the displacement is left where it is to get larger or smaller as fortune dictates, it will sometimes take the latter course. Even so, the longer the protrusion lasts, the more time it has to stretch the posterior longitudinal ligament, perhaps irretrievably, thus enhancing the likelihood of further attacks. The prevention of eventual pressure on a root or the spinal cord is clearly the reduction of the displacement when it first appears. In other words, reduction now, repeated as the years go by as often as proves necessary, affords the best—indeed the only—hope of preventing attacks of pain increasing in severity and duration and leading to eventual crippledom in old age. Elderly patients often attribute the earliest paraesthesia due to osteophytic cord pressure to painting a ceiling or merely going round an exhibition, looking upwards. They should therefore be warned against keeping the neck extended for any length of time, and at the theatre should prefer the dress-circle to the stalls.

# Reduction by Manipulation

In his book on *Cervical Spondylosis* (Brain & Wilkinson 1967), no less an authority than Lord Brain maintains that the chief use of manipulation of the neck is 'to reduce an intra-articular displacement . . .' Since cervical spondylosis is secondary to changes in the disc, and the symptoms, especially in the early stages, stem from minor degrees of disc protrusion, we have here clear confirmation that the prophylaxis and treatment of choice in cases not too advanced is manipulative reduction. It is the first treatment to be considered, no less so at the neck than at, say, the knee. Unless some contraindication exists, manipulative reduction should be attempted within the hour. It is my habit to carry this out as soon as the diagnosis is established; for, in the early case, waiting some hours or a day may make a great difference to the reducibility of the protrusion. This should be pointed out to patients who, usually because of some important engagement, wish to defer treatment.

## Contraindications

The manipulator's hand is sensory as well as motor. He perceives the end-feel in time to alter the manoeuvre he had contemplated. Bone-to-bone indicates that further forcing in that direction is useless. Crisp resistance calls for smart overpressure. Muscle spasm springing into play to protect the joint or a soggy end-feel both warn against manipulation. Hence the first contraindication may appear during the first manoeuvre. Laymen's techniques are different and my experience is that they do not have the benefit of end-feel in singling out the unsuitable case.

Evidence of an *upper motor neurone lesion* shows that manipulation is unsafe; and it will fail. I have tried on two patients, at the request of the doctor and the orthopaedic surgeon looking after them. They were made no worse but certainly no better, and cases have been reported of tetraplegia after manipulation in disc lesions of this type. However, a central posterior protrusion may exist not yet large enough to interfere with conduction along the pyramidal tracts. In such a case, the symptom is usually pins and needles in

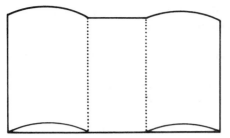

hands or feet, or both. A patient with a cervical disc lesion with this *symptom*, but no *sign* as yet of pressure on the spinal cord, may be treated by an attempt at manipulative reduction. It must then be most carefully carried out with *a maximum of manual traction and a minimum of articular movement.* In particular, rotation must be avoided during the manipulation. It is in this type of case that manipulation under anaesthesia is apt to make the condition worse, since the common manoeuvre is rotation. Chriopraxy is also dangerous; osteopathic methods are unsuccessful but less harmful. Oscillatory techniques may help a little, but the best hope of reduction lies in really strong manual traction. Since this method of treatment is the one least practised, those who regard manipulation as unsuited to this type of case are, in general, right, the more so since disc lesions that have been aggravated by ill-chosen measures, particularly under anaesthesia often prove difficult to reduce, and even harder to keep reduced, afterwards.

In *basilar ischaemia* (see p. 74) it is important to adopt the correct technique—strong traction with little or no rotation. If, at full rotation, bruising causes traumatic spasm where the atlas compresses the vertebral artery, cerebral damage or even death may result.

Inquiry should be made for *drop-attacks.* In patients with congenital ligamentous laxity at the occipito-atlantoid joint or a deformed odontoid process (Ford 1952), the instability may be such that the vertebra suddenly shifts far enough to occlude both vertebral arteries (Harrison 1820; Nagler 1973). In consequence the patient is apt, for no apparent reason, to fall to the ground without losing consciousness and be unable to get up again for a minute. In such cases, the excessive elasticity of the neck can be felt as manual traction is begun and leads to immediate relaxation of the pull. Drop attacks provide an absolute bar to manipulation. They should lead instead to radiography at the extremes of flexion and extension of the neck, followed by arthrodesis. Manipulation is unwise if a patient is on anticoagulants. Dabbet et al. (1970) describe an extensive thoracic haematoma compressing the spinal cord following chiropractice during warfarin administration. Surgical evacuation of the clot led to recovery. This event reveals how specific chiropractice actually is, for the patient was suffering from sciatica. In rheumatoid arthritis, forced movements aggravate the pain and are dangerous if ligamentous laxity has supervened.

## Criteria of Reducibility or Not by Manipulation

Four questions must be answered. How large is the protrusion? Is it central, unilateral or bilateral? Do the articular movements affect it? How long has it been present?

Central and bilateral displacements require strong traction and slight articular movement for their reduction; these cases are unsuited to osteopathy and chiropraxy; oscillatory techniques achieve their effect slowly but may help. Unilateral displacement is best dealt with by strong movement during traction, and if there is no root pain, osteopathy and chiropraxy, i.e. manipulation without adequate traction, may well succeed, though more sessions are usually required. Evidence of pressure on the spinal cord shows manipulation to be dangerous.

The larger the protrusion the more marked the neurological signs. A root palsy shows the herniation to be larger than the aperture whence it emerged. Therefore, it cannot be put back, but the vain endeavour is not dangerous. Pins and needles as an isolated phenomenon do not preclude manipulation.

If several of the neck movements set up or markedly increase the scapular aching, the displacement clearly lies where the articular movements influence it. Such 'good' neck signs suggest reducibility. If the neck movements set up pain in the upper limb, reduction is always difficult and often impossible. Pain felt at one side of the upper neck and caused by a cervical disc lesion at the second and third level nearly always proves more difficult to abolish than when an apparently identical displacement exists at the fourth to seventh levels, setting up pain in the lower neck and scapular area. If the ordinary manipulations do not secure reduction, the technique suitable for a central displacement may succeed.

The time factor also comes into play, but only from the moment that unilateral root pain has become established. As long as the pain is cervicoscapular only, there is no time limit to successful manipulative reduction. After two months of unilateral root pain reduction can seldom be secured by manipulation, but this limitation does not apply when the root pain is bilateral.

Osteophyte formation and attrition of one or more discs do not contraindicate an attempt at manipulative reduction. It is true that ligamentous contracture makes traction less effective, the patient's age makes him less tolerant of discomfort; but the endeavour is perfectly safe. Less is done at one sitting and post-manipulative soreness is apt to last a couple of days instead of some hours; moreover, it cannot, at really stiff cervical joints, be abolished by a lateral glide. Hence it is best to see the patient two or three times in all at weekly intervals. But the treatment of a cartilaginous displacement within an osteoarthrotic cervical joint is identical with the same condition in a joint devoid of osteophytosis. In fact, reduction has been successfully achieved in patients over 80 years old.

It should be noted that none of these criteria relates to the presence or not of diminished joint spaces or osteophyte formation on the radiograph.

The possibilities are:

1. Scapular pain without root pain. Good or bad neck signs without neurological weakness. Reducible in one or two sessions.
2. Unilateral scapular pain with root pain. Good neck signs; no neurological deficit. Almost certainly reducible.
3. Unilateral scapular pain with root pain. Neck movements hurt down the upper limb as well as in the scapular area. No neurological weakness. Probably irreducible.
4. Bilateral scapulobrachial discomfort with paraesthetic hands and/or feet. Fair neck signs, no neurological deficit. About half are reducible in up to four sessions.
5. Unilateral root pain followed by scapular pain. Symptoms begin at the hand and slowly progress upwards to the scapular area. Such primary posterolateral protrusions, as at the lumbar spine, are irreducible. *N.B.* Cervical neuromas often begin this way.
6. Unilateral scapular pain with root pain. Good neck signs and minor paraesthesia only. Sometimes reducible, especially if the brachial pain has lasted less than a month.
7. Unilateral scapular pain with root pain. Poor neck signs and major root palsy. Certainly irreducible. This fact was confirmed by Wilkinson (1974) who stated that in cervical radiculopathy the nucleus cannot be restored to its original position by traction or manipulation.
8. Unilateral scapular pain and root pain of more than six months' standing. Fair neck signs and a recovering root palsy. One manipulation will often restore full and painless movement to the neck, abolishing the scapular ache. The root pain is unaltered there and then, but slowly begins to ease some days after the manipulation. Two or three sessions at fortnightly intervals are required. In these cases, the manipulation appears to restart the mechanism of spontaneous cure which normally would have become complete in four months.
9. Unilateral scapular pain persisting for months after a root pain has ceased. Only one neck movement elicits the discomfort. Irreducible.
10. Paraesthetic hands and/or feet. Neck flexion evokes the symptoms. Gait not spastic. Plantar response: flexor. Usually reducible.
11. Swift progression. Scapular pain one day followed by root pain and paraesthesia the next day. Good neck signs and no neurological weakness yet. Very seldom reducible.
12. Elastic recoil. Rarely manipulation is confidently started in a patient with signs suggesting that reduction by manipulation will prove simple. When this is attempted a rubbery rebound is felt when the extreme of passive rotation is reached. No matter how often this movement is forced, apparent full range being achieved each time, no increase in the active movement is found when the patient sits up. When manipulation fails in this rare type of primary nuclear displacement, it is wise to pass on at once to sustained traction in bed.
13. Paraesthetic hands and/or feet with extensor plantar response. Irreducible.

## Gross Deformity

Acute torticollis in patients aged under 30 should be treated differently from other disc lesions, since this is the only cervical protrusion that consistently behaves in the nuclear manner. On examination one side flexion and the rotation movement towards the same side are grossly limited. Manipulation consists in carrying out, during strong traction, the movements of rotation and side flexion *only* in the painless direction. If this is repeated several times, the patient's pain will be much diminished, he can sit up and hold his head in the neutral position, but the range of movement in the two very restricted directions will not have increased. He is then lain on a couch and the head is gradually pushed more and more over towards the unobtainable side flexion. It may take an hour of repeated small shiftings by the physiotherapist to achieve this end. The same has then to be done for rotation. Hence it may well be three hours in all before a full and painless range of movement is restored to the affected cervical joint. An alternative in these acute cases is oscillatory treatment to the affected joint while the patient lies prone, as first put forward by Récamier in 1838 (*percussion cadencée*). My father, Edgar Cyriax, used to vibrate with his fingertips. Maitland uses his thumbs for manual oscillation. In either case the patient should be seen the next day, since some degree of relapse is common. The youngest patient I have encountered requiring manipulation was aged 4 and my physiotherapist was able to restore full painless range in one session.

Curiously enough, acute torticollis in patients aged over 30 can be treated in the ordinary way; indeed the disorder is, at that age, no longer caused by a *nuclear* protrusion, nor so severe. The deformity is less pronounced; the limitation of movement in the two directions is less extreme; there is no particular tendency to recurrence the next day.

Gross side flexion deformity with scapular pain calls for manipulation repeatedly in the line of the deformity until the neck can be held painlessly in the mid-position. A most dangerous treatment—far worse than doing nothing—is to push the head over the other way during anaesthesia. Gross intractable fragmentation of disc substance, severe root pain or pressure on the spinal cord often results.

Patients who are forced to hold their chin on their chest, hardly able to extend the neck at all, have a herniation lying posteriorly and centrally. Manipulation in such cases must be very gradual, involving a great deal of traction without, at first, an attempt being made to extend the neck; otherwise the manipulation carries with it the risk of increased posterior protrusion with damage to the spinal cord.

## Anaesthesia

Manipulation of the neck is widely regarded as dangerous. This is correct when laymen's techniques are used, since little or no traction is employed. Indeed, Maigne insists that it is safe only to manipulate the neck osteopathically in the direction that does not hurt. He is right, particularly when one remembers that only a local examination by palpation of the neck is considered sufficient by lay manipulators. This view also applies when manipulation is carried out under anaesthesia. But the fact that manipulation with little or no traction and without the benefit of the patient's cooperation may well have unfortunate results is no reason for avoiding manipulation carried out with proper safeguards on suitable cases. Manipulating the cervical joints under anaesthesia is equivalent to crossing the street with the eyes shut: no argument at all against crossing the street.

General anaesthesia is strongly contraindicated; for a set manipulation is not performed. What to do next, whether to repeat a manoeuvre or avoid it, whether to stop or go on, depends on re-examination after each manoeuvre. When it appears to be required, i.e. because the displacement proved irreducible in its absence, it will be found that those protrusions that could not be reduced without anaesthesia cannot be reduced with anaesthesia either. Anaesthesia leaves the manipulator wholly in the dark, depriving him of that most essential adjuvant—the patient's cooperation. In fact, adequate relaxation can be readily secured without anaesthesia, for as soon as adequate traction is applied, the patient's pain ceases. Hence he automatically relaxes.

## Manipulative Technique During Traction

All cervical manipulation is carried out during traction (see Volume II). This has a fivefold effect: (1) The cessation of compression on the displacement enables it to recede slightly; this stops the pain and the patient is happy to relax his neck muscles. (2) The posterior longitudinal ligament is rendered taut. (3) The loose fragment has room to move. (4) The subatmospheric pressure produced at the joint induces suction. If, then, anything moves, centripetal force ensures that it moves towards the centre of the joint and away from its posterior edge. (5) It distracts the surfaces of the facets, disengaging them. The fact that manipulation is carried out in slight extension—never in flexion, not in *much* extension—ensures that more space exists at the front than the back of the joint; this too encourages the intra-articular fragment to move forwards, thus ensuring that the spinal cord is not touched as the fragment shifts. Slight extension also prevents undue tension on the posterior longitudinal ligament during the traction. It is important to avoid the lay methods of manipulating the neck, since they involve crowding the joints together: what osteopaths call 'locking the facets'. Disengaging them by traction allows for more movement at the affected joint. In any case, Bihaug (1974, personal communication), experimenting with a cadaveric spine from which the muscles but not the ligaments had been removed, found it anatomically impossible to lock the facets.

Strong traction is applied and maintained for a second or two until the manipulator feels that he has taken up all the slack in the joints of the neck. Traction is maintained and the required movement is pressed home until a small click is felt. This may occur long before full range is reached, particularly during rotation. The patient sits up and the result on the pain is reported by the patient and on the range of movement noted by the manipulator. If this manoeuvre has helped, it is repeated; if it has not, another technique is tried, and so on, the result being evaluated after each attempt. Cervical reduction does not take place with one resounding thud, as at the lower lumbar spine; it involves a series of small clicks. If no click is felt, nothing has been achieved; but a click does not mean that any benefit has necessarily resulted. It is only when it is followed by improved symptoms and signs that it is shown to have been significant. After each manoeuvre, the conscious patient sits up and moves his neck; the manipulator assesses the effect on the range of movement and the patient on the degree of pain.

If the pain and tender spot have shifted, the patient is asked to point out their new situation. It is a good sign when a pain felt in the upper thorax moves upwards and medially. With this knowledge of the effect of each step, the manipulator can see at once if any particular manoeuvre has done good, has had no effect, or has done harm. Decision on the next step depends partly on this knowledge, and partly on the end-feel. It is quite possible in difficult cases to spend the whole of the first session in finding out what particular manoeuvre helps—and there may be only one. At the patient's next attendance, this particular technique may be repeated even a dozen times. It is my view that only the patient's active cooperation renders manipulation in cervical disc lesions simple, effective and really safe. When the manipulator feels that, at the extreme of rotation, bone meets bone, it is no use continuing forcing in that direction. During side flexion, the feeling of coming up against a leathery block also indicates that no more can be expected from that manoeuvre.

*No* exercises 'to maintain range' follow manipulative reduction, for the same movements as the manipulator carried out during traction have the opposite effect of that intended when repeated with centrifugal force acting on the joint.

The failure of manipulation in what appears a thoroughly suitable case raises the question of an error in diagnosis. Since nuclear protrusions are rare, pulmonary neoplasm, occipital arteritis, myeloma, chordoma, or an intraspinal neuroma must be reconsidered.

In 1955 an experiment was made to find out how much pull I exerted when reducing a cervical disc displacement. The maximum was found to be 140 kg. Miss Moffatt, then my senior physiotherapist at St Thomas's, reached 100 kg.

Radiography was carried out before and during a few seconds' fairly strong manual traction on the neck. It showed that traction increased each joint space by 2.5 mm—in other words, almost doubled the distance between the bones. No wonder cervical disc lesions are not difficult to reduce so long as the traction is adequate. Dr P. Flood's report was:

> Two anteroposterior films were taken. The first before pull was applied and the second while you pulled on the head. In the preliminary film the distance between the upper surface of the first dorsal vertebra and the upper surface of the fourth cervical vertebra is on measurement 7 cms; during pull this distance is increased to 8 cms. In order to avoid magnification the position of the spine relative to the film was, as far as was possible, similar in both cases. This is confirmed on measurement of the transverse width of the spine which does not vary by more than a millimetre.
>
> The increase of 1 cm over the distance of the bodies of the lower 4 cervical vertebrae must therefore be due to opening of the intravertebral spaces (see Plate VII).

The importance of adequate traction was emphasized by Varma et al.'s results (1973). They found that a pull of 14 kg maintained for as long as two minutes produced only 2 mm increase in the distance between the second cervical and the first thoracic vertebra. This amounts to a mere 0.34 mm increase at each joint space, compared with 2.5 mm after a few moments' proper manual pull.

*Novice's Routine.* A suitable routine for the novice would be as follows, evaluation following each step. The neck is never manipulated in flexion.

1. Rotation half the way towards the painless side.
2. Full rotation towards the painless side.
3. Rotation three-quarters of the way towards the painful side.
4. Full rotation towards the painful side.
5. Side flexion towards the painless side.
6. Lateral gliding.

Many variations are imposed by what happens at each manoeuvre, and greater and lesser degrees of extension can be used during the preliminary traction. Obviously, if one technique is found to help, it is repeated, perhaps many times at slightly different angles. If a manoeuvre does harm, or shoots pain down the patient's arm, it is avoided. If two or three manoeuvres are without effect, or increase symptoms, manipulation is abandoned.

*Osteopathy.* The main school of manipulation in France is headed by Dr R. Maigne, who manipulates only in the *direction indolore.* As far as this applies to osteopathic manipulation, of which he is a past master, this is doubtless excellent teaching. However, this restriction does not apply to the orthopaedic medical type of manipulation during traction, since a centripetal force is now acting on the joint during each manoeuvre. Indeed, it is very often rotation during traction in the painful direction that proves the most effective. Nor does the converse hold; for, even if Maigne's restriction is observed, harm may nevertheless result if manipulation is attempted in really unsuitable cases.

Patients are often met with who have received manipulation for months, even years, from a layman. Though it is true that osteopathic or chiropractic manipulation, without adequate traction, takes more sessions of treatment to achieve its effect than the orthopaedic physician's methods, the fact remains that what can be shifted by manipulation does so almost at once. What has not begun to move after two orthopaedic medical or six of layman's attempts clearly cannot be benefited thus, and alternative methods of treatment must be considered. Four sessions of treatment for posterolateral, and eight for posterocentral, protrusions are my maximum, even in cases where osteopathy or chiropraxy had already failed.

*Mobility Tests and Specificity.* Those who think on osteopathic lines go to great trouble to feel for hypermobility and hypomobility and to localize the lesion to one particular cervical joint. This is a praiseworthy intention, but the question arises whether it is feasible in practice. Testing mobility would afford an excellent guide to the level of the lesion if it were always at the joint with limited movement at which the fault lay. Both on myelography and at laminectomy it is by no means always found that the protrusion lies at the joint where the greatest attrition of disc-substance is seen. Moreover, when osteopaths examine a patient within a few minutes of each other, their palpatory findings show no correspondence whatever (Schiötz 1958). In 1973 I attended a demonstration at which five senior physiotherapists, all well versed in mobility tests, examined the same painful neck. The stiffness was held to lie at the second, fourth, fifth and sixth cervical, and at the second thoracic levels respectively, and there was no agreement whether the restriction was rightward or leftward. I feel sure that, had this patient been manipulated by any of these five physiotherapists using what they regard as specific technique (i.e. affecting one joint only), he would have been put right; for it is not possible to move one spinal joint without affecting those adjacent. Clearly (luckily for those who employ them), specific manoeuvres are much less specific than they believe. On the other hand, the methods that I have devised, though universally criticized in osteopathic circles for their lack of specificity, are involuntarily specific. They do not rest on choice of level by fallible palpatory findings. Each unaffected joint moves as far as it will, but the internally deranged joint is blocked. Hence the final manipulative thrust inevitably falls at the correct level. In consequence, my manipulative techniques have been found by those who have tried both at least as successful as osteopaths'. This makes nonsense of the time required by osteopaths to teach students (in England, four years) since my methods can be learnt by physiotherapy students in a few months. It is not elegance, impressiveness, specificity or technical difficulty by which manipulative techniques should be judged, but effectiveness and safety. My methods must be tested against osteopaths' on a basis of which gets the patient well quicker.

## Maintenance of Reduction

If a loose body in a joint has moved once, it can move again. Patients with only cervicoscapular pain often describe a number of previous attacks, and others are to be expected unless the patient is careful about the posture of his neck, especially at night. A recurrent displacement should be reduced again at once. The patient must be warned that the longer a protrusion is left unreduced, the more ligamentous stretching results and the greater the likelihood of recurrence and the eventual supervention of root or cord pressure. Even if previous attacks were self-limiting, there is no guarantee that this will be so again in the present attack. Hence, immediate complete reduction is the first line of defence.

Recurrence is not to be expected after root pressure that is allowed to run its full course untreated. By contrast, if reduction succeeds in cases of root pain, the position is the same as in scapular pain—namely, the protrusion has gone back to its original bed and what has shifted once can obviously shift again.

## Postural Maintenance

The endeavour is to keep the joint as still as possible in the neutral position. The neck should be moved smoothly, and the extremes of range avoided, certainly for long at a time. Only one pillow—better, one shaped like a butterfly—should be used at night. A two-thickness pillow, thin in the centre for lying supine, and thick at both ends for occupying the greater distance between ear and shoulder, is useful for restless sleepers (see Fig. 31). Postures that involve keeping the neck fixed, e.g. reading, writing, sewing, should be altered by raising the object on a thick cushion. A typist can put her papers almost vertically above her machine on a music stand placed behind it. Her eyes are then level with her reading matter. Moreover, manual dexterity is diminished during considerable rotation of the neck (Wyke 1973). There is thus everything to be said against craning the neck to look at papers on the table beside the typewriter.

## A Collar

It occasionally happens that reduction, though fully achieved, proves very unstable. This is most apt to occur in protrusions of some years' standing and after ill-advised manipulation under anaesthesia.

A moulded plastic collar is made; being transparent, it is remarkably inconspicuous. It must support the mandible well, and the occipital piece must not tend to push the head forwards. When careful trying-on shows that the collar fits, the patient's disc lesion is reduced again and the collar applied while he remains lying on the couch. It must be worn by day for three or four months. Then it should become possible to discard it gradually. It would naturally be an advantage if it were also worn at night for the first few weeks, but it is rare to meet a patient who can sleep in it. If the displacement recurs during the night, reduction by manipulation must be repeated.

In the mushroom phenomenon a weight-relieving collar is required, consisting of two plastic hinged circles, one applied to occiput and chin and the other to the root of the neck. Four bottle screws hold the two halves apart and can be adjusted to maintain a suitable distracting force.

It is well to realize that wearing a collar does not bring about reduction, nor does it often ease the pain in a patient awaiting spontaneous recovery of root pain with radicular weakness. Collars have a bad name with patients because they are so often prescribed *before* reduction. The only exception is when the dura mater has become adherent to the posterior longitudinal ligament and neck flexion overstretches the spinal cord.

## Suspension at Home

A patient with recurrent trouble may find that daily suspension keeps him comfortable. The apparatus is installed at his home and he gives himself ten minutes' traction every day (see Volume II). Others find that they can restore movement caused by a recent and minor subluxation by active movement while the head is floating. The patient lies supine in a warm bath, only his nostrils projecting above the surface of the water. The weight of the head is now borne by the water; hence compression strain on the joint ceases. The head is now moved voluntarily into the position previously unattainable, and held there for some time. If this manoeuvre is carried out early enough, reduction often ensues.

## Operative Fixation

Arthrodesis is, of course, successful in the maintenance of reduction, so long as it is done when no displacement sufficient to cause symptoms is present. It is the only really effective treatment for the mushroom phenomenon, avoiding compression of the joint during the time the neck bears the weight of the head.

## The Avoidance of Exercises

Movement of the neck during the time that the weight of the head is borne on the cervical spine may well have the opposite effect of the same movement carried out during traction. In the one case centrifugal, in the other centripetal, force is acting on the joint. Most patients after manipulative reduction are advised, even by osteopaths, to perform exercises. The effect is the reverse of that intended. Many patients, particularly those attending hospitals, are given exercises (often after heat or massage) without reduction. This is most unkind, for the symptoms can only increase if, during weight-bearing, the edge of the joint is forced by muscular action against the displacement that blocks movement. No one advises exercises before reduction of a torn meniscus at the knee. The same applies at a spinal joint.

## Dangers of Cervical Manipulation

The dangers of medical treatment are usually assessed in relation to the harmful effects likely to accrue when the work is carried out under the best auspices. No one warns against the dangers of appendicectomy when carried out in a cottage by candlelight. The important results are those of competent surgeons working under ideal conditions. A great deal is heard about the dangers of manipulating the joints of the neck, without any reference to the operator or the cases selected. This is quite unrealistic; the dangers and successes must be assessed by the results obtained at an efficient hospital properly staffed, not what happens when any comers are manipulated cheerfully by laymen or when anaesthesia is used.

The first chiropractic disaster to be recorded was by Blaine in the USA in 1925. Pratt-Thomas and Berger described three more cases (1947). These were followed by reports from Kunkle et al. (1952), Lièvre (1953), and Schwartz et al. (1956). Ford and Clark (1956) encountered five cases of brain damage, of which two proved fatal owing to thrombosis of the basilar artery. Four of the manipulations were performed by chiropractors, the fifth by the patient's own wife. Bénassy and Wolietz (1957) described the case of a man of 61 who developed quadriplegia and died after five chiropractic adjustments. Then Green and Joynt (1959) met with two more patients with damage to the brain-stem following chiropractice; neither died. A further fatal case was reported by Smith and Estridge in 1962; Pribeck's (1962) patient recovered. In Miller's case the spasticity was permanent but the patient survived (1964). It is interesting to note that none of these cases followed manipulation by an osteopath and that the age of the patients ranged from 28 to 55 with a mean of 35. It is clear, therefore, that vascular disease is not a predisposing factor. Indeed, in the four cases that came to autopsy, the arteries were found normal. Krueger and Okazaki (1980) report the case of a fit young man of 25 who died after a chiropractic manipulation. Full post mortem details of thrombosis of the vertebral arteries are set out together with 51 references to reports of similar accidents. From their studies on cadavers, de Kleyn and Nieuwenhuyse (1927) had already discovered that the vertebral circulation could be occluded during extension and side flexion of the neck. This is a frequent chiropractic manoeuvre, but is a posture avoided in the methods advocated by myself. Angiographic research by Bauer et al. (1961) showed that, in all cases in which kinking of the vertebral artery was seen when the neck was held symmetrically, this was increased to the point of occlusion on full rotation. Here lies the reason for the clinical observation that I had made in 1948—that in elderly patients with central neckache appreciable rotation during manipulation must be avoided.

I have had three complications. A man of 65 with a disc lesion causing pain in the scapular area and upper limb was manipulated with due care as regards rotation. Then side flexion away from the painful side was carried out and his leg on that side became spastic with extensor plantar response. He recovered fully in a week. Then there was a woman of 76 with right-sided neckache. This was slightly eased by her first manipulation, rather more by a second, but this was followed by two days' inability to write. There was no incoordination; the pen would not form the words and she brought the piece of notepaper for my inspection. A third patient's neckache was abolished by one session of manipulation but he had numbness of the pinna and circumauricular area for a week, presumably the result of a third cervical sensory palsy. The fact that we have had no lasting trouble after manipulation may be because our technique is different from laymen's, or merely because the misfortune is such a rarity. There are estimated to be 16 000 manipulators in the USA who must be regarded as likely to manipulate not less than one neck each day. If five cases have occurred in ten years, this risk works out at about one in ten million manipulations, and is no argument against manipulative reduction in suitable cases. As a safety measure, Smith and Estridge recommend that, before the neck is manipulated, the head should be rotated and extended, if vertigo or sensory disturbances appear, the attempt should be abandoned.

## The Danger of Not Manipulating

Manipulation of the neck is usually done by laymen with little or no training and no knowledge of what lesion they are proposing to affect, or by surgeons under anaesthesia. It is rightly regarded by most doctors, in these two sets of circumstances, as dangerous. I wholeheartedly agree. But this applies to all effective manoeuvres; they are dangerous when wrongly performed or when unsuitable cases are chosen.

These facts must not be allowed to discredit manipulation of the cervical joints by trained persons, in suitable cases, during traction and without anaesthesia. Bad results in poor circumstances do not preclude good results when due care is taken. When the indications for treatment are considered, it is usual to weigh the dangers of action against the dangers of inaction. Contemporary medical literature is littered with warnings against manipulation of the cervical spinal joints, particularly when X-rays show osteophytosis, without due attention to other aspects of the question: what is likely to happen if manipulation is withheld? Manipulation can relieve pain, perhaps of years' standing, that might well have continued for a lifetime, and it can reduce a disc lesion that is slowly enlarging, or by ligamentous traction is drawing out an osteophyte. In either case, the spinal cord is menaced and eventually pressure may lead to thrombosis of the anterior artery, whereupon not even laminectomy can help. Left where it is (the standard procedure in Britain) such a cervical protrusion can lead not only to pain but to crippledom. Since paraplegia from cervical disc lesion and consequent osteophytosis is by no means rare, it is worth contemplating an even greater danger—leaving the early minor displacement unreduced. The time for quick and simple reduction is missed, and the displacement left to get larger or smaller, to raise osteophytes by ligamentous pull or not as fortune dictates. There comes a time when manipulation is no longer any use; later still, it may become dangerous. When the patient has died, post-mortem studies show that the pressure on the spinal cord could not *then* have been relieved by manipulation. To argue from this that manipulation should not have been used early on involves casuistry unworthy of our profession. The harm caused by not manipulating may not show for some or many years, but if the right moment has been missed the harm done may be irretrievable. This delay obscures the connection between the missed opportunity and the later disablement, but this does not make the situation any less real, nor any more excusable.

## Prolonged Traction

### Head Suspension

This measure is used far too often. Numerous cases with neck symptoms receive endless traction, either with no result or with some benefit after 10 or 20 sessions, whereas one or two manipulations would have given full relief.

Suspension has its indications, but they are few and infrequently encountered.

*For Early Nuclear Protrusions.* These are rare, and manipulation is powerless to effect reduction. When the attempt is made, full range is achieved with a soft end-feel, but when the patient is re-examined the limitation persists unaltered. Suspension is substituted and should succeed in three to six daily sessions.

*For Stability.* Manipulative reduction has succeeded but by next morning the case has relapsed. Manipulative reduction is repeated, but with the same relapse next day. After the third reduction, the patient is treated by suspension, say, daily for a week, in order to attempt to secure a more stable position of the loose fragment.

*For Reduction.* An extremely nervous patient may be unable to bear the idea of manipulation. If a genuine slight disc displacement is present, daily suspension for two or three weeks may achieve what could have been done in a few minutes by manipulation.

Small posterocentral displacements in patients not too elderly, presenting with a minimum of articular signs, may also benefit in the long run.

*Prophylaxis.* Patients with a very unstable fragment of disc can often be kept free from trouble by head suspension at home for ten minutes daily, usually for years on end.

Suspension is unsuited to the elderly or to patients so heavy that the neck cannot stand such weight, or when the dura mater is adherent to the cervical spine. However, the real contraindication is trying in vain to reduce a cervical disc lesion by traction alone, when this can be effected quickly and easily by manipulation during traction. My advice to a physiotherapist who has been asked to give neck suspension to an obviously reducible cervical disc lesion is to carry out 'passive movements during suspension' and do her best that way.

### Long Traction

This is seldom indicated. It can be used for patients with severe pain in the arm, not controllable by drugs, and preventing sleep. The patient lies on a sloping couch; a collar is placed round his neck and a 7–10 kg weight attached over a pulley. After a few minutes' traction, the brachial pain ceases and the patient falls asleep. He can then stay so for as many hours as is convenient. When he walks out of the hospital, his pain returns to its former pitch, but he is rested. This method can therefore be used in severe root pain while spontaneous resolution is awaited; it does not alter the displacement nor expedite cure but, by affording sleep, makes the patient more able to tolerate the pain.

### Traction in Recumbency

This is the method of choice in patients with the following conditions.

*A Nuclear Protrusion.* This is rare, but is encountered between the ages of 20 and 30. Scapular pain results, reproduced by rotation of the neck towards the painful side; the active movement is 45° limited, whereas all the other movements are of full range and either quite or nearly painless. When rotation is carried out passively during traction, full range is easily achieved, but when the patient sits up, the limitation of active movement is unaltered. The neck is then manipulated in the same direction again, rather harder, and the elastic recoil characteristic of a nuclear protrusion is felt. Such a displacement can go on for many years unchanged, and the only remedy is sustained traction in bed.

*A Disc Displacement with Root Pain but no Root Palsy.* Though neurological signs are absent, the displacement has proved irreducible by manipulation. The patient is then told that he must await spontaneous recovery, due four months after the onset of the brachial pain. He avers very reasonably that he cannot endure such severe pain for so long. Continuous traction in bed is then the alternative, but should not be initiated without warning the patient that it is quite an ordeal. It should not be prescribed for root pain with a root palsy, nor for ordinary cartilaginous disc lesions; it is very seldom successful. Traction, however prolonged, fails to reduce many cartilaginous displacements and I have on a number of occasions easily reduced a displaced fragment of annulus causing severe scapular pain in patients who had had up to a fortnight's fruitless traction in bed elsewhere.

*Posterocentral Protrusion.* Soon after an injury to the neck, usually a whiplash, a disc protrusion may bulge out the posterior longitudinal ligament enough to impinge on the spinal cord and cause pins and needles in hands, feet or both. In a young patient with a short history irreducibility by manipulation cannot yet be due (as in the elderly) to the protrusion consisting of a bony osteophyte. Reduction by sustained traction in bed must be attempted.

Traction in bed is best carried out in hospital, because the patient requires full nursing day and night. He cannot feed himself or move his head appreciably. The principles of treatment are to give the patient enough drugs to prevent his feeling the mandibulo-occipital pain of the collar and that down his upper limb and never to allow the traction to abate for one moment. The well-intentioned nurse who tries repeatedly to adjust the collar, meanwhile relieving the traction, ruins the success of this method. No one may touch the harness or weights. So long as the severe brachial pain continues, it overshadows all else and the patient is kept well drugged. Heroin is much preferable to morphine unless cyclizine (50 mg) or promethazine (25 mg) are added; otherwise vomiting may make removal of the harness imperative. A dipipanone preparation containing cyclizine is useful.

Traction of 5–6 kg day and night is maintained during heavy sedation until the brachial pain ceases—usually in 20–40 hours. Traction is then diminished in force and after two days the patient is allowed to lie without weights. At the end of three or four days he sits up for short periods. Hence, even in the most satisfactory case in which all pain ceases at the end of 24 hours, five days in bed are the least that can be hoped for; more often seven days elapse before the patient is fit to go home. As soon as the pain ceases and the stronger analgesics are no longer required, the patient makes every sort of complaint about the collar and indeed every aspect of his treatment; he becomes difficult and may need several visits a day. Not being in any way ill, he has plenty of will-power; hence traction in bed, although often effective, should be undertaken with great reluctance. (For details of apparatus, etc., see Volume II.)

## Awaiting Spontaneous Recovery

It is curious that, however long a disc protrusion exerts pressure at or near the midline, no tendency to spontaneous recovery is manifest at any spinal level. However, in acute torticollis or lumbago, recovery seldom takes more than a week or two. A disc lesion causing chronic central or unilateral neckache or scapular pain can continue indefinitely. If the bulge is wide enough to give rise to bilateral scapular or bilateral brachial pain, with or without pins and needles in the hands, there is the same likelihood of continuance. If the bulge moves a little to one side, giving rise to unilateral scapular pain, there is still no tendency to recovery. It is quite useless, therefore, to predict that unilateral or bilateral neckache or scapular pain of some months' standing will ever cease; it may or it may not. Once the displacement has moved posterolaterally, compressing the dural investment of the nerve root with consequent brachial pain, spontaneous cure in 3 to 4 months becomes extremely probable. The more marked the palsy, the more quickly the pain abates. Full strength will almost certainly have returned to the muscles by, say, three to six months after the symptoms ceased. The only exception is an eighth root palsy which may take up to six months to disappear and may occasionally leave a patient with a permanently weak thumb.

The normal course of unilateral root pain due to a cervical disc lesion is intermittent scapular pain for some or many years. Then increasing scapular pain comes on followed by pain in the upper limb. This becomes severe in the course of a week and pins and needles are apt to begin in the fingers corresponding to the dermatome. The pain remains severe, much worse at night, for four to six weeks, then begins to ease. In severe root palsy, the pain has often eased after two months, and very seldom lasts longer than three months. When the protrusion is smaller, and unilateral pain without muscle paresis results, cessation of pain may well take the full four months. (The time must be reckoned from the onset of brachial pain, not of scapular aching.) As stated above, when the root is bilateral, with merely some aching in the arms and pins and needles in the hands as the important symptom (acroparaesthesia), there is no limit to the duration of symptoms.

During the period of unavoidable root pain pending spontaneous cessation, not much can be done. The possibilities are as follows.

## Explanation

The patient who is told he has a displacement that cannot be put back naturally expects that he will suffer his present pain for life. Hence, learning that the symptoms subside in the end affords considerable reassurance, and the time when relief may be expected to begin can be foretold with considerable accuracy by merely assessing the severity of the root palsy.

The ordinary course of events is quite different, and has unfortunate repercussions against the medical profession. The patient starts his brachial pain; he sees his doctor and is given analgesics with only temporary benefit. After a month he goes to hospital where he is told he has a 'slipped disc', he is given either physiotherapy, traction or a collar; the pain continues unchanged. After a month of this 'treatment' (i.e. two months in all), he presumes that the medical profession cannot help him and he goes to a lay manipulator who treats him two or three times a week for another month. During this (the third) month, his symptoms slowly abate spontaneously, but both he and the layman ascribe the relief to the manipulative treatment. This series of events must not be allowed to continue for it gives futile manipulation and laymen a gratuitous and undeserved advertisement.

The prognosis should be explained to the patient, he should be seen fortnightly until the forecast has been fulfilled. This continued interest in the patient by the physician prevents him from going elsewhere to waste his time and money. Moreover, watching to see what the degree of root palsy demands in length of time needed for the pain to stop increases the physician's prognostic accuracy. It is this unrealized spontaneous recovery that has led to belief in the efficacy of every sort of treatment for what used to be called 'brachial neuritis'. Massage, electrotherapy, salicylates, vitamin B—all appear successful if persisted in for long enough. It is the fashion nowadays to put patients into a collar while they are awaiting spontaneous recovery from a cervical disc lesion causing root palsy. This measure neither diminishes immediate symptoms nor hastens eventual cure, and it entails the patient enduring the additional and pointless discomfort of the collar.

This view of the uselessness of all treatment in established root palsy has been emphasized in succeeding editions of this book since 1954. It was confirmed by Nichols (1965) who reported a trial on 493 patients divided into 5 groups and treated respectively by (*a*) traction, (*b*) a collar, (*c*) advice on posture, (*d*) physiotherapy and (*e*) placebo tablets. At the end of a month, 80% of the members of group (*c*) were relieved, as were 75% of groups (*a*), (*b*) and (*d*) whereas only 56% of group (*e*) were better. Clearly, treatment has no effect on established unilateral root paresis, which ceases spontaneously whatever is or is not done. Nichols draws the modest conclusion that physiotherapy does not materially affect the eventual course of cervical spondylosis. He is right, but that does not imply that logical treatment in cases without root paresis is without value. St Thomas's offered to join in this investigation, but my suggestion was declined by his committee.

## Analgesics and Posture

The pain at night is severe and minor analgesics like aspirin are useless. Pethidine, methadone (Physeptone) or one of the stronger drugs of this sort are required. There is one posture that considerably eases the nocturnal pain: sleeping with the affected arm elevated. This relaxes the nerve root and many patients can get off to sleep with their hand on their head.

## Manipulation

This helps in two sets of circumstances, even when a root palsy is present.

*Marked Articular Signs.* Usually, by the time that root pain has continued for two or three months, the articular signs become inconspicuous. An occasional case is encountered of marked limitation of movement in some directions persisting with considerable scapular pain evoked at the extreme of range. In this event, one reason for the patient's broken sleep is scapular pain waking him each time he turns in bed. One session of manipulation, even in the presence of a root palsy, can be relied on to restore a full and almost painless range of movement to the neck without, unfortunately, affecting the root pain. Much better nights often follow.

*Overdue Root Pain.* A patient may have had an attack of unilateral root pain which has not resolved in the normal three to four months. It is rare for an attack of brachial pain due to a cervical disc protrusion not to subside spontaneously, but such a case may be encountered, lasting, say, a year or two. The articular signs do not amount to much and, had the root pain been of a month or two's standing, manipulation would be quite useless. In fact, after the lapse of six months it is often effective, but in a different way. It appears to afford no benefit then and there; yet a few days later brachial pain, of say a year's duration, begins to ease. A second manipulation a fortnight later leads to disappearance of the pain in the upper limb. It is difficult to understand exactly what has happened, but the aborted mechanism of spontaneous recovery has clearly been restarted.

## Injection at Nerve Root

This is not so difficult as it would appear. Any patient with scapulobrachial pain with or without a root palsy, is suitable. It is true that the pain will go spontaneously in four months, but it will be severe for up to two months.

If manipulation fails or is considered not worth trying, the injection follows at once. The palsy tells the physician at which level the disc lies; if not localized, tenderness is usually clear and pressure anteriorly often reproduces the scapulobrachial symptom recognizably. A 2 cc syringe is filled with either 2 cc 2% procaine, or 1 cc procaine 1 cc steroid suspension. A thin needle 2.5 cm long is fitted. The physician's thumb identifies the lateral edge of the transverse process and presses on the nerve root, which lies close under the skin, just behind the posterior edge of the sternomastoid muscle. The needle is inserted until it meets bone and a quarter of the syringeful is injected, aiming at a point 1.5 cm from the midline. Then the rest follows at three adjacent sites. The injection reproduces the discomfort.

After a few minutes, pain ceases. If it returns, cortisone is added to the next injection. The injection is repeated at whatever intervals prove necessary, e.g. once or twice a week for two or three weeks.

## Epidural Local Anaesthesia

Root pain that has lasted say a year and has shown no tendency to resolve spontaneously, and is not helped by manipulation, is a rarity. Epidural local anaesthesia is then called for; 10 ml of 1:200 procaine are injected at the required level and the root pain ceases within a few minutes. It does not return to its previous intensity, and should disappear after two to four inductions at, say, fortnightly intervals.

# Laminectomy

Myelopathy results from advanced cervical spondylosis leading to ischaemia (Stookey 1940). Blood flow along the surface of the spinal cord becomes obstructed by increasing pressure; finally thrombosis of the anterior spinal artery supervenes. Once this has happened, it is too late to operate. Since laminectomy stops further progression of the disorder, but seldom affords much improvement, it is better performed early than late. However, cervical laminectomy is not without danger; for during the operation, the fall in blood pressure together with the flexion of the neck may provoke thrombosis of the anterior spinal artery, and the reported results mostly claim not more than 50% success. The indications are: (*a*) Advancing spastic paresis. If the myelogram shows one large indentation, the result of removal of the posterior osteophyte at laminectomy is better than cases with smaller protrusions at several levels. Most surgeons regard three as a maximum. (*b*) Advancing weakness of the hand, i.e. progressive muscular atrophy. (*c*) Sudden bilateral advance of paralysis of the brachial nerve roots, such that root conduction is being lost at the rate of, say, a level a day. In such emergencies in elderly patients, whose general condition is poor, decompression without any attempt to deal with the lesion lying in front of the spinal cord may prove the only practicable measure. It is important that no exercises should follow the operation since Adams and Logue (1971) have shown that the smaller the range of movement at the cervical joints, the better the prognosis.

Osteophytic root palsy demands removal of part of the facet or grinding away the bony outcrop with a dental burr.

## TREATMENT OF CAPSULAR DISORDERS

The degree of osteoarthrosis must be assessed clinically, not by radiography.

Post-traumatic stiffness of the cervical joints comes on after immobilization, especially if the patient has lain unconscious for some days, unable to move his neck. The manipulation consists of a quick jerk at the extreme of the possible range, rupturing adhesions (see Volume II). Traction is not required.

Traumatic osteoarthrosis in middle-aged patients often appears uninfluenced by treatment, but since many of these patients are claiming compensation it is difficult to be sure whether or not this condition really causes discomfort, apart from limited range.

In *osteoarthrosis* of the upper two cervical joints, capsular contracture is present and leads to considerable limitation of movement. Rotation and side flexion manipulations are performed, but now they are carried out during traction with the slow strong pressure calculated to stretch out a tough structure. As a result, not only is the pain in the upper neck abolished, but the matutinal occipitofrontal headache also disappears. There is no upper age limit to manipulation, which can be safely carried out after the age of 80. However it is often best to force only one movement at a session; hence the really elderly patient may have to come two or three times for as much treatment as, had he been 10 years younger, could have been carried out at one session.

The stiffness of *spondylitis ankylopoetica* can be temporarily offset by the same gradual stretch. Sooner or later, the manipulator feels bone hitting bone when forcing is attempted; if so, the contracture is too advanced to benefit. *Rheumatoid arthritis* of the cervical joints is best treated by a collar and indomethacin. Manipulative stretching is contraindicated. Subluxation requires arthrodesis.

### Arthrosis at a Facet Joint

Capsular stretching and capsular desensitization both afford considerable improvement. Troisier advocates deep massage to the capsule of the joint.

Manipulation is carried out by gradual capsular stretching during traction, and is reasonably successful. The range is not much increased, but the ache when the extremes are reached is largely abated.

If manipulation affords a mediocre result, considerable relief can be obtained by infiltration of the affected facet joint with triamcinolone. The choice between the third and fourth joint is made by palpation for tenderness. If necessary, both joints can be injected.

*Arthritis.* When rheumatoid or spondylitic arthritis attacks one or two facet joints, intra-articular triamcinolone is called for.

*Technique of Injection.* The patient lies prone with his neck fully side flexed towards the painless side. This posture distracts the articular processes and widens the joint space. A 1 ml syringe equipped with a thin needle 3 cm long is used and the insertion made 2 cm from the midline. If the tip strikes bone directly, it is impinging against the lamina. It is then partly withdrawn and inserted obliquely lateralwards. If it is felt to traverse a thick fibrous layer and then strike bone, the posterior ligament has been pierced and the needle has reached the joint. A few drops are then injected at several adjacent points, some intracapsular, some intra-articular. One or two infiltrations suffice.

## TREATMENT OF MUSCLES

Painful scarring at the occipital insertion of the semispinalis capitis muscle may follow the prolonged rest in bed necessitated by concussion. This results in headache, elicited by the resisted neck movements. The treatment is deep massage there (see Volume II): permanent relief is obtained in two to six sessions of proper friction.

It is a curious fact that a patient who receives deep massage to the muscles overlying a joint which is the site of internal derangement may temporarily recover a full range of active movement, though nothing else has been done. As a result, massage to the semispinalis capitis muscle at the requisite level may also be ordered as a means of securing localized relaxation of muscle before manipulative reduction is attempted.

## TREATMENT OF LIGAMENTS

I am not at all sure in what circumstances ligamentous disorders occur at the neck. The following are the views of my colleague, R. Barbor.

The ligamentum nuchae becomes affected in three circumstances:

1. As the ligamentous component of a 'whiplash injury'.
2. As a chronic strain following repeated internal derangement at a cervical intervertebral joint.
3. As an occupational stress when the patient has to hold his neck in a flexed position for long periods.

In all these cases, stretching the ligament causes discomfort or pain, and there is abnormal tenderness to palpation usually between C5 and C6, or C6 and C7 spinous processes.

The treatment consists of intraligamentous injection of dextrose sclerosant solution mixed with a local anaesthetic agent on one to three occasions.

This should be followed by the patient maintaining a full range of movement at the cervical joints twice a day until all discomfort has ceased.

*Technique of Injection.* The patient sits on a chair and leans forward to rest the forehead on a table. In this position the cervical spine is flexed so as to facilitate palpation of the ligamentum nuchae at the lower two cervical levels.

A 2 ml syringe is used and a flexible type 5 cm medium fine needle, filled with 1 ml of 2% procaine and 1 ml of P2G, dextrose sclerosant solution.

The skin is sterilized and the needle inserted just above the seventh cervical spinous process and is injected at, and to either side of, the spinous process. The needle is partly withdrawn: skin and needle are then pulled upwards and the process repeated about the sixth spinous process. The ligamentoperiosteal attachments are infiltrated at both levels through one skin puncture.

CHAPTER 8

# THE JAW, THE THORACIC OUTLET, THE STERNOCLAVICULAR AREA

## THE TEMPOROMANDIBULAR JOINT

When this joint is affected, the patient himself nearly always supplies the diagnosis. It should not be forgotten that a painless stiffness of the joint may be the first symptom of tetanus.

The temporomandibular joint is essentially one in which both the bone and the socket move.

The joint space is divided horizontally into two compartments by the meniscus. At the upper, the meniscus glides to and fro on the temporal bone; at the lower the mandibular condyle hinges on the meniscus. On opening the mouth fully the condyle and meniscus move forward together, i.e. the mandible and its socket move as one on the temporal bone.

The patient is asked to open and close the mouth, to deviate the mandible to right and left and to protrude it forwards. He then clenches his teeth and attempts to open the mouth against the examiner's resistance under his chin. The joint is then palpated while the patient opens and shuts his mouth and deviates each way. The examiner's finger should be placed just below the zygomatic process when opening is examined, and in the external auditory meatus when the jaw closes.

Whether or not each condyle of the mandible moves forwards or not on to the articular tubercle can be felt, together with any click or crepitus.

### Clicking Jaw

This is due to a momentary luxation of the intra-articular meniscus. It can usually be relieved by so strengthening the muscles of mastication that they hold the jaw steady. To this end, resisted exercises are practised, i.e. opening the mouth, protrusion and lateral deviation. There is seldom any need to give a resisted exercise to the muscles that close the jaw; for these the patient maintains for himself by chewing. If dislocation of the meniscus takes place during the exercises, this must be prevented by the physiotherapist's finger pressing against the side of the jaw while the movements are resisted with the other hand.

### Fixed Dislocation of the Meniscus

When this occurs the patient finds himself suddenly unable to open his mouth more than 1 cm. Full closing of the jaw is painless. Lateral deviation towards the affected side is usually painless and may be the position of ease.

Manipulative reduction without anaesthesia usually succeeds. The operator inserts his thumb and presses downwards on the molar teeth on the affected side. The point of the patient's chin is cupped between the operator's fingers and palm. During strong disengagement of the temporal bone and the mandible, this is rocked backwards and forwards, in alternate deviation laterally. The click is felt (see Volume II). If the endeavour fails, under general anaesthesia, the patient's jaws are merely forced apart with a dental gag until the meniscus slips home (Fig. 32). Reduction by this means presented no difficulty even in a case of two years' standing.

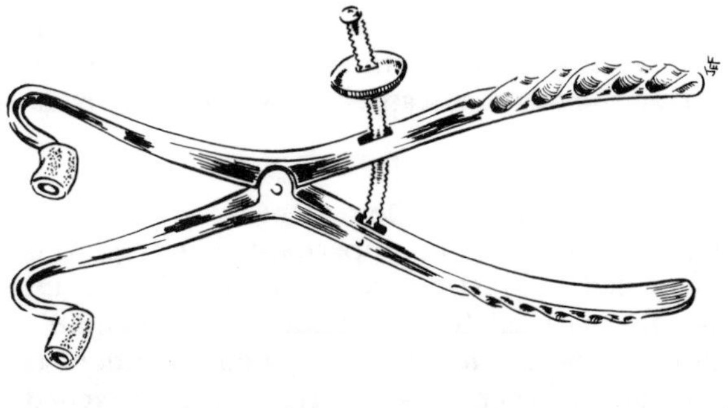

**Fig. 32.** A dental gag for reducing a dislocated meniscus in the temporomandibular joint.

## Osteoarthritis

If this causes symptoms, there is pain on, seldom limitation of, the extreme of each movement. Crepitus is felt. Treatment consists of deep friction to the capsule of the joint followed by forcing movement.

## Sympathetic Arthritis

A day or two after the extraction of molar teeth, the patient may notice increasing difficulty in opening his mouth. On examination, movement is limited in every direction and the bone in the region of the tooth socket is tender. This type of sympathetic irritation of the joint appears analogous to that occurring in connection with any abscess near the extremity of a bone.

Spontaneous cure of the arthritis may take two or three weeks. Treatment is seldom required, but must be directed to the dental sepsis, not the joint.

## Non-specific Arthritis

Occasional cases are seen of arthritis of one temporomandibular joint for no apparent reason.

In the course of some weeks the patient develops increasing pain in the cheek and inability to open the mouth. This may remain slight, but may also progress to the point where opening beyond 1 cm is impossible; it may go on for months unchanged. Eating is painful and if much limitation is present the patient has to live on slops.

No clear cause is discernible. Gonorrhoeal ankylosis is a disease of the past, and neither Still's disease nor ankylosing spondylitis is present. In some cases, monarticular rheumatoid arthritis is apparently responsible, since triamcinolone injected once or twice into the joint is curative. It should always be tried, even if the sedimentation rate and other tests are negative (as they so often are when only one large joint is affected). When the arthritis complicates widespread rheumatic disease elsewhere, the diagnosis is obvious.

*Technique of Injection.* The patient lies on his side, with the affected joint uppermost. The zygoma is identified and just below, level with the tragus, the physician can feel the condyle of the mandible moving as the mouth is opened as much as possible and then closed. A thin needle attached to a syringe containing 0.5 ml of triamcinolone suspension is inserted at the base of the tragus and pointed slightly forwards, aiming at the space left behind when the condyle has shifted anteriorly as far as possible by the patient opening his mouth as wide as he can. The needle becomes intra-articular at about 1 cm.

*Stretching.* If triamcinolone has no effect, the only alternative is stretching the joint first with a Hallam's gag, then with a dental gag. It is remarkable that this treatment should be effective, but it is. Within a couple of months, full, painless movement is often restored, without tendency to recurrence.

When arthritis at the temporomandibular joint proves refractory to all treatment, arthroplasty is a satisfactory operation.

## Ankylosis

This is apt to follow a rheumatoid, septic or, in times past, a gonorrhoeal infection.

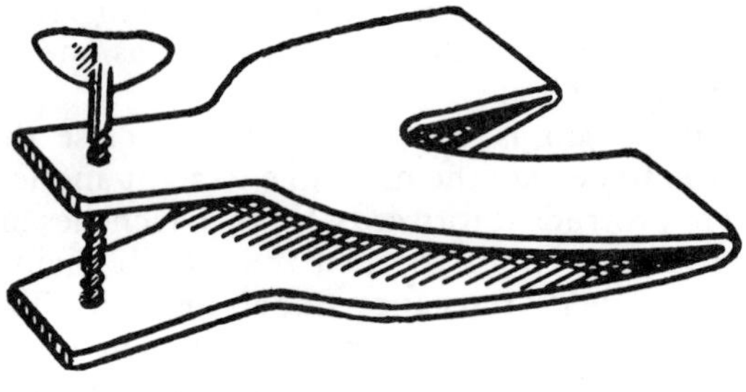

**Fig. 33.** Hallam's gag for forcing movement slowly at the temporomandibular joint.

If the ankylosis is unsound, Hallam's gag may be used so long as enough space exists between the teeth for the introduction of the steel plate. It is opened by turning a screw and bears on all the front teeth (Fig. 33). He suggests that pressure should be exerted in this way for 20 minutes every three hours. Arthroplasty is a most satisfactory operation for intractable limitation of movement. It should not be performed too late in cases of Still's disease, for lack of growth of the mandible from disuse leads to unsightly facial deformity. Condylotomy is usually performed with Ward's (1961) technique of blind division with a Gigli saw. Banks and MacKenzie followed up 211 such cases for up to 20 years and found half had remained well and a further one-third were improved.

### Pain Arising in the Pterygoid Muscles

Rarely, the track of a local anaesthetic injection for dental purposes in this area becomes secondarily infected. Seward (1966), in hospital practice, estimates this occurrence as only two or three times in 100 000 injections. A day or two after the visit to the dental surgeon, pain in the cheek and stiffness set in. The history of a local anaesthetic injection is clear, and examination shows limitation of jaw opening. But clenching the teeth hurts, as does resisted deviation towards the painful side. If these resisted movements hurt, the patient's temperature should be taken and treatment by antibiotics is called for at once.

Intermittent claudication of the pterygoid muscles occurs in giant-cell arteritis. Cortisone must be started without delay for fear of blindness from involvement of the opthalmic artery.

### Loss of Molar Teeth

The patient complains of a constant deep burning pain inside the temple and the upper part of the cheek, not necessarily made worse by eating. Examination reveals pain at the extremes of all movements at the temporomandibular joint, and loss of all the molar teeth, on the same side as the painful joint, on the opposite side, or on both sides.

The arthritis is caused by excessive upward pressure of the mandible against the articular fossa of the temporal bone, due to loss of the distance-maintaining apposition between the molar teeth of the mandible and maxilla (Costen 1936). Dentures restoring the proper distance between the jaws lead to the disappearance of the pain in a few weeks, and have also proved efficacious in trigeminal neuralgia occurring in the edentulous (Blair & Gordon 1973). It has been pointed out by Shore et al. (1979) that during cervical traction, when carried out on patients with missing posterior teeth, the distracting force is borne by pressure on the condyles of the mandible. This may set up trouble in the temporomandibular joints preventible by a splint giving enough thickness to divert the strain to the posterior part of the mandible.

### Hysteria

Obviously, patients, especially adolescents, wishing to draw attention to themselves by a reluctance to eat or speak, readily develop difficulty in opening the mouth. They are apt, however, to describe too diffuse a pain, extending perhaps all over the head and face, and to hold the neck stiffly as well. The circumstances attending the onset may ring false.

Examination of the jaw in an uncooperative patient is difficult, for he may merely hold his jaw closed and allege such pain that he cannot open his mouth. It is wise, therefore, to test the resisted movements of the neck first and to palpate indifferent spots (e.g. the maxilla) for tenderness in suspicious cases. Except in tetanus, gross limitation of movement does not come on suddenly on both sides at once; moreover, in subluxation of the meniscus at least 1 cm of opening range is always retained.

The result of treatment often proves conclusive, persuasion aided by gentle forcing restoring range in a few minutes.

## THE THORACIC OUTLET SYNDROME

It has long been recognized that pressure on a nerve, if sustained or severe, sooner or later interferes with the parenchyma; the signs of loss of conduction characterizing a lower motor neurone lesion appear. If, however, the pressure is slight or intermittent, conduction may not become impaired, even after many years of symptoms. Hence intermittent pressure on a nerve trunk may never result in the development of the neurological deficit that would be expected sooner or later to clarify the diagnosis. Yet the patient's sensations, particularly his complaint of pins and needles, indicate that a nerve is affected. This is often the situation at the thoracic outlet in middle-aged women. The nerve recovers by night as fast as it is compressed by day, no loss of conduction ever supervening.

The thoracic outlet syndrome is an affection of the brachial plexus, not the nerve roots. The patient therefore experiences no symptoms at the base of the neck where the lesion lies, but only those referred to the distal part of the upper limb. The nerves derived from the eighth cervical and first thoracic roots, i.e. the lower trunk, are affected alone. The mere discovery, therefore, of neurological signs at or above the seventh cervical level, excludes pressure at the thoracic outlet as the cause.

There are two main types of pressure at the thoracic outlet: that associated with a cervical

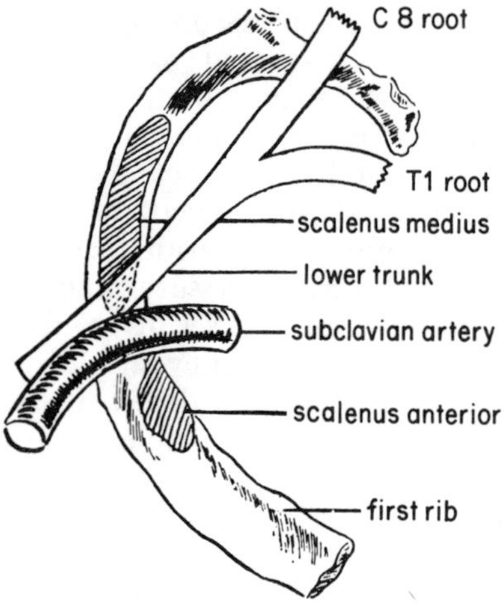


**Fig. 34.** The anatomy of the thoracic outlet. (*After Rogers*).

rib and that associated with the first rib. Cervical ribs show, of course, by X-rays, but it must be remembered that patients with every gradation of bony abnormality, from unusually long transverse processes at the seventh cervical vertebra to large cervical ribs, may have no relevant symptoms at all. By contrast, a strong fibrous band in the position of a cervical rib but without ossification does not show radiologically, but can cause just as much trouble as a bony rib.

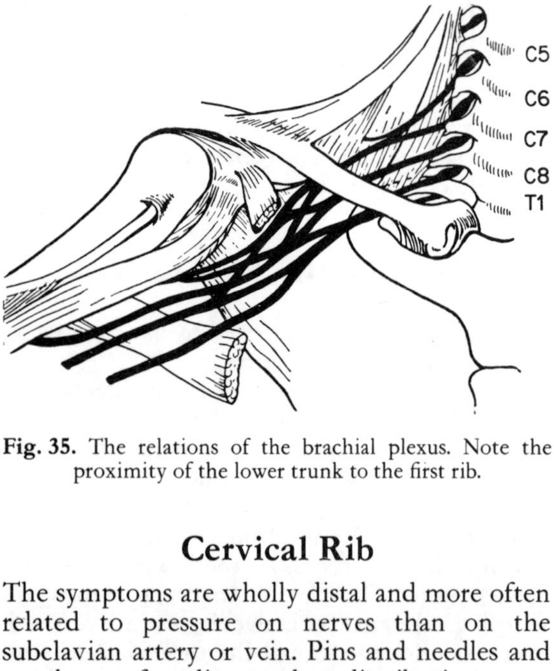


**Fig. 35.** The relations of the brachial plexus. Note the proximity of the lower trunk to the first rib.

## Cervical Rib

The symptoms are wholly distal and more often related to pressure on nerves than on the subclavian artery or vein. Pins and needles and numbness of median or ulnar distribution, more often the latter, are commonly the first symptoms. The complaint is usually bilateral, but often more severe on one side than the other. The patient, who is usually in his twenties or thirties, notices that carrying anything heavy or even wearing a winter overcoat brings on the paraesthesia in the hands. Sometimes he states that dependence of the arm for any length of time is followed by aching in the hand, which remains white and cold for some hours. This can be confirmed objectively, and indicates pressure on the subclavian artery. If the pressure is exerted on the subclavian vein, the hand may become oedematous and, less often, cyanosed for hours or days. Occasionally, he is concerned to see that, albeit painlessly, bilateral wasting of the abductor pollicis brevis muscle has slowly become complete over a period of years; the patient then attends merely to find out the cause of the alteration in the contour of his thenar eminence.

On examination, scapular elevation and holding the arms up for a while bring on the pins and needles but alleviate the vascular signs. Approximation of the scapulae draws the clavicles backwards and often stops the radial pulse, but this is not uncommon in normal individuals. Passive depression of the scapulae by the examiner seldom has any effect, but making the patient carry a weight for some time may increase or bring on the symptoms. Palpation at the root of the neck anteriorly may reveal a unilateral increase in the ease with which subclavian pulsation is felt. By contrast with these scapular findings, the movements of the neck are free and painless and examination of the upper limb usually reveals no abnormality until the hand is reached, when ulnar or median weakness sooner or later becomes detectable. In early cases no abnormality is necessarily found.

Radiography shows the cervical ribs. It must be borne in mind that supernumerary ribs, visible by X-rays, do not necessarily cause symptoms.

In due course, in cases of median development, wasting of the abductor pollicis brevis muscle begins to show itself. In cases of ulnar development, the hypothenar and interosseous muscles weaken. Cutaneous analgesia is seldom a prominent feature. After some years, all the small muscles of the hand and the flexor digitorum profundus to the fourth and fifth fingers may become very weak.

## Pressure exerted by the First Rib

### Acute Onset

Rare cases occur of pressure at the thoracic outlet arising suddenly. A young person, after carrying a heavy weight for some distance—usually a suitcase on a journey—suddenly feels faint and develops pain in the chest and upper limb. Within a few minutes the hand and forearm blanch, but, since breathing usually hurts, consequent shallow respiration often leads to the patient's immediate admission with a provisional diagnosis of spontaneous pneumothorax. The radial pulse and warmth and colour return to the upper limb within a few hours.

Even more uncommon are attacks of severe, momentary pectoral pain caused by sudden impingement of the clavicle against a prominent costochondral junction of the first rib. If the diagnosis is confirmed by local anaesthesia and the attacks are severe and frequent, osteotomy of the clavicle is warranted.

## Slow Onset

When the pectoral girdle droops during middle-age and subjects the lower trunk of the brachial plexus to pressure from the first rib by day, the symptoms are altogether different. Moreover, the radiograph reveals no extra rib, though a fibrous band is suggested when the seventh cervical transverse process projects as far as the thoracic instead of being 1 cm shorter.

The patient, nearly always a middle-aged woman, complains that each night she is woken two or three hours after falling asleep (i.e. between 1 and 3 a.m.) by severe pins and needles in both hands. She soon learns that if she lets her arms hang over the edge of the bed, or if she sits or stands up, the symptoms quickly subside. She falls asleep again, and the same thing may happen some hours later, or she may then sleep uninterrupted until the morning. Often the hands feel numb on waking; if so, the patient has difficulty for the first half-hour with small actions such as turning on the light; for she cannot feel the switch between her fingers. By day, she is little troubled unless she carries a heavy weight on one arm, e.g. a shopping-basket, which soon brings on the pins and needles. These are seldom confined to any one part of the hand; they usually affect all five digits equally, on both aspects or within the palm. After some months or years, nocturnal pain begins in the hands and forearms, later still reaching to the shoulders. The patient sometimes comes to realize that the more she exerts herself by day, the more pain she will have that night; she may also notice that after a few days in bed with, say, influenza or while on a lazy holiday, her nocturnal symptoms disappear. The hands do not change colour. Sometimes the paresthesia is purely unilateral. Rarely, patients present themselves with pain in the arm and forearm without pins and needles in the hand. If so, psychogenic pain is closely simulated, but the absence of exaggeration when the patient is examined makes the organic nature of the pain obvious and suggests the thoracic outlet as a possible source of pain.

The paraesthesia is a release phenomenon; it comes on only when the day's constant downward strain is taken off the pectoral girdle, i.e. at night, when the relief from the weight of the upper limb on lying down allows the lower trunk of the brachial plexus to move upwards out of contact with the first rib. Recovery takes some time after a whole day's compression, and it is therefore some hours before the paraesthesia appears and reaches an intensity that wakens the sleeping patient. Since the nerves recover each night, no signs of a lower motor neurone lesion may ever become manifest, even in those patients who have had severe nocturnal symptoms for several years.

Examination of all the movements of the neck and upper limb reveals full power and full painless range, except that sustained elevation of the scapula and of the arms brings on the symptoms. If a patient appears to be suffering from compression at the outlet, these two postures should be maintained for several minutes, since the pins and needles and/or pain never come on instantly. If these two tests fail, the patient should lie supine with the arms above her head for five or ten minutes. Throughout the examination, it is the negative response to all the diagnostic tests, combined with a positive response to one or other of these ways of lifting the lower trunk of the brachial plexus off the first rib that, together with a suggestive history, enables a firm diagnosis to be made.

### *Differential Diagnosis*

1. Bilateral protrusion of the seventh cervical intervertebral disc: acroparaesthesia. The symptoms nearly always begin at the scapulae; there is discomfort on moving the neck, and the muscles affected are different.
2. Central cervical disc lesion. Pressure on the spinal cord may give rise to pins and needles in the hands only, but they usually appear in the feet as well quite soon. The paraesthesia comes and goes in a wholly irregular way, most marked by day. Movement of the cervical spine is limited and bilaterally uncomfortable. Neck flexion may bring on the pins and needles in the hands.

3. Pulmonary sulcus tumour (Pancoast). Horner's syndrome is present: severe weakness of the small muscles of the hand (they are all affected) comes on rapidly. The radiograph of the apex of the lung is diagnostic. In advanced cases, erosion of the first and second ribs is also visible, and the patient may be hoarse owing to paralysis of one vocal cord.
4. Friction on the ulnar nerve at the elbow.
5. Compression of the median nerve in the carpal tunnel.
6. Compression of the ulnar nerve at the wrist.
7. Ischaemic fingers in Raymond's disease.
8. Blotchy red hands in liver disease.

# Treatment

## Operation

When cervical ribs set up marked signs of pressure on the brachial plexus or the subclavian artery, operation is usually indicated, especially in younger patients. If the obstruction is fibrous, not bony, the radiograph is misleadingly negative. Nevertheless, exploration of the outlet is warranted, especially in cases with vascular symptoms, in order to avoid the development of thrombosis, or later of a subclavian aneurysm. Unless operation is done early in vascular cases, gangrene of the fingers or ischaemic contracture may supervene (Hébréard 1817; Raynaud 1888; Rob & Standeven 1958). Many different mechanical abnormalities exist. Hence the surgeon exposes the outlet and examines the relationship of the first rib and its muscles to the artery and the lower trunk of the brachial plexus, planning any subsequent operation according to what is found at the time.

## Conservative Treatment

In the middle-aged patients who provide the majority of sufferers from pressure at the thoracic outlet, conservative treatment is usually very effective. Within two or three weeks the patient loses her long-standing symptoms and, as long as she keeps to her regimen, remains well. After a time, the nerves lose the heightened sensitiveness resulting from repeated bruising; some months later the patient finds that she can relax her precautions a good deal. If she suffers relapse, she knows its cause and it remedy.

Treatment requires the patient's cooperation and comprises the following.

*Explanation.* It is important to make the patient understand the mechanism by which her pain is produced. If she takes it as a release phenomenon, she bears with it until it ceases, realizing that the presence of pins and needles characterizes recovery and implies that she has adopted an eventually beneficial postion. In the absence of such guidance, she unwittingly makes herself worse by, logically enough, avoiding such postures as bring on her unpleasant symptoms. Once she realizes that her pain is abolished by renewed compression of the nerve, she can appreciate why she must reverse her attitude. Otherwise she merely postpones her symptoms voluntarily, and has to suffer the more each night in consequence.

*Elevating the Scapulae.* It is quite useless merely to give exercises to the trapezius muscles. In the first place, these muscles are extremely strong in all healthy individuals. In the second place, strengthening a muscle in no way hinders it from fully relaxing when not in use. The patient must learn to keep her shoulders very slightly shrugged all the time, in other words, to maintain a slight constant postural tone in the trapezii. This habit can be inculcated; exercises to make the muscles contract and than relax miss the point altogether. Before lifting anything heavy she must shrug her scapula right up and maintain it so all the time that she is carrying the weight. So far as possible, she must avoid wearing an overcoat. A basket on wheels is a great help to the housewife. Provision of domestic help fully relieves some patients, as study of the history may indicate.

*The Armchair.* Each evening, after supper, she must sit in an armchair with her arms adducted

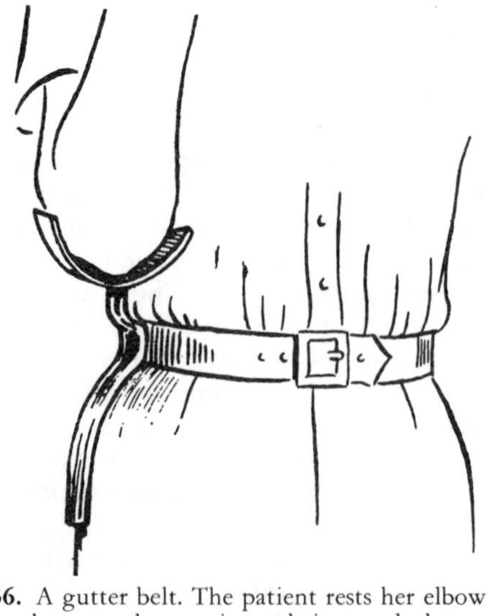

**Fig. 36.** A gutter belt. The patient rests her elbow on the gutter whenever the arm is not being used, thus relieving the pectoral girdle of the weight of the upper limb.

to her sides and the forearms so supported on the arms of the chair that the scapulae are held well up without effort on her part. After a while, this posture results in the appearance of the familiar symptoms. She remains seated thus until the paraesthesia has ceased, however long this may take—at first often 20 to 30 minutes, later only a few minutes. The nerve trunk having now recovered, she can go to bed, free from fear of being woken.

*Support.* Occasionally, it is wise to take the downward strain off the thoracic outlet. In unilateral cases, a sling can be worn bearing on the other shoulder only. In bilateral cases, it is necessary to provide a belt with adjustable gutters supporting the upper forearm (Fig. 36). The patient rests her elbow on the gutter all the time that the arm is not in active use.

*Raising the Trapezius Muscles.* The operation devised by Cockett should be employed in resistant cases. The trapezius muscles are detached from the spinous processes of the cervical vertebrae and then sutured back again higher up, thus providing the scapulae with a permanent brace.

## SUBCLAVIAN OCCLUSION

The chief symptom is intermittent claudication in the arm, i.e. pain after continuing hard work for a while. Hence, the patient complains of an increasing ache in whatever muscles he has been using most strongly, whereas the examiner finds no lesion when he makes the patient contract each muscle momentarily. It is the pain brought on by persistent exertion that suggests thrombosis of the subclavian artery, and a negative examination makes it the more probable. The diagnosis is made when the radial pulse is found absent. The aortogram reveals the exact state of affairs.

If, as the result of vigorous use of the arm, the brachial demand for arterial blood becomes so great that the pressure in the circle of Willis rises above that in the subclavian artery, blood is drawn to the arm from the cerebrum. Reversal of blood flow in the vertebral artery occurs when the subclavian stenosis lies proximal to the origin of the vertebral artery. In these cases, in addition to the increasing discomfort, exertion of the arm makes the patient feel faint from diminution in the blood flow to the brain. This was the first example of the 'steal syndrome' to be described (Reivich et al. 1961).

## RARE CAUSES OF SCAPULOCLAVICULAR PAIN

A number of conditions exist in which the movements of the neck and scapula both hurt, sometimes of the arm too. Such a multiplicity of painful movements suggests psychoneurosis, but the following conditions must be eliminated before such an attribution can be confidently made.

### Cervical Disc Lesion

The pain is in the upper scapular area, and is brought on in the usual way by some but not others of the active and passive neck movements. However, in acute cases, testing the scapular and arm movements against resistance may hurt too, since the scapula must be fixed by contraction of the scapulovertebral muscles before the arm can be pushed hard in any direction, thus compressing the spinal joint. But the pain is felt at the base of the neck, not the arm. There is occasionally a painful arc. A patient with really acute torticollis may be unable to get his arm up voluntarily above the horizontal. Resisted lateral rotation at the shoulder and resisted flexion at the elbow may also cause pain, but again in the scapular area.

The diagnosis is immediately clarified by reducing the cervical displacement by manipulation; then the same arm and scapular movements are tested again. If, as often happens, they no longer hurt, the cervical displacement is shown to be responsible for the whole syndrome. All patients, therefore, who clearly possess a cervical disc lesion, and perhaps also trouble in the scapular area or arm, should be treated thus. After manipulative reduction, it becomes clear if they arose from transmitted stress or because two lesions are present.

### Fractured First Rib

Since this is usually a stress fracture, there is no history of trauma, merely the unprovoked appearance of pain at the root of the neck. The neck movements hurt, expecially side flexion away from the painful side, when the scalenes pull on the rib adjacent to the fracture. Resisted side flexion towards the painful side is also painful for the same reason. Raising the arm is painful and often cannot be carried out beyond the horizontal, but full passive elevation is seldom more than uncomfortable. Since a fractured rib unites in two months, this disorder need be considered only when the history is short—a few weeks. The radiograph is diagnostic.

## Clay-shoveller's Fracture

This is a stress fracture, caused by unaccustomed exertion, usually digging, by an unfit person. The pain is central at the base of the neck and active and passive flexion and extension of the neck prove painful. However, elevation of each scapula also hurts and again the arms cannot be actively elevated beyond a small amount of abduction.

This time the pain is central and the inability bilateral, and again spontaneous recovery takes two months; hence this diagnosis need be considered only in short-lived cases. The seventh cervical or first thoracic spinous process is tender. The radiograph is diagnostic.

## Costocoracoid Fascia

### Idiopathic Contracture

This is a very uncommon cause of limited elevation of the arm. The symptom is gradually increasing, upper pectoroscapular pain on one side only. It is provoked at first only by full elevation of the arm. After a year or two elevation becomes slightly limited, and any prolonged reaching upwards leads to some hours' or days' increased aching.

The syndrome is difficult to recognize, because the symptoms suggest a cervical disc lesion and the signs, unless carefully studied, suggest a psychogenic disorder. The key to the condition is the discovery of slight painful limitation of elevation of the scapula.

Examination of the neck movements reveals that active side flexion away from, and resisted side flexion towards, the painful side hurt at the root of the neck. Upward movement of the scapula, active or passive, is painful at its extreme and slightly limited. Resisted elevation is painless. Forward movement of the scapula is usually full and painful; backward, full and painless. Since the patient seldom asks advice for the first year or so, by the time he is seen, active and passive elevation of the arm has become about 10° limited by pectoroscapular pain; but passive movements at the glenohumeral joint are neither restricted nor painful. All the resisted shoulder movements hurt a little at the base of the neck.

This curious pattern occurs only in contracture of the costocoracoid fascia. When inspection of the range of elevation of both scapulae together discloses limitation on the painful side, this rare condition is brought to mind. One cause is dense adhesions at the apex of one lung such as occurs in long-standing tuberculosis. However, not all cases show such a shadow. Follow-up for several years reveals no ultimate cause, nor any tendency to spontaneous recovery; indeed the contracture tends to become very slowly worse. My youngest patient had had it for a year when she was first seen aged 23. It does not appear to start after the age of 50.

### Traumatic Fasciitis

Occasionally, these symptoms and signs come on after trauma. If so, a deep breath also hurts and pneumothorax is suspected, but the radiograph excludes this disorder. I regard these cases as caused by a small haematoma lying beneath the costocoracoid fascia. No treatment avails, and spontaneous resolution takes about three months. I have encountered one case in which the fibrosis was permanent.

### Treatment

Conservative treatment is vain. Forcing elevation of the arm brings on increasing aching for several days; no benefit follows. If the cause is tuberculous fibrosis at the apex of the lung, forcing is contraindicated since it might well disturb the healed area. The patient must just accept that he cannot lift his arm right up.

So far only one patient has accepted operation. She was a secretary and typing made her upper pectoral area ache so severely that she could not go on. In 1967, my surgical colleague D. R. Urquhart exposed the fascia, which appeared quite normal and divided it and the pectoralis minor muscle. She retained some 5° limitation of elevation a year later, but is symptom-free and works well.

## Basal Pulmonary Neoplasm

Some early cases can be mistaken for a shoulder lesion. The neoplasm interferes with the diaphragm and pain at the point of the shoulder results. When it begins to erode the chest wall, the pectoralis major protects the ribs by going into spasm when the arm is elevated. Hence, pain at the point of the shoulder and limitation of elevation of the arm beyond the horizontal result. The neck and scapular movements may cause slight discomfort, but the range of both is full. The passive range of movement at the shoulder joint is full and painless, thus forming a strong contrast with the fact that the arm cannot be lifted even passively above the horizontal, in the presence of a fully mobile scapula. When the agent responsible for this restriction is sought, the pectoralis major can be seen to contract and prevent further movement.

The radiograph of the lower lung reveals a large shadow.

## Subclavian Muscle

This muscle is occasionally strained, especially in patients with a lax sternoclavicular joint. The pain is felt accurately at mid-clavicle, and may be brought on slightly by passive elevation of the scapula, but is severe when the patient presses his pectoral girdle downwards against the examiner's resistance applied to the elbow, while the arm is approximated to the patient's trunk.

However long the symptoms have continued, deep massage to the muscle affords permanent relief.

# STERNOCLAVICULAR JOINT

This joint possesses some 60° range of elevation, 60° of rotation and 30° of forward movement, the range being limited by the fact that the trapezius and rhomboid muscles are at full stretch, restraining the scapula.

The joint may be sprained as the result of a fall and any capsular stretching that occurs there is permanent. The weight of the upper limb makes the medial end of the clavicle ride upwards, after capsular rupture, as far as the costoclavicular ligament permits. A permanent prominence is then visible. Subluxation is common also in osteoarthrosis and (rarely) after a bacterial infection.

The patient himself supplies the diagnosis, for the pain is felt exactly at the joint and does not radiate. Movement at the joint produced by the active scapular movements usually evokes slight discomfort, but the main discomfort appears at the extreme of each movement of the humerus at the shoulder: a more powerful way of straining the joint. Adduction of the arm across the chest hurts most and in recent sprains may prove painful enough to be limited. On palpation, the joint is prominent and tender. In osteoarthrosis, the joint may appear swollen and feel soft in a manner more suggestive of rheumatoid arthritis, but this finding need not arouse alarm. Syphilis is said to have a special predilection for the inner end of the clavicle, but this appears no longer so.

### Treatment

*Recent Sprain.* A sling should be worn for a couple of days to relieve the joint of the weight of the upper limb and triamcinolone injected as soon as the patient is seen. Recent and chronic cases respond equally well. Subsequent instability, provided that it is painless, is of no inconvenience to the patient. Exercises are contraindicated since the sternoclavicular joint is dependent for stability on ligaments alone; hence movements only cause further stretching. Moreover, no adhesions can form in a joint about which no muscle exists that could hold it too still.

*Chronic Cases.* Pain follows exertion (the joint is already osteoarthrotic or subluxated), and may continue indefinitely in spite of the avoidance of exertion. One injection of triamcinolone into the joint abolishes the symptoms, but the patient must permanently restrict exercise thereafter, otherwise pain will return and a further intra-articular injection will be required.

## Posterior Sternoclavicular Syndrome

This is a rare condition. For no apparent reason, a middle-aged patient develops unilateral pain at the *posterior* aspect of the neck, which continues unchanged for years. The pain is not severe, but constant, worse on using the arm. There is no discomfort anteriorly in the region of the sternoclavicular joint.

On examination, the neck movements, passive and resisted, do not hurt, but scapular elevation is painful at its extreme, passively as well as actively. There is no scapulothoracic crepitus. No weakness or pain is revealed when scapular elevation is tested against resistance. Full elevation of the arm is difficult to achieve because of pain felt at the base of the neck, whereas full abduction at the glenohumeral joint is painless. Examination of the rest of the upper limb reveals no abnormality. The anterior sternoclavicular ligaments are not tender. Thus nothing draws attention to the sternoclavicular joint. Patients are apt to receive treatment intended to restore full elevation to the arm, but this increases the symptoms. Yet 1 ml of triamcinolone injected into the posterior sternoclavicular ligament, either through the joint or by approaching the back of the joint from above, relieves the condition, apparently permanently.

## SCAPULOTHORACIC CREPITUS

When one or other scapula—sometimes both—is actively moved up and down against the thorax, painless crepitus may be palpable. Occasionally, a loud creaking audible across the room is provoked. If the scapulae are abducted, the crepitus on movement ceases. The condition is clearly due to roughening of the posterior thoracic wall just beyond the lateral edge of the iliocostalis muscle.

When the crepitus occurs in young people, there may be concern lest the crepitus prove the precursor to 'rheumatism'. Explanation that the crepitus is permanent and insignificant is usually all that is necessary.

Occasionally the patient complains of considerable scapular aching after exercise. Typists, gymnasts and physiotherapists may become scarcely able to work. In such cases, the area whence the crepitus originates must be outlined by discovering just how far the scapula need be abducted for the crepitus on movement to cease. The roughened area now lies just medial to where the vertebral border of the upper scapula lay. Deep massage must be given to this spot. The patient feels no special tenderness here; the physiotherapist cannot feel any crepitus as she gives the massage; hence the spot must be found mathematically. The crepitus on scapular movement does not cease; yet say 20 such treatments largely or wholly abolish the ache, even when it is of many years' standing.

The patient may begin to develop a tic, moving his scapula repeatedly so as to elicit the crepitus; this naturally increases the ache, though he imagines that the action provides temporary relief. Advice to resist this habit suffices.

Should massage fail and the symptoms warrant, excision of the upper inner angle of the scapula affords permanent cure, but I have only once met sufficient disability to warrant this.

CHAPTER 9

# EXAMINATION OF THE SHOULDER: LIMITED RANGE

The shoulder is the most rewarding joint in the whole body. It possesses the salient merits of honesty and curability. When some movement is found painful or limited, the significance of this finding is seldom equivocal, and with regularity implies what on anatomical grounds it ought to imply. Moreover nearly all lesions of the joint and of adjacent soft tissues are tractable and, once relieved, seldom recur. It is a fact therefore that most patients are rapidly *cured*. When the trouble taken to establish a precise diagnosis is matched by equal accuracy in reaching the tissue at fault, patient and physician derive great satisfactions. Since, too, problems at the shoulder can be solved only clinically, diagnosis is open to every clinician, whether he has access to hospital facilities or not. Indeed, the consultant is no better off than the family doctor when it comes to a painful shoulder, the more so since treatment necessitates merely a syringe and a pair of hands. My advice, therefore, to all physicians faced with a painful shoulder is: 'do it yourself'.

It is true, as always, that difficult cases exist, perhaps a double lesion or a pattern hard to interpret. When this happens, local anaesthesia is invaluable in confirming or disproving a tentative localization. If one lesion is singled out, it should be dealt with and, when it has recovered fully, further examination identifies the second disorder. In general, it is best to treat the joint first, since signs thought to incriminate some other tissue often disappear as the joint recovers.

Many doctors regard disorders at the shoulder as uninteresting, undiagnosable and incurable, but tending to recover in the end. Nothing could be further from the truth; for many shoulder lesions persist unchanged for years and nearly every one is fully, often permanently, relievable.

## PAIN

Symptoms arising from the tissues at the shoulder are seldom felt at the shoulder itself. The exception is the acromioclavicular joint. This is developed within the fourth cervical segment and cannot, therefore, refer pain to the arm. All the other common lesions at the shoulder affect structures derived largely from the fifth cervical segment.

How far the pain is referred depends on the severity of the lesion. For example, in slight arthritis or tendinitis, the pain is usually felt at the upper arm only, whereas the same lesion, if more intense, leads to radiation of pain as far as the wrist. This extended reference is an error of perception occurring in the sensory cortex. Precise delineation of the extent of the pain has two values: (*a*) it outlines the dermatome and thus shows within which segment to look for the lesion; (*b*) it indicates the severity of the pathological process.

Whatever the disorder at the shoulder may be, the pain is apt to be felt in the same place except for the ache at the point of the shoulder that suggests a lesion of the acromioclavicular joint. For example, whether arthritis, bursitis or tendinitis is present, the lesion lies in a structure of largely fifth cervical derivation; hence fifth cervical reference is common to each. Furthermore, the same lesion, when its severity alters, may at different times give rise to pain at different sites; for the symptoms are confined only by the segmental boundaries.

No matter what the position of an articular or para-articular lesion at the shoulder, if it is severe, the patient feels a deep burning ache running down the anterolateral aspect of the arm and the radial side of the forearm. He has little idea of its source; if he indicates an exact point, he is usually wrong. Whenever such diffuse pains are met with in the upper limb, examination of the entire forequarter is always required. Nor must the examiner stop when one disorder has been identified, for combined lesions are fairly common in this area.

## PRESENT-DAY MISCONCEPTIONS

There are a number of important errors in current medical thought on the shoulder leading to difficulty in correctly interpreting the clinical findings. The most important error is to ascribe capsular lesions to disorder of the tendons about the joint. This is considered below.

### Tendinous Lesions Thought to Cause Limitation of Movement

There is a widespread belief that limitation of movement at the shoulder can result from tendinous lesions. Limitation of *active* movement can, of course, be due to, say, supraspinatus tendinitis, when so painful an arc exists that the patient cannot by his own efforts get the arm beyond the horizontal. But full passive elevation relaxes the supraspinatus muscle and can always be obtained. Hence, tendinous lesions do not limit the *passive* range of movement, and it is the passive movement, not the active, that informs the examiner what is the true range. Tendinitis leading to capsulitis is a neat idea, but bears no relation to what is found on clinical examination of painful shoulders. Another notion is that degenerative change in the biceps and supraspinatus tendons leads to subsequent arthritis; this theory creates a pleasant unity, but is without justification. Tendinous and capsular lesions at the shoulder are quite separate, and each may be present for years without affecting the other; they do not merge, however long the patient is kept under observation.

*Bicipital tendinitis* is held by many authorities to be the forerunner of a 'frozen shoulder'. In fact, the tendon of the long head of biceps does not move during abduction of the humerus, the bone gliding under the stationary tendon. Were the tendon to become inflamed or fixed to bone, it is conceivable that limitation of abduction of the humerus might in theory result; but passive abduction could not become restricted. If the tendon is frayed, degenerated or chronically inflamed, the only symptom would be pain on resisted flexion and supination of the forearm.

More recently orthopaedic surgical opinion has accused the *rotator cuff* as the primary lesion in a frozen shoulder. This alternative is equally mistaken. In fact, the muscles about any joint do not go into spasm spontaneously. They do so to protect the joint, and it is here that the primary lesion lies. In any case, no lesion (short of ossification) of any tendon can give rise to limitation of passive movement, the characteristic finding in arthritis of the shoulder. Were the rotator cuff to contract, the pull of the subscapularis and infraspinatus muscles would cancel each other out, but no tendon lies inferiorly to counterbalance the pull of the supraspinatus tendon. Hence, did the 'rotator cuff syndrome' exist, it would lead to fixation of the shoulder in full abduction—the exact contrary of what actually happens.

The idea that tendinous disorders can limit movement at the shoulder has arisen in three ways:

1. Because limitation of active movement, in spite of its ambiguity, is taken at its face value. If active movement is limited, either joint range is restricted or the muscle will not move the arm properly. Hence, if the examiner does not then test the passive movement, he is misled. No one denies that tendinous lesions can lead to limitation of the voluntary range, but they cannot restrict the range on passive testing.
2. Because of the difficulty often experienced in distinguishing between the earliest stage of an arthritic shoulder and a tendinous lesion.
3. Because injury to both the capsule of the shoulder joint and the supraspinatus tendon is fairly common. As a result of the tendinous lesion, the patient has considerable pain on attempting active abduction. He therefore avoids this movement and the damaged shoulder joint develops post-traumatic adhesions. Thus a traumatic supraspinatus tendinitis, accompanied initially by a full range of movement at the shoulder joint, may later lead to a joint at which true limitation of movement from disuse has supervened.

### 'Periarthritis'

Presumably 'periarthritis' can only mean that some tissue about a joint, rather than those forming it, is at fault. This word is unhelpful, for it fails to answer the vital question—which of the periarticular structures is affected? At the shoulder, the condition to which the term 'periarthritis' is least ill-suited is subdeltoid bursitis, which should be described as such.

The false concept of 'periarthritis' has arisen from a mistaken belief in the diagnositic value of radiography. Limitation of movement at the shoulder associated with normal X-ray appear-

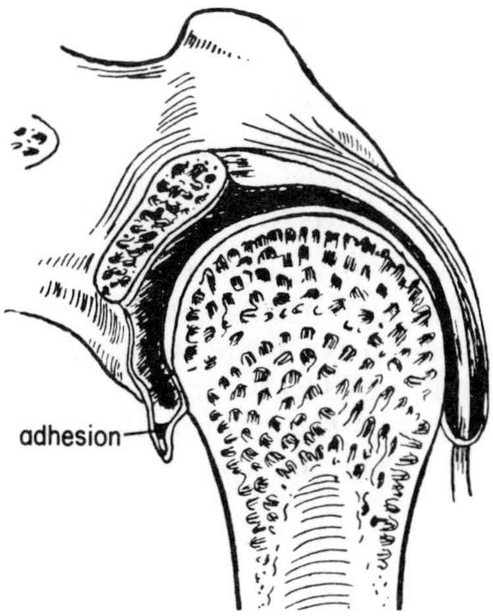


**Fig. 37.** Coronary section of the shoulder. A dense adhesion has formed at the inferior aspect of the joint, binding together the capsular fold. (*After Neviaser*).

ances has been thought to exclude a diagnosis of arthritis. This is not true. Many types of arthritis at other joints continue for a long time without showing any radiological changes and yet are unhesitatingly and correctly ascribed as arthritis, e.g. traumatic or rheumatoid arthritis of the fingers, traumatic, gonorrhoeal or rheumatoid arthritis at the knee and gouty arthritis of the foot. The fact that what had, on negative radiological grounds, been called 'periarthritis' was a capsular lesion meriting the term arthritis, was finally proved by Neviaser (1945). He dissected post-mortem, or inspected at operation, 63 shoulders with limited movement on clinical examination. He found that the capsule of the joint, instead of showing the normal laxity, was tight, closely applied to the head of the humerus and under such tension that it gaped widely when incised anteriorly. He found the densest adhesions between the two capsular surfaces (Fig. 37) inferiorly, thereby limiting abduction. His conclusions were that the lesion was not a 'periarthritis', but thickening and contracture of the capsule which microscopy showed to be the site of reparative inflammatory change. He suggested 'adhesive capsulitis' as a suitable term. These findings provide clear pathological confirmation of the views, then based on clinical considerations only, expressed in the original edition of this book. Viessel (1949) carried out arthrography with pyelosil on three cases of frozen shoulder and also found 'a degree of obliteration of the inferior joint recess'. The concept of an inferior capsular fold with adhesions had already been put forward in 1888 by Penny, who broke them down under chloroform anaesthesia and published a drawing almost identical with Neviaser's.

J. H. Young confirmed this finding (1952) by post-mortem dissection. Capsular contracture was the only lesion in six cases of blocked shoulder opened by de Sèze et al. (1959). Reeves (1966) found a marked reduction of the volume of fluid that was injectable at constant pressure in arthritic shoulders, less so when the lesion followed trauma.

### 'Frozen Shoulder'

The patient states that his shoulder is stiff and painful; he has noted that he cannot move it properly. The doctor confirms the limitation of movement and announces that the shoulder is 'frozen'. When asked what that implies, he replies 'limited movement at the shoulder joint'. Hence, 'frozen' means 'limited range'. The change in wording adds nothing to the patient's statement, and indicates no diagnosis. No one would be satisfied with a diagnosis of 'frozen' knee or elbow; it is well recognized that more than one cause of limited movement exists at these two joints. This is so also at the shoulder. Hence the term describes a symptom—stiffness.

## Possible Sources of Shoulder-Arm Pain

The preliminary examination singles out pain referred to the shoulder from elsewhere, e.g. diaphragm. Radiography identifies lesions of the bones. When these two possibilities have been excluded, pain felt in the shoulder and upper limb should be sought at the following 12 sites:

| | |
|---|---|
| Capsule of the shoulder joint | C5 |
| Subdeltoid bursa | C5 |
| Subcoracoid bursa | C5 |
| Acromioclavicular joint | C4 |
| Costocoracoid fascia | ? |
| Subclavian artery | ? |
| Supraspinatus tendon | C5 |
| Infraspinatus tendon | C5–6 |
| Subscapular tendon | C5–6 |
| Subclavius muscle | C5 |
| Biceps tendon | C5–6 |
| Triceps muscle | C7 |

# EXAMINATION OF THE SHOULDER

## History

The object of taking a history is twofold. First, to help decide whether or not the source of pain is likely to be in the shoulder region. Second, to assist further in assessment when the conditions that cause limitation of movement at the shoulder are encountered. In these cases, the answers to the questions set out below help to determine the stage that the lesion has reached. By contrast, if a tendon is found at fault, none of the points raised in the history is relevant.

Nine questions are enough:

1. Where is your pain? If the patient indicates the point of his shoulder, a lesion of the acromioclavicular joint is suggested; pain felt anywhere in the arm is common to all the other possible lesions.
2. Was there any injury? If later examination shows the capsular pattern, this suggests traumatic arthritis.
3. What is your age? Age is relevant to the distinction between the different types of arthritis at the shoulder.
4. How long have you had it? If the capsular pattern is present after a day's pain, palindromic rheumatism is suggested. Chondrocalcinotic arthritis recovers in about a month. Duration longer than that suggests monarticular rheumatoid arthritis. Acute subdeltoid bursitis leads to gross limitation of movement in a few days; the non-capsular pattern is present, and spontaneous recovery takes six weeks.
5. Have any other joints been affected? An affirmative answer suggests rheumatoid, psoriatic or lupus erythematosus arthritis or that complicating ankylosing spondylitis. Gout is rare at the shoulder and in most gouty patients with shoulder trouble the lesion there is unconnected.
6. Has your pain spread? The farther down the upper limb the pain goes, the more severe the lesion. Radiation to the arm excludes a lesion of the acromioclavicular ligaments.
7. Can you lie on that side at night? If not, and the capsular pattern is present, treatment by forcing movement is inappropriate.
8. Is there pain by day even when your arm is kept still? If there is, forcing is contraindicated.
9. Have you ever had an operation? This and questions about visceral function are relevant only if the pattern for malignant invasion at the shoulder emerges.

## Examination: First Part

The first question is: does the pain felt at the shoulder arise from the tissues about the shoulder? The second is: if the shoulder is at fault, which of the structures there contains the lesion? The first part of the examination decides the former point, and since any patient with armache is complaining of pain felt within a dermatome between the fourth cervical and the second thoracic, these segments must be fully examined. The first stage of the examination, therefore, consists of a quick survey from neck to hand. If the lesion is found to lie within the shoulder area, this is then examined more carefully. If the pain is found to be referred to the shoulder from some other moving part, examination is concentrated there. If no abnormality, i.e. neither limited movement, pain nor weakness is found at all, the lesion clearly lies outside the moving parts, and conditions like angina or diaphragmatic pleurisy are brought to mind. If all the movements, or a number of contradictory movements, are stated to hurt, the question of a psychogenic disorder arises.

The examination proceeds as follows, the patient being asked, as he performs each movement, if it hurts and, if so, where, while the examiner notes if weakness is apparent on any of the resisted movements:

| | |
|---|---|
| Neck | active flexion |
| | extension |
| | both side flexions |
| | both rotations |
| | resisted rotation (C1) |
| Scapula | resisted elevation (C2, 3, 4) |
| Shoulder | active elevation (C5) |
| Elbow | passive flexion and extension |
| | resisted flexion (C5 and C6) and extension (C7) |
| Wrist | resisted flexion (C7) and extension (C6) |
| Thumb | resisted extension (C8) |
| Finger | resisted adduction of fourth and fifth fingers (T1) |

If this examination shows that the lesion lies about the shoulder, this is examined in detail. However, if abnormality is detected on movements other than those of the shoulder, the lesion is shown to lie elsewhere.

# Examination: Second Part

## The Twelve Movements

Is is just as important to carry out not more than 12 movements as to test not less than 12. Too few movements means incomplete examination, but too many muddle the examiner, expecially if he attributes significance to impure movements that test two structures simultaneously. When the arm is brought away from the side in the coronal plane, the amount of movement of which the arm is capable is referred to as *elevation*. This is possible through 180°. The amount of movement existing in this direction between the scapula and the humerus is called *abduction*. This is possible through 90°.

Since combined lesions are not uncommon at the shoulder, the fact that there is limitation in every direction must not lead the examiner to omit trial of the resisted movements. A fall on the shoulder may, for example, damage the fifth cervical nerve root as well as the joint; partial rupture of the supraspinatus tendon may set up a secondary subdeltoid bursitis; myopathy may result in capsular contracture from disuse; neoplasm may invade both joint and tendons, and so on. Hence, the *resisted movements must be examined even in cases in which the discovery of limitation of range makes the diagnosis appear obvious.*

Normally, however, capsular lesions are uncomplicated and trial of the resisted movements does not set up pain or show weakness. This fact provides clear evidence that, as at other joints, there is no primary lesion of the muscles in arthritis at the shoulder.

*Active Elevation.* The patient is asked to bring his arm up as high as he can and is asked what he feels. His active range of movement and statement on pain are noted for correlation later.

Patients do not know how the arm gets up to full elevation; most imagine that 180° of movement are present at the shoulder joint. In fact, the first 90° of elevation take place at the scapulohumeral joint. The next 60° result from rotation of the scapula. The last 30° involve adduction of the humerus, the surgical neck crossing in front of the coracoid and acromion processes which rotation of the scapula has now made to point upwards instead of forwards. This knowledge is important in detecting psychogenic limitation of active elevation. If the scapula is mobile and its muscles intact, even if the shoulder is ankylosed, 60° of active elevation must be attainable by scapular movement alone.

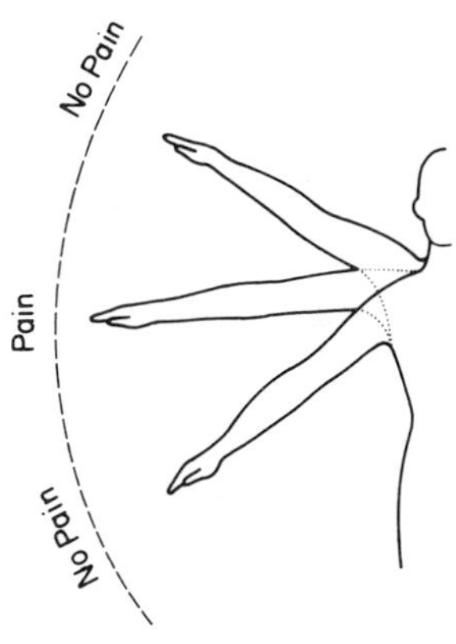


**Fig. 38.** A painful arc at the shoulder. As the arm passes the horizontal, pain is elicited. It disappears as this point is passed in either direction.

*Passive Elevation.* The examiner pushes the patient's arm up as high as possible and notes (*a*) whether full elevation is obtainable; (*b*) if it hurts; and (*c*) if active and passive elevation correspond in range or not. During passive elevation and the two passive rotations, there is an opportunity to note the end-feel. This may be important both in diagnosis and deciding treatment. If pain comes on well before the extreme of range is reached, and the end-feel is soft, subdeltoid bursitis is suggested. If full range is present, all extremes hurting, a hard end-feel characterizes a capsular lesion. If the point when pain comes on and the extreme of the possible range lie very close together, the capsule is probably at fault. By contrast, when chronic bursitis, tendinitis or an affection of the acromioclavicular joint causes pain at the extremes of full range, the hard capsular end-feel is absent and overpressure results in increased pain but no more resistance than that of the normal joint. There is a characteristic free feel to the extreme of full elevation of the normal joint which has a strong positive significance and is easily identified after a little experience.

*Painful Arc.* This applies only when 90° of abduction range at the shoulder joint is present, passively or actively. The patient is asked to bring his arm up outwards and to state if, at any point in the upward movement, he feels an ache, and if so, if it disappears again. Pain starting at the horizontal and continuing until full elevation is reached is not an arc. If the pain disappears above the horizontal but returns at full elevation, an arc is present. It is pain abating on either side of the painful point that has diagnostic significance. Since the abductor muscles draw the head of the humerus upwards and medially, an arc is usually best elicited on voluntary movement. However, an arc is an arc, whether felt on the way up only, down only, or both, active or passive.

A painful arc can often be seen, the arm faltering momentarily in its upward sweep at about the horizontal. Alternatively, the patient may have learnt how to avoid it by bringing his arm forwards into the sagittal plane before the horizontal is reached. So severe an arc, that active elevation stops at the horizontal and the patient uses his other hand to push the arm up farther, suggests calcification in bursa or tendon.

*Scapulohumeral Range of Abduction.* The examiner fixes the lower angle of the scapula with his thumb, applying the heel of his hand to the patient's mid-thorax, and lifts the elbow outwards with his other hand until he feels the scapula start to move. He notes the amplitude of this angle (normal 85 to 100°).

*Passive Lateral Rotation.* The patient bends his elbow to a right angle and the examiner holds the forearm pointing straight forwards. The humerus is now rotated outwards, first on the good, then on the affected side. The range is usually 90°, occasionally a little more in the young, and often 10 to 20° less in the elderly. If the restriction is due merely to age, it is painless and bilateral.

If lateral rotation is limited, the angle by which this falls short when the two sides are compared is estimated, and the examiner tests for the capsular end-feel. Whether the pain appears before or at the extreme of range, and whether or not overpressure increases the pain, are all noted.

*Passive Medial Rotation.* The normal range, starting from the forward position of the forearm (as above) is 90°. The examiner rotates the patient's humerus inwards and notes if full painless, full painful, or limited range is present, and in the latter case assesses the amplitude of this limitation.

Rarely a painful arc exists on medial rotation (never on lateral); if so, a tender structure is being pinched. It is important that the physician should not be too tender-hearted when medial rotation is rested, or he will stop at the arc and suppose that medial rotation is limited. If so, misdiagnosis is inevitable.

*Resisted Adduction.* The patient's elbow is brought a few centimetres from his thorax and he is then asked to pull his arm to his side as hard as he can. The examiner prevents all movement by placing one hand on the inner side of the patient's elbow, and the other on the patient's near flank. The patient says whether pain is evoked or not, and, if so, where. The examiner notes the strength of the muscles.

**Schematic Examination of the Shoulder** (prepared by R. Barbor)

| Thirteen movements | Arthritis (capsulitis) | Chronic sub-deltoid bursitis | Acromioclavicular joint strain | Supraspinatus tendinitis | Infraspinatus tendinitis | Subscapular tendinitis | Adductor strain | Biceps tendinitis |
|---|---|---|---|---|---|---|---|---|
| Active elevation | + | – | – | – | – | – | – | – |
| Passive elevation | + | – | + | ± | – | – | + | – |
| Passive scapulohumeral abduction | 30°* | – | + | – | – | – | – | – |
| Passive lateral rotation | 60°* | – | + | – | – | – | – | – |
| Passive medial rotation | 5°* | – | + | – | – | – | – | – |
| Passive adduction | – | – | ++ | – | – | ± | – | – |
| Painful arc | – | + | – | ± | ± | ± | – | – |
| Resisted abduction | – | – | – | ++ | – | – | – | – |
| Resisted adduction | – | – | – | – | – | – | + | – |
| Resisted lateral rotation | – | – | – | – | ++ | – | – | – |
| Resisted medial rotation | – | – | – | – | – | ++ | + | – |
| Resisted extension of elbow | – | ± | – | – | – | – | – | – |
| Resisted flexion of elbow | – | – | – | – | – | – | – | + |

* Limitation in these proportions = capsular pattern.

*Resisted Abduction.* The patient pushes his elbow laterally as hard as he can; the examiner holds the elbow so strongly that the shoulder joint does not move. Pain is reported; strength noted.

*Resisted Lateral Rotation.* The patient bends his elbow to a right angle, the forearm pointing forwards. Keeping his elbow well into his side actively, he tries to rotate the arm outwards against the examiner's pressure, applied to the patient's lower forearm (not his hand), so strongly that the shoulder joint does not move. Pain is reported; strength noted.

*Resisted Medial Rotation.* The same as for lateral rotation, except that the resisted movement takes place towards the trunk.

*Resisted Extension of the Elbow.* The patient's elbow is bent to a right angle; he then presses his forearm down against the examiner's resistance applied to his lower forearm (not the hand). Pain is reported; strength assessed.

*Resisted Flexion to the Elbow.* The same as for resisted extension, except that the patient flexes his elbow.

## MOVEMENT AT THE SHOULDER

The normal range of movement of the arms is a matter of dispute. Clearly, the general belief—90° at the shoulder joint and 90° at the scapula—when the arm is moved from its dependent position to full elevation, is incorrect; for inspection shows that the vertebral border of the scapula never lies horizontally when the patient's arm is held vertically upright. The actual mechanism is as follows: from the adducted position to the horizontal position the arm moves at the scapulohumeral joint. At 70°, the greater tuberosity of the humerus is approaching the acromion, at 80° it lies immediately beneath and the head of the humerus moves slightly downwards as the tuberosity passes under the coraco-acromial ligament. At 90°, the tuberosity has moved beyond the arch and engages against the upper edge of the glenoid labrum. This is how a painful arc comes about (Fig. 39).

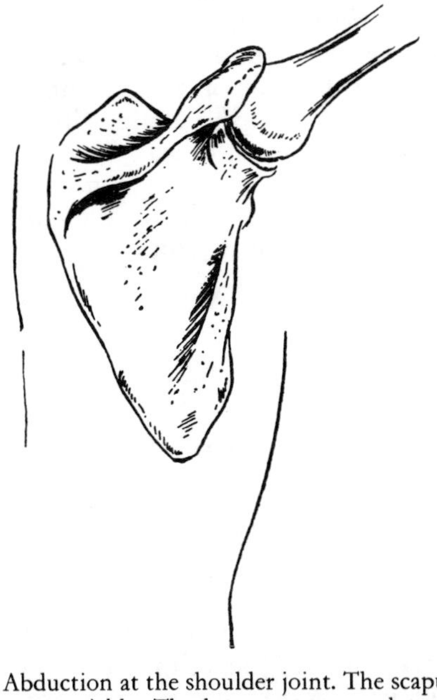

**Fig. 39.** Abduction at the shoulder joint. The scapula does not move appreciably. The humerus moves through 90°, until the abduction movement is stopped by engagement of the greater tuberosity against the glenoid fossa.

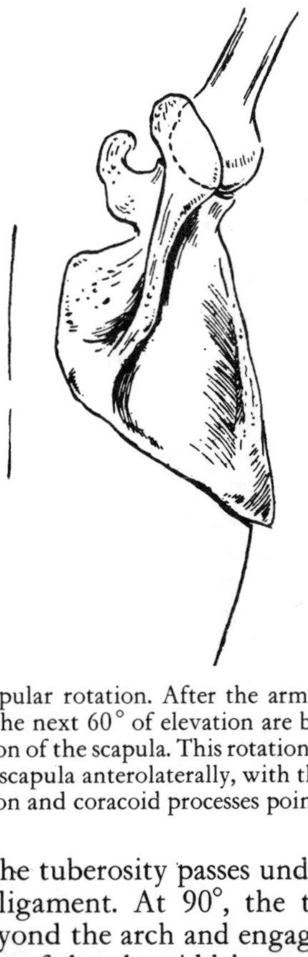

**Fig. 40.** Scapular rotation. After the arm has reached the horizontal, the next 60° of elevation are brought about by active rotation of the scapula. This rotation brings the lower angle of the scapula anterolaterally, with the result that the acromion and coracoid processes point vertically.

The next 60° of elevation are performed by rotation of the scapula by the serratus anterior and the upper half of the trapezius muscle. In doing so, the lower angle of the scapula moves well forward, and the whole bone now lies tilted so that the coracoid and acromion processes lie pointing vertically (Fig. 40). At the same time the clavicle, being attached to the acromion, has

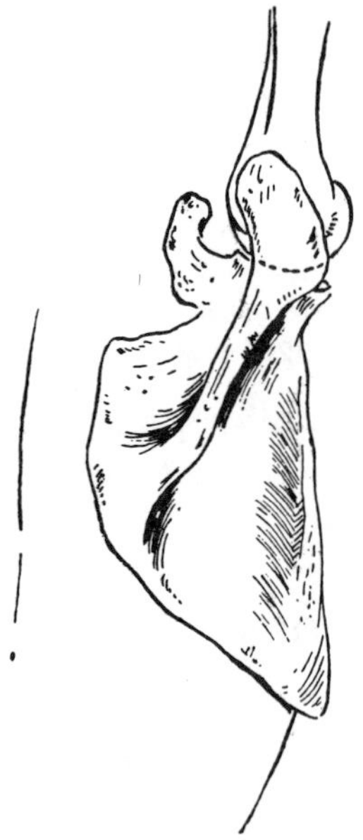

**Fig. 41.** The final stage of elevation of the arm. During the last 30° of elevation the scapula does not move. The neck of the humerus glides past the coraco-acromial arch by a movement of adduction, which can now be carried out in the vertical instead of the horizontal plane on account of the rotation of the scapula.

to rotate also. It possesses about 60° range of rotation at the sternoclavicular joint. The last 30° of elevation now take place as a result of adduction of the humerus (Fig. 41), largely owing to contraction by the pectoralis major muscle. The coraco-acromial ligament no longer hinders the movement when the scapula has rotated fully, for the surgical neck of the humerus can now glide along it anteriorly.

The range of rotation at the shoulder joint is 180°. It is best measured from the mid-position (i.e. the forearm pointing straight forwards) and the humerus is then normally capable of being turned 90° medially and laterally.

## Psychogenic Disorders at the Shoulder

The outstretched arm affords somatic evidence of welcome; by contrast, revulsion is evinced by withdrawal, characterized by the arm held close to the side. Since the position of the arm is closely connected with the emotions, patients with a distaste for their circumstances or their company readily develop inability to abduct the arm, holding it rigidly adducted.

In the detection of limited movement at the shoulder joint of hysterical origin, exact knowledge of the sequence described above is essential. Moreover, even if the shoulder joint is completely fixed, 60° of abduction can always be obtained by scapular rotation. If the scapula was found normally mobile during the preliminary examination, this is the minimum range of abduction possible. The patient has no idea of these facts. Hence, gross inconsistencies are quickly detected.

A common self-contradictory situation is as follows: The patient can raise his arm voluntarily only to the horizontal. Since 60° of this movement is scapular he can possess only 30° range of abduction at the shoulder joint. But passive abduction may reveal 90° scapulohumeral range. Further examination may show the serratus anterior and supraspinatus–deltoid muscles to be perfectly strong when tested against resistance. The patient's limitation of elevation can result only from unwillingness, due to either psychoneurosis or malingering.

A malingerer, if middle-aged, who keeps his arm firmly to his side or wears a sling for some weeks, soon develops genuine limitation of movement at the shoulder. This should be remembered when gross inconsistencies are found in conjunction with an immobilizational arthritis at the shoulder joint.

# INTERPRETATION

When the patterns that emerge on clinical examination come to be interpreted, there are four main divisions:

1. Limited passive movement; capsular pattern.
2. Limited passive movement; non-capsular pattern.
3. Full passive range; one resisted movement hurts.
4. Full passive range; one or more muscles are weak.

## The Capsular Pattern

The presence of the capsular pattern indicates arthritis. At the shoulder there exist 90° range of abduction, 90° range of medial rotation and 90° range of lateral rotation. The capsular pattern is: so much limitation of abduction, more limitation of lateral rotation, less limitation of medial rotation. In the very early case, therefore, arthritis may show itself as isolated restriction of lateral rotation. Probable proportions are:

| Arthritis | Abduction limited by | Lateral rotation limited by | Medial rotation limited by |
|---|---|---|---|
| Slight | 10° | 30° | Full and painful |
| Medium | 45° | 60–70° | 10–15° |
| Gross | 70–80° | 90–100° | 30° |

An interesting confirmation of this pattern was provided by Reeves (1966) who illustrates an arthrogram of an arthritic shoulder which shows 'less restriction of posterior distribution of dye than anterior'. Clearly, if the anterior aspect of the capsule is more contracted than the posterior, lateral rotation will be more limited than medial rotation. The pattern is the same whatever the cause of the arthritis, which has to be decided on the criteria set out below. Moreover, the stage that a capsular pattern has reached is often as important as its nature, in particular when treatment is considered; the end-feel is very informative in this respect.

There are 12 separate disorders characterized by limitation of movement at the shoulder joint in the capsular pattern.

## Traumatic Arthritis

A minor injury is reported by a middle-aged or elderly patient. After the immediate pain has ceased, he feels little or nothing for some days, then the upper arm begins to hurt, first on certain movements only; later, a constant ache sets in, soon spreading down to the elbow. Untreated, the pain and limitation of movement continue to get worse for four months. Then the pain begins to ease and at the end of a year full painless movement has returned spontaneously to the joint.

This is an avoidable condition, but is rarely prevented. Since it occurs so seldom before the age of 45, and never before the age of 40, except with fractures, prophylaxis is not necessary under that age. What is so often apt to happen is that, when the radiograph of the sprained shoulder shows no bony injury, the patient is merely reassured. No instructions on movement are given. In consequence, a traumatic arthritis leading to increasing pain and limitation of movement is allowed to develop. There comes a moment after three to five weeks when the joint has become so irritable that an attempt to treat it by stretching the capsule out aggravates the disorder, whereas, in the early stage, maintenance of mobility would have prevented the onset of the arthritis.

No muscular wasting occurs in traumatic arthritis, and in the common uncomplicated case, the resisted movements show that the muscles are not involved.

## Immobilizational Arthritis

When an elderly patient's arm is put in a sling for any reason, e.g. Colles's fracture, limitation of movement of the capsular pattern is apt to come on quite quickly and lead to a painful arthritis indistinguishable from a traumatic arthritis, except by the history. The active maintenance of range from the first is all that is required in prophylaxis.

## Hemiplegia

Nearly all patients develop a stiff shoulder after a stroke. This is very difficult to treat, but simple to prevent. Prophylaxis consists merely in moving the arm passively up into full elevation as from the first day. The spouse or the nurse must carry this movement out at least once a day until the patient has recovered enough control to do it for himself, at first using his good arm to push the arm up in the same way as he is enjoined to move his elbow, wrist and fingers.

If the shoulder has been allowed to stiffen, the pain from the capsular contracture may become severe and interfere with sleep, in the end causing more distress than the hemiplegia itself. The physiotherapist must try to stretch the joint out as best he can. Adequately done, this hurts, and elderly patients bear pain badly. If this proves impracticable, the distraction technique must be tried. If this fails, an intra-articular steroid injection may ease the pain, securing a better night's rest. Spontaneous subsidence of pain with permanent stiffness takes six to twelve months.

## Frozen Shoulder

I am becoming increasingly doubtful of the existence of this disorder. At first, I regarded freezing arthritis as common; later as rare. Until 1970, all patients with unprovoked arthritis at the shoulder, i.e. limited movement in the capsular pattern, proving refractory to intra-articular hydrocortisone were regarded as suffering from 'freezing arthritis'. But I then started using triamcinolone in these resistant cases, and found the response excellent. In my last 100 cases I have had only two that neither hydrocortisone nor triamcinolone abated (one responded dramatically to the distraction manipulation; the other proved intractable). Search for another variety of steroid suspension might well have relieved that solitary case.

The term 'frozen shoulder' is obsolete; it is merely a synonym for 'stiff shoulder'. An interesting alternative arises from work by Bulgen et al. (1976). They found that 42% of patients with a 'frozen shoulder' had HLA–B27 in their blood, but only 10% of controls. Tests for antinuclear antibodies and rheumatoid factor were all negative, which suggested a seronegative arthritis similar to that occurring in ankylosing spondylitis. This may be so, but even an untreated 'frozen shoulder' seldom fails to recover full range in the end, the opposite of the final fixation by spondylitis.

## Monarticular Rheumatoid Arthritis

Since all tests for rheumatoid disease are nearly always negative in this condition, which very seldom spreads to other joints, rheumatologists disapprove of my label 'rheumatoid'. For them I offer an alternative name: *steroid-sensitive arthritis.*

Traumatic and monarticular rheumatoid arthritis are about equally frequent in civilian practice. No age is exempt from rheumatoid disease, but the common incidence is 45–60 years old. It is certainly not a degenerative condition, for the elderly appear immune (over 70). The normal course of the arthritis is spontaneous recovery in one to two years. Both shoulders are seldom attacked at once, but recurrence at the other joint within two to five years does occur.

For no apparent reason, a middle-aged patient begins to feel an ache at the shoulder on moving the arm. There is no pain when the arm is kept still. Examination reveals almost a full range of movement at the shoulder joint, each extreme hurting when tested passively; the resisted movements are painless. After a month or two, the pain on movement becomes more severe and spreads as far as the elbow; a constant aching sets in, worse at night and worse still if the patient lies on that side in bed. Limitation of movement at the shoulder joint of the capsular type is now apparent. At the end of three months the pain has become constant, interfering with sleep, and reaches to the forearm and wrist. Severe pain on jarring the joint may compel the patient to wear a sling. Limitation of movement at the joint is now obvious. In slight cases this may never amount to greater restriction of the range of abduction than 45 or 60° (with corresponding restriction of both rotations); if so, the disorder is apt to last a year. If movement continues to decrease so that abduction eventually becomes 80° limited, spontaneous recovery may well take two years. The shoulder scarcely ever becomes truly 'frozen', complete fixation of the joint being a great rarity. Sometimes the arthritis neither progresses nor remits, 10 or 20° limitation of abduction having developed and stayed unchanged for say six months. (These are the cases that recover with only two or three intra-articular injections.)

In mild cases the pain is at its worst after three or four months and is easing after six months and has ceased (except on passive stretching of the capsule) after eight months. During the next four months, the movement returns spontaneously and after a year the patient is cured. I use 'cured' advisedly, for a second attack at the same shoulder is very seldom met with. Arthritis at the other shoulder some years later is sometimes encountered, but never amounts to much, since the patient, knowing what it is and remembering the immediate relief from injection into the joint, comes for treatment within a few weeks and is soon well. In severe cases, the distressing pain may last until 12 months from the onset of symptoms; if so the restriction may take two years to subside entirely. However, once the pain has ceased, the patient is quite content to await spontaneous return of range. Only a very few continue with a painless stiff shoulder indefinitely. As the arthritis lessens in degree, the ache leaves the forearm and is felt in the upper arm only, and only if the shoulder is pushed to the extreme of the possible range. Lying on that side ceases to hurt. It will be noted that the pain and limitation of movement come on together, increasing for three or four months. Then the severe ache continues for another six months, then dwindles, but the restriction of range does not alter. During the final period, movement slowly returns.

Examination reveals limited movement in the capsular pattern throughout. Though the deltoid muscle is visibly wasted in the more severe cases, the resisted movements remain strong and painless.

## Rheumatoid-type Arthritis

This group includes the arthritis that complicates psoriasis and lupus erythematosus. In these diseases the pain and restriction are apt to go on indefinitely; yet both respond well to treatment by intra-articular steroids. Though in long-standing cases the range may not fully return, the patient is not aware of stiffness.

The same applies to the arthritis that is apt to occur in ankylosing spondylitis; the pain ceases but movement is apt to remain limited.

In osteitis deformans no local treatment avails and, if pain warrants, arthroplasty is required. Reiter's disease remains intractable too, but seldom lasts more than a year. Gout may attack the shoulder late in the evolution of the disease. Phenylbutazone or indomethacin is effective.

In palindromic rheumatism the limitation of movement lasts only a few days and in chondrocalcinosis a month. The former type of transient arthritis was first described by Hench and Rosenberg in 1944 and in 1959 Ward and Okihiro followed up 140 cases for five years. They found that the attacks ceased spontaneously in only 7.8% and that rheumatoid arthritis developed later in 36% of all cases. In the remainder, the attacks continued and in 2% lupus erythematosus had supervened. Huskisson (1976) found that D-penicillamine 250 to 750 mg daily stopped the attacks. Hardo (1981) has contributed a good review of palindromic rheumatism.

*Polymyalgia Rheumatica.* The common cause of what is misnamed polymyalgia rheumatica is bilateral monarticular rheumatoid arthritis at the shoulders. If it so happens that a raised sedimentation rate is found in conjunction with pain from the base of the neck to the forearms, the diagnosis is apt to be 'polymyalgia'; if the sedimentation rate is normal, 'cervical spondylosis' (which is bound to be symptomlessly present in any elderly patient). The limitation of movement is apt to be missed and a disorder easy to relieve if allowed to continue.

## Osteoarthrosis

Osteoarthrosis at the shoulder joint is usually symptomless. The patient is aware of crepitus on movement of years' standing and a tendency to minor ephemeral aching after considerable exertion. Primary osteoarthrosis causing symptoms is uncommon, but the presence of this degeneration makes the joint very apt to develop a superimposed traumatic arthritis after quite a slight, often indirect, strain on the joint or merely some overuse. Alternatively, quite a brief period of immobility, e.g. rest in bed after a coronary thrombosis, may set up a similar condition. Myopathy and hemiplegia have the same effect. Hence, it is open to argument whether what is called osteoarthrosis of the shoulder in these circumstances often merits the term; for the arthrosis is usually brought to light by the injury or the immobilization. Osteoarthrosis at the shoulder is not necessarily connected with osteophyte formation visible on the radiograph. Many shoulders affording such X-ray evidence possess a full and painless range of movement; others with pain, capsular contracture and marked crepitus on movement, are found normal on X-ray examination. Moreover, the presence of an osteophyte does not protect a patient against tendinitis or bursitis. It is thus a clinical diagnosis only.

The first pointer to osteoarthrosis, other than the patient's age, is gained on examination of the painless shoulder which is found to be the site of symptomless osteoarthrosis. The characteristic finding is slight limitation of elevation, such that the patient's arm, instead of reaching his ear, lies forward of this line, level more with his nose. Rotation is of full range and painless. Crepitus is palpable on movement, showing articular cartilage at the glenoid fossa to be fragmented.

Examination of the passive movements at the affected shoulder reveals the capsular pattern, combined with palpable crepitus. The resisted movements are painless.

## Shoulder–Hand Syndrome

This is a variety of monarticular rheumatoid arthritis occurring in an elderly patient. After the age of 60, pain in the arm and marked limitation of movement at the shoulder joint sets in. At the same time, the hand on the same side becomes stiff and the skin of the fingers undergoes trophic change. The ordinary capsular pattern is present at the shoulder joint; in addition, movement at the wrist, metacarpophalangeal and interphalangeal joints becomes markedly limited. Often the stiffness is such that it prevents the patient from gripping things in his hand at all. The fingers are shiny and red, and the skin atrophic; the nails may cease to grow. Recovery is uncertain. J. H. Young's post-mortem dissection (1952) of a shoulder showing this syndrome revealed the same inferior capsular adherence as Neviaser described in freezing arthritis.

It has been suggested that the shoulder–hand syndrome is in some way connected with taking large doses of phenobarbitone, but cases certainly occur without any such drug having been ingested.

## Bacterial Arthritis

Bacterial arthritis is uncommon, whether septic, gonorrhoeal or tuberculous; in tuberculosis, by the time the patient is first seen, destruction of part of the articular surface of the humerus is already established, and permanent ankylosis unavoidable.

## Bony Block

Patients with tertiary syphilis or syringomyelia may develop painless limitation of movement at the shoulder. When the joint is forced, a bony block is felt, but no pain is evoked. The radiograph shows huge osteophytic outcrops, engagement of which clearly restricts range. Examination of the nervous system reveals the cause of the neuropathic arthropathy, usually syringomyelia.

Displacement of a fractured tuberosity under the acromion also leads to a bony block, but there is a history of severe injury. Again, the radiograph is diagnostic.

## Secondary Neoplasm

Invasion of the upper humerus and glenoid area by secondary malignant deposits affects the joint and the adjacent muscles. Hence the signs are dual: marked limitation of movement at the shoulder joint, accompanied by severe muscular weakness and pain when the resisted movements are attempted. The muscle wasting is greatly in excess of any attributable to the arthritis, and follows a bizarre pattern, not conforming to any one neurological lesion nor being confined to any one muscle. X-ray examination is confirmative.

Localized warmth felt at part of the scapular area may prove the first sign of a malignant deposit eroding bone. Within at most a week or two or this observation, a palpable tumour will have appeared and erosion of bone will be visible on the radiograph.

*Exception.* There exists an incomprehensible shoulder lesion that I have encountered twice. A youngish patient develops a painful shoulder and within a week has marked limitation of movement in the capsular pattern. All the muscles round the joint become rapidly wasted and weak; the resisted movements are all very painful. This is the pattern for neoplasm. Yet the radiograph is normal, but the sedimentation rate raised (40–60). By a week later, movement at the joint is all but lost and the weakness now includes the flexors and extensor of the elbow.

All investigations proved negative in the first; the second had *Salmonella* antigens in the blood. After two months the pain began to abate and full recovery was established in six months. There has been no relapse.

## Primary Neoplasm

This occurs chiefly in young patients, in whom the slightest causeless limitation of movement at the shoulder should lead at once to study of the radiographic appearances. If the tumour originates from the shaft of the humerus, the first symptom may be pins and needles in the hand associated with fixation of the biceps and triceps muscles, leading to limitation of movement at the elbow. Chronic afebrile osteomyelitis and sarcoma are sometimes indistinguishable radiologically; biopsy or the response to penicillin may then be required to establish the diagnosis.

## Haemarthrosis

After a slight injury the joint becomes painful quickly and the capsular pattern is found present on examination. When this happens in a young man, almost the only cause is haemophilia.

# THE RADIOGRAPH

There are few joints where the radiographic appearances afford so little assistance as at the shoulder. Usually nothing abnormal is seen, even after the shoulder has been the site of severe arthritis for months. Traumatic capsulitis, no matter how long-standing, does not give rise to radiographic change.

Monarticular rheumatoid arthritis is often associated, at first, with a normal picture; later, slight general decalcification may be seen. Osteophyte formation may be seen but may be symptomless. Huge osteophytes limit movement, of course, at times all but painlessly. It should not be forgotten that osteophyte formation at the shoulder does not protect a patient against other lesions, to which all the symptoms may be attributable.

Calcification may appear in the subdeltoid bursa, but even a large area of calcification of the bursa is consistent with full and painless function at the shoulder joint; by contrast, many cases of bursitis display no calcification. Often, only one shoulder has been hurting, but the calcification is bilateral. Small calcified nodes may be seen at various places, most often in the supraspinatus tendon, but do not usually cause symptoms; on the other hand, large deposits in the tendon do cause pain, both at the arc and on active abduction. *Deposits should be regarded as significant only when they correspond in situation with the lesion already determined by clinical examination.*

Tuberculosis, neuropathic arthropathy, primary and secondary neoplasm, dislocation, fracture, osteoma, bone abscess, chondromatosis, osteitis deformans—it is conditions like these that show on the radiograph, whereas all the common causes of pain arising at the shoulder fail to show. Hence, radiography provides no short cut to diagnosis.

## CLINICAL STAGES OF CAPSULAR LESION

The division of capsular lesions at the shoulder into acute, subacute and chronic has proved unsatisfactory, in so far as these words can be used equally well to describe how recent or how severe the lesion is. It so happens that soon after an injury, the capsulitis is acute in the sense that it is recent, but chronic in the sense that the lesion is not yet severe and responds well to active treatment. Equally, after some months, the inflammation may become acute, i.e. severe, when the passage of time clearly warrants the designation chronic. This nomenclature has, therefore, been abandoned and the stages merely numbered. Severe, moderate and mild are not satisfactory alternative qualifications; for a lesion leading to little pain but marked limitation of movement at the shoulder clearly cannot be termed 'mild' even though, like a recent capsulitis associated with little restriction of range, it responds well to active treatment.

### First Stage

This stage is present:

1. When the pain is confined to the deltoid area or at least does not extend beyond the elbow.
2. When the patient can lie on the affected side at night.
3. When there is no pain except on movement.
4. When the end-feel is elastic.

### Second Stage

Should the above criteria be satisfied only in part, the capsulitis is in the second stage. For example, a patient may have pain confined to the shoulder and yet be unable to lie on the affected side at night.

### Third Stage

When the following criteria are satisfied, the arthritis is in the stage when all active measures directed to the joint are harmful. It is at this stage that intra-articular triamcinolone is so valuable.

1. Severe pain extends from the shoulder to the forearm and wrist.
2. The patient cannot lie on the affected side at night.
3. The pain is greatest at night, and persists even when the arm is kept still.
4. The end-feel is abrupt.

As stated above, the *second state* of capsular lesions comprises those cases in which a mixture of these two sets of criteria exists. When the cause of the capsular lesion is clearly traumatic, an arthritis in the second stage can often be cautiously treated as if in the first stage; when the onset is unprovoked, the opposite holds. When this uncertainty exists the deciding factor on whether to stretch or not is the end-feel.

## THE NON-CAPSULAR PATTERN

The presence of limitation of passive movement in other than the capsular proportions shows that a lesion other than arthritis is present. This cannot be a tendinous lesion, since it is anatomically impossible for a tendinous lesion of itself to limit passive range, although pain on voluntary movement may deceptively restrict the active range. Those who test the range of passive, as well as active, movement cannot be deceived by this reluctance. The causes of limited movement in the non-capsular pattern are acute subdeltoid bursitis, pulmonary neoplasm, capsular adhesion, subcoracoid bursitis, contracture of the costo-coracoid fascia, fracture of the first rib, clay-shoveller's fracture, and psychogenic limitation.

## Acute Subdeltoid Bursitis

The bursa exists to provide two gliding surfaces that enable the greater tuberosity to slip smoothly under the acromion; otherwise the two projections would catch against each other. It has two parts: subacromial and subdeltoid. The subacromial part covers the superior aspect of the supraspinatus and infraspinatus tendons, extending medially as far as the acromioclavicular joint line. The subdeltoid part reaches about 2 cm below the greater tuberosity, covering the entire outer aspect of the uppermost part of the humerus.

*Swift Onset.* A distinguishing feature is the speed of onset. A patient who, without injury, in the course of two or three days, loses almost all capacity to abduct the arm is almost certainly suffering from acute subdeltoid bursitis. Since it is apt to recur at two to five year intervals, on the same or the other side, there is often a history of previous attacks, subsiding in about six weeks. The only other disorders are septic arthritis, a febrile disease, and palindromic arthritis which lasts only three days.

*Age.* There is scarcely any limit. My youngest patient was a girl aged 17 who had three previous attacks during two years. Acute bursitis is very uncommon after 65.

*Non-capsular Pattern.* In acute bursitis, 60° limitation of abduction is usually associated with little limitation of either rotation. This is very different from arthritis when 60° limitation of abduction would correspond to some 90° limitation of lateral rotation. When so much limitation of abduction is present, the characteristic painful arc cannot be elicited; hence lack of the normal articular proportions provides a physical sign of the first importance.

*No Muscle Spasm.* Another distinguishing feature is that, the joint not being involved, the range is limited by the patient's declaring that he cannot, because of increasing pain, allow further movement; there is no involuntary muscle spasm at all. If the examiner continues to move the joint on, the patient voluntarily brings his arm down again by using his own muscles; this takes place at a variable point, depending upon how much he will let himself be hurt at any particular moment. By contrast, in a capsular lesion, however often the movement is attempted, muscle spasm occurs at the same point and no amount of forcing without anaesthesia increases the range.

*Disproportionately Limited Active Abduction.* Another feature is the fact that the range of active abduction may be limited to say 10° at a time when the passive range in this direction is, say, 30° or even 45°. Apparently the abductor muscles, on account of their intimate relationship to the bursa, are inhibited from any but slight contraction in the acute stage. Unless this fact is kept in mind, severe bursitis may be mistaken for a psychogenic disorder.

*Palpation.* Palpation for tenderness follows. In acute subdeltoid bursitis, the tenderness is very obvious when the two sides are compared. Exceptionally, unilateral thickening of the bursal wall may be felt, and even less often fluctuation may be detected. If so, aspiration shows whether blood or clear fluid is present.

*Painful Arc.* In acute bursitis, this valuable sign is lacking, but, as the patient recovers his range of abduction, the painful arc eventually appears, thus confirming the diagnosis retrospectively.

## Pulmonary Neoplasm

This may cause pain felt at the shoulder with limitation of elevation at the shoulder—a very deceptive pair of facts. Muscles have only one pattern of response; any serious lesion is apt to produce spasm in nearby muscles. For example, a Brodie's abscess at the upper tibia sets up muscle spasm limiting movement at the knee joint; appendicitis causes rigidity of the abdominal muscles, and so on.

If the neoplasm interferes with the diaphragm, pain will be felt at the fourth cervical dermatome, i.e. at the deltoid area. If it encroaches on the ribs, stretching the muscle attached to the ribs leads to sympathetic spasm, i.e. of the pectoralis major. When the shoulder is examined, the patient is unable to lift his arm beyond the horizontal, and passive elevation beyond this level is impossible because of pain and spasm. By contrast, the scapula is mobile, and a full range of passive movement is present at the shoulder joint without muscle weakness. This may suggest psychogenic limitation, but further examination shows otherwise. The reason for inability to elevate the arm is involuntary spasm of the pectoralis major muscle.

The diagnosis of pulmonary neoplasm is now obvious and confirmed radiologically. The patient is apt to come with a radiograph of the shoulder and the apex of his lung, just missing the lower lung field.

The same signs are also found in contracture of the pectoral scar after radical mastectomy but there is no pain.

## Capsular Adhesion

It is surprising how seldom injury to part of the capsule of the shoulder joint results in one localized patch of capsular scarring. Although this does occur, subsequent traumatic arthritis with increasing limitation of movement in *every* direction is much the commoner result.

The history of injury is clear; often it is of a reduced dislocation. The patient's immediate post-traumatic pain ceases, but the deltoid area goes on aching during exertion for months or years afterwards. The condition persists, tending to get neither better nor worse.

Examination of the passive movements reveals a non-capsular pattern. Elevation is of full range and painful; medial rotation is of full range and painless; lateral rotation is limited in range and painful. Such a finding might suggest a lesion of the subdeltoid bursa, but for the absence of the painful arc. After a dislocation, the scarring in the capsule lies anteriorly, hence it is lateral rotation that becomes limited in range. Examination of the resisted movements shows that the muscles are not involved.

A similar pattern emerges many months after complete rupture of the infraspinatus tendon. Since the patient has lost the capacity voluntarily to rotate his arm laterally, he finally loses part of this movement, even when attempted passively, from localized capsular contracture. The range of abduction and medial rotation is not affected. When resisted lateral rotation shows the infraspinatus muscle to be powerless, the cause of the localized contracture becomes obvious.

Lateral rotation is also limited alone in subcoracoid bursitis, but in such a case passive adduction is painful at its extreme and, when the arm is elevated to the horizontal, the limitation of lateral rotation disappears.

## Subcoracoid Bursitis

This is also rare, and confusingly enough gives rise to isolated limitation of lateral rotation, as does the anterior capsular contracture due to trauma, or after rupture of the infraspinatus muscle.

Differential diagnosis rests on:

1. The absence of a history of a severe injury to the front of the joint.
2. The absence of the capsular feel and of spasm limiting the amount of lateral rotation range. In consequence, the patient can, by disregarding the pain, allow rather more movement.
3. If the humerus is abducted to the horizontal, a full range of lateral rotation can be achieved in bursitis, but not, of course, without pain. In capsular contracture, it is unattainable whatever the position of the arm.
4. Passive adduction hurts at the extreme of range.

## Contracture of the Costocoracoid Fascia

This is a very uncommon cause of limited elevation of the arm. The symptom is gradually increasing upper pectoroscapular pain on one side only. It is provoked at first only by full elevation of the arm. After a year or two, elevation becomes slightly limited and any prolonged reaching upwards leads to increased aching for some hours or days.

The syndrome is difficult to recognize; for the symptoms suggest a cervical disc lesion and the signs, unless carefully studied, suggest a psychogenic disorder. The key to the condition is the discovery of slight limitation of elevation of the scapula.

## Fracture of the First Rib

This may be a stress fracture, without history of trauma. The pain is at one side of the base of the neck and is brought on by the neck and scapular movements. Voluntary elevation of the arm stops at the horizontal, but a full passive range exists at the shoulder. The radiograph is diagnostic.

## Clay-shoveller's Fracture

This is usually a traction fracture. The pain is at the centre of the lower neck. Though the neck movements scarcely hurt, the patient can hardly abduct either arm actively at all. The passive range is full. The radiograph shows avulsion of the tip of the spinous process of the seventh cervical or first thoracic vertebra.

## Acromioclavicular Joint

At the extreme of each passive movement at the shoulder, the acromioclavicular ligaments are more strongly stretched than on full active movement of the scapula. Scapular movement may well prove painless yet the extreme of every passive shoulder movement may hurt, passive adduction usually the most. Patients with a lesion at the shoulder joint complain of pain in the arm, whereas disorders of the acromioclavicular joint give rise to purely local symptoms. Thus pain confined to the point of the shoulder elicited by the passive shoulder movements, associated with a full range of movement at the shoulder joint, draws attention to the acromioclavicular joint even if the scapular movements have proved painless. None of the resisted movement hurts.

## Psychogenic Limitation

The shoulder joint is closely connected with emotional tone. The outstretched arm is a symbol of pleasure and welcome; the arm held into the side expresses repugnance. Hence, those who feel withdrawn from the world or view it with disgust readily develop an inability to abduct the arm. This is therefore common in endogenous depression or conversion hysteria. But the patient does not realize that, even if the shoulder joint is ankylosed, mobility of the scapula permits 60° of abduction and that the arm must be capable of this amount of abduction unless the scapula has also become fixed. Hence, detection of psychogenesis is simple if the range of voluntary and passive elevation is contrasted with the range of passive abduction at the scapulohumeral joint. In organic disability, the range of passive elevation equals the passive scapulohumeral range plus 60°.

The large number of patients who have carried off this psychogenic conversion undetected, and have in consequence enjoyed years of treatment, confirms the diagnostic importance of comparing the responses to active, passive and resisted movement.

CHAPTER 10

# EXAMINATION OF THE SHOULDER: FULL RANGE

The causes of limitation of movement at the shoulder have been dealt with in Chapter 9. The presence of a full range of movement at the shoulder excludes arthritis and acute bursitis, and concentrates attention on the tendons and on chronic bursitis.

*For the diagnosis of a tendinous lesion,* it is essential that *a full range of passive movement should exist at the joint.* Some discomfort may be elicited at one or more extremes of range, but the range is *full.* Hence there is all the difference in the world between 1° of limitation of movement and full range, and no effort must be spared to be sure, even at the expense of hurting the patient. There is not necessarily a full range of *active* movement, since a patient may be prevented by severe pain on using an injured muscle, or by a painful arc on abduction or medial rotation, from achieving more than partial movement. It is then *passive* testing that demonstrates that the range is full. This is the basis of the divergence of opinion between orthopaedic surgeons and myself; for they often make a diagnosis of tendinous lesion in the presence of limited range. Agreement on the different significance of the active and passive ranges of movement would quickly resolve this situation.

During the first part of the examination (outlined in the previous chapter) lesions of the moving parts referring pain to the shoulder will have been detected. Visceral pain must also be considered if the examination from neck to fingers is negative. For example, diaphragmatic pleurisy may set up pain felt at the shoulder on deep breathing and coughing, and myocardial pain may be felt in one or both upper limbs, without any pain in the chest. In such a case, exertion unconnected with use of the arm (e.g. walking upstairs) brings on the symptoms and examination of the upper limb reveals no abnormality. If continued exertion of the arm sets up claudicational pain in the arm and shoulder, subclavian occlusion should be suspected. If so, the radial pulse is absent.

It is when the movements of the shoulder prove painful, but a full range of passive movement is present, that attention is paid to pain evoked by a resisted movement. These are tested one by one—abduction, adduction, lateral rotation, medial rotation at the shoulder, followed by flexion and extension of the elbow. Care should be taken to have the patient's arm near the mid-position and to resist the contraction so strongly that no movement of the joint takes place.

Lesions simultaneously affecting every muscle about the shoulder joint do not, in my experience, occur except in neoplasm; if so, the passive range is also very limited. If every resisted movement hurts in the presence of full passive range then there is nothing wrong with the muscles being tested. The scapula has to be fixed by contraction of the vertebroscapular muscles before any strong movement of the arm can be begun; hence, pain on all resisted movements suggests a severe lesion in the cervicoscapular area; alternatively, psychoneurosis. When pain on every resisted movement accompanies pain on every passive movement, the question of psychogenic or assumed disability comes very much to the fore. Alternatively, there may be constant pain to which the patient refers each time, since he fails to realize that the question is one of *aggravation* by movement. Renewed explanation is therefore required.

In the first place, resisted abduction, adduction, medial and lateral rotation are tested. If one movement proves painful, each of the others should still be tried for the reason adduced above—that the response to pain produced by one resisted movement can be regarded as significant only if others are stated not to hurt. Alternatively if one movement is found weak, it is by discovering what other movements are or are not weak that a diagnosis is reached. If one resisted movement hurts, a group of muscles is thereby incriminated; various subsidiary movements are then tested to show which individual of that group is at fault. The movements may be tried in any order, but they must *all* be tried.

## EXAMINATION

### Resisted Abduction Movement

The term 'abduction' cannot be properly applied to positions of the arm after it has passed the horizontal and, to avoid ambiguity, will be reserved for movement away from the body *below* the horizontal. The movement is resisted by the examiner's hand placed at the outer aspect of the patient's elbow (Fig. 42).

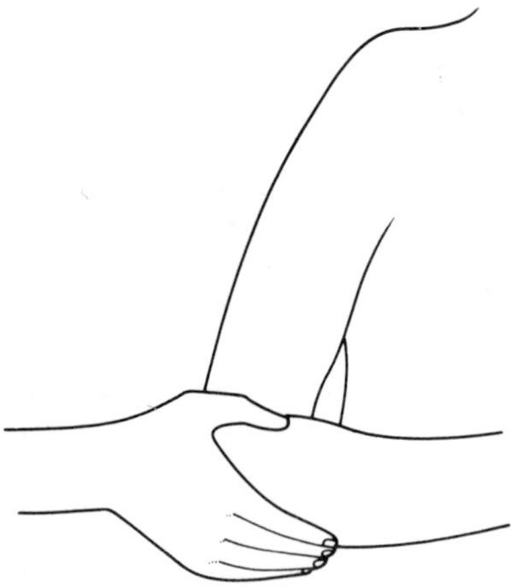

**Fig. 42.** Resisted abduction of the arm. The patient pushes his elbow away from his side while the examiner's hand resists the movement so strongly that none can take place.

In theory, pain on a resisted abduction movement can arise from the supraspinatus or the deltoid muscle. Apart from direct injury, complete recovery from which is usually swift, lesions of the deltoid muscle do not occur. Hence, pain on the resisted movement towards abduction incriminates the supraspinatus muscle. To be quite sure, the patient's arm is held passively at the horizontal by the examiner, who resists a forward and backward movement; this elicits pain from the anterior and posterior fibres of the deltoid muscle in turn. If, as expected, neither of these movements hurts, the fault lies with the supraspinatus muscle.

The position of the lesion within the supraspinatus muscle is then identified as in Fig. 43.

1. A painful arc exists. This shows the lesion to lie superficially near the tenoperiosteal junction, just medial to the greater tuberosity of the humerus.

   If the painful arc is more marked when the abduction movement is carried out in medial rather than lateral rotation of the arm (i.e. palm down or palm up), additional information is afforded. If the arc is more marked when the arm is brought up palm-upwards, the lesion lies at the anterior aspect of the tenoperiosteal junction; if palm-downwards hurts more, the posterior part of the tendinous insertion is singled out. A painful arc evoked when the arm is brought up forwards, absent when it is elevated outwards, indicates the anterior edge of the tendon.

   The mere presence of a painful arc exculpates the deltoid muscle; it does not lie between tuberosity and acromion and thus cannot be pinched.
2. Full *passive* elevation of the arm hurts. This implies tenderness of that part of the tendon which is pinched between the greater tuberosity and the glenoid rim, i.e. the deep aspect of the tenoperiosteal junction. If this sign is found together with a painful arc, the lesion clearly traverses the distal end of the whole tendon. The fact that full *active* elevation hurts has no localizing significance; for during this movement the supraspinatus muscle is contracting and pain will be elicited wherever the lesion in the muscle happens to lie.
3. The absence of a painful arc and of pain elicited on full passive elevation suggests a lesion of the supraspinatus at the musculoten-

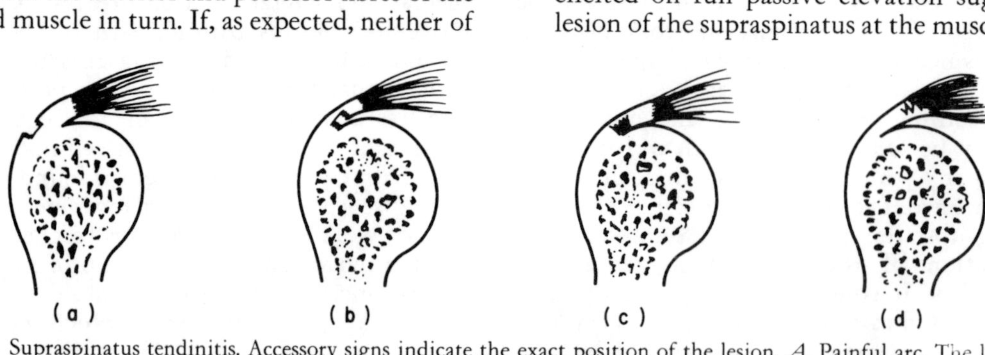


**Fig. 43.** Supraspinatus tendinitis. Accessory signs indicate the exact position of the lesion. *A*, Painful arc. The lesion lies superficially at the tenoperiosteal junction. *B*, Pain on full passive elevation: the lesion, lies deeply at the tenoperiosteal junction. *C*, painful arc and pain on full passive elevation: the lesion traverses the distal end of the tendon. *D*, Neither a painful arc nor pain on full passive elevation: the lesion lies at the musculotendinous junction.

dinous junction, since the belly itself is very rarely affected. Tenderness of the musculotendinous junction may be sought, and the two sides compared, deeply within the angle formed by the clavicle and the spine of the scapula while the arm is passively supported horizontally. However, local anaesthesia should always be used to verify this diagnosis; for an occasional case of tendinitis at the tenoperiosteal junction unexpectedly fails to show either of the two appropriate localizing signs.

In spite of the intimate relation of the supraspinatus tendon to be subdeltoid bursa, a resisted abduction movement is painless in even acute bursitis.

Weakness of abduction occurs in: (*a*) rupture of the supraspinatus tendon; if so, the power to initiate abduction is lost and a painful arc is present on passive elevation; (*b*) partial rupture of the supraspinatus tendon; voluntary abduction is possible but weak and painful; (*c*) suprascapular nerve palsy; (*d*) axillary nerve palsy; (*e*) fifth cervical root palsy; (*f*) malignant deposit in the acromion.

## Resisted Adduction Movement

The arm is brought a short distance away from the body and the adduction movement resisted by pressure against the inner side of the elbow (Fig. 44). The muscles responsible are the pectoralis major, latissimus dorsi and the two teres. Pain, except when it arises from the axillary portions of the pectoralis major or latissimus dorsi muscles, is usually correctly appreciated by

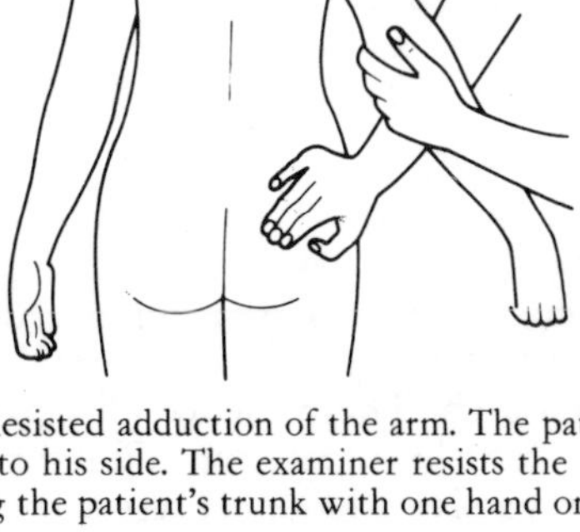

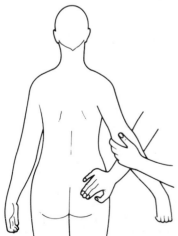

**Fig. 44.** Resisted adduction of the arm. The patient draws his elbow to his side. The examiner resists the movement, steadying the patient's trunk with one hand on his hips.

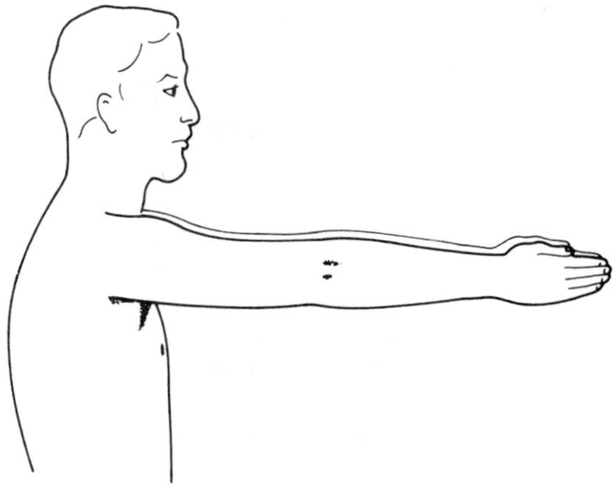

**Fig. 45.** Resisted horizontal adduction of the arms. The patient is pressing his palms together. Pain arising from the pectoralis major muscle is most easily elicitated in this way.

the patient at the anterior or posterolateral aspects of the thorax respectively. When the patient's sensations are no guide and an adduction movement hurts, the next part of the examination is to ask him to bring his arm first forwards then backwards against resistance. If the former hurts, the pectoral muscle is at fault and confirmation may be sought by asking him to press his hands together as in Fig. 45. If the backward movement hurts, the fault lies in one of the other three muscles. The teres muscles may be differentiated by the fact that the major is a medial, the minor a lateral, rotator of the humerus. The lattisimus dorsi and teres major muscles, being identical in function, cannot be distinguished by any test. In fracture of an upper rib anteriorly, testing the pectoralis major muscle hurts at the upper part of the thorax, and full elevation of the arm also pulls painfully on the broken bone.

Palpation follows when the pectoralis major muscle is affected. The fibres just below the lateral half of the clavicle or those at the lower extent of the outer edge are the probable sites.

If the lesion lies at the pectoral insertion at the bicipital groove the pain evoked by resisted adduction is felt at the shoulder and upper arm. The latissimus dorsi muscle is usually affected at the upper part of the outer edge.

Weakness of adduction is found in severe cervical seventh root palsy as the result of weakness of the latissimus dorsi muscle. The pectoralis major usually escapes.

### Long Head of Biceps

There exists one lesion that gives rise to incomprehensible signs—strain of the origin from the glenoid of the long head of the biceps muscle. Localized pain is felt in the region of the acromioclavicular joint. It is elicited only by resisted adduction of the arm; all the other passive and resisted movements are found painless. Resisted flexion and supination at the elbow do not hurt. In such a case, the resisted adduction movement may be found painful when it is tested with the elbow kept in extension, and not when kept flexed. This suggests the constant length phenomenon and draws attention to the long tendon of the biceps at its glenoid origin.

## Resisted Lateral Rotation Movement

The patient's arm must be kept at his side with the elbow held at a right angle and the movement resisted by pressure applied just above the wrist (Fig. 46). If the pressure is applied at the hand, the response to resisted wrist extension complicates the picture, and the examiner, who may think he is testing the infraspinatus muscle alone, may in fact, be eliciting pain from a tennis elbow.

Patients are very apt to abduct the arm when asked to rotate it outwards; this must be avoided, otherwise a supraspinatus tendinitis may be mistaken for an infraspinatus tendinitis. If resisted lateral rotation hurts alone, infraspinatus tendinitis is present. If a resisted adduction movement also hurts—which is very uncommon—the teres minor muscle is inculpated. A painful arc on elevation occurs with infraspinatus tendinitis, when the lesion lies at the distal and superficial fibres of the tendon, i.e. where it can be pinched between tuberosity and acromion. In the absence of a painful arc, there is no way of telling which part of the tendon is affected except by palpation for tenderness supplemented by local anaesthesia. Palpation is carried out in the position for massage of the tendon (see Volume II).

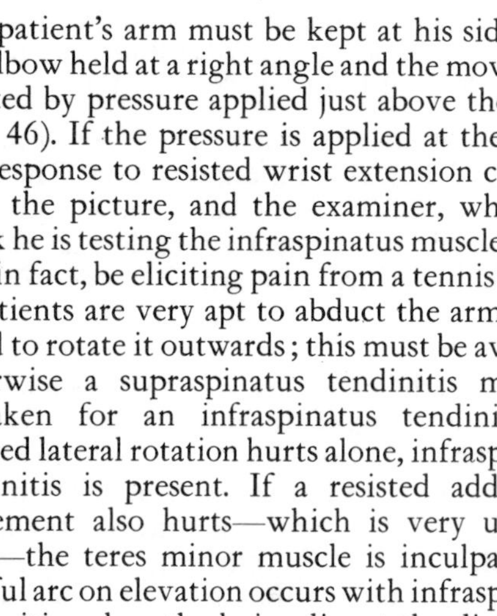

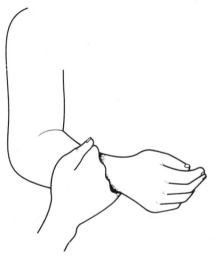

**Fig. 46.** Resisted lateral rotation of the arm. Keeping his elbow at his side, the patient pushes his wrist away from his body. Note that the examiner's hand is placed at the lower forearm, avoiding pressure on the patient's hand. The patient's forearm is supported by the examiner's fifth finger. No abduction movement is allowed to occur.

It is not uncommon for pain to be evoked both by resisted abduction and resisted lateral rotation, even when correctly carried out. In such cases, a double lesion is usually present, and both tendons require treatment. Occasionally, however, this combination characterizes chronic subdeltoid bursitis. (I call it 'Skillern's bursitis', after the physiotherapist who first pointed this out to me.) Before a confident diagnosis of two tendinous lesions is made, therefore, it is well to palpate the subdeltoid bursa for a tender spot and, if one is found, induce local anaesthesia there diagnostically. A painful arc is common to all three lesions; hence this finding is no help. In tendinitis, since the supraspinatus is affected twice as often as infraspinatus, the former should be infiltrated with triamcinolone first, on statistical grounds. In some cases, both movements become painless a few days after this single injection.

In rupture of the infraspinatus tendon, painless weakness with a painful arc at first is very noticeable. After a year or two, the arc ceases but some 30° of the range of lateral rotation at the shoulder becomes lost. The infraspinatus muscle is weak and wasted in suprascapular palsy and in some cases of neuralgic amyotrophy.

## Resisted Medial Rotation Movement

This movement (Fig. 47) provides information about pain arising from the subscapularis, pectoralis major, latissimus dorsi and teres major muscles. The last-named three muscles are all adductors, whereas the subscapularis muscle is a weak abductor. It suffices, therefore, to show the absence of pain on a resisted adduction movement to demonstrate that the subscapularis is the muscle affected. If a lesion of this muscle has thus been shown to exist, two further localizing signs should be sought.

1. A painful arc. If this is present, the lesion is at the uppermost part of the tenoperiosteal junction, since only the top of the lesser tuberosity can engage against the coraco-acromial arch. The presence of a painful arc also serves to exculpate the adductor muscles.
2. Pain on passive adduction across the front of

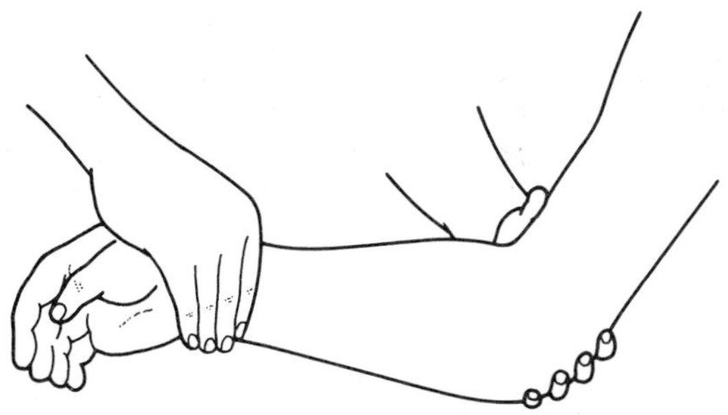

**Fig. 47.** Resisted medial rotation of the arm. The patient pulls his forearm towards his trunk. The examiner steadies his elbow and resists the movement by pressure against his wrist.

the chest. At the extreme of this movement the lower part of the lesser tuberosity is squeezed against the coracoid process. This shows the lesion in the tendon to lie at the humeral insertion at its lower extent. Lesions in the subscapular belly appear not to occur.

Complete rupture of the tendon is rare and leads to great painless weakness on resisted medial rotation.

## Resisted Forward Movement

When pain is elicited by this movement alone, the lesion has on each occasion been found to lie at the upper extremity of the coracobrachialis muscle. In theory, resisted adduction should also hurt; in practice, it does not do so.

## Resisted Flexion and Supination at the Elbow

Though parts of the biceps and triceps muscles lie at the shoulder, they control the elbow. Hence no examination of the shoulder muscles is complete until the resisted elbow movements have been tested. If pain is felt at the shoulder and examination of the passive and resisted shoulder movements is negative, the resisted elbow movements must be tested. Pain brought on at the shoulder by resisted flexion and supination at the elbow arises from the biceps muscle, probably the tendon of the long head; trouble at the short head is very uncommon indeed. Unless, as is rare, a painful arc exists, there is no way of finding out which part of the long tendon is affected except by palpation for local tenderness.

A snapping long head of biceps seldom causes clinical tendinitis.

## Resisted Extension at the Elbow

When this hurts in the upper arm, it should not be assumed that the lesion necessarily lies in the triceps muscle; for it may well arise when a tender structure lies between the acromion and the head of the humerus. Strong contraction of the triceps muscle forces the humerus upwards, and thus pinches painfully any lesion lying between these two bones. It then provides another way of eliciting tenderness when a painful arc is present.

If no painful arc is found, the upper part of the belly of the triceps is palpated for tenderness. A lesion here is a real rarity and requires confirmation by local anaesthesia before it can be accepted.

## Local Anaesthesia

Whenever possible, all diagnoses based on the indirect evidence afforded by which movements prove painful, and which do not, should be confirmed by local anaesthesia.

Indeed, it is by trial and error over the past 30 years that I have taught myself the proper interpretation of these similar but not identical patterns.

# PAINFUL ARC OF MOVEMENT

A painful arc must be regarded as an accessory sign, indicating whereabouts in a tissue already identified as the culprit the tender point lies. It is not to be thought of as primary, e.g. 'the painful arc syndrome'. Once the tissue at fault has been singled out, the arc shows which part *of that structure* is affected, namely the pinchable part. Since the acromion itself is very seldom tender inferiorly, the discovery of a painful arc implies tenderness of a structure lying between the acromion and humeral tuberosities. The lesion is pinched when the prominent tuberosity passes under the arch, i.e. at 80° of abduction (Fig. 48).

The pain is elicited better on active than on passive movement and is usually greater on the way upwards than downwards. Since the pain is due to pressure of one or other tuberosity towards the coraco-acromial arch, it is greatest when the abductor muscles are contracting and the head of the humerus is held well lodged against the arch. Once the arm has passed beyond the horizontal in either direction, the pain ceases abruptly. A

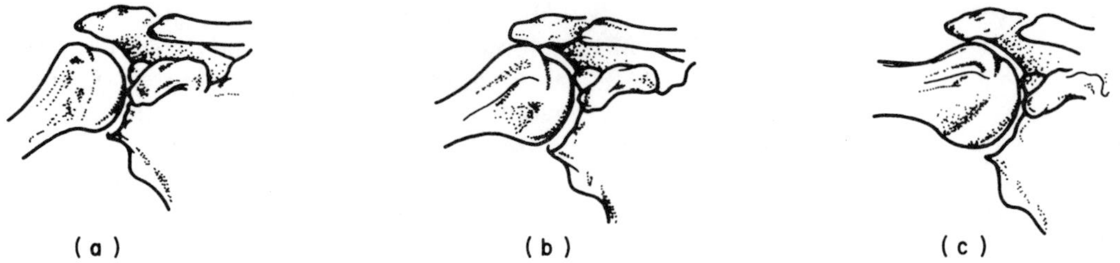


**Fig. 48.** The mechanism of a painful arc at the shoulder. *A*, No pain. At 70° of abduction the humeral tuberosity is approaching the acromion. As yet no pain is felt. *B*, Pain. At 80° of abduction the tuberosity lies under the acromion. If a tender structure lies between the two bones, it is now painfully squeezed. *C*, No pain. At 90° of abduction the tuberosity has passed the acromion and the painful pinching eases.

painful arc can sometimes be obviated by bringing the arm up forwards instead of outwards. Many patients have learned this for themselves and may be seen, as the proposed movement reaches the horizontal, to bring the arm forwards and rotate it outwards so as to minimize the painful pressure. Sometimes the painful arc appears solely on the upwards, less often only on the downwards, passage of the arm. Rarely, there is a painful arc on medial rotation of the arm; if so, it can happen that the patient stops medially rotating his arm when he reaches the arc, and apparent limitation of range results. The examiner who, when testing passive range, stops too soon because of the strong ache, is also misled. Since limited range has so different a significance from a painful arc, firm pressure, even if it does hurt the patient, must be used in such an instance to make sure.

A painful arc nearly always indicates tenderness of a structure lying between the acromion and one or other humeral tuberosity. It is only rarely that the arch itself is tender, as the result of a severe sprain at the deep fibres of the acromioclavicular joint, or rarely, malignant invasion of the acromion. The possible causes of a painful arc are thus as follows:

## Supraspinatus Tendinitis

This is by far the commonest cause and implies tenderness at or very near the greater tuberosity, either from strain of, scarring in, calcification in, or rupture of, the supraspinatus tendon. In the first two instances, the power of abduction is full and this movement is painful when resisted. The radiograph reveals nothing. In the last, all power of initiating abduction is lost and the presence of a painful arc discoverable only on a passive elevation movement; the radiograph is normal. Calcification is of course clearly visible radiographically (Plate IX/2), and is suggested clinically by a *very* painful arc.

## Subdeltoid Bursitis

If this causes a painful arc, the bursitis is localized; for in acute bursitis pain prevents movement long before the arc is reached. The affected part of the bursa can remain tender for years. In such cases there is a painful arc, with or without pain at the extreme of each passive movement; none of the resisted movements hurts. Often there is *only* an arc. This finding differentiates chronic bursitis from lesions of the supraspinatus, infraspinatus or subscapular tendon, all of which are characterized by pain elicited by the appropriate resisted movement. Many authorities regard bursitis and tendinitis at the shoulder as identical or, at least, indistinguishable. This is by no means so, if the examiner tests the function of each tendon by the appropriate resisted movement.

Calcification may be visible lying in the bursa at a point below the insertion of the tendon (Plate IX/1). A deposit lying higher up cannot be ascribed to any one structure by examination of the X-ray picture; clinical examination is required.

## Infraspinatus Tendinitis

A painful arc is often associated with pain on resisted lateral rotation. If so, the lesion in the infraspinatus tendon lies at the uppermost part of the tendinous insertion at the humeral tuberosity.

## Subscapular Tendinitis

In this case, the painful arc is associated with pain on a resisted medial rotation movement. The presence of the painful arc singles out the upper extremity of the tendinous insertion at the lesser tuberosity.

PLATE I

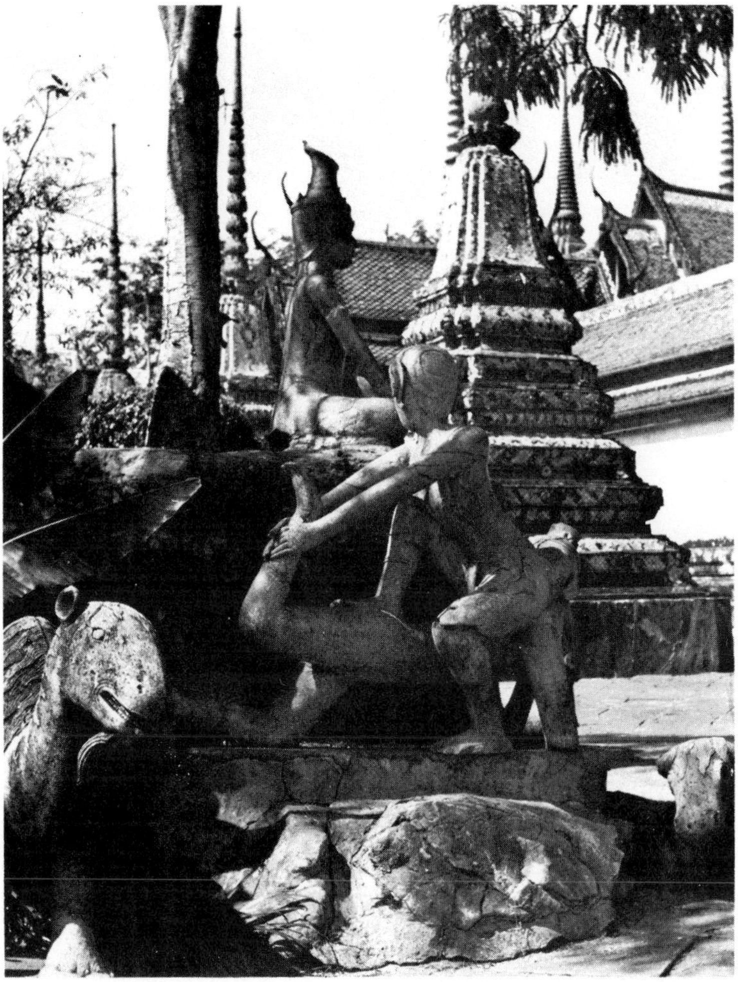

Reduction of a lumbar disc lesion by manipulation shown in an ancient Buddhist temple in Bangkok, Thailand, regarded as being 2000 years old. *(Photograph by Dr K.L. Mah; by courtesy of Doctors Only)*

PLATE II

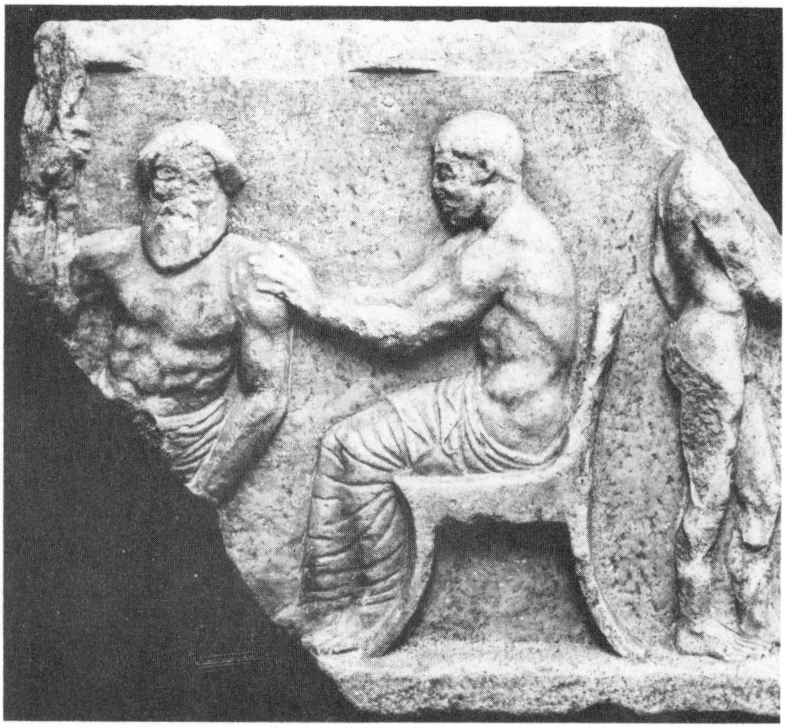

Fig. 1. Massage to the shoulder show in a relief at the museum in Cyrene Libya, thought to be 2000 years old *(By courtesy of the Curator of th Department of Antiquities)*

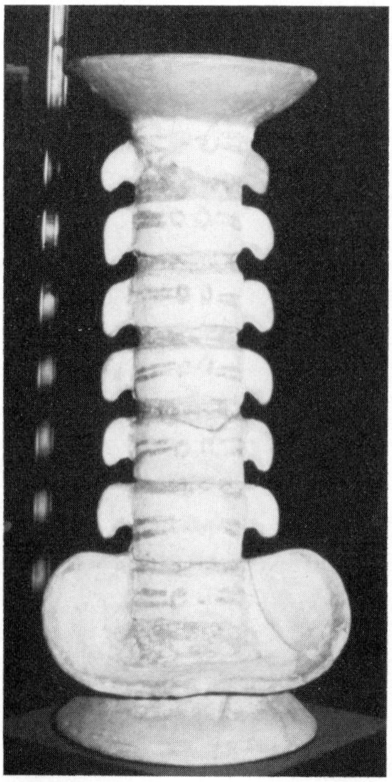

Fig. 2. A vase in the Museo Naciona de Antropologia in Mexico City. It wa made by the Olmecs, who inhabite Mixteca-Oaxaca from 900 BC . It bel ongs to the Monte Alban period, 30 to 100 BC , when ceramics wer beautifully finished and knowledge o anatomy was amazing. Note the clea depiction of the intervertebral discs 1700 years before the earliest Euro pean description. *(By courtesy of C. Foa and C. Watson II)*

PLATE III

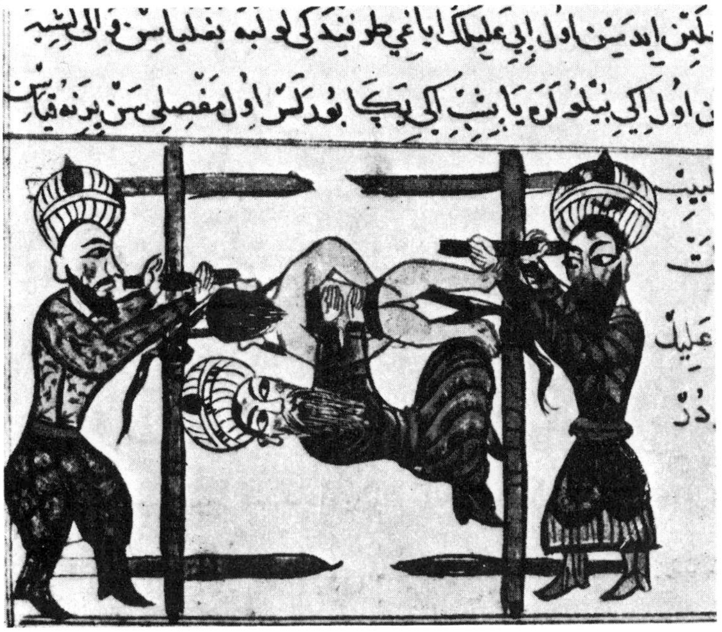

Fig. 1. Manipulation during traction in medieval Turkey, shown in an illustration from *Le Premier Manuscrit Chirurgical Turc de Charaf-Ed-Din* (1465). *(By permission of the British Museum)*

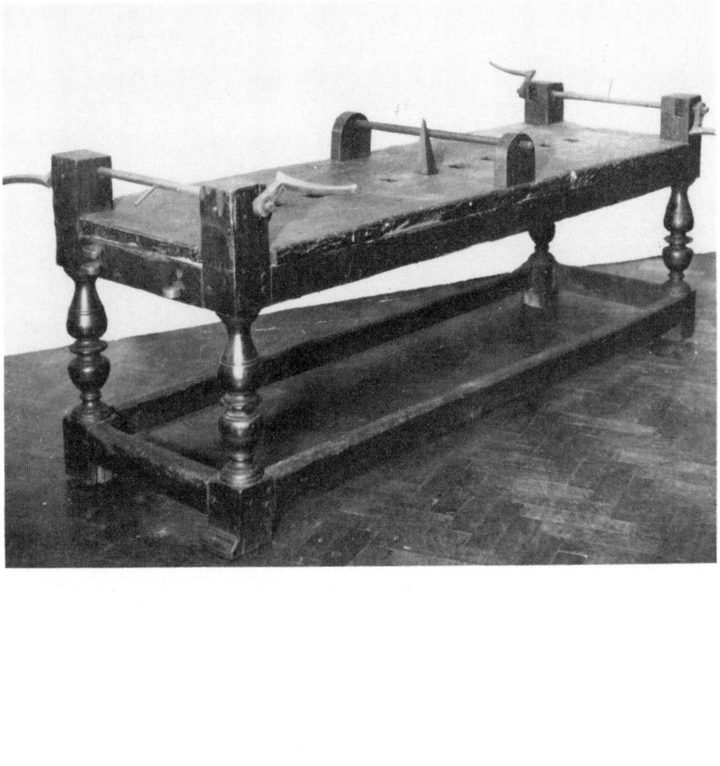

Fig. 2. A medieval traction couch as used by Hippocrates and illustrated in Guidi's *Chirurgia* (1544), discovered in 1923 near Urbino, Italy, and now in the Wellcome Historical Museum. *(By courtesy of the trustees of the Wellcome Historical Museum)*

PLATE IV

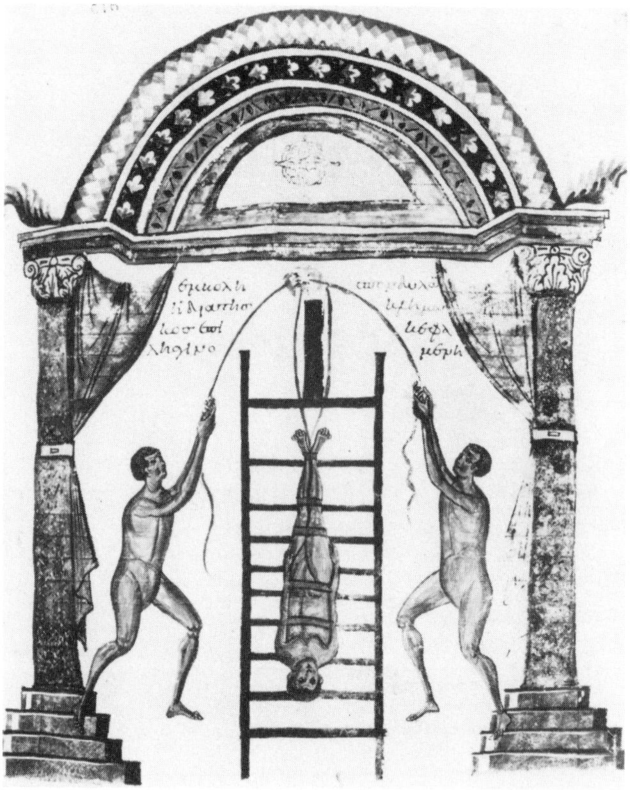

Fig. 1. Correction of dislocation of the spine by 'succussion', from a ninth-century Greek manuscript in the Laurentian Library, Florence – a commentary by Appolonius of Kitium on the Hippocratic treatise on dislocation.

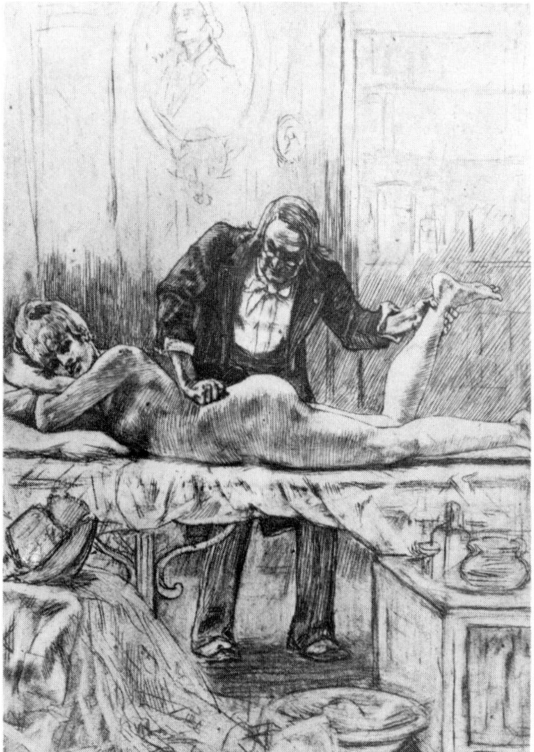

Fig. 2. An etching by Felicien Rops entitled 'Massage'. Unintentionally, it depicts the way in which the third lumbar nerve is stretched by prone knee flexion.

PLATE V

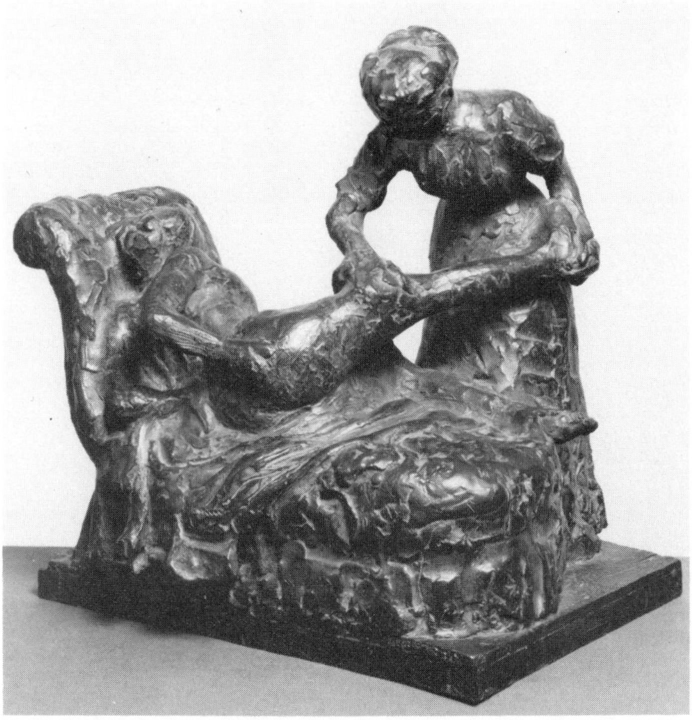

Fig. 1. A statuette by Degas depicting a physiotherapist testing straight-leg raising in a patient with pain in the right buttock. *(By courtesy of the Ny Carlsberg Glyptotek, Copenhagen)*

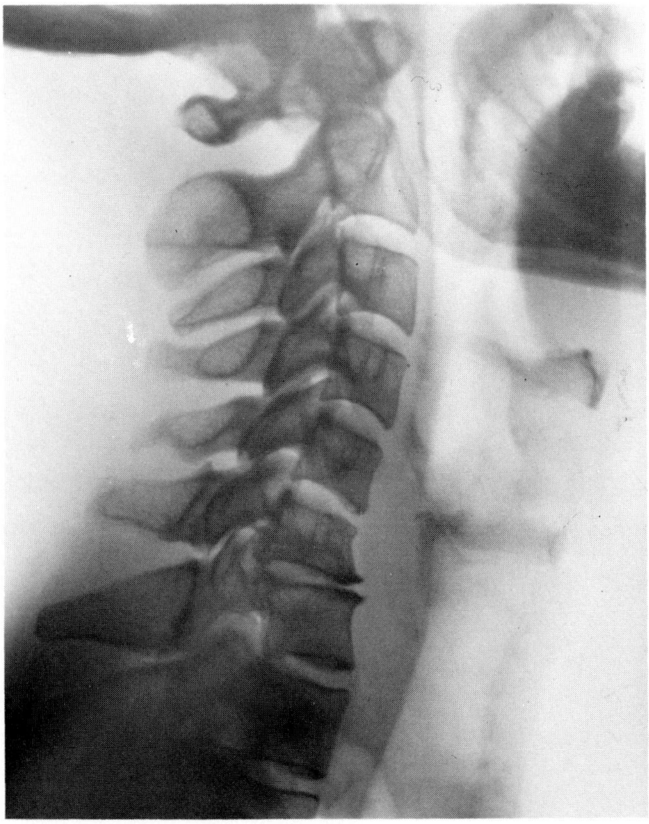

Fig. 2. Sixth cervical disc lesion. Lateral view of the cervical spine, showing marked narrowing at the sixth cervical joint. This contrasts with the normal space above and below. The patient had a seventh root palsy.

PLATE VI

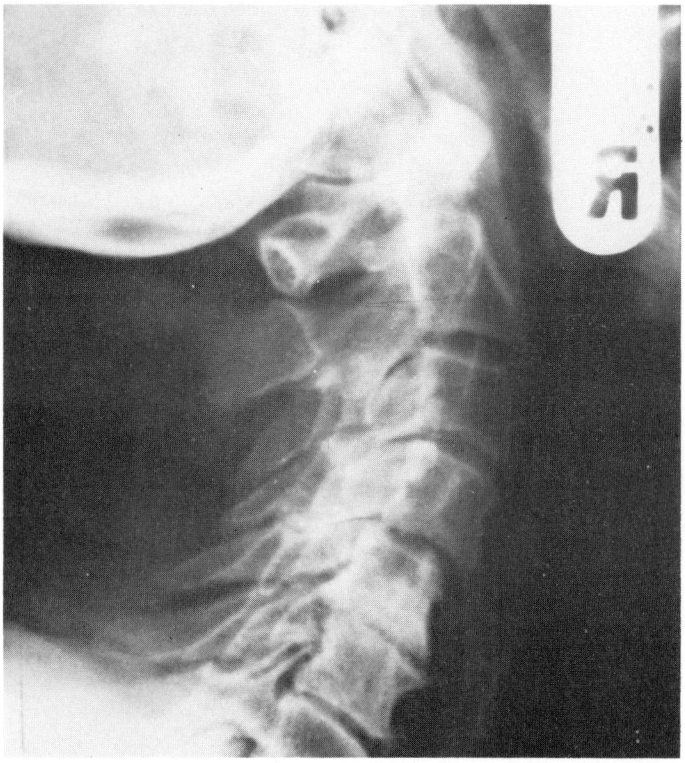

Fig. 1. Osteophytic compression. A man of 68 had three years' tingling at the right thumb due to compression of the sixth cervical root. No root paresis was detectable.

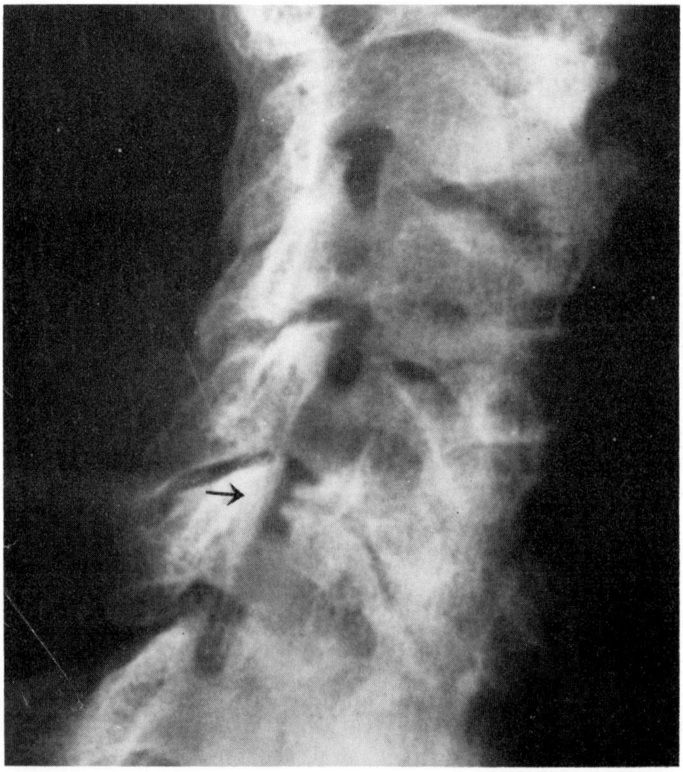

Fig. 2. Osteophytes encroaching on the fifth cervical foramen. The patient, aged 68, had a sixth cervical root palsy

PLATE VII

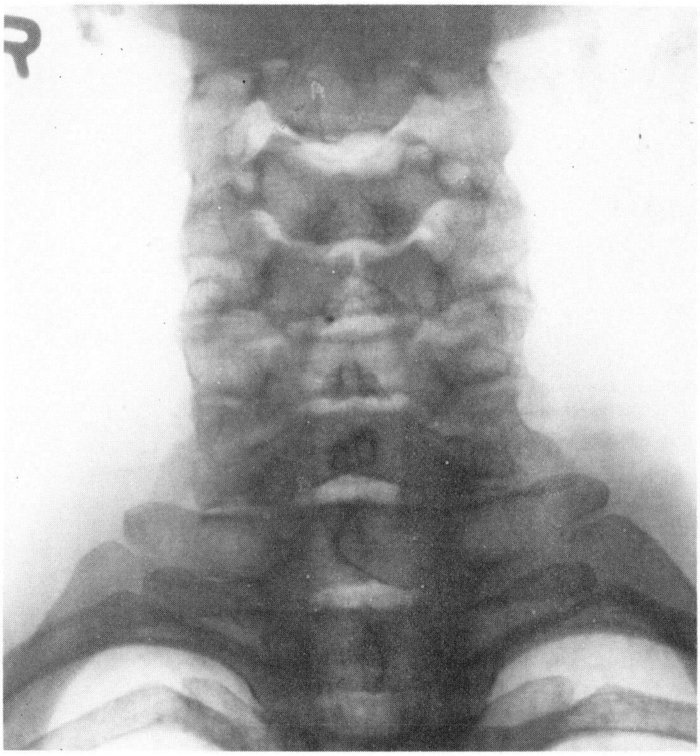


Fig. 1. Radiograph of the cervical spine taken before traction.

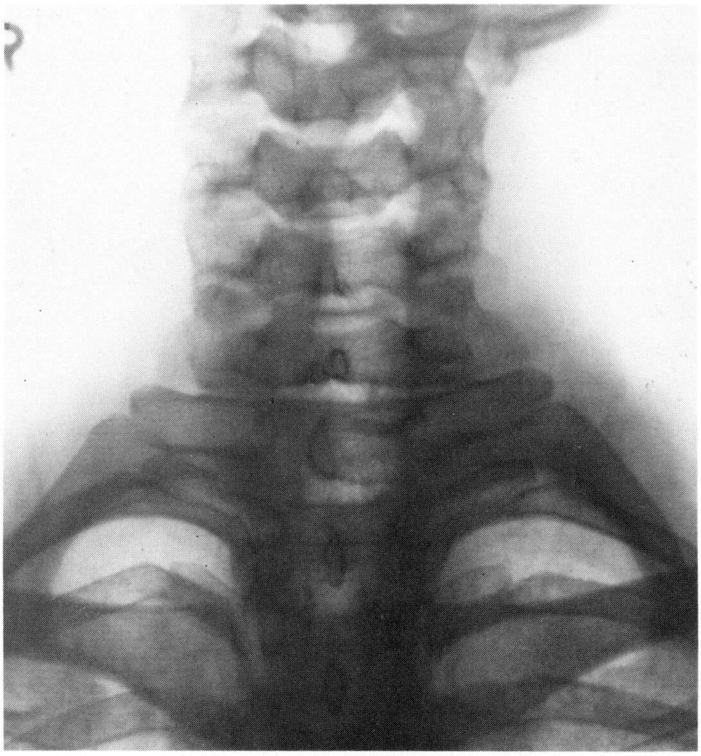


Fig. 2. The same subject after several seconds' manual traction. The distance between the upper border of the first thoracic vertebra and the lower border of the fourth cervical has been increased by 1 cm, i.e. 2.5 mm per joint.

PLATE VIII

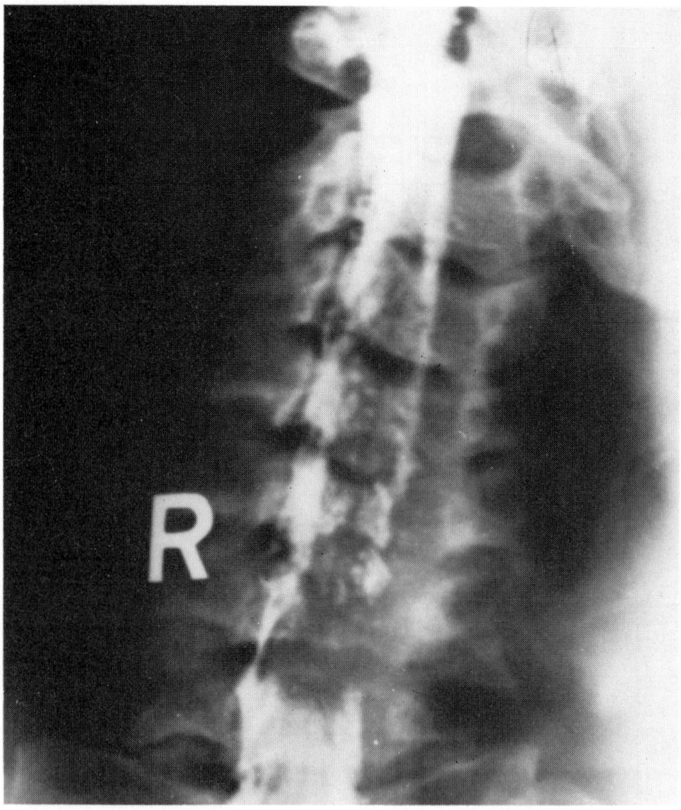


Fig. 1. A cervical myelogram of a sixth cervical disc lesion, taken 4 months after the onset of brachial symptoms, when root pain had almost ceased. Note the unilateral arrest of contrast medium at the sixth level.

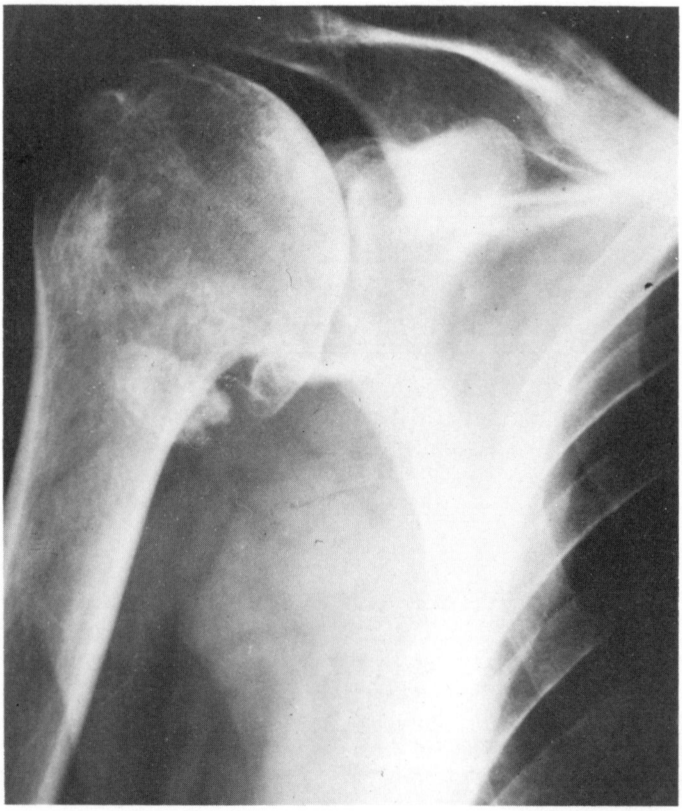

Fig. 2. Osteoarthritis of the shoulder with a loose body. The patient, a man aged 68, had had repeated twinges in his upper arm for 3 years.

PLATE IX

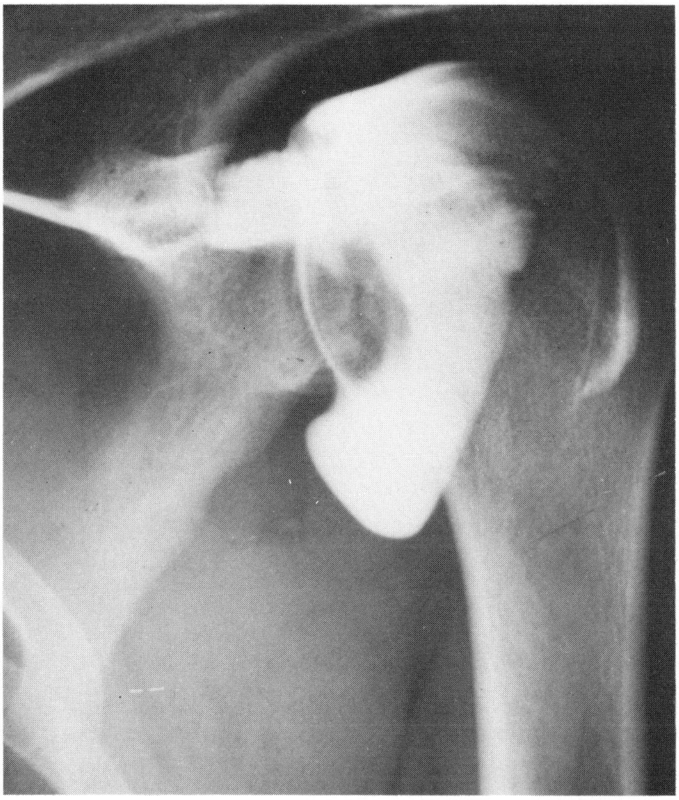

Fig. 1. A normal arthrogram of the shoulder. The articular cavity is outlined, together with the subcoracoid and bicipital bursae.

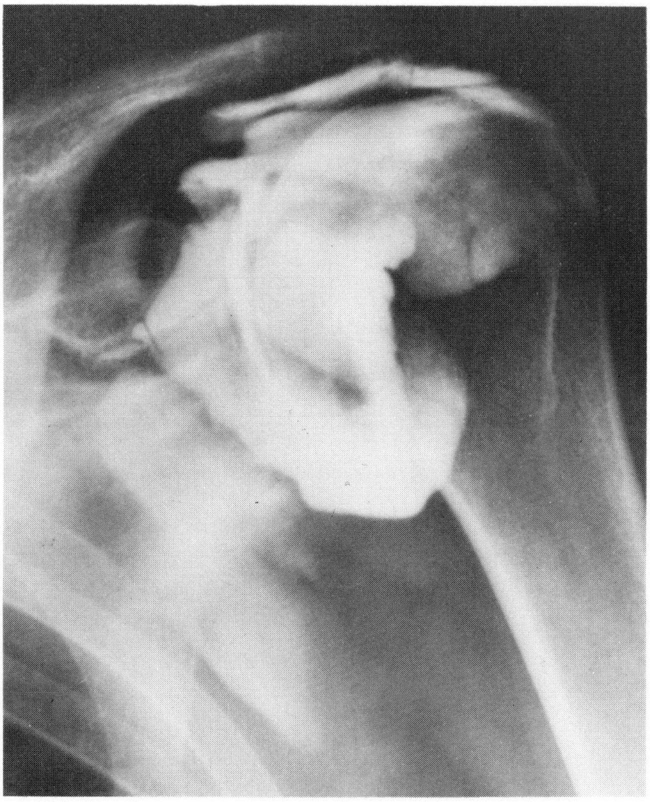

Fig. 2. Arthrogram of a ruptured supraspinatus tendon. The contrast medium, injected into the joint, has passed through the gap, outlining the subdeltoid bursa.

PLATE X

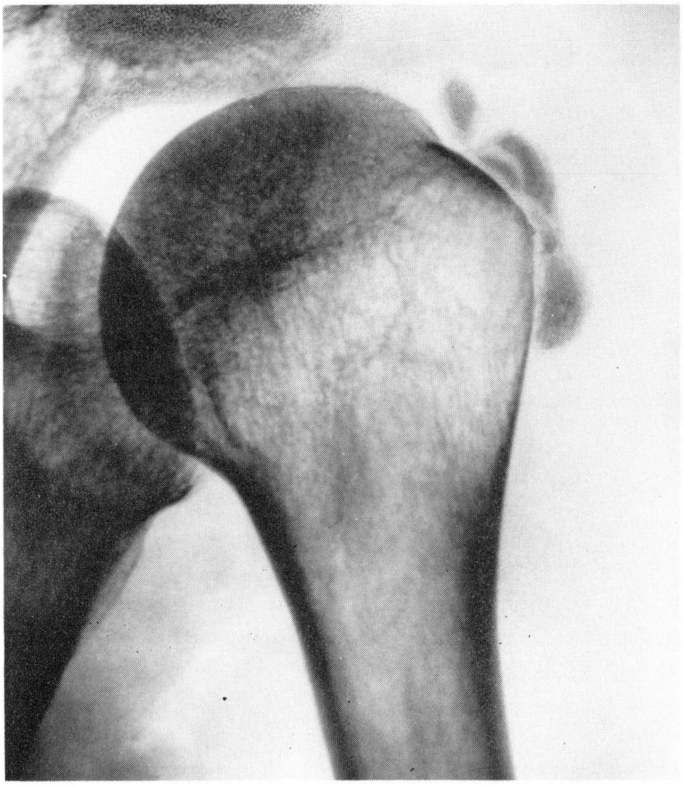

Fig. 1. Calcification in the subdeltoid bursa of a woman aged 33, who had suddenly developed brachial pain four days previously. Marked limitation of movement of the non-capsular pattern was present.

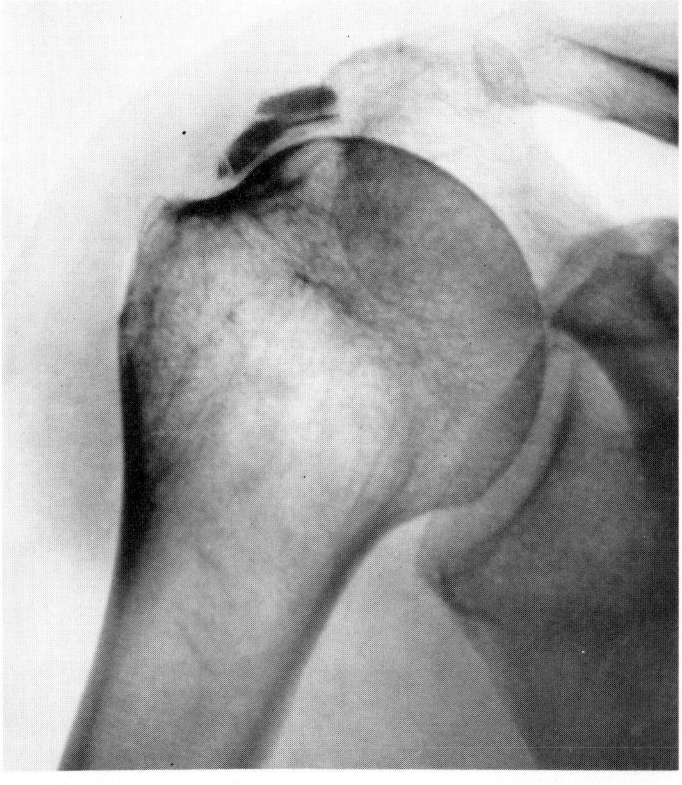

Fig. 2. Calcification in the supraspinatus tendon. The clinical signs of tendinitis were present.

PLATE XI

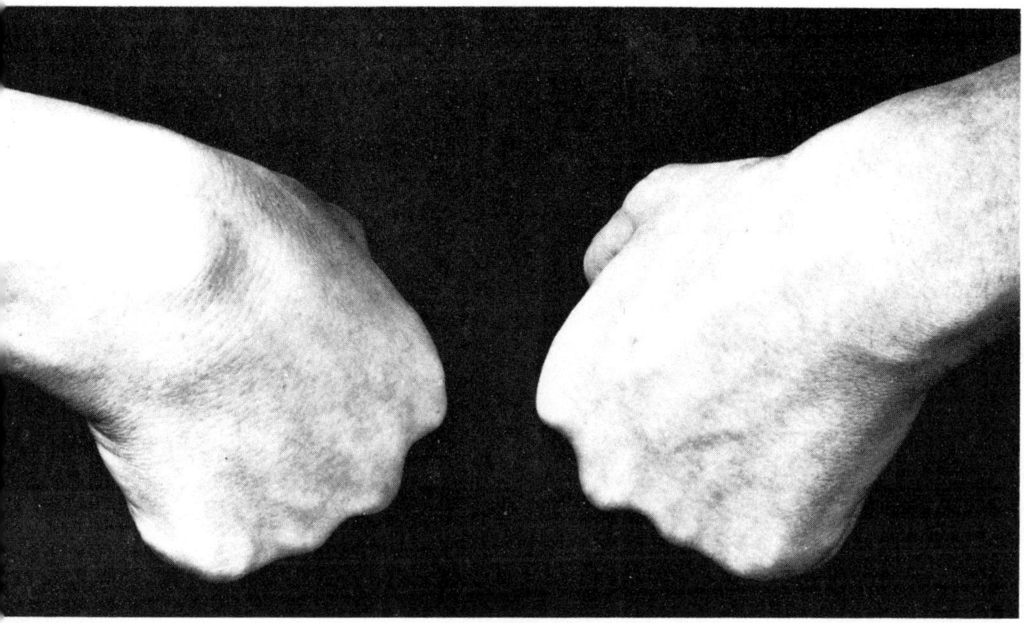

ıbluxation of the capitate bone. The radiograph showed no displacement

PLATE XII

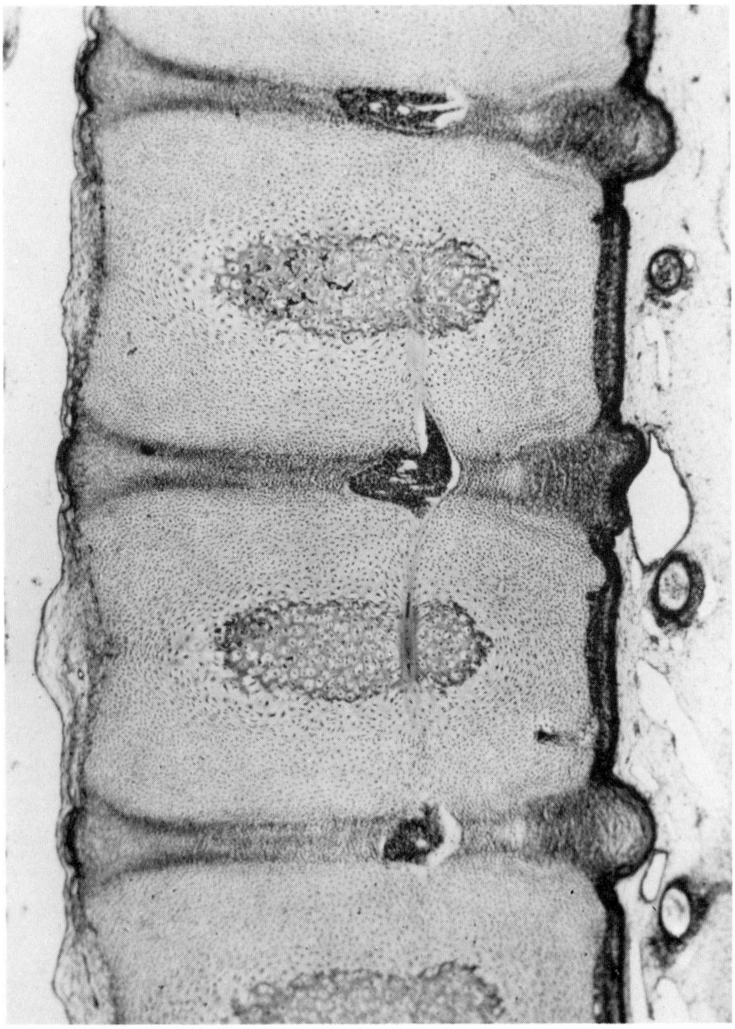

Development of the discs. A photomicrograph of a 64 mm human embryo.

PLATE XIII

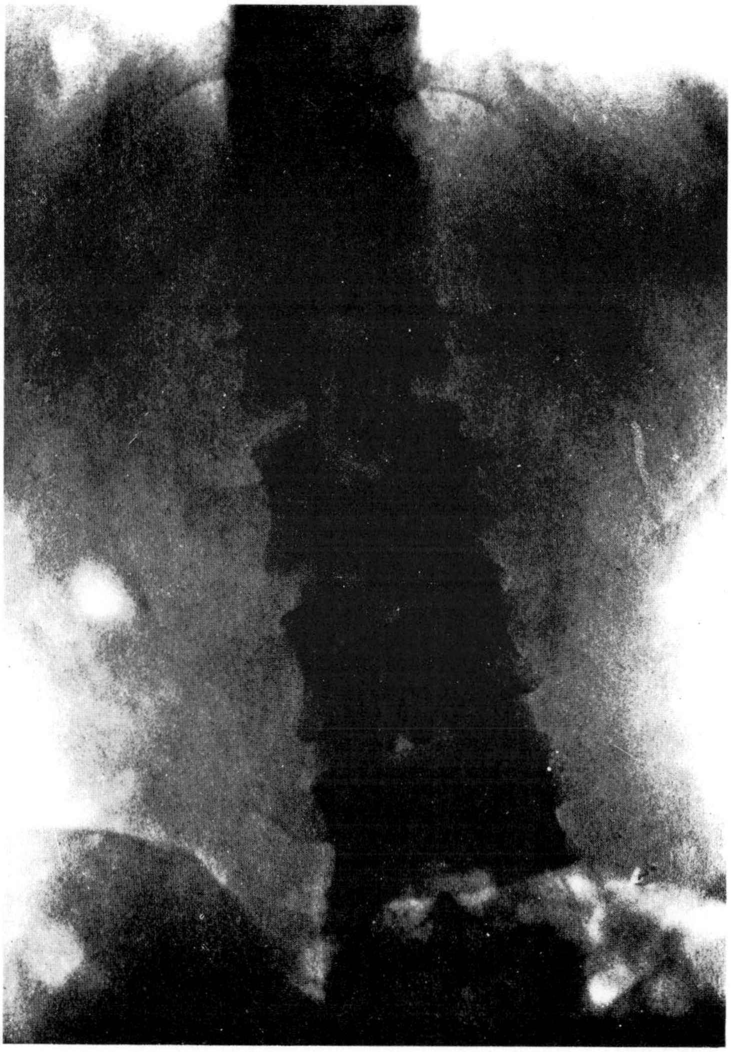

Attempted side flexion towards the patient's left does not even result in the spine reaching the vertical position. The block clearly lies at the left side of the fourth lumbar intervertebral joint, and a large cartilaginous fragment lying here was removed at operation.

PLATE XIV

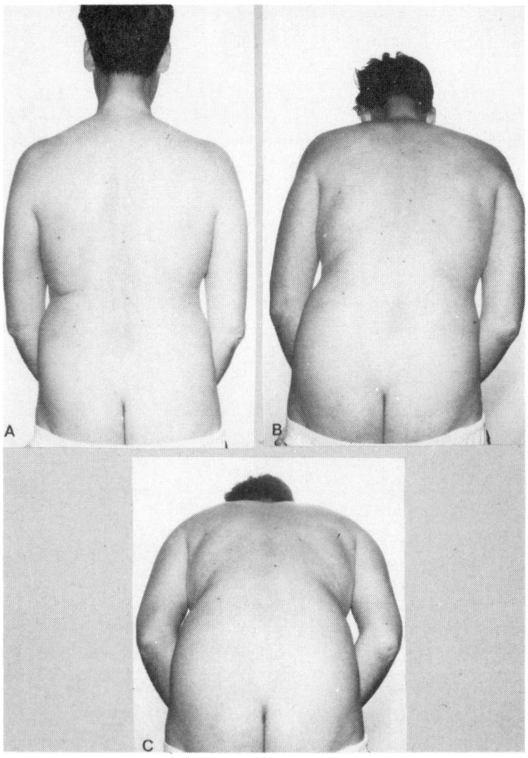


Fig. 1. Momentary deviation at the arc. A, Erect: no deviation. B, Deviation to the right at half range. C, Full flexion: once more symmetrical.

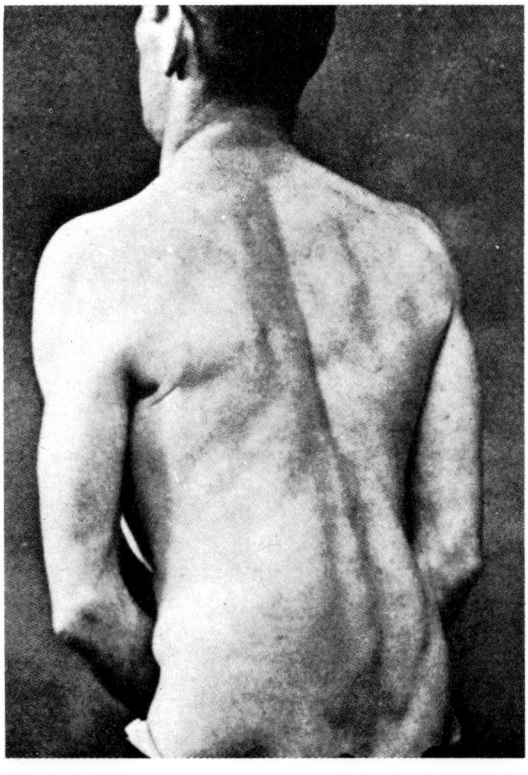

Fig. 2. Marked lumbar kyphosis caused by posterior protrusion of part of a low lumbar intervertebral disc with left-sided sciatica. The patient is bending backwards as far as he can.

PLATE XV

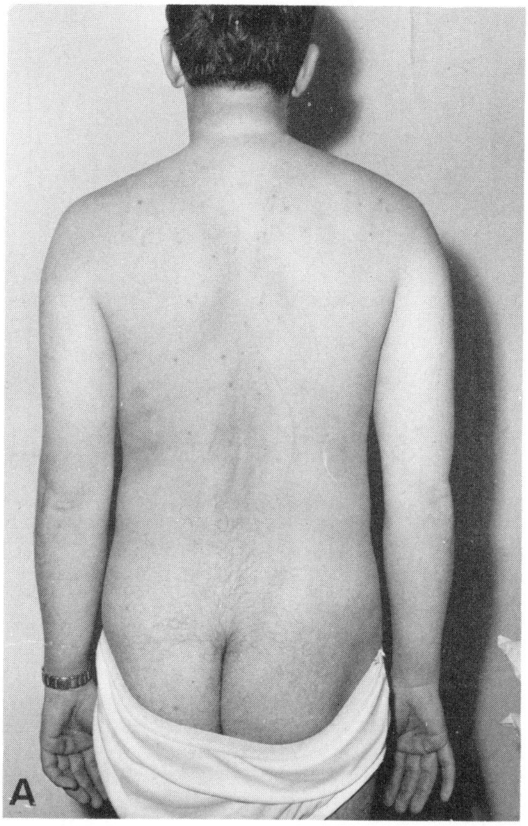


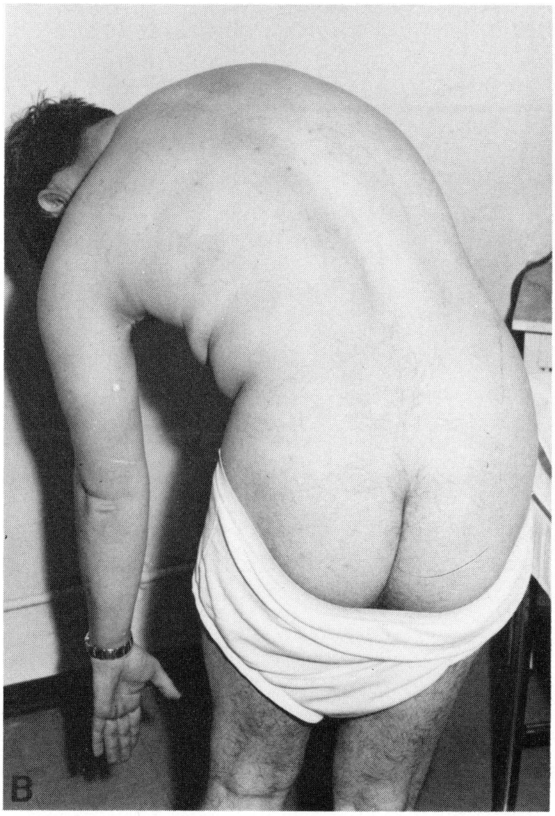


A patient with left-sided sciatica. A, Upright: symmetrical posture. B, Attempted flexation: he reaches to half range with gross leftward deviation.

PLATE XVI

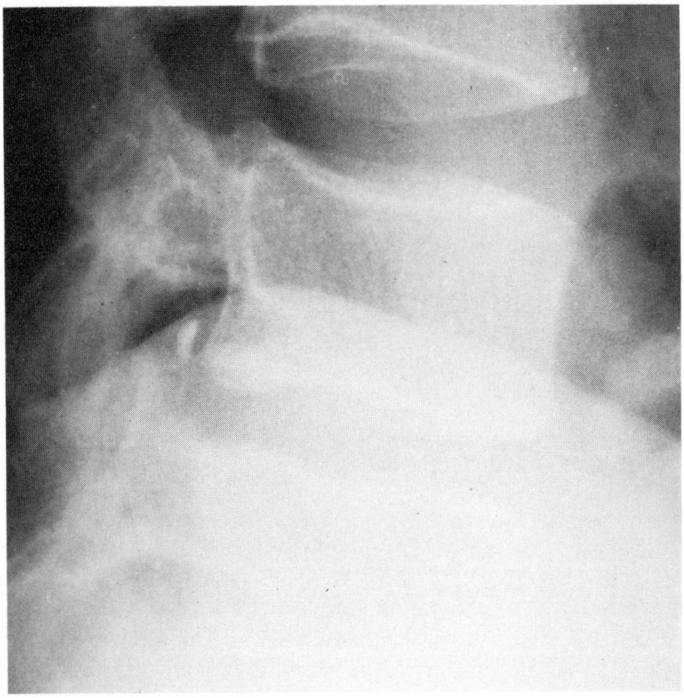

Fig. 1. Calcified posterior longitudinal ligament. It has been raised from the vertebral body by a large disc protrusion causing sciatica.

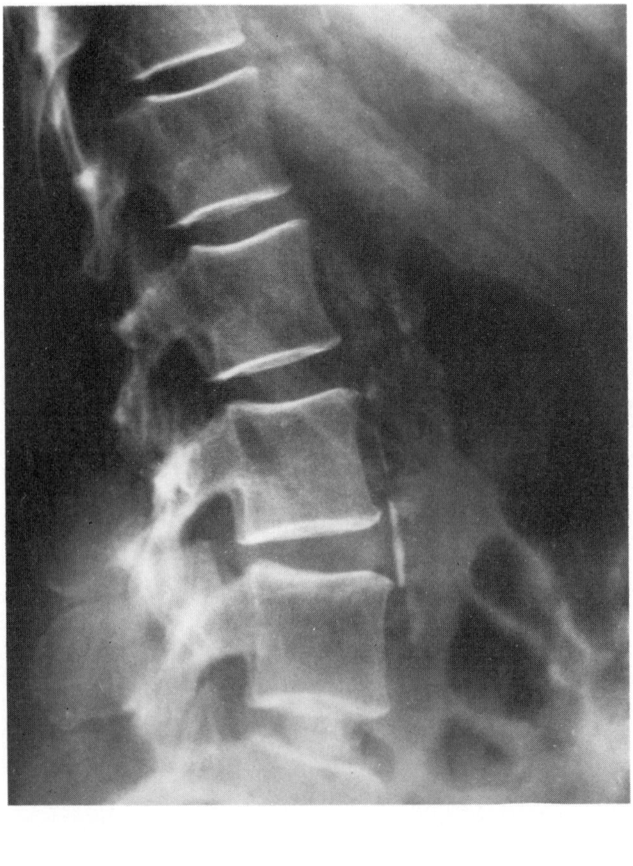

Fig. 2. Calcified nucleus. The size of the pulpy nucleus is clearly shown at the fourth lumbar level.

## Biceps Tendinitis

The intra-articular extent of the long head of biceps is very seldom affected, the tendon being usually at fault where it lies in the bicipital groove. Here it cannot be pinched. However, intracapsular bicipital tendinitis is identified when the arc is associated with pain elicited by resisted supination of the forearm and resisted flexion at the elbow. The passive and resisted movements of the shoulder are all painless.

## Sprain of the Inferior Acromioclavicular Ligament

This is also rare. The painful arc is associated with the pattern suggesting that the acromioclavicular joint is at fault. It is not easy to differentiate chronic strain of the inferior acromioclavicular ligament from long-standing subdeltoid bursitis, since, both are lesions of adjacent inert tissues. The fact that the scapular movements set up localized aching and that the extreme of passive adduction at the shoulder joint hurts, suggests the acromioclavicular joint, but only local anaesthesia settles the matter.

## Metastases in the Acromion

Secondary neoplasm of the acromion alone is rare. It causes tenderness of the bone itself, demonstrated indirectly by the existence of a painful arc and detectable superficially by palpation. Localized warmth is found when erosion of bone is proceeding rapidly.

The action of the supraspinatus muscle is grossly impeded. Hence, pain and marked weakness on testing abduction, associated with bony tenderness, leads to immediate radiography.

## Capsular Laxity at the Shoulder

After a dislocation or sprain, residual capsular laxity at the glenohumeral joint may give rise to momentary subluxation of the head of the humerus as the arm moves upwards towards the horizontal position. At about 80°, it clicks back into place, perhaps with some discomfort. The examiner can see the momentary arrest of the movement and feel the click. This is not a true painful arc, but the resemblance may be close, and its spurious nature must be recognized.

Localized erosion of cartilage at the upper part of the humeral head also gives rise to a false arc. Again the momentary arrest on active elevation can be seen, this time accompanied by the coarser crepitus of bone against bone, audible and palpable.

## Cervical Disc Lesion

An extraordinary occasional finding in disc lesions with pain in the scapulohumeral area is the presence of a painful arc as the affected arm is elevated. Patients with pain in the region of the shoulder often believe that they cannot move the arm away from the side; this is merely another manifestation of the common, deep-rooted idea that function is necessarily impaired at a painful member. Most can be gradually persuaded fully to elevate the arm actively but when the arm passes the horizontal, the muscular effort is at its greatest and some secondary tautening of the cervical muscles takes place, leading to such pain that the arm falters, and a false localizing sign appears. This phenomenon has created the mistaken idea that certain neck conditions give rise to disorders occurring at—not just pain felt in—the shoulder. Osteopaths even claim cure of various types of shoulder trouble by manipulating the neck. Since differential diagnosis is sometimes difficult, it is easy to see how this error arose. In a case of this sort, showing indefinite signs at both the neck and the shoulder, manipulative reduction at the neck should be performed at once until a full and painless range has been restored. The shoulder should then be examined again and, in many instances, the previous signs at the shoulder will be found to have disappeared.

# SUBCLAVIAN OCCLUSION

In this disorder, claudicational pain comes on after the arm has been powerfully used for some time, accompanied by a feeling of weakness. If the brachial artery dilates enough, and the thrombosis lies proximal to the root of the vertebral artery, the direction of flow through this artery becomes reversed and after strong exertion the patient feels faint.

Examination of the muscles and joints of the upper limb reveals no disorder, since exertion has to be continued for some while before a concentration of the products of muscular metabolism is reached enough to cause pain. But the history of pain coming on in the arm after a time, accompanied by weakness, in a patient with normal joints and muscles, should lead to palpation of the radial pulse. This is absent and arteriography reveals the state of affairs.

## SUBDELTOID BURSITIS

Six types of bursitis occur.

### Acute Diffuse Bursitis

If an afebrile patient, because of increasing pain, loses all capacity to abduct his arm actively in the course of a few days, much the likeliest cause is acute subdeltoid bursitis. In dislocation, there is a history of trauma and the deformity is obvious. In pathological fracture the limitation of movement is immediate. Palindromic rheumatism recovers in three days.

Acute bursitis is an uncommon condition, occurring equally in men and women. It is self-limiting within six weeks, and apt to recur at intervals of two to five years. The cause is unknown and injury plays no part in the aetiology. At the earliest stage, which lasts only a day, a painful arc can be elicited; after that the range of abduction becomes too restricted for this point to be reached. It is then limitation of movement of the non-capsular pattern that draws attention to the bursa. The usual finding is marked limitation of abduction with very little restriction of lateral rotation: the reverse of the findings in arthritis; moreover, the capsular feel is absent. This pattern leads to palpation of the bursa, the whole of which is exquisitely tender.

The bursitis takes two or three days to become really acute. First an ache sets in at the shoulder; pain soon spreads down the arm to the wrist; after three days it becomes severe and constant. The patient's sleep is now disturbed, and he soon finds that he can barely move his arm at all. After seven to ten days of severe pain, the symptoms abate somewhat; at the end of two or three weeks there remains only an ache, and active abduction may have reached half-range. At the end of four to six weeks the patient has fully recovered. When he is nearly well the painful arc appears again for the last week.

### Acute Bursitis with Calcified Deposit

Judging by the literature, calcification of the bursa occurs less often in England than in the USA and, when it is met within this country, the patient is often of mid-European descent.

The onset is sudden and unprovoked. Within a few days the patient finds himself unable to move the arm appreciably because of severe pain spreading from the shoulder to forearm and wrist. The pattern of limitation is noncapsular; the capsular end-feel is absent; the bursa is very tender and the radiograph reveals quite a large area of calcification. There is often a smaller similar shadow at the other (symptomless) shoulder. The disorder recovers rather more quickly than acute bursitis without a deposit, usually in a month. There is some tendency to recurrence. After recovery the calcification remains, sometimes disappearing spontaneously after several years. The sequence of events is so similar to that in gout, that blood uric acid estimations were carried out in a small series of cases. However, the highest figure obtained was 4 mg and some were low normal levels (under 2 mg).

### Haemorrhage into the Subdeltoid Bursa

In my experience this occurs only in old age. The haemorrhage was apparently spontaneous in all cases except one in which the bleeding was secondary to rupture of the supraspinatus tendon. The complaint is of swelling and pain. Visible bruising is occasionally present. The bursa is prominent and tense; fluctuation is easily detectable. Aspiration reveals blood. In long-standing cases, fibrous clots can be felt to move about inside the bursa.

The range of movement is limited more by the bulk of the fluid than by the bursitis; it is slight, but after a period of immobilization owing to pain, greater limitation due to capsular contracture may well supervene. Recurrent haemorrhage into the bursa after aspiration suggests haemangioma.

### Chronic Localized Bursitis

Chronic localized bursitis does not result from an acute bursitis that has not resolved completely; it is a separate entity. It is quite a common cause of painful shoulder.

The onset is gradual and apparently causeless; the pain may continue for years. Sometimes the radiograph shows a calcified deposit; more often no abnormality is revealed. Men and women are attacked at ages ranging from 15 to 65. Rarely, localized bursitis is the result of direct contusion. If so, thickening of the bursal wall is visible and palpable and there may be a small effusion.

The pain is felt in the lower deltoid area and examination discloses a painful arc and often nothing else. Sometimes, in addition, though the passive range is full, every extreme is uncomfortable. No resisted movement hurts. This finding implies that of the four tissues tenderness of which commonly give rise to a painful arc—the supraspinatus, infraspinatus, and subscapular tendons, the subdeltoid bursa—it is none of the tendons, since each resisted movement is painless. There remains only the bursa.

The question is now which part of the bursa is affected. Half of it lies under the acromion and out of finger's reach. The subdeltoid moiety is palpated for tenderness and, if such an area is found, it is anaesthetized with 10 ml of 0.5% procaine. After five minutes, the patient is asked to elevate his arm again and to state whether the arc has been abolished or not. All diagnoses of subdeltoid bursitis are tentative, until confirmed by this test.

If none of the accessible part of the bursa proves to be tender, the lesion must lie subacromionally. Again local anaesthesia must be used to decide the diagnosis (especially in incomprehensible bursitis, p. 151). The same amount of solution as before is introduced with a 5 cm needle deeply between the acromion and the tendons, and the patient declares the result a few minutes later.

Spontaneous painless effusion into the bursa may, as happens at other joints, complicate severe rheumatoid arthritis; doubtless it would give rise to a painful arc if the arthritis at the shoulder did not prevent movement to that point.

## Crepitating Bursitis

Patients are seen, usually a year or two after a subdeltoid bursitis with effusion has subsided, complaining of creaking at the bursa on moving the arm and some aching in the deltoid area after exertion. (No treatment appears to make any difference, but the disability is very minor.)

### 'Adhesive bursitis'

This is an alleged entity copied from one textbook to another. In my experience, it does not occur and inquiry from surgeons who operate on shoulders shows that they do not encounter bursal adhesions either.

## Incomprehensible Bursitis

Patients are rarely encountered who have pain felt at the shoulder arising only during, and for some hours after, considerable exertion. They can carry on in spite of the pain, which is disagreeable but not disabling, and persists for years.

Examinations shows one of four patterns.

1. Full range; both passive rotations hurt; full elevation is painless; there is no arc; the resisted movements do not hurt.
2. Full range with discomfort at extremes; painful arc; resisted abduction and lateral rotation both hurt.
3. A changing pattern of pain on resisted movement. Full painful range of passive movement. The resisted movements hurt in an erratic way, the response being pain, then not, when the test is repeated. Slight arc.
4. Slight limitation of passive abduction alone or passive medial rotation alone. The resisted movements are painless or all equally painful. No arc.

It cannot be explained how these signs signify bursitis, but infiltration of the affected area of the subdeltoid bursa is immediately curative after every other known treatment has failed. If no part of the subdeltoid bursa is found tender, local anaesthesia has to be induced under the acromion repeatedly until the right spot is found.

## INTERPRETATION OF PATTERN

### Summary of Significant Findings

**Full range**

| | | |
|---|---|---|
| Pain on resisted abduction | deltoid | anterior fibres—pain on forward movement from the horizontal<br>posterior fibres—pain on backward movement from the horizontal |
| | supraspinatus | unaffected by forward or backward movement |
| Pain on resisted adduction | pectoralis major | pain on swinging forwards |
| | teres minor | pain on lateral rotation |
| | latissimus dorsi and teres major | pain on swinging backwards<br>pain on medial rotation |
| Pain on resisted lateral rotation | teres minor | pain on adduction |
| | infraspinatus | no pain adduction or abduction |
| | supraspinatus | pain on abduction |
| Pain on resisted medial rotation | subscapularis | no pain on adduction |
| | pectoralis major<br>latissimus dorsi<br>teres major | pain on adduction |
| Pain on resisted flexion | coracobrachialis | |
| Painful arc | muscular | supraspinatus—pain on resisted abduction<br>infraspinatus—pain on lateral rotation<br>subscapularis—pain on medial rotation |
| | inert | mild chronic subdeltoid bursitis<br>ruptured supraspinatus—loss of voluntary abduction<br>acromioclavicular joint—localized pain and tenderness |

**Limited Range**

| | |
|---|---|
| Capsular pattern | traumatic capsulitis—history—no radiographic change<br>osteoarthrosis—age, crepitus, other shoulder too<br>monarticular rheumatoid arthritis—no trauma—spontaneous onset of 'frozen shoulder'<br>bacterial arthritis—great wasting, radiographic change |
| Non-capsular pattern | acute subdeltoid bursitis—site of tenderness, disproportionate limitation of abduction, calcification<br>subcoracoid bursitis—disproportionate limitation of lateral rotation ceasing when arm horizontal<br>anterior capsular adhesion—disproportionate limitation of lateral rotation persisting when arm horizontal<br>secondary neoplasm—bizarre pattern, radiographic change<br>neoplasm of lung—radiographic change, Horner's syndrome, weak fingers |
| Bony block | neuropathic arthropathy—no pain, radiographic change, WR, syringomyelia<br>displacement of fractured tuberosity under acromion—pain, recent injury, radiographic change |

## MUSCULAR WEAKNESS IN SHOULDER AND ARM

If a patient cannot reproduce actively a movement of which his joint can be shown by passive testing to be capable, one or more muscles must be out of action, either from intrinsic or nervous defect. Alternatively, the disorder may be psychogenic. In many cases, although the voluntary movements are not limited in range, trial of the resisted movements displays weakness. On the whole, weakness is much easier to detect than wasting; for inspection of the serratus anterior and spinatus muscles, except in thin subjects, is difficult; even at the deltoid muscle a minor degree of wasting is surprisingly difficult to see. Naturally, the examination for weakness must continue from scapula to hand; for if the lowest cervical or first thoracic root or the lower trunk of the brachial plexus is involved, it is only examination of the hand that affords the clue. The test for winging of the scapula must not be forgotten. There are eleven possible findings.

## Painless Weakness of the Deltoid Muscle

This may result from traumatic compression of the axillary nerve, usually by the head of the humerus when it dislocates. The bony displacement may have been momentary only; hence, there may not be clear history of dislocation. A patient with a powerless deltoid but with a strong supraspinatus muscle possesses a full range of active elevation, but he cannot bring his arm backwards from the horizontal position. Gross wasting of the deltoid is usually obvious and a patch of cutaneous analgesia is found at the mid-deltoid area. An interesting sign in the early case is involuntary spasm of the trapezius muscle, lasting a week or two. The scapula is thus kept elevated, relieving tension on the axillary nerve. In such a case, full side flexion of the neck away from the weak side is apt to hurt in the area of cutaneous analgesia at the upper arm.

Treatment consists merely of making sure that the patient uses his supraspinatus muscle so as to maintain a full range of movement at the shoulder joint pending recovery of the deltoid muscle. This often takes six months.

## Painless Weakness of Deltoid, Biceps and Both Spinatus Muscles

This combination characterizes a lesion of the fifth cervical nerve root. It may result from a *fourth cervical disc protrusion*. If so, some of the cervical movements give rise to scapular pain. If the cause is a *traction palsy*, there is a history of an accident depressing the shoulder girdle and the cervical movements are of full range and painless.

Myeloma may result in monoradicular weakness, but is usually bilateral. Secondary neoplasm sets up widespread weakness involving two or more roots, usually bilateral. In neuroma, the weakness may be too great for a mere disc lesion or it may affect the muscles relevant to more than one root. In gradual osteophytic compression of the root, pain is slight or absent.

No treatment avails in a disc lesion that has already caused a root palsy. Spontaneous recovery must be awaited; this takes three to four months for the root pain and six to eight months for the return of muscle power, from the onset of the pain in the upper limb, not from when the scapular ache began. In traction palsy there is little discomfort, and the muscles recover in about six months. If necessary, the patient is taught meanwhile to maintain a full range of movement at the shoulder joint. Residual weakness is rare. A fifth cervical root palsy caused by encroachment on the fourth intervertebral foramen is best treated surgically by drilling away the osteophyte.

## Painless Weakness of the Supraspinatus Muscle Alone

This results from rupture of the supraspinatus tendon. The disorder may come on insidiously without a history of trauma, since the tendon can degenerate slowly, parting gradually until it finally gives way altogether. Alternatively, a strain or a fall on the shoulder may be responsible. The diagnosis suggests itself when a middle-aged patient suddenly loses all power to abduct his arm. In this circumstance, the deltoid is powerless to act as an abductor; for its contraction merely moves the head of the humerus upwards into the hiatus left superiorly by the gap in the supraspinatus tendon. As the head of the humerus must move downwards as abduction proceeds, the deltoid cannot work alone and all power of active abduction below the horizontal is lost. When he tries, rotation and elevation of the scapula, combined with lateral flexion of the trunk away from the affected side, give rise to an apparent range of at most 20°. On inspection, the deltoid muscle is not wasted. Passive elevation is full—except in neglected cases—and a very pronounced painful arc is discovered as the examiner lifts the patient's arm past the horizontal. After the arm has been passively raised just above the horizontal, past the arc, voluntary elevation once more becomes possible and the patient now has no difficulty in bringing his arm right up by using his deltoid and serratus muscles.

Radiography is often confirmative, since the gap between acromion and head of the humerus can be seen to be much narrowed, the bone having subluxated upwards into the gap left by the parted tendon.

The above description applies to cases seen within the first month or so of the occurrence of the rupture. Since the condition is almost confined to the middle-aged or elderly, capsular contracture from disuse soon sets in. In such cases the picture is complicated by the addition of limitation of movement in the capsular proportions from immobilizational arthritis.

Wasting of the supraspinatus muscle belly is detectable at the end of some weeks, and is permanent.

## Painful Weakness of the Supraspinatus Muscle Alone

This implies a partial rupture of the supraspinatus tendon and is difficult to differentiate from uncomplicated tendinitis. Supraspinatus tendinitis is clearly present, but marked weakness as well as pain becomes apparent when the abduction movement is attempted against resistance. If, in such a case, local anaesthesia destroys the pain but leaves the weakness unaltered, mere unwillingness to perform a painful movement can be ruled out. There is no particular tendency for a painful partial rupture to become complete, at any rate within some years. Malignant invasion of the acromion also leads to pain and weakness of abduction of the arm.

## Painless Weakness of the Supraspinatus and Infraspinatus Muscles

This is likely to come to light only if the power of resisted lateral rotation movement of the two arms is compared. Pain constantly day and night lasting three weeks is felt in the scapular area and upper arm. No movement of the neck, scapula or upper limb affects it. Voluntary movement of the arm is not lost because the deltoid and teres minor muscles remain in action. Except in fat subjects, wasting of the supra- and infraspinatus muscles can be detected on inspection and palpation. The cause is neuritis involving the suprascapular nerve alone. No treatment is required; recovery is spontaneous and seldom takes more than four to five months.

The lesion is occasionally traumatic. If an injury results in severe traction on the arm pulling it away from the trunk, the suprascapular nerve may be caught against the edge of the bony notch it traverses at the upper border of the scapula. Rarely, the nerve is ruptured completely and permanent palsy results.

Bilateral painless disappearance of the spinatus muscles suggests myopathy. If so, the serratus anterior muscles are often also affected. Since the cases of myopathy usually seen by an orthopaedic physician occur in middle-aged patients, secondary limitation of movement may have occurred at the shoulders as a result of capsular contracture from disuse. The wasting, if perceived at all, is then ascribed to arthritis. The great wasting and weakness contrast strangely with the small degree of limitation of movement; moreover, in uncomplicated arthritis the muscles are not clinically weak.

## Painless Weakness of the Serratus Anterior Muscle

This weakness is detected when the patient is asked to elevate his arm actively, whereupon 45° limitation of elevation is found, whereas passive elevation is full and painless. This means that there is a full range of voluntary movement at the shoulder joint but that active rotation of the scapula is defective. When the patient is asked to lean forward with his arms stretched out in front of him and to push against a wall, winging of one scapula at once becomes apparent. The cause is a long thoracic nerve palsy—another manifestation of neuritis. Most patients suffer two or three weeks' constant aching in the scapular region and upper arm unaffected by movement, but the neuritis sometimes comes on painlessly. Spontaneous recovery is the rule, and takes four to eight months. No treatment is necessary.

Occasionally the palsy follows direct or indirect trauma to the nerve. In one case a horse had trodden on the patient's scapula (and a year later no recovery had begun), and in another the scapula had been wrenched away from the body laterally and recovery began six months later.

Partial weakness of the serratus anterior muscle is occasionally detectable (with some difficulty) in a cervical disc lesion resulting in a sixth cervical root palsy. A suggestion of winging is perceptible; voluntary elevation of the arm is lacking in only the final 5°.

Bilateral painless disappearance of the serratus anterior muscles characterizes myopathy.

## Painless Weakness of the Trapezius Muscle Alone

The history and clinical picture resemble those of long thoracic neuritis. Sometimes painlessly, sometimes with up to three weeks unilateral scapular aching, the arm becomes weak and heavy. The patient finds he cannot raise his arm fully and examination shows 10° limitation of voluntary elevation, with a full passive range. This is a lesser degree of restricted voluntary elevation of the arm than is found in long thoracic neuritis, where it usually amounts to 45°. Testing the serratus anterior muscle shows that the scapula does not wing. The neck and arm movements are painless and strong. Active approximation of the scapulae causes the vertebral border of the scapula to project from the chest wall. The examiner, by hooking his finger round the prominent edge of the bone, can pull the scapula laterally however much the patient tries to prevent him. The sternomastoid muscle is not affected.

The cause is spinal accessory neuritis. Spontaneous recovery takes some six months.

Paralysis of one trapezius muscle ever since an operation for tuberculous glands in childhood with accidental division of the spinal accessory nerve is no longer encountered.

## Painless Weakness of the Infraspinatus Muscle Alone

The cause is rupture of the infraspinatus tendon; it is rare. The patient is middle-aged or elderly, and has suffered some accident or overstrain involving the shoulder. In the early case, examination reveals a painful arc accompanied by great weakness of lateral rotation of the arm; if the teres minor muscle escapes, the movement can just be performed actively; if not, the active movement is completely lost. After many months, the remnants of the tendon still attached to the tuberosity lose their tenderness and the painful arc ceases. The weakness is permanent, and leads to painless capsular contracture anteriorly; as a result, after a year or two 30 to 45° of passive lateral rotation range have been lost, abduction and medial rotation remaining of full range.

Treatment consists of infiltrating the remnants of the infraspinatus tendon with triamcinolone to abolish the arc, and showing the patient how to maintain the range of lateral rotation by using his other hand daily to rotate the arm outwards.

## Painless Weakness of the Subscapular Muscle Alone

This too is rare and results from rupture of the subscapular tendon. The history is of trauma followed by weakness at the shoulder. Examination shows a painful arc and great weakness of medial rotation of the arm. It is remarkable, considering the strength of the pectoralis major, latissimus dorsi and teres major muscles, how little power remains when medial rotation is tested. The weakness is permanent, but the painful arc on elevating the arm usually disappears within a month or two. The patient should be shown an exercise to strengthen the intact medial rotator muscles and how to maintain a full range of movement at the shoulder. Triamcinolone injected at the lesser tuberosity desensitizes the tender tendinous remnants and should be carried out at once in all cases with a painful arc.

## Weakness of the Triceps and Forearm Muscles

This is nearly always due to protrusion of the sixth cervical intervertebral disc, setting up a seventh cervical root palsy. The pain may be concentrated at the scapula and arm, rarely it is confined to the pectoral area, but on examination the scapular muscles, the shoulder joint and the muscles controlling it are all normal. By contrast the neck movements set up the thoracic pain. The triceps muscle may be weak alone, or in conjunction with the flexors of the wrist and the adductors of the arm. The triceps jerk is seldom affected.

## Weakness of the Biceps and Forearm Muscles

This finding characterizes a sixth cervical root palsy. The loss of power of flexion and supination at the elbow is often minor but is accompanied by clear weakness of the extensor muscles of the wrist. The biceps and brachioradialis jerks are usually sluggish or absent. The only common cause is a fifth cervical disc lesion.

Examination shows that the neck, but not the scapular or shoulder, movements increase the pain felt in the scapular area.

## Neuralgic Amyotrophy

The first symptom is central neckache, then pain in both arms, then concentrating in one upper limb only. The pain is severe and takes from four to six months to cease completely. Pins and needles are seldom experienced; if they are, they occupy the fingers segmentally relevant to the muscles most severely affected.

The affected muscles are completely paralysed from the outset and the weakness is of individual muscles, irrespective of segmental origin. The infraspinatus muscle is often involved, sometimes bilaterally, whatever other muscles are found weak.

## SNAPPING SHOULDER

This is nearly always the result of subluxation of the long head of biceps. As the result of rupture of the transverse humeral ligament, the tendon slips in and out of the upper end of its groove. It is almost invariably painless, and in most snapping shoulders the cause of pain and the snapping are unrelated, although the patient naturally associates the two.

## RECAPITULATION

A few unusual patterns are listed here for speedy reference:

1. *Passive elevation is full, but active elevation is limited.*
   Ruptured supraspinatus
   Fifth cervical root palsy
   Suprascapular neuritis
   Long thoracic neuritis
   Spinal accessory neuritis
   Clay-shoveller's fracture
   Fractured first rib
2. *Passive elevation is limited but there is 90° abduction range at the scapulohumeral joint.*
   Contracture after radical mastectomy
   Basal pulmonary neoplasm
   Contracture of the costocoracoid fascia
   Ankylosis of the acromioclavicular joint
3. *Passive lateral rotation is limited alone.*
   Anterior capsular scar (old dislocation)
   Subcoracoid bursitis
   Ruptured infraspinatus tendon
4. *Full range with incomprehensible pattern*
   Probably localized subdeltoid bursitis

## CHRONOLOGY OF LIMITED MOVEMENT

Only approximate periods can be given.

### Three Days

Limited movement of capsular pattern. Frequent recurrence. Spontaneous recovery in three days.
Palindromic rheumatism

### One Month

Limited movement of capsular pattern. Spontaneous recovery in one month.
Chondrocalcinosis (pseudo-gout)

### Six Weeks

Limited movement of non-capsular pattern. Recurrence each two to five years at either shoulder. Spontaneous recovery in six weeks.
Acute subdeltoid bursitis

### One Year

Limited movement of capsular pattern. Spontaneous recovery in one year.
Traumatic arthritis or minor attack of rheumatoid arthritis; Reiter's arthritis

### Two Years

Limited movement of capsular pattern. Spontaneous recovery in two years.
Monarticular rheumatoid arthritis

### Indefinite Limitation

Limited movement of capsular pattern. Spontaneous cessation of pain in two years, with, often permanent, residual limitation of movement.
Arthritis complicating ankylosing spondylitis, psoriasis, lupus erythematosus or osteitis deformans

## STATISTICAL ANALYSIS

The frequency of lesions at the shoulder was determined by analysing 150 consecutive cases.

| | |
|---|---|
| Traumatic arthritis | 40 |
| Monarticular rheumatoid arthritis | 36 |
| Supraspinatus tendinitis | 29 |
| Subdeltoid bursitis | 23 |
| Infraspinatus tendinitis | 8 |

| | | | |
|---|---|---|---|
| Acromioclavicular strain | 6 | Freezing arthritis* | 5 |
| Subscapular tendinitis | 6 | Bicipital tendinitis | 2 |

## ACROMIOCLAVICULAR JOINT

When this joint is affected, usually after a fall on the shoulder, the patient complains of pain exactly at the site of the joint. There may be a slight aching also in the upper deltoid area, but such reference is uncommon and does not deceive; for when asked to indicate whence the pain springs, the patient places one finger on, or very close to, the joint. Rarely, the inferior aspect of the capsule bears the brunt of an injury. If so, the pain at the joint is sometimes felt to travel as far as the mid-arm and a painful arc may then occur on abduction at the shoulder. Hence a puzzling picture emerges, very similar to that of localized subdeltoid bursitis. Local anaesthesia has to be employed to clarify the diagnosis; for tenderness cannot be elicited either at the deep aspect of the joint or at the subacromial part of the bursa. Since they are both inert structures lying in contact and beyond reach of the examiner's finger, differentiation is difficult.

If any movement at the acromioclavicular joint hurts at the point of the shoulder, diagnosis is simple. But it often happens that no scapular movement hurts; it is only when the extremes of passive movement at the shoulder are tested that pain is evoked. These, surprisingly enough, appear to strain the joint more effectively than do the scapular movements. A useful distinction is to test full passive adduction of the arm across the front of the upper thorax. This is often the most painful movement when the acromioclavicular joint is affected, but causes little discomfort in chronic subdeltoid bursitis. If the posterior acromioclavicular ligament is severely strained, passive adduction of the arm may become so painful as to appear limited. Another difficulty is the very earliest stage of arthritis at the shoulder, when full range at this joint is still retained with merely pain at extremes. The site of the pain helps, for glenohumeral capsular pain is rarely felt at the point of the shoulder. The end-feel is also useful diagnostically; it is normal at the shoulder when the acromioclavicular joint is at fault. Moreover, in arthritis at the shoulder, passive testing discloses that it is the extreme of lateral rotation, not of adduction, that hurts most.

Severe stretching of the acromioclavicular joint leads to laxity and a tendency to subluxation, which may be visible and is usually easily palpable. Recurrent subluxation soon becomes a painless clicking; its degree is limited by the length of the conoid and trapezoid ligaments. It does not constitute an appreciable disability in itself, and in any case the capsular laxity is permanent. Osteophyte formation at the acromioclavicular joint leads to prominence of the ends of the bones; these may be slightly tender. Such osteoarthrosis seldom causes more than some temporary aching after exertion, but is a common radiographic finding in elderly patients. It is thus usual to find patients credited with a lesion of the acromioclavicular joint on the strength of misapplied X-ray findings, although the most cursory examination would have revealed, for example, limitation of movement at the shoulder joint. No degree of arthritis at the acromioclavicular joint can affect the range of movement at the shoulder joint. In advanced ankylosing spondylitis, fixation of the acromioclavicular joint occasionally becomes complete. The arm can then be raised only to the horizontal, but a full range of passive movement is found at the scapulohumeral joint. Examination of the scapular movements then shows that rotation and elevation are not possible, i.e. that the limitation of elevation of the arm is dependent on fixation of the scapula.

Puzzling signs may accompany strain of the conoid and trapezoid ligaments, such as may continue to cause pain after a fractured clavicle. The extremes of all passive scapular and arm movements often bring on discomfort felt at mid-clavicle. None of the resisted movements hurt, including depression of the scapula, thus exculpating the subclavius muscle. Tenderness should be sought along the anterosuperior edge of the coracoid process, while the patient holds the scapulae well approximated, so as to bring the process into prominence. If nothing is found there, a lesion at the ligamentous insertion on the inferior aspect of the clavicle can be identified only by local anaesthesia. Once the right spot is singled out, one steroid infiltration should suffice.

*These figures date from before my use of triamcinolone.

## Treatment

Since no muscle effectively spans the acromioclavicular joint, the patient cannot voluntarily stabilize it after a sprain. Even less can he hold it too still, in such a way as to lead to the formation of post-traumatic adhesions. Hence this joint is always treated by rest rather than movement.

### Recent Case without Subluxation

All that is required is to get rid of the post-traumatic inflammatory reaction. Triamcinolone is therefore injected, care being taken to deal with the inferior aspect of the joint no less than the rest. The patient should be symptom-free after two days and fit then to return to full activity.

Although the bones lie so superficially, the joint line is tiny and difficult to palpate except in thin subjects. The right spot is thus difficult to identify, and it assists to have the patient's arm, his elbow by his side, held in full lateral rotation by an assistant, so as to distract the clavicle from the acromion as far as possible.

The area of tenderness lying superiorly and anteriorly is mapped out and infiltrated all over, using 2 ml of triamcinolone suspension.

The inferior acromioclavicular ligament is now injected by putting a 2.5 cm needle vertically into the joint and pushing on it until the resistance of the ligament is encountered on the far side. A drop is injected at half a dozen different places along the ligament, by altering the angle of the needle at each little withdrawal and reinsertion.

Occasionally, the trapezoid and conoid ligaments require infiltration. If so, the clavicular insertions are most readily reached by fully elevating the arm. This rotates the clavicle until its inferior surface faces forwards and 2 ml of triamcinolone can be injected in a linear manner over 3 cm, starting just medial to the joint line.

### Recent Case with Subluxation

In addition to the steroid injection, relief from tension is required. The arm should, therefore, be supported in a sling for a few days, so that its weight does not pull the clavicle and acromion apart. Strapping should be applied from the lower sternum, passing over the joint and reaching the lower ribs behind (Fig. 49) and kept on for ten days. Exercises are contraindicated except that, as always, a full range of movement is maintained daily at the shoulder joint if the patient is more than 40 years of age.

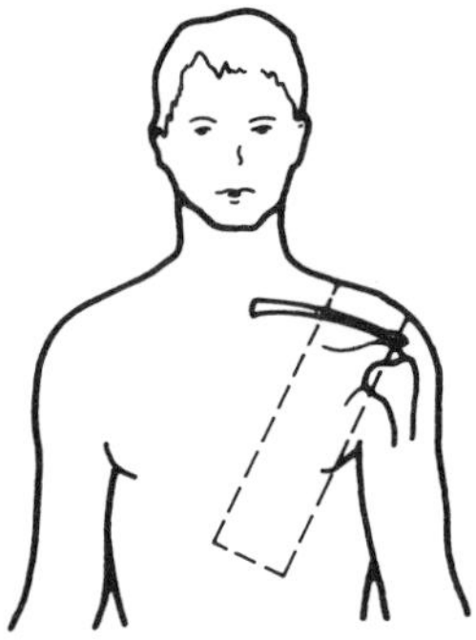

**Fig. 49.** Strapping for the acromioclavicular joint. The strapping passes from the lower ribs, over the joint, to the lower scapular area.

Naturally enough, the laxity of the ligament persists indefinitely, but so long as there is no pain, there is no appreciable disability.

### Osteoarthrosis

The shoulder is apt to ache after overwork, e.g. digging, and sometimes after a spell of overuse goes on aching. Such a persistent ache can be dispelled by an injection of triamcinolone, but the condition of the joint has not been altered and the patient must be warned that further exertion will lead to relapse.

CHAPTER 11

# THE SHOULDER: TREATMENT*

The shoulder is a most rewarding joint when accurate diagnosis is followed by accurate treatment, since an effective remedy exists for nearly every disorder. In the past, many conditions at the shoulder were considered incurable. This was, and in part remains today, a justified view; for how to arrive at an accurate diagnosis at the shoulder was not known, and the diagnostic methods set out in the previous two chapters are still not practised widely enough. In consequence, even today, many easily curable conditions remain uncured. Patients are told they will recover without treatment in a year, which often proves a most inaccurate prognosis in arthritis, and even more so in tendinitis which may go on indefinitely. Further difficulty arises from the general but erroneous belief that tendinous lesions cause, or by extension to adjacent structures result in, limitation of movement. Clearly, if the earliest stage of arthritis is mistaken for tendinitis, it is logically assumed that the later supervention of marked limitation of movement results from extension of the alleged tendinitis. This notion, unfortunately, is widespread, undisputed and based on excellent authority—yet false. Clinical perseverance and determination to assess the function of each moving tissue in turn and abide by the interpretation that applied anatomy warrants are the first essentials. Precise injection technique is equally important; for the shoulder is *the* part of the body where nearly every lesion responds well to accurately placed steroid infiltrations. No less indispensable is a physiotherapist fully conversant with frictional techniques for the tendons at the shoulder and in the manoeuvres involving stretching and distraction. Given such collaboration, there should be next to no failures.

## GENERAL PRINCIPLES

Treatment at the shoulder is a pleasure. The abiding problem is diagnosis. Once the right lesion has been singled out, almost every disorder is quickly relievable.

The objects of treatment are as follows.

### To Restore a Full Range of Painless Mobility at the Joint

There are four different approaches:

*Intra-articular Triamcinolone.* In recent traumatic arthritis, the injection may of itself suffice, the range returning spontaneously as the injections allay the synovial inflammation. If not, once the joint enters the stage when active treatment is indicated, stretching out should begin. In monarticular rheumatoid arthritis, the injections are enough in themselves. Stretching out is contraindicated.

*Stretching out the Joint.* This entails gradual and repeated forcing by the physiotherapist. The capsule is first rendered analgesic by the increased local circulation that follows short-wave diathermy. It is then stretched out two or three times a week until the range has been restored.

*Distraction of Humerus from Glenoid.* When the joint is unsuited to passive stretching, distraction may be indicated (see Volume II).

*Manipulation under Anaesthesia.* This is rarely required. When real indications exist, it is made much more quickly effective by injecting triamcinolone into the joint the day before. The post-

*A film on diagnosis and treatment at the shoulder has been made by Hirschfield and Cyriax for the manufacturers of triamcinolone in Germany. An accompanying explanatory leaflet by Cyriax has been translated into German and published as a short book. Doctors or physiotherapists wishing to show the film should contact Dr D. Chalmers, Director of Medical Affairs, E. R. Squibb & Sons Ltd, Regal House, Twickenham, Middlesex, England.

manipulative reaction is thus largely avoided and after-treatment shortened and simplified.

*N.B.* It will be noted that no mention is made of heat, diathermy and exercises. Though these measures are universally prescribed, they are worse than useless; for they fob patients off with the idea that they are receiving treatment and thus prevent the employment of swiftly successful methods.

### To Restore Painless Function of a Tendon

There are two approaches. One is to break down unwanted scar tissue by deep friction given across the fibres of the tendon. The other is to leave the scar tissue in being, but to remove the traumatic inflammation from it by infiltrating the lesion with triamcinolone suspension.

### To Abolish Tenderness of a Bursa

Procaine and triamcinolone can both be used for this purpose.

### To Get Rid of Calcified Material

Repeated infiltration with 2% procaine dissolves a deposit; alternatively, it can be removed by operation.

## CAPSULE OF SHOULDER JOINT

### Prophylaxis of Stiffness

This is most important, for stiffness at the shoulder is often as easy to prevent at the time as it is troublesome to put right afterwards. For example, when a middle-aged or elderly patient's upper limb is kept in a sling for some time for any reason, and no instructions are given about moving unaffected joints, the immobilization imposed on the shoulder joint is purely wanton. The same applies after hemiplegia.

Post-traumatic adhesions are very apt to form at the inferior aspect of the joint (see Fig. 37, p. 129) where damaged folds of lax capsule lie in contact so long as the patient keeps his arm to his side. Since this is what he naturally does in order to avoid pain, treatment by early movement is essential after any sprain of the capsule of the shoulder joint in any patient over 40. The joint movement is maintained passively; active repetition follows.

### Fracture

Examination of the shoulder in cases of united fracture of the surgical neck of the humerus shows that, when treatment by movement is not instituted at once, stiffness supervenes rapidly from traumatic arthritis. Hence, in this type of fracture it is not the broken bone that governs treatment, but the damage done to the joint by a force sufficient to break bone. Any bruised shoulder, whether associated with a simple fracture or not, should be taken seriously and treated by immediate movement. In fracture of the surgical neck, movement must of necessity be given passively for the first week. Since it is movement at a joint, however induced, that prevents stiffness, passive movements are strongly indicated. During the first few days after an injury, the passive movement may be possible over quite an ample range at a time when no

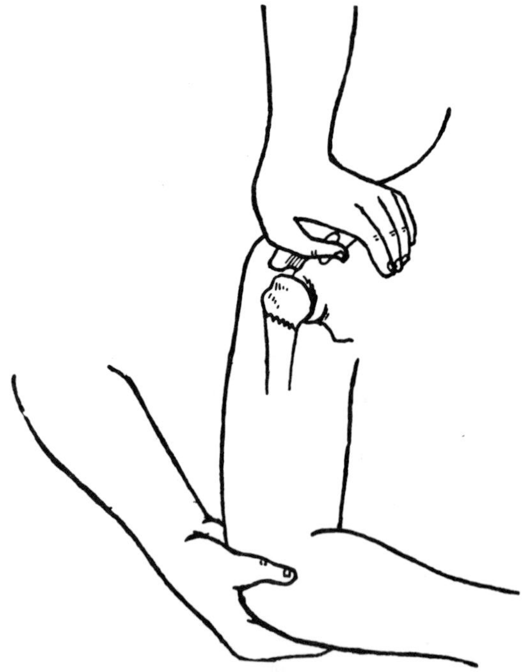

**Fig. 50.** Passive movement at the shoulder in a recent fracture of the surgical neck of the humerus. The bone ends are kept opposed by pressure exerted upwards from the elbow while the shoulder is held down. In this way a good range of movement can be maintained at the shoulder joint pending the return of active movement.

amount of encouragement induces much active movement. For the first fortnight after fracture of the surgical neck of the humerus, abduction is the principal movement to maintain. Rotation is more likely to occur at the site of the fracture than at the shoulder joint, and should therefore be avoided. When the abduction movement is carried out, the physiotherapist must place one hand on the shoulder and the other under the elbow (Fig. 50) and press the fractured ends together. In this way the humerus is made to move in one piece as the physiotherapist abducts it; there is very little pain, and movement at the joint, not at the fracture line, is secured.

## Treatment of Arthritis

Treatment depends on the type and stage of arthritis present.

When two disorders coexist at the shoulder, the capsular lesion always takes precedence. Until full movement has been restored, little advantage accrues from treating, for example, a tendinous lesion.

### Immobilizational Arthritis

If the arm is put in a sling for any reason, stiffness of the shoulder must be prevented from the outset. The older the patient, the sooner immobility leads to an arthritis. In recent hemiplegia, the patient cannot use his muscles to move the shoulder and the range has to be maintained passively until voluntary movement returns.

From the first, the patient must take the arm out of the sling night and morning and move the shoulder joint through its full range. If stiffness has already set in, the shoulder must be stretched out daily by the physiotherapist until the full range is restored. If the arthritis has got to the stage when such stretching is no longer effective, triamcinolone must be injected into the joint. Unsuitability for stretching is signalled by three criteria: the patient cannot lie on that side at night, he is in pain even when the arm is kept still and the ache spreads to the forearm.

After fracture the same stiffness results until the shoulder joint is stretched out by the physiotherapist a little more each day until the full range has been regained.

### Traumatic Arthritis

This can be avoided by early gentle forcing of the joint, which leads to rapid restoration of the full range of movement. Once limitation has set in, stretching by the physiotherapist remains successful if the signs of activity are absent, i.e. there is no pain when the arm is kept still, no reference of pain below the elbow, the patient can lie on that side at night and the end-feel is elastic. If these signs point to a degree of irritation contraindicating active treatment, the ordinary method of stretching aggravates symptoms but distraction by the physiotherapist is indicated (see Volume II). Better however, is triamcinolone injected into the joint to allay the inflammatory reaction at the synovial membrane. If the first injection relieves, the second is given as soon as its effect is passing off. Others are given at whatever intervals prove necessary. Since the intention is to keep the joint continuously under the influence of the steroid, the next injection is given *just before* relapse is to be anticipated. Hence intervals of a week, ten days, a fortnight, three weeks and a month are a likely sequence. More than four or five injections are seldom required. The pain subsides, and the joint enters the first stage again. If the range has increased spontaneously as the result of the intra-articular steroid injections, they are kept up until it is clear that recovery will continue spontaneously. If the joint reaches the first stage but no increase in range results from the injections, stretching is cautiously begun by the physiotherapist. If the joint tends to flare, triamcinolone is repeated and the forcing postponed for a few weeks. If all goes well, treatment can usually cease before full range has been quite restored, final resolution occurring spontaneously. Repeated intra-articular injection of a steroid suspension has never, in my experience (since 1953), caused an arthropathy, since it is not a weight-bearing joint. The techniques involved in entering the shoulder joint are described in Volume II.

### Osteoarthrosis

The presence of osteophytes and the crepitus indicating roughening of the surface of cartilage cannot be altered by any treatment. But the cause of pain is capsular contracture which may come on as the result of the degenerative process itself, but much more often results from minor injury or even mere overuse, e.g. sawing wood for some hours. Osteoarthrosis makes the joint very susceptible to outside influences, which easily evoke a traumatic arthritis superimposed on the symptomless osteoarthrosis.

Steroid injections have no effect on osteoarthrosis without a secondary traumatic element. The only effective treatment is gradual stretching of the joint. But the joint may not be in the first stage, in which case little can be done except wait until time has brought the joint into a treatable condition. Alternatively, the patient may be, as so many old people are, intolerant of any uncomfortable treatment; the disorder is then intractable. However, the results are good in those cases that can be treated actively.

### Monarticular Rheumatoid Arthritis

Even when fully within the first stage, this condition provides a permanent contraindication to forcing movement at the joint, whether by the physiotherapist after heat or, even worse, under anaesthesia. It is the existence of this condition that is the major reason for the gradual abandonment of mobilization under anaesthesia for what is almost always misdiagnosed as a 'frozen shoulder'. No one would force movement, still less under anaesthesia, at a hot and swollen rheumatoid knee or wrist; neither should this be performed at the shoulder, even though the capsule lies too deep for the heat and swelling to be detectable.

Intra-articular steroid therapy is strongly indicated; indeed, it provides the only treatment. All other measures are harmful, as no one knows better than I from the futile attempts that I made to help before hydrocortisone became available in 1952. The relief of monarticular rheumatoid arthritis at the shoulder affords one of the most dramatic results in all orthopaedic medicine. The patient, pale, miserable and worn out by months of constant pain and lack of sleep, finds that 24 hours after the first injection his pain when the arm is kept motionless has ceased, and that he can turn and lie on that side at night and sleep without difficulty. He comes again some days later, scarcely recognizable as the wan creature of the previous week. The joint is injected again. The principle is to repeat the injection just *before* it begins to relapse. A likely sequence is 7, 7, 10, 14, 21 days' interval between injections; six to ten will probably be required in all and, when the patient is doing well on monthly or six-weekly injections, they can be stopped. Though pain ceases, except when the joint is stretched, as from the first injection, increase in range is seldom noted for the first month or two, and is apt to begin only after, say, the fourth injection. The patient is asked to return at once if the interval between injections has been misjudged, the pain beginning to reappear before the allotted period has elapsed. Since monarticular rheumatoid arthritis tends eventually to recur at the other shoulder, the patient is warned—though he scarcely needs the advice—to come at once if either shoulder troubles him again.

Psoriatic arthritis at the shoulder responds well and quickly to intra-articular triamcinolone. The arthritis complicating lupus erythematosus takes a larger number of injections and the range may not be fully restored even though pain ceases; the same applies to the arthritis complicating ankylosing spondylitis.

Whatever happens to the range of movement, in all these different types of arthritic shoulder, pain is relieved and stays away as from the first injection.

For the three-day attacks of arthritis due to palindromic rheumatism, no prevention had been devised until Huskisson (1976) found that D-penicillamine in a dose of 250 mg daily was effective even in cases of three to eight years' standing.

## Recurrent Dislocation

When the humerus dislocates anteriorly this aspect of the capsule becomes overstretched.

R. Barbor (personal communication 1972) has carried out sclerosis at this area of the capsule in four cases, using 4 ml of the sclerosant solution and 6 ml of procaine. The front of the capsule was infiltrated with 10 ml of this mixture on two to five occasions, and the patient was asked to use his arm gently for two months afterwards, so as to give the fibrosis time to become complete.

The results were: a professional footballer who dislocated his shoulder at each weekly match reported freedom from recurrence a year later; a bricklayer who suffered almost daily dislocations which he was able to reduce himself had had no further trouble by nine months later. The fourth patient was untraced.

Operation can be relied upon to stop recurrent dislocation. of these, Bonnin's transplantation of the tip of the coracoid process appears to me the most logical.

## STRETCHING THE SHOULDER

This is not so simple as it sounds. If the physiotherapist does too much, she provokes a reaction that leads to a diminished range of movement, whereas if she is too gentle, she achieves nothing. Considerable judgement and care are required.

Heating the joint capsule by short-wave diathermy is a useful preliminary to forcing, since the temporary increase in circulation acts as an analgesic. The patient lies on the couch and the physiotherapist notes the range of passive movement, paying great attention to the end-feel. Discomfort is, of course, evoked when the arm is pushed towards the extreme of the restricted range. If sustained pressure can be felt to coax a little further movement from the joint, without increasing this pain or provoking the abrupt onset of muscle spasm, the joint should respond well to stretching. Again, this is likely to succeed if the resistance to movement begins before any pain is elicited. If, by contrast, pain and spasm come on sharply together, the experienced physiotherapist will refuse to force the joint, probably stating merely that it does not 'feel right'; for these sensations imparted to the hand are difficult to put into words. Assuming that she finds the end-feel satisfactory, she next forces the arm up for a few moments, then brings it down again. If the pain ceases at once it is clear that treatment can be reasonably strenuous; if it continues, a cautious start must be made. Her first treatment is fairly gentle, and at the patient's next visit she asks him for how long he was sore afterwards and assesses anew the range of passive movement. He should experience increased aching for one or two hours after the forcing, the symptoms then returning to their previous level. This period of exacerbation is her criterion, and she adjusts the vigour of her treatment to secure this result. This rule is a great safeguard; for not all shoulders respond well to forcing, even when fully within the first stage. If she finds the patient is still suffering from increased pain a day or two after his first treatment, it is clear that forcing has been ordered in error and that an injection of triamcinolone into the joint should be substituted. By contrast, if she provoked no lasting reaction at all, she must press harder, at times with great strength and persistence, to get her result.

This applies as much to the physiotherapist's after-treatment of mobilization under anaesthesia as to the gradual stretching out that is required in recent traumatic or immobilizational arthritis (to prevent adhesions forming), long-standing traumatic or immobilizational arthritis (to break adhesions) and osteoarthrosis.

If the physiotherapist is asked to increase range at a shoulder which the symptoms show to be in the third stage, or if she unexpectedly provokes an excessive reaction after her first gentle treatment to a shoulder in the first stage, it is clear that the ordinary way of stretching a shoulder out is inapplicable. The suitable technique in such a case is distraction of the humeral head from the glenoid fossa (see Volume II).

*Long-standing Cases.* After many days' vigorous forcing of movement by the physiotherapist without apparent effect, a loud crack may be heard as a discrete band parts. Thereupon, the range of movement increases and the pain diminishes. After an interval the same happens again. Thus, in these cases, the shoulder recovers by a series of sudden improvements punctuating stationary periods.

### Manipulation under Anaesthesia

This should be undertaken with caution, forethought and unwillingness. Occasionally in long-standing traumatic arthritis or osteoarthrosis *in the first stage*, it becomes immediately clear that fractional mobilization under general anaesthesia is required. In others the physiotherapist reports at the end of two or three weeks that even strenuous treatment is without effect on the range of movement or the pain. If so, forcing under anaesthesia should be carried out at once. The day before the manipulation, 2 ml of triamcinolone are injected into the joint, to diminish the otherwise severe reaction. A small amount of intravenous anaesthetic given quickly suffices, since only half a minute's relaxation is necessary. The patient lies supine on the couch. The operator brings the patient's arm up as far as it will go without forcing, allowing it to rotate so that his hand is pressing on the medial aspect of the elbow (see Volume II). Quite gentle sustained pressure suffices, the operator continuing his pressure until one large band of adhesions is heard to part; *no more should be attempted, and no endeavour is made to force either rotation.* This was an empirical finding, but now that Reeves has shown that stretching out rotation is apt to rupture the stretched capsule and tendon, the inadvisability of forcing these movements rests on a sound theoretical basis.

Reeves (1966) exposed two shoulders at operation and watched the effect of manipulation. Abduction was obtained when the inferior aspect of the capsule of the joint ruptured close to the glenoid attachment. He then forced lateral rotation and saw the subscapular tendon and the front of the capsule rupturing together. Curiously enough, there was no bleeding. A post-manipulative arthrogram showed the contrast material leaking out from the tear and tracking down the shaft of the humerus.

The physiotherapist's after-treatment is vigorous and lasts several weeks, i.e. until the full active range is retained between treatments.

It should be clear from the above remarks that *nothing is easier than to force movement at the shoulder joint under anaesthesia, whereas to know when to carry this out and, in particular, when to abstain requires great judgement.*

Manipulation has no effect in acute or chronic subdeltoid bursitis; a full range is found to exist under anaesthesia but the symptoms and limitation of movement remain unaltered when the patient regains consciousness.

## Operation

Intractable continuing arthritis at the shoulder is very uncommon. If all treatment fails and time brings no relief, arthrodesis affords a satisfactory solution. The patient retains 60° of abduction by rotating his scapula and becomes fit for quite heavy work once more.

Lettin and Scales (1972) have described two successful cases using the Stanmore cobalt–chromium prosthesis for severe long-standing rheumatoid arthritis. Relief of pain was immediate and a year later the shoulder joint was comfortable with increased movement. Reeves uses a prosthesis consisting of a metallic ball attached to the scapula and a plastic socket fixed to the humerus.

# THE SUBDELTOID BURSA

## Localized Bursitis

Every diagnosis of localized subdeltoid bursitis is tentative, since the signs are so often closely mimicked by minor degrees of tendinitis. Hence, confirmatory local anaesthesia is always required. The accessible portion of the bursa is palpated for tenderness, and the chosen spot infiltrated with 5 or 10 ml of 0.5% procaine solution, the amount depending on the size of the tender area. If no tender spot can be found, and the signs indicate that subdeltoid bursitis is undoubtedly present, the conclusion must be drawn that the affected area lies in the half of the bursa beyond fingers' reach, i.e. under the acromion. A longer needle is now used to infiltrate the bursa here. In either case, after waiting five minutes for the local infiltration to take effect, the patient is examined again to determine if the signs, in particular the painful arc, have ceased. If the right spot has been chosen, no movement now causes pain; if the diagnosis of bursitis is mistaken, or if it is correct but the wrong spot has been infiltrated, the symptoms persist. The procedure must then be tried again at another part of the bursa.

The diagnostic injection also provides the treatment. A couple of infiltrations at the correct spot with procaine solution are usually curative. If they fail, 5 ml of triamcinolone suspension are used, and, as the result of the previous diagnostic local anaesthesia, the exact spot to inject is known in advance. One, at most two, such infiltrations are always curative.

No physiotherapy has the slightest effect on subdeltoid bursitis. Manipulation is futile, for there is already a full range of movement at the shoulder joint.

Contusion of the bursal wall by a direct blow requires no treatment; recovery is spontaneous.

## Acute Bursitis

The severe pain lasts seven to ten days; hence the treatment described below is called for only if the bursitis has lasted less than a week. Since it is a recurrent condition, patients soon learn when an attack is beginning and should attend at once for repetition of treatment.

In acute subdeltoid bursitis the whole accessible bursal wall is very tender; it may even be somewhat swollen. The patient lies in bed, the entire area is mapped out and the skin marked to define the edge. He is now given a strong analgesic, e.g. morphine. The entire area is now infiltrated, a drop at each point, with 5 ml of triamcinolone suspension. Another 5 ml are then injected all over the subacromial extent of the bursa, and the morphine repeated two or three hours later. The next morning the patient wakes with rather a sore shoulder but with virtually no pain. Most of the movement has returned and he is able to go about his business. A few days later, if any aching persists, some small point missed during the diffuse infiltration may need injecting with, say, another 2 ml of the suspension. The obvious alternative is steroid phonophoresis.

This treatment aborts an attack but does not, of course, diminish the tendency to further bouts, which are apt to recur at intervals of two to five years. If the patient is seen after ten days, a sling should be worn for a week or two by day. By night, the patient is repeatedly woken because in bursitis involuntary muscle spasm is absent (unlike arthritis). Hence each time he moves in bed, his arm is shifted into the painful range. A figure-of-eight bandage round the thorax and the arm avoids this phenomenon and should be applied each night. Butazolidine 200 mg three times a day is particularly suited to acute bursitis and may be continued for a week.

## Bursitis with Calcification

### Acute Episodes

Although symptomless for years at a time, calcification renders a patient liable to attacks of acute bursitis; if so, severe pain accompanied by little or no movement at the shoulder joint results from a subdeltoid bursitis of sudden onset which reaches its maximum in three days. The treatment is the same steroid infiltration as for acute bursitis without calcification.

### Persistent Pain

If calcification gives rise to persistent symptoms—and a small shadow on the radiograph is no guarantee that it causes whatever symptoms attributable to the shoulder the patient may have—local anaesthesia is the treatment of choice. Whether the acid solution dissolves the deposit or acupuncture liberates it—indeed, the two actions may be combined—is uncertain, but the results are usually good. If 5 ml of a 2% solution of procaine are used, two or three infiltrations often suffice; weak solutions work less quickly. Radiotherapy is said to abolish pain and to lead to disappearance of the deposit, but did so in only one of a trial series of ten cases thus treated. Spontaneous disappearance of the deposit and of the symptoms may take place in the course of two or three years. This is not invariable, and deposits have persisted for up to seven years. Removal of the deposit at open operation is not often required, but is very successful.

## Rheumatoid Bursitis

This causes a prominent swelling at one or both shoulders and fluctuation is easily detectable. Bursae may also be swollen elsewhere. The symptoms are rarely due to the bursitis, but to associated rheumatoid arthritis at the shoulder joint. Aspiration can be performed and triamcinolone injected, but little benefit accrues.

## Haemorrhagic Bursitis

Aspiration, perhaps more than once, is all that is required. Immediate return of the blood after aspiration occurs in angioma.

# SUBCORACOID BURSITIS

Triamcinolone should be injected in the region of the bursa. Three or four infiltrations are often required, since great accuracy in the placing of the injection is unattainable. Nevertheless, they must be continued until the patient is well; for the condition may last many months, showing little tendency to spontaneous cure within the first year.

The tip of the coracoid process is identified. A spot 2 cm below this point is chosen and a needle 5 cm long long inserted backwards and medially, tangentially to the curve of the process and aiming at its base. When it strikes bone at the neck of the scapula, it is pulled back 1 cm. The area hereabouts is infiltrated with 2 ml of triamcinolone suspension by a series of withdrawals and reinsertions at a slightly different angle.

# TENDONS AND MUSCLES

General principles apply at the shoulder. Tendinous lesions respond to triamcinolone, which disinflames the painful scar; massage breaks up the scar tissue itself and is also effective, but is more painful and takes longer. Lesions of a muscle belly are rare at the shoulder, but when they do occur, deep transverse massage is quickly curative. No other treatment exists.

Nowadays athletes may refuse injections of steroid suspensions into tendons for fear of rupture later. This has not happened to any of my patients over the last 25 years, but the technique that I recommend—about 20 tiny droplets injected along the whole affected area of tendon, about 1 ml in all—bears little resemblance to the injection of a larger quantity all in one spot and with a thicker needle. This might well have a disrupting effect on the tendon locally.

## Supraspinatus Tendon

### Tendinitis

This common lesion often shows no tendency to spontaneous recovery, and cases of many years' standing are encountered. Hence this otherwise trivial lesion may make a man permanently unfit for heavy work or unable to follow his favourite sport. Yet, cure is simple.

The tendon may be affected at:

1. The superficial aspect of the tenoperiosteal junction, anteriorly or posteriorly.
2. The deep aspect of the tenoperiosteal junction.
3. The musculotendinous junction.

At the tendon, triamcinolone is the treatment of choice; the alternative is deep massage which is naturally more effective when the superficial rather than the deep fibres of the tendon are affected. At the musculotendinous junction, only massage avails (see Volume II). Local anaesthesia is required in diagnosis, since only a few supraspinatus lesions lie at this point, but it affords no lasting benefit. Surgical removal of the acromion used to be carried out for supraspinatus tendinitis, but is now out of date; for it abolishes the painful arc leaving the tendinitis unaltered. It thus helps only a little. It also has the unintentional merit of improving access for the physiotherapist's finger, and has thus facilitated cure both of infraspinatus and of supraspinatus tendinitis with greater ease than in unoperated cases. The position of the arm during injection is the same as for massage (see Volume II).

### Partial Rupture

Difficulty arises when the tendon contains a button-hole gap. This is suspected when the resisted movement is both painful and weak. When the needle is inserted, the expected resistance is lacking and the intact strips of tendon on either side must be sought. Introducing triamcinolone into the tear is useless; it is the intact remnants that are the source of pain.

### Calcification in the Tendon

The first approach is to ignore the calcification and merely inject the tendon itself in the ordinary way, since the lesion may be adjacent to the area of calcification and not due to the deposit at all. But a large deposit may cause symptoms; if so, an endeavour must be made to get rid of it. No notice need be taken of tiny nodes visible radiographically; they have no significance.

Local anaesthesia should be induced at the deposit once every week or two until the symptoms cease; two to four infiltrations of 5 cc 2% procaine usually suffice. The acid solution of procaine hydrochloride dissolves the deposit which becomes absorbed.

In the event of the injections failing, removal of the deposit at open operation is curative.

### Complete Rupture

The immediate objective is to get rid of the painful arc. To this end triamcinolone is injected into the tendinous remnants at the humeral tuberosity to destroy their sensitivity. As soon as the arc ceases, the patient should be shown how to initiate the abduction movement of the arm by placing his hand against the outer side of his thigh and then giving a twitch to his hip and simultaneously bending his trunk over to the opposite side. The supraspinatus muscle alone initiates abduction; this manoeuvre swings the arm outwards to the point where the action of the deltoid muscle becomes effective and, since a painful arc no longer halts the movement, he can elevate his arm fully. If the rupture is of some standing, secondary capsular contracture from disuse may have supervened. If so, the physiotherapist must stretch the joint out until the full range is restored. Permanent loss of power of abduction is inevitable, but return to all but heavy work is possible within a few weeks. A patient with a light job need not take time off work at all.

Since supraspinatus rupture affects chiefly the elderly, surgery is seldom indicated. If it is decided upon, exposure of the belly usually shows that contracture prevents direct suture of the tendinous remnants. If so, the belly is freed and slid along the fossa until the proximal end of the torn tendon can be fixed into a cavity prepared for it in the humeral tuberosity. Debeyre (personal communication, 1968) followed up his cases for six years and reported 45% cures, 25% improvement and 30% failures.

## Infraspinatus Tendon

Triamcinolone should be injected into the affected part of the tendon, or deep massage given at that point.

The patient lies prone, propped up on his elbows (see Volume II). The body weight now forces the scapula to a right angle with the humerus, thus uncovering the tuberosity. The tendon is identified below the lateral aspect of the spine of the scapula and followed along to the humeral head. If a painful arc exists, the lesion lies distally and superficially; if there is no such localizing sign, the tendon is palpated for tenderness. If no part of the tendon is more sensitive than another, the first point to try is the deep aspect of the tenoperiosteal junction (see Volume II).

## Subscapular Tendon

Massage at the subscapular tendon is more painful and less successful than at the spinatus tendons. It is thus a fortunate circumstance that triamcinolone is particularly effective here. Indeed, a small investigation of the results of steroid injection in subscapular tendinitis showed that one single infiltration of triamcinolone gave relief in every instance, whereas at the other tendons the first injection cured only half of all cases. The technique involved is discussed in Volume II.

## Recurrent Tendinitis

It sometimes happens that the recovery from supraspinatus, infraspinatus or subscapular tendinitis proves temporary, the symptoms returning after some months after the steroid injection. If so, the first approach is to try to get rid of the scar by deep friction. The second is to give several injections each timed a fortnight or so before the recurrence is due. If these two measures fail, the tendon can be infiltrated with the same hypertonic glucose solution as is used for the lumbar ligaments. The intention now is to provoke denser fibrous tissue—a stronger scar. The patient must expect a week's considerable soreness after the injection.

## Bicipital and Pectoral Tendon

Tendinitis of the long head of biceps, even of years' standing, recovers with two to four sessions of transverse friction. Therefore, no alternative treatment seems worth considering. Strain of the tendinous insertion of the pectoralis major at the edge of the bicipital groove is also best treated by deep friction, but recovers more slowly. However, infiltration with a steroid all along the edge would clearly prove very difficult technically.

When the bicipital tendon is affected at its insertion at the uppermost point of the glenoid, triamcinolone is injected there (see Volume II).

## Pectoralis Major and Latissimus Dorsi Bellies

Local anaesthesia usually has a good lasting therapeutic effect on lesions of the belly of these two muscles; should it fail, deep massage is quickly effective.

## Contracture of the Costocoracoid Fascia

This is a disorder for which no conservative treatment exists. Stretching the arm into elevation causes several days' increased pain, but does no permanent good or harm. In one case, operative division of the costocoracoid fascia and the tendon of the pectoralis minor, kindly carried out by my surgical colleague D. R. Urquhart, proved curative.

If the contracture is secondary to apical fibrosis of the lung, it is best left alone.

# SUBLUXATION OF THE HUMERAL HEAD

When a false painful arc occurs at the shoulder as the result of subluxation upwards of the head of the humerus during abduction, the patient must be taught how to depress the bone as the arm goes up. He can avoid the upward movement by using his pectoralis major and latissimus dorsi muscles; the physiotherapist teaches him how to do this.

CHAPTER 12

# THE ELBOW

There is no line of demarcation between the shoulder and elbow regions. Pain in the arm may originate at the shoulder with reference downwards, or less often at the elbow with reference upwards. Most pains indicated by the patient at the elbow or forearm have a local origin, since at the more distal part of the upper limb the capacity for correct localization is good. If he describes the pain as occupying an ill-defined area, it is almost certain that a pain referred from above is present. If the slightest doubt exists, the patient is examined from neck to fingers.

Once it is clear that the elbow region is at fault, the joint and the muscles about it are tested by ten movements.

1. Four. Passive extension, flexion, pronation, supination—full range, limited range, painful, painless.
2. Four. Resisted extension, flexion, pronation, supination—strong, weak, painful, painless.
3. Two. Resisted flexion and extension at the wrist—painful, painless. The muscles that perform these two movements arise from the humeral epicondyles and a lesion in either often causes pain felt at the elbow although the tissue affected is not functionally a part of the elbow (i.e. tennis and golfer's elbow).

## PAIN ON PASSIVE MOVEMENTS

The passive range of flexion, extension and rotation is ascertained and the end-feel noted. When extension is tested, the hard end-feel of the normal joint or of arthritis contrasts with the soft end-feel of an impacted loose body. If the passive, but not the resisted, movements hurt, the joint is affected. If the passive movements are painless, but one, or two compatible, resisted movements hurt, the trouble lies in the muscles thus singled out.

Early arthritis at the elbow shows itself as an isolated affection of the humero-ulnar joint. Passive flexion and extension are limited, but rotation is of full range and painless, showing that the radiohumeral and radio-ulnar joints are not involved. It is only in advanced arthritis that rotation is also limited. The *capsular pattern* at the elbow is rather variable, flexion is usually rather more restricted than extension, but sometimes the degrees of limitation are nearly equal. A 10° limitation of extension would correspond to about 30° limitation of flexion; 30° limitation of extension would correspond to perhaps 45° even up to 80° limitation of flexion, with this degree of arthritis some restriction of rotation would be beginning. Palpation of the joint may reveal warmth, effusion, synovial thickening, crepitus, or clicking.

Pain felt at the wrist on the extremes of passive rotation of the forearm incriminates the lower radio-ulnar joint.

The following types of articular disorder occur.

## CAPSULAR PATTERN

### Traumatic Arthritis

This shows itself in the humero-ulnar joint. After an injury of any severity to the elbow, flexion and extension are markedly limited and painful, but rotation is full range and painless. In other words, an arthritis exists at the humero-ulnar joint but not at the radiohumeral and radio-ulnar joints. Should rotation be painful in a patient with an acute traumatic arthritis at the elbow, the head of the radius is almost certainly chipped or cracked. The radiograph is then diagnostic.

The interesting question of the relationship between traumatic arthritis of the elbow joint and traumatic *myositis of the brachialis muscle* arises. On the one hand resisted flexion of the forearm does not hurt in traumatic arthritis; hence, there is nothing to suggest a lesion of the brachialis muscle. Moreover, flexion is limited, not merely painful at its extreme—a point at which a tender part of the muscle might lie squeezed between humerus and ulna. These two findings suggest that the brachialis muscle is not involved in traumatic arthritis. On the other hand, two conflicting facts emerge, both of which suggest that there is some connection. These are:

1. Traumatic arthritis may later lead to myositis ossificans. If the late stage is an obvious affection of the brachialis muscle, what was the early stage?
2. In traumatic arthritis, resting the elbow in flexion in due course restores the range of extension at the joint. This position rests the brachialis muscle and, were an irritative lesion present, should let this subside. Analogy with other joints suggests that, in a purely articular disorder, fixation in flexion is not likely to lead to an increase in the range of extension. However intra-articular steroid quickly abates traumatic arthritis; such an injection could not influence a lesion of the brachialis muscle. This finding has considerable medicolegal import, since it proves that myositis and traumatic arthritis are unrelated phenomena, though an injury may provoke either, occasionally both.

## Treatment

*Rest in Flexion.* Whether the lesion is of the joint or of the brachialis muscle may not yet be agreed, but there is no difference of opinion on the treatment, which is *rest in flexion.* The elbow is immediately immobilized in flexion by a collar-and-cuff bandage. If full flexion is no longer attainable at the patient's first attendance, the elbow is held as flexed as possible, and flexed more daily until full flexion is achieved. This position is held for, say, a fortnight; then the elbow is rested in slightly less flexion. If, three days later, examination shows the range of flexion to remain full, the forearm is allowed to drop a little farther.

Enough range at the elbow is usually regained after six weeks to enable the patient to wear a sling instead of collar-and-cuff bandage. At the end of two or three months, a full range of painless movement has returned to the joint.

Efforts to speed recovery by massage, exercises or, worse, passive stretching of the joint defeat their own ends. They lead to irritation of the joint and increased limitation of movement. They are widely regarded as encouraging the development of myositis ossificans, and it would be scarcely possible to defend a medicolegal action were this 'treatment' given and a bony mass found later.

*Triamcinolone.* Rest in flexion is still widely practised but is in fact out of date. All that is required is two intra-articular injections of 2 ml of triamcinolone suspension, the first on the day the patient is seen. The arm kept in a sling for a few days; and the second given seven days later. In about a fortnight the joint has recovered. If there is any blood in the joint, it is aspirated first.

There are many approaches to the elbow joint. A simple technique is for the patient to lie prone on a couch, his arm by his side and the forearm supinated. During full extension of the elbow the groove between the humerus and the head of the radius is easily felt posteriorly, and a 2 cm thin needle can be accurately introduced between them.

## Myositis Ossificans

It is widely believed that myositis ossificans results from improper treatment of a damaged elbow, i.e. by neglect of rest in flexion. My view is that the development of the bony mass is determined by the nature of the original injury. If the brachialis tendon is torn, rest in flexion, even from the outset, will not necessarily prevent ossification. If it has not been torn, improper treatment postpones recovery and increases pain, but does not cause myositis; a number of such cases have been encountered, some of whom had received quite strong manipulation from bonesetters.

In established myositis ossificans of the brachialis muscle, only a little movement to either side of the right angle is possible. Rotation is also markedly limited. The bony tumour is sometimes palpable and is shown clearly by X-rays.

No treatment avails, but the bony mass may disappear spontaneously in the course of two years. Excision of the bony mass seldom helps.

## Osteoarthrosis

This may come on for no apparent reason in late middle-age and is often bilateral. Alternatively, it may follow fracture involving an articular surface. Quite often the only symptoms are aching after considerable exertion and inability fully to extend the joint. Examination shows 5–10° limitation of extension and 10–20° limitation of flexion, the movement ending abruptly with the sensation of bone-to-bone. Coarse crepitus is often palpable. Forcing is uncomfortable rather than painful. This discomfort and the slight limitation of movement differentiate osteoarthrosis from the gross painless limitation of neuropathic arthropathy. In the latter, the radiograph is diagnostic. By contrast, X-ray evidence of osteoarthrosis at the elbow is compatible with full range and painless function at the joint.

As a rule no treatment is required. If overuse has superimposed a traumatic arthritis, an intra-articular injection of triamcinolone suspension is indicated.

## Monarticular Rheumatoid Arthritis

When other joints are also affected, the rheumatoid or spondylitic origin is clear. In acute or subacute monarticular rheumatoid arthritis, the joint is warm and the capsule thickened; this is best detected by palpation over the head of the radius laterally. Marked limitation of flexion, some limitation of extension and, in due course, some limitation of rotation supervene in the untreated case. The end-feel is hard and the wasted muscles spring into spasm when the extreme of the possible range is reached. After some years of arthritis a characteristic silken crepitus becomes palpable on movement, quite different from the coarse grating of osteoarthrosis. Decalcification and, later, erosion of cartilage are visible on the radiograph. Distinction should be made between involvement of the joint in Reiter's disease, psoriasis, gout, spondylitis, or lupus erythematosus.

Intra-articular triamcinolone is the only effective treatment and can be repeated as often as necessary. I have never encountered steroid arthropathy in a joint that does not bear weight. The injection stops the pain but does not usually increase the range of movement much. In the late stage of rheumatoid disease, relief from pain with maintenance of function usually follows synovectomy with, if necessary, removal of the radial head.

# NON-CAPSULAR PATTERN

## Loose Body in the Joint

A displaced loose body jams the joint, either preventing full extension but leaving flexion full and painless or preventing flexion and leaving extension full and painless. When extension is limited by the displaced fragment, the end-feel is characteristically soft; in all other disorders of the elbow joint it is hard.

### In Adolescence

From the age of 14, osteochrondrosis dissecans, less often a chip fracture into the joint, leads to exfoliation of a fragment of bone covered by articular cartilage. These loose bodies are often multiple and two to six fragments may be encountered at operation. They have three effects.

*Attacks of Internal Derangement.* The young patient describes sudden twinges at irregular intervals and attacks of sudden fixation of the joint that gradually subside in a few days. It is curious that, although the joint usually locks suddenly, it does not unlock equally suddenly with a click, as happens at the knee. The range of movement returns by itself gradually in a few days; in due course, this series of events is repeated.

*Growth of the Loose Body.* In a growing adolescent, the loose body may grow too. The fragment, whose osseous nucleus may have been 1 mm across at radiography at 14 years of age, may become a centimetre across five years later. It then jams the joint increasingly, and should be removed. The loose body is covered with cartilage and is thus always considerably larger than the shadow on the X-ray photograph.

*Osteoarthrosis.* If the loose bodies are left inside the joint, even though they cause no trouble, slight limitation of movement soon sets in at the elbow joint, and by the time the patient is 18 or 20, osteophyte formation has begun to show radiographically. There may well be 5° limitation of extension and 10° limitation of flexion at the elbow, permanently.

If, in the absence of obvious trauma, an adolescent complains of trouble at the elbow, this diagnosis suggests itself; for it is the common cause at that age. If the joint is locked at the time the patient attends, the mere fact this came on suddenly and is known to be transitory is significant; examination shows the non-capsular pattern and a soft end-feel. For the first couple of years nothing may be discernible between attacks, but the history is clear and the radiographic appearances confirmatory. By the age of 20, slight limitation of movement appears, due to osteoarthrosis, now with a hard end-feel between attacks, but a soft end-feel when extension is additionally blocked by the displaced fragment. Loose body formation is the only non-traumatic cause of osteoarthrosis in a young person; this fact alone suggests the diagnosis.

Manipulative reduction seldom presents difficulties and should be carried out (see Volume II). But removal is advised, since recurrence is very probable and, in any case, osteoarthrosis is a strong likelihood unless operation is done early. Admittedly, such osteoarthrosis is not at all painful, but limited extension at the elbow may interfere with a man's games or a girl's piano playing.

### In Adults

The patient complains of attacks of pain at the elbow. If a loose body becomes impacted, it may cause a constant ache or pain whenever the elbow is exerted; if so, the trouble is regularly ascribed to a tennis elbow. If such an elbow is manipulated in Mills's manner, a severe traumatic arthritis may be provoked. The distinction is therefore important.

There are two possible sites for the fragment. If the loose body lies in the triangle between humerus, ulna and radial head, it limits extension, while flexion is full and painless. Extension has a soft end-feel, and the limitation does not exceed a few degrees. If it lies between the coronoid process and the anterior aspect of the humerus, it limits flexion, extension being free and painless. Flexion has a hard end-feel, but is not as painful as in arthritis; it just will not go, since the coronoid process is engaged against the loose body. Flexion may be anything from 45 to 70° limited, at a time when extension is unaffected; a very clear non-capsular pattern.

When the attacks begin in middle age, osteoarthrosis does not supervene (at any rate within ten years) even if the bouts of internal derangement continue. At this age too, many loose bodies are purely cartilaginous (presumably chip fractures) and do not show on X-ray. Hence, if they show, well and good; if not, the diagnosis need not be altered; the fragment merely does not contain a bony centre. But to many, pain at the elbow and a normal radiograph in middle age suggests tennis elbow: an ascription easily disproved by clinical examination.

A loose body limiting extension can usually be reduced, i.e. shifted to a part of the joint where it no longer blocks movement and lies silently (see Volume II). If the attacks are not too frequent, this is all that need be done. If the patient prefers, and X-ray examination shows its position (and how many are present), removal is a satisfactory operation. Elderly patients' elbows do not take kindly to being opened; hence, removal is best avoided for fear of marked postoperative stiffness. Manipulative reduction must be carried out each time derangement occurs.

A loose body limiting flexion cannot be shifted by manipulation; hence treatment is removal or nothing, depending on the patient's age and preference. If nothing is done, the loose body may, it seems, become slightly embedded; in one patient with 60° limitation of flexion the day after the shift, there was only 30° ten years later.

## Osteoarthrosis with a Loose Body

Osteoarthrosis is often complicated by the presence of one or more loose bodies, displacement of which gives rise to attacks of pain seldom lasting more than about a week. These attacks are not abrupt, they come on in the course of hours and subside even more gradually. The history is indicative; an elderly patient complains of slight, long-standing aching in the elbow, punctuated by attacks during which the elbow loses most of its movement. Between bouts, examination reveals merely the osteoarthrosis (see p. 169). During an attack, gross limitation of recent onset usually of the non-capsular pattern makes the diagnosis clear. The radiograph is confirmative; for the loose body has a bony nucleus. However, it should be remembered that not all elderly patients with loose bodies in the elbow suffer attacks of internal derangement.

Manipulative reduction should be carried out (see Volume II).

## Sprain of Upper Radio-ulnar Joint

This is a rare cause of pain at the elbow. Examination shows that passive supination evokes the discomfort; the other passive movements do not and resisted movements at elbow and wrist are painless. The patient is always regarded as suffering from tennis elbow.

One, or at most two injections of triamcinolone into the elbow joint are curative within a few weeks. Untreated, or aggravated by active measures, the disorder is apt to last several years.

It should be remembered that in bicipital tendinitis occurring at the radial tuberosity, full passive pronation squeezes the tender tendon against the shaft of the ulna. Passive pronation hurting alone must thus not be regarded as an articular sign unless—unexpectedly—bicipital tendinitis is absent.

Limitation of passive pronation alone is a rare and curious articular sign. It appears to continue indefinitely and intra-articular steroids have no effect. I am not at all sure what the lesion is in these cases and regard it as incurable.

R. Clark of Ohio wrote to me in 1980 to say that his daughter had had a painful elbow, with limitation of pronation as the only sign. Radiography and all tests proved negative. Finally, exploration revealed a neoplasm which was resected.

Bilateral limitation of extension and supination since childhood can result from the subluxation of the hypoplastic radial head that characterizes the patella–nail syndrome. If so, the thumb nails are absent and the patella tiny.

## Ligamentous Sprain

Sprains of either collateral ligament set up traumatic arthritis; they do not show as an isolated lesion. Calcification in either collateral ligament giving rise to slight limitation of movement is rare, and is not amenable to active treatment. The radiographic appearances are diagnostic.

## Pulled Elbow

I have never met with a case myself. It occurs when children are pulled along by the hand too forcibly. The disorder is confined to children less than 8 years old. In 100 children with pulled elbow studied by Illingworth (1975) none was older than 6. The radius is displaced vertically downwards; this is best shown on a radiograph not of the elbow but of the wrist (which has been shown to me). The resulting articular disturbance at the elbow and the lower radio-ulnar joint naturally gives rise to limitation of movement and Magill and Aitken (1954) state that extension is 20° limited and that forcing is met by rubbery resistance. Corrigan (1965) states that the child holds his elbow fixed at a right angle. Reduction is immediately secured by rotating the forearm rapidly to and fro, while pushing the radius upwards towards the humerus by pressing the elbow against a wall; the click of reduction is felt on full supination.

# PAIN ON RESISTED MOVEMENT

If the passive movements show the joint to be normal, and the preliminary examination shows the region of the elbow to contain the lesion, the elbow is held at mid-range and the effect of resisted flexion, extension, supination and pronation is reported. The examiner must apply the resistance with his hand on the patient's lower forearm, for, should the movement be resisted by pressure against the hand, pain will also be elicited from the muscles controlling the wrist joint.

Pain may be felt or weakness discovered on resisted movement, always associated, except in rare double lesions, with full range at the joint.

## Resisted Flexion

When this hurts a lesion of the biceps or brachialis muscle exists. If, as is to be expected, it is the former, there is pain on resisted supination. Moreover, resisted flexion with the forearm fully pronated is performed only by the brachialis muscle, hence a bicipital lesion causes pain on resisted flexion only when the forearm is held actively supinated. When the biceps is affected, the lesion may lie at one of four sites.

### Biceps Muscle

*At the Long Head of Biceps.* The tendon is nearly always affected at the upper part of its extent in the groove on the humerus, and the patient states that the pain is felt at the shoulder. The only way to find out which part of the tendon is involved is by palpation for tenderness along its course. Local anaesthesia affords no added precision. Finding the right point is vital; for cases of even ten years' standing, that have resisted every treatment, are permanently cured after three or four sessions of deep massage, given to the exact spot (see Volume II).

If the tendon has been strained at its origin from the edge of the glenoid, a steroid injection provides the only treatment (see Volume II).

Rupture of the long head of biceps causes no symptoms then or later, merely a round ball of muscle at the lower part of the biceps belly appearing when the elbow is actively flexed.

Clinical testing does not even reveal any weakness of the muscles flexing the elbow.

*In the Belly of the Biceps.* When a few muscle fibres at the posterior aspect of the belly, pain in the arm on certain movements results which may persist for months or years. Spontaneous cure usually takes two years in patients who avoid straining the muscle during this time; in those who continue at heavy work the symptoms may go on indefinitely.

The area of tenderness at the back of the belly must be sought by pinching the deep aspect of the muscle between finger and thumb; palpation from in front is no help. When the probable site of the lesion has been found, local anaesthesia should always be used as confirmation; for exact localization is otherwise difficult. The injection sometimes does lasting good in recent cases, and in any case shows the physiotherapist exactly where to give the deep massage. This is quickly effective (see Volume II).

*At the Lower Musculotendinous Junction.* The pain is felt at the lower arm and palpation confirms its site. Local anaesthesia is usually required to confirm the diagnosis, but has no therapeutic value. Without deep friction, a lesion at this point in the muscle is apt to go on hurting indefinitely; for it has occurred at a point where the natural mobility of muscle is restricted by the presence of tendinous strands. The patient's active efforts merely strain the muscle afresh; there is no alternative to proper massage.

*At the Lower Tenoperiosteal Junction.* At this level the position of the pain is distinctive and a localizing sign exists. The patient complains of pain felt to start at the centre of the front of the elbow, radiating down the front of the forearm as far as the wrist. Resisted flexion and supination elicit the pain; so does full passive pronation at the elbow joint, especially when this is held flexed. This sign indicates that tenderness is evoked by pressing the tuberosity of the radius against the ulna; in other words, that the lesion in the tendon lies at the tuberosity. One infiltration with triamcinolone is usually curative. The alternative treatment is deep friction, but it is painful and takes several weeks (see Volume II).

*Ruptured Biceps.* A middle-aged physiotherapy graduate of mine has written to me that she suffered a complete rupture of the tendon of biceps from the radius. She felt a sudden painful twang at the elbow and lost the capacity to supinate the forearm. She could not feel the biceps tendon move. After ten days it was sutured and by six months later her arm was reasonably strong again. I have never encountered such a case.

*Weakness of the Biceps Muscle.* This occurs in fifth and sixth cervical root palsies; in the former, in conjunction with weakness of abduction and lateral rotation in the arm; in the latter, together with weakness of the extensors of the wrist.

### Brachialis Muscle

If resisted flexion hurts but resisted supination does not, the lesion must lie in the brachialis muscle. The tender spot is difficult to discover, and is usually at the lowest part of the muscle under the biceps tendon. Since steroid injections show that traumatic arthritis of the elbow is not a lesion of the brachialis muscle, the stigma attaching to massage of this muscle has been lifted. Even so, it would be unwise for medicolegal reasons, to give massage to this muscle, unless a full passive range of movement was present at the joint, or it might be falsely alleged that the limitation of movement was the result of the massage—a notion that some present opinion would support. In fact, massage to the affected area in a lesion of the belly is quickly curative.

## Resisted Extension

### Triceps Muscle

Lesions of the triceps are uncommon. If this muscle is affected, the usual site of the lesion is the musculotendinous junction; deep massage is quickly curative. If the tendon itself or the tenoperiosteal junction is affected, infiltration with 1 or 2 ml of triamcinolone suspension is indicated. If the olecranon is fractured, pain is severe and accompanied by gross weakness and marked articular signs at the elbow joint.

Pain felt near the shoulder on resisted extension at the elbow has the same significance as a painful arc. When the triceps contracts, the humerus is pulled upwards towards the scapula. If a tender structure lies between the humeral head and the acromion, this upward movement may pinch it and cause pain, especially in subdeltoid bursitis.

Weakness of the triceps muscle occurs in two disorders:

*Radial Palsy.* This is usually due to pressure from a crutch or sleeping with the inner side of the

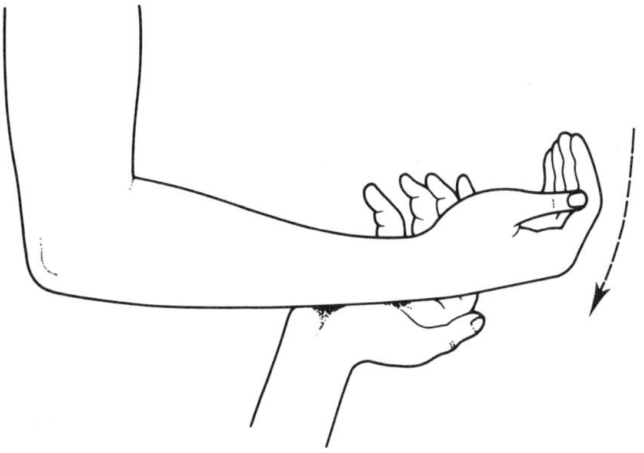

**Fig. 51.** Resisted extension at the elbow joint. The examiner resists the movement by pressure directed upwards at the patient's lower forearm.

arm pressed against an edge ('Saturday-night paralysis'). If so, extension of the hand is even more obviously weak; wrist-drop may result. By contrast with the obvious weakness, there is no pain.

*Seventh Root Palsy.* In sixth cervical disc lesions, the triceps may be found weak in isolation, or in conjunction with the flexor muscles of the wrist. The pain is severe, the weakness by comparison is slight. The neck movements set up scapular pain.

## Resisted Supination

If this movement hurts, resisted flexion must also be tested. If this hurts too, the biceps muscle is at fault (see above). If flexion against resistance is painless, the *supinator brevis* muscle is at fault. This ascription is confirmed if resisted supination hurts while the elbow is kept actively in full extension, thereby obviating contraction of the

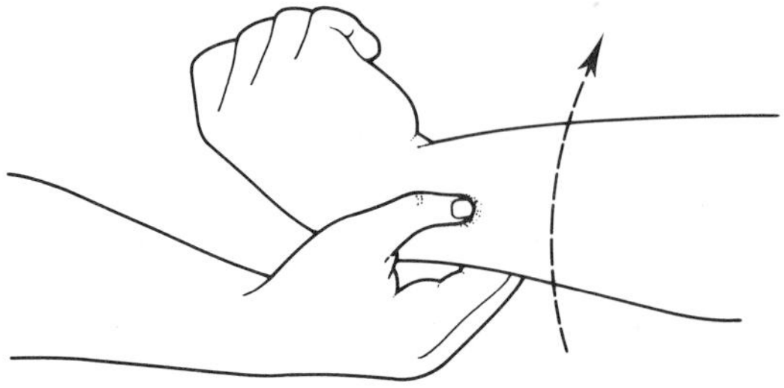

**Fig. 52.** Resisted supination at the elbow joint. The examiner resists the supination movement by pressure exerted at the lower forearm.

biceps muscle. Local anaesthesia induced at the muscle posteriorly between the upper radius and ulna confirms the diagnosis and is occasionally followed by lasting relief. If, as more often happens, the pain returns, deep massage soon brings about full recovery (see Volume II).

## Resisted Pronation

The common cause of pain on resisted pronation is a golfer's elbow. The origin of the pronator teres muscle merges with the common flexor tendon. Hence strain here deceptevely gives rise to pain on resisted pronation as well as on resisted flexion at the wrist. This should therefore be tested.

Very rarely, the lesion actually affects the belly of the pronator muscle. The tenderness is usually at its mid-point and a few sessions of adequate deep massage are curative.

Incapacity to perform alternate rotation movements of the forearm quickly is a most useful early sign in paralysis agitans. The first few rotations can be carried out fairly rapidly; after that, the affected forearm flags and finally stops.

# BURSITIS AT THE ELBOW

## Olecranon Bursa

Pain at the elbow may occur in the absence of any pain on passive or resisted movement. The pain may be provoked by leaning the elbow on a table, or on a flexion movement at the elbow only when a coat is worn. This is typical of olecranon bursitis, and tenderness should be looked for about the tip of the olecranon. A blow may induce haemorrhage into the bursa. Palpable thickening of the bursal wall may or may not be present, but it is very sensitive to pressure. Rheumatoid disease, gout, and chondrocalcinosis xanthomatosis affect this bursa.

*Septic Olecranon Bursitis.* As the result of a local abrasion of the skin, cellulitis at the back of the elbow may result. This involves the olecranon bursa which may fill first with clear fluid; eventually sepsis may set in and pus require evacuation. Miners refer to this condition as 'beat elbow'. In the earliest stage, when heat or redness of the skin are not yet obvious, confusion may arise, since resisted extension of the elbow is painful.

## Epicondylar and Radiohumeral Bursae

Two other bursae may give rise to vague symptoms at the elbow—the superficial epicondylar and the radiohumeral. Epicondylar bursitis in my experience, is always secondary to rheumatoid arthritis of the elbow joint. One bursa formed a large painless swelling which aspiration showed to contain 15 ml of fluid. In another, an area of calcification 1 cm across was shown on the radiograph. In none of the cases was an appreciably degree of pain mentioned. Radiohumeral bursitis can be detected only if calcification has made it visible on the radiograph and even then the distinction between this condition and calcification in the radial collateral ligament is by no means clear. Bursal affections have been mistaken for tennis elbow, but as no pain results from resisted movements at the wrist joint, examination distinguishes tennis elbow immediately.

Aspiration followed by protection is called for. When the bursa contains blood, aspiration suffices. Septic bursitis requires wide incision and antibiotics.

When tenderness or swelling persists, a bursa may be excised. According to Carp (1932), the radiohumeral bursa can be burst by manual pressure against the head of the radius.

Large round swellings attached to the posterior aspect of the shaft of the ulna about 4 cm below the olecranon occur in tophaceous gout, rheumatoid arthritis and xanthomatosis. If they cause annoyance, surgical removal is indicated. Multiple xanthomas gradually disappear on prolonged treatment with clofibrate, which reduces the plasma level of cholesterol and trigycerides.

# NERVES AT THE ELBOW

## Ulnar Nerve

Friction against the sheath of the ulnar nerve at the medial humeral condyle gives rise to little or no aching at the elbow, but to paraesthesia at the fourth and fifth fingers (Panas 1978). In recurrent dislocation of the ulnar nerve, the patient feels something go out and in at the elbow with a paraesthetic twinge. Structural abnormalities at the elbow, such as the cubitus valgus that may occur developmentally or as the result of a malunion of a condylar fracture, may cause friction here on account of the altered stresses on the nerve. Some cases result from a fall on the elbow, bruising of the nerve sheath setting up an irritability that elbow flexion habits may now maintain. Many cases are postural, the patient sleeping with his elbow bent up under him, or he may hold a telephone receiver to his ear for hours on end, or enjoy lying with his hands at his occiput. Wadsworth and Williams (1973) have entitled this disorder the cubital tunnel syndrome, and point out that the arcuate ligament, under which the nerve passes, runs from a fixed point at the medial epicondyle to a movable one—the olecranon. The nerve is thus subject to compression during elbow flexion. An uncommon cause of ulnar paraesthesia is a loose body displaced medially at the posterior aspect of the joint.

Examination in the first place reveals that the patient is not suffering from (*a*) a seventh cervical disc lesion; (*b*) first rib pressure on the lower trunk of the brachial plexus; (*c*) a ganglion in connection with the flexor carpi ulnaris tendon; (*d*) occupational pressure on the ulnar nerve at the proximal part of the palm.

An old injury to the elbow is soon apparent when the joint is examined. If the joint itself is normal, the elbow should be kept bent for some time; this may bring on the pins and needles. Unfortunately, no such test as stretching the nerve by a full radial deviation movement of the hand, while the elbow is kept fully flexed has proved helpful in diagnosis. Friction on the nerve trunk is suggested by finding tenderness of the nerve sheath; the two sides must always be compared. Thickening, especially in cases of recurrent dislocation, may be great enough to produce a spindle-shaped swelling of the nerve at the back of the elbow. Local anaesthesia provides the only satisfactory diagnostic criterion in early cases; in late cases, an ulnar palsy makes the diagnosis obvious.

If ulnar neuritis occurs apparently causeless, it should be remembered that such monoeuritis may result from diabetes or leprosy. In the latter case, the swelling of the nerve continues well above the humeral groove.

### Treatment

*Avoidance of Postural Strains or Pressure.* Keeping the elbow bent for any length of time, or resting the inner side of the flexed elbow on the arm of a chair or on a desk while writing, must be avoided. A cushion under the forearm to raise the elbow off the desk may suffice. The substitution of a hard for a soft arm to the chair enables the olecranon to bear all the weight of the arm. It is important to study the patient's daily routine and to explain to him which of his activities is maintaining the pressure.

*Traimcinolone.* An injection of triamcinolone suspension about the nerve desensitizes its sheath and can afford lasting relief, as long as conduction has not yet become impaired and structural changes are absent at the elbow. After the injection the patient must avoid the postural strains or minor traumas that originally caused the disorder.

The injection must be made not into the nerve but about it, since it is the extenal surface that is primarily affected. The patient lies prone, his arm by his side, palm on couch. The condylar groove is identified and a site 2 cm from it chosen. A needle 4 cm long is inserted horizontally and guided towards the groove. It reaches the edge of the bone and is then manoeuvred so as to lie deeply within the groove, between nerve and bone. Since the needle passes parallel to the nerve it will push it aside rather than enter it. One millilitre is injected here.

*Anterior Transposition of the Nerve.* When the frictional element is due to structural changes at the elbow, undue stress on the nerve cannot be avoided. Thus, in cubitus valgus deformity, transposition is called for without too much delay. Indeed, once ulnar weakness has begun, there is no point in waiting for it to become more severe before operating.

## Medial Cutaneous Nerve of Forearm

This nerve becomes superficial at mid-arm and supplies the skin from the inner aspect of the elbow as far as the wrist. It crosses over the median basilic vein at the elbow and is subject to trauma there by extravenous injections of pentothal. Numbness lasting some months results, but pain and hypersensitivity of the skin at the anteromedial extent of the forearm may continue for up to a year.

# TENNIS ELBOW

By tennis elbow is meant a lesion, situated near the elbow, of the extensor muscles controlling the wrist. Hence, the movement that hurts the *elbow* is resisted extension of the wrist (Fig. 53).

The condition is frequently misunderstood. Its notoriety with the public is due to the ease with which the layman arrives at a correct diagnosis, its frequency and its refractoriness to treatment. A tennis elbow may be provoked by any exercise involving repeated and forcible extension movements at the wrist—not necessarily tennis—and bears this name only because it was first described as a tennis player's disability. Indeed, in Coonrad and Hooper's (1973) thousand cases, only 5 % occurred in tennis players. Rarely, a direct injury to the epicondyle sets up a traumatic periostitis that the repeated irritation of muscle-pull prevents from subsiding.

## Historical Note

The tennis elbow syndrome has been recognized for a century and received its name more than 90 years ago. Renton (1830) described a patient with a pain along the outer forearm increased on using the hand whom he cured by inserting needles into the brachioradialis muscle. Runge mentions another case (1873). In an article on writer's cramp—from which he distinguished it—he cited a case of two years' inability to write associated with tenderness on the lateral condyle of the humerus. As rest for three months and electrical treatment had no effect, he cauterized the skin over the tender area and rested the elbow

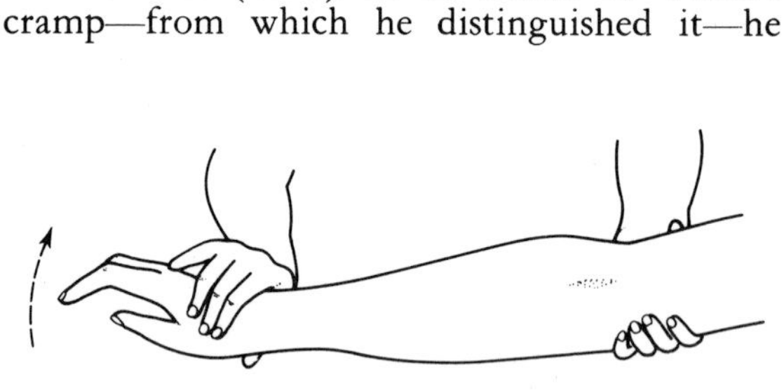

**Fig. 53.** Resisted extension at the wrist. When the elbow is held in extension, the wrist movement is resisted by the examiner's hand pressing on the dorsum of the patient's hand.

until the ulcer had healed; this took six weeks. The patient was now well, and remained so a year later. Runge ascribed the cramp to a traumatic inflammation of the periosteum in this position due originally to a forcible supination effort and kept chronic by the continual pull of the extensor muscles attached to the lateral condyle.

The condition was first named by Morris (1882), who called it 'lawn tennis arm' and noted its similarity to rider's sprain. An annotation in the *Lancet* (1885) drew attention to the number of sufferers from 'tennis elbow' whose plaintive letters had recently appeared in the lay press. Remak (1894) and Bernhardt (1896) agreed that it was a periosteal tear due to occupational overuse of the extensor muscles arising from the lateral condyle; the latter had collected 30 cases. Coudere (1896) called it a ruptured epicondylar tendon: Féré (1897) 'epicondylalgie'; Franke (1910) 'epicondylitis'. Osgood (1922) suggested radiohumeral bursitis, thereby incriminating the bursa described by Monro in 1788. Schmidt (1921), on the other hand, believed the fault to lie in the superficial epicondylar bursa, first described by Schreger in 1825. On the whole, English writers have called it 'tennis elbow' while continental authors have preferred 'epicondylitis'. The former name is preferable, since in by no means every tennis elbow does the lesion lie at the epicondyle.

In my paper on tennis elbow (Cyriax 1936), I collected no less than 26 different lesions to which the condition had been attributed by 91 authors during the previous 63 years. To this list can now be added another. In 1972 Roles and Maudesley put forward the concept of 'radial tunnel syndrome' thus reviving the description of 'radial neuritis' of Winkworth (1883). They relieved 35 of 38 hitherto intractable patients by operative release of the radial nerve in its passage between the brachioradialis muscle, the extensores carpi radialis and the radiohumeral joint. In the cases they describe, the outstanding sign was pain felt at the elbow on resisted extension of the long finger.

## Pain

Pain starts at the outer side of the elbow when, as in nine patients out of ten, the lesion lies at the common extensor tendon; and the patient has usually found for himself that the epicondyle is tender. The pain is referred along the back of the forearm often as far as the wrist and the dorsum of the hand. Occasionally, the long and ring fingers also ache. Rarely, there is no pain in the forearm, the pain spreading up from the elbow to the shoulder. The pain is brought on by grasping and lifting—indeed, by any exertion involving extension of the wrist; sometimes there is also a constant ache, worse at night, with stiffness of the elbow on waking.

At the moment when he gives himself a tennis elbow, the patient feels nothing. Some days after the causative exertion, he notices an ache in the forearm on certain movements. This gets worse and after a fortnight he cannot take a backhand stroke at all. It is thus not the tear in the tendon that causes pain; the symptoms result from the painful scar that forms later. Tennis is by no means the only cause of tennis elbow; a right-handed golfer gets a left-sided tennis elbow in the same way as a tennis player with a strong forehand drive can give himself a golfer's elbow. Using an axe, a hammer, a fishing-rod or even scouring pots and pans can strain the extensor muscles enough to lead to post-traumatic scarring. A curious feature of tennis elbow is sudden twinges, so severe that the grip is rendered momentarily powerless involuntary; the patient drops even a light object held in the hand, e.g. a teacup.

## Examination

My youngest patient was a nurse of 23; Boyd and McLeod's survey of 871 patients included one of 19, whereas Coonrad and Hooper's youngest in a series of a thousand cases was 27 years old. However, the common age for a tennis elbow is 40–60; it is thus highly probable that any patient old enough to suffer from this disorder will have X-ray evidence of 'cervical spondylosis' as well. Hence the view has been expressed that tennis elbow is a result of such 'spondylosis'. No one denies that pain in the elbow can arise from the neck, but it is impossible for pain in the elbow evoked by wrist movements to have such an origin. Hence clinical examination distinguishes the two sources.

Whatever the type of tennis elbow, on examination, although the elbow hurts, there is nothing amiss at the joint or the muscles controlling it. The negative signs are that passive movement of the elbow is of full range and painless and the resisted movements of the elbow are of full power and painless. The positive sign is that the pain at the elbow is reproduced on resisted extension, but not resisted flexion, at the wrist.

Care must be taken that the elbow is held in full extension while the resisted wrist movements are tested, otherwise a false negative result may be obtained. In the ordinary tenoperiosteal variety, the pain is such that the patient often winces and lets his hand go when asked to extend it vigorously against resistance. Further examination shows that resisted radial, but not ulnar, deviation hurts. If the fingers are held flexed actively so that the extensor digitorum is thrown out of action, the extension movement at the wrist still hurts. In this way it can be proved that the only muscles at fault in tennis elbow are the extensores carpi radialis. If, as is usual, the tenderness is at the epicondyle itself, the extensor carpi radialis brevis is at fault, since the longus is inserted higher up.

Two facts warn that one of the unusual sorts of tennis elbow may be present:

1. No wince: the patient can hold his wrist extended against strong resistance feeling pain insufficient to make the muscles give way.
2. A history lasting longer than a year in a patient under 60 years of age.

## Palpation

When it has been established by selective tension that a tennis elbow is present, precision is lent by search along the radial extensor muscles for tenderness. The origin of the longus is palpated above the epicondyle along the supracondylar ridge; then the brevis at the anterior aspect of the epicondyle; then the tendon level with the joint line and over the head of the radius; finally, the uppermost extent of the muscle bellies. When tenderness is sought here, it must be remembered that the brachioradialis muscle lies superficially and is always tender in normal people. Since it is a muscle not involved in extension at the wrist, such tenderness must be ignored and palpation confined to the muscles lying deeply to it (Fig. 54).

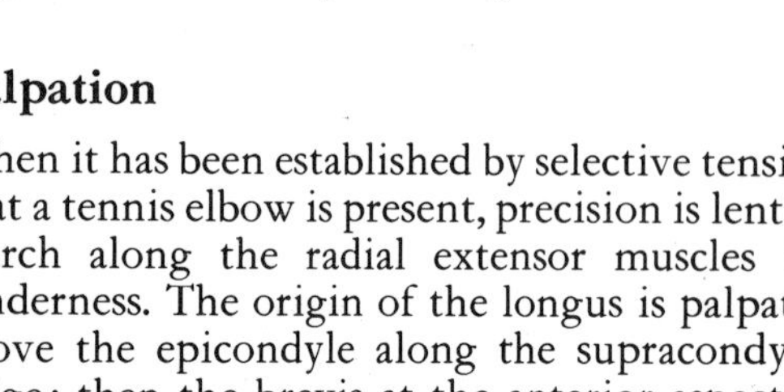

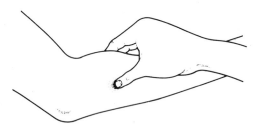

**Fig. 54.** Palpation of the bellies of the extensor muscles in the upper forearm. Since pressure of the muscle bellies against the radius is normally painful, the palpation must be carried out in the manner shown.

Palpation usually identifies the lesion at (*a*) the anterior aspect of the lateral humeral epicondyle, at the origin of the common extensor tendon from the bone, i.e. the tenoperiosteal junction—90 %; (*b*) the upper extent of the muscle belly, level with the neck of the radius—8 %; or (*c*) the supracondylar origin of the extensor carpi radialis longus or the part of the extensor tendon lying level with the head of the radius—1 % each.

Double lesions can occur in tennis elbow; the findings on palpation are then very difficult to interpret and diagnostic local anaesthesia may become imperative. Alternatively, the more obvious of the two lesions can be treated and the forearm muscles then examined again.

It should be remembered that, in cases of the tenoperiosteal variety, *associated tenderness* of the type well recognized in 'styloiditis radii' may be found at the *back* of the lateral humeral epicondyle. Since the patient's pain is elicited by a resisted extension movement at the wrist and no part of this extensor mechanism is attached to the posterior aspect of the epicondyle, tenderness here represents no relevant lesion.

In tennis elbow, the radiograph is normal.

# Pathology of Tennis Elbow

The muscular and tendinous types are examples of ordinary overstrain such as may occur anywhere. On the other hand, the far commoner tenoperiosteal type is an injury to which no exact parallel exists elsewhere in the body. Much evidence has been brought forward (Cyriax 1936; Garden 1961) to show that the usual lesion is a tear between the common extensor tendon and the periosteum of the lateral humeral epicondyle. Examination of the resisted wrist movements shows clearly that the trouble lies in one of the radial extensor muscles of the wrist. Since the tenderness is at the epicondyle, the fault cannot lie at the origin of the long radial extensor muscle, which is attached to the supracondylar ridge. Hence the tear lies at the origin of the extensor carpi radialis brevis muscle. In the early stages, just as often as the tear begins to unite, so often does the patient, by using his hand, pull the healing surfaces apart again. The result, as might be expected, is that a painful scar forms at the tenoperiosteal junction with self-perpetuating inflammation there. This view, first expressed in 1936, was confirmed by McKee (1937), when operating on cases of tennis elbow. My view was confirmed afresh by Coonrad and Hooper (1973) who operated on 39 patients, in 28 of whom a macroscopic tear was visible, as is clearly shown in their operative photographs. Lymphocytic infiltration and scattered areas of fine calcification were found on microscopy of excised tendon. Mills' attribution of tennis elbow to a lesion of the orbicular ligament was revived by Newman and Goodfellow (1975). They regarded fibrillation of the head of the radius as one cause of resistant tennis elbow. Division of the ligament and removal of abnormal cartilage from the radial head had good results in 19 out of 20 cases. In such cases testing resisted extension at the wrist would not have hurt.

The onset of a tennis elbow is always slow. This shows that the minor tear in the tendon is not itself a source of appreciable pain. It is only when endlessly repeated attempts at union have broken down again and again during daily use of the hand that chronic inflammation sets in at the scar and causes the symptoms.

### Spontaneous Cure

In patients with a tenoperiosteal tennis elbow, recovery seldom takes more than a year if the patient is under 60 years, two years if he is older. The uncommon varieties, with the lesion above or below the epicondyle, show no such tendency and often go on indefinitely. At the tenoperiosteal junction, a second attack is rare, and freedom from recurrence for as long as 25 years has been reported (Cyriax 1936). In Boyd and Macleod's series of 871 cases, the recurrence rate was only 3 %. Injection of any steroid inhibits the mechanism of spontaneous cure. Hence it is not uncommon for patients to remain well after an injection for some months and then to need another, and so on for several years. Left untreated, the tennis elbow would have got well by itself in 12 months.

Spontaneous cure appears to result, in a case of tenoperiosteal tear, from a gradual widening of the gap between the two edges. Finally, the two surfaces cease to lie in apposition and tension on the scar ceases. The gap now fills with fibrous tissue and heals with *permanent lengthening*. In consequence much strain no longer falls on that part of the tendon connected to the extensor carpi radialis brevis muscle. Recurrence is prevented by this structural alteration. Moreover, several muscles are attached here; hence slight permanent lengthening of the section of tendon relevant to only one muscle does not weaken the power to control the wrist.

## Treatment

The different types of tennis elbow need different treatment. This fact is by no means widely appreciated, all tennis elbows being regarded as requiring treatment directed to the epicondyle, owing to the idea that there exists only one type of tennis elbow—tenoperiosteal. This is the common variety, it is true, but there are three other positions for the lesion, accounting for 10 % of all cases.

### Tenoperiosteal Variety

This is the common site for the painful scar. Three different approaches exist:

1. To stop the inflammatory process within the scar by means of a steroid infiltration.
2. To separate the two surfaces which the scar joins, by means of manipulation or tenotomy.
3. To engulf the scar in a mass of further and more extensive scarring, by means of a sclerosant infiltration.

Before treatment, the patient, if less than 60 years old, should be told that spontaneous cure is highly probable within a year. He may, if he knows this, prefer merely to wait, sparing his elbow as much as possible meanwhile.

*Injection of Triamcinolone.* Since hydrocortisone was first suggested for tennis elbow (Cyriax & Troisier 1952), there have been many cases in which various steroids have been injected without success; yet an injection of triamcinolone suspension has proved curative. It is clear, therefore, that many different techniques exist, some of them unsatisfactory. Dingle et al (1978) showed that when a steroid suspension with a liposome covering is injected into an animal's inflamed joint, the effect lasts longer and is fifty to five hundred times more than the same dose without the liposome envelope. This encouraged me to write to them offering to try this preparation on tennis elbow, but so far permission has not been obtainable for human use.

Hydrocortisone is not the steroid of choice. It is successful, but causes two days' severe after-pain, whereas triamcinolone is just as effective and sets up much less discomfort, for only 12–24 hours. The injection procedure is described in Volume II.

*Manipulation.* The intention is to pull apart the two edges of the tear and thus relieve the painful scar lying between them from tension, imitating the mechanism of spontaneous recovery. This allows the self-perpetuating post-traumatic inflammation to subside, and healing with permanent lenthening. Henceforth the intact part of the tendon takes all the strain, thus affording protection against the recurrences that are sometimes a problem when steroids are used. The method is that described by Mills in 1928. His intention was to shift the annular ligament, which he regarded as out of place, in fact, it applies the greatest possible stretch to the extensor carpi radialis muscles, and, carried out with a sharp jerk, tends to open the tear in the tendon and abolish tension on the tender scar by converting a tear shaped like a V into separation of the torn surfaces, i.e. a U (see Volume II).

*Sclerosis.* When a tenoperiosteal tennis elbow keeps recurring, sclerosis is called for. The intention is now reversed—no longer the removal of inflammation in the scar by steroid infiltration, but provoking dense adhesions engulfing the scar by the irritant effect of hypertonic glucose.

It is given in the same way as the injection of triamcinolone, but the patient is warned to expect severe soreness for two days and some exacerbation lasting two weeks. One injection is usually enough; if it is not followed by success, a second is unlikely to help.

*Tenotomy.* If a tenoperiosteal tennis elbow proves incurable and goes on for several years, the only treatment left is tenotomy (Hohmann 1926). This appears to cure about half of all cases submitted to open division. Garden (1961) lengthens the extensor carpi radialis tendon just above the wrist rather than at the epicondyle. Newman and Goodfellow (1975) opened the elbow joint in 25 patients with resistant tennis elbow and found abnormality of the cartilage covering the head of the radius in 20 instances. Division of the orbicular ligament and removal of the fibrillated areas afforded a good result in 19 cases. These successes give further point to my contention (1936) that all operations on the outer aspect of the elbow, on whatever pathological premise they are based, are curative.

Subcutaneous tenotomy under local anaesthesia is very simple. The skin over the epicondyle is infiltrated with 1 ml of 2% procaine and another 1 ml is used for the common extensor tendon. After a minute, resisted extension at the wrist is tested; if the correct spot has been infiltrated, this movement has become quite painless. The tenotome is then thrust through the skin and the tendon divided down to the bony epicondyle across its whole width. Mill's manipulation is then carried out to ensure complete separation of the two cut ends.

This little operation is not always successful although it is difficult to understand how division—open or closed—can fail. However, a happy result in these failures is that a lesion hitherto refractory to steroids becomes amenable, and cure results from one or two further injections of triamcinolone.

*Cock-up Splintage.* Distraction by muscle pull of the two edges of the tear can be prevented by immobilization of the wrist (not the elbow) in full extension in a splint or in a plaster cast; the elbow must not be included. This treatment is worth a trial if the history is short, say a month or less. The plaster splint should be retained until attempted extension of the hand against the resistance of the cast is painless. If this is not being achieved by the end of two months, the immobilization is hardly worth continuing. The only theoretical objection is that, since healing occurs without any permanent lengthening, the patient may develop a tennis elbow again later, but this also applies to steroid injections. It is a matter of some importance to professional tennis players.

Cock-up splintage is sometimes called for in the treatment of tennis elbow in patients so neurotic that they cannot stand active measures.

## Muscular Variety

Local anaesthesia is the treatment of choice. Even though the patient may have had pain for five or ten years, two to four weekly injections into the right spot nearly always permanently cures. The great difficulty is to find the right spot and infiltrate it thoroughly (see Volume II).

## Tendinous Variety

The lesion lies in the body of the tendon, level with the head of the radius. Adequate massage is effective in four to eight sessions, however long the symptoms have lasted.

## Supracondylar Variety

When the origin of the extensor carpi radialis longus at the supracondylar ridge above the epicondyle is at fault, two to four treatments by deep massage always cure (see Volume II). This is the easiest tennis elbow to relieve; unfortunately, it is seldom encountered.

## GOLFER'S ELBOW

This is the lesion of the common flexor tendon at the medial epicondyle. In the right-handed, golfer's elbow occurs at the right elbow in those who play golf; at the left elbow the lesion produced by golf is a tennis elbow. Again, those who play tennis with a strong forehand drive can develop a golfer's elbow—and both disorders affect those who play neither game. The names are useful to indicate the condition, but they should not be given aetiological weight; they are justified only historically.

Golfer's elbow is less common than tennis elbow. In Coonrad and Hooper's (1973) series it was 317 tennis elbows to 22 golfer's. It is much less disabling. The pain is felt clearly at the inner side of the elbow and does not radiate far, seldom beyond the ulnar side of the mid-forearm. Severe pain on using the flexor muscles and paralysing twinges—both common in tennis elbow—are seldom experienced.

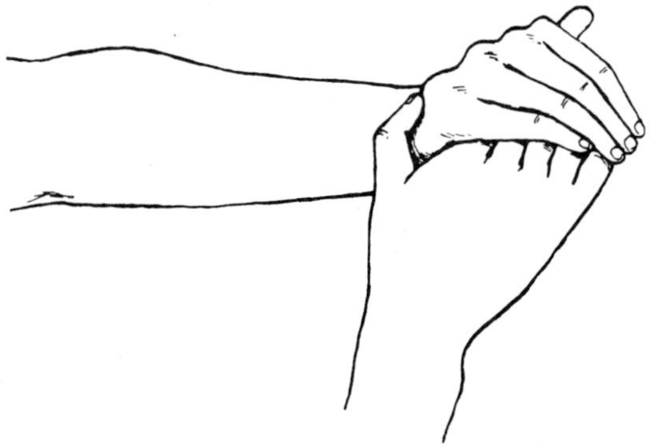

**Fig. 55.** Resisted flexion at the wrist. The patient flexes his hand at the wrist against the resistance of the examiner's hand. The elbow is kept extended.

### Examination

The signs are:

1. A full range of painless movement at the elbow.
2. All resisted movements at the elbow are painless except, occasionally, pronation, since this muscle takes origin from the common flexor tendon.
3. Resisted flexion, but not extension, of the wrist sets up pain at the elbow. Rarely, flexion of the fingers rather than of the wrist elicits the symptoms best.

*N.B.* The movement should be tested while the elbow is held extended, or a false negative result may be obtained.

### Treatment

The tenoperiosteal tear is best treated analogously to tennis elbow by a *local injection of steroid suspension*, thereby transforming a painful into a painless scar. The alternative is *deep localized massage* breaking up the scar tissue; this is not followed by manipulative stretching as in tennis elbow. Manipulation is without effect and in any case unnecessary; for the massage suffices. Indeed, tennis elbow is the only tenoperiosteal tear in the body insusceptible to massage alone, and the only one where manipulation has any effect. When the musculotendinous junction of the wrist-flexor group is at fault, the only successful treatment is adequate massage (see Volume II).

## ISCHAEMIC CONTRACTURE

Permanent contracture (Volkmann) of the flexor muscles of the forearm results from persistent spasm of the brachial artery, caught against the edge of the humeral shaft in supracondylar fracture of the humerus. The elasticity of the muscle bellies is largely lost and extension of the fingers remains possible only after the wrist has been flexed—the constant length phenomenon. Resisted flexion of the fingers does not hurt.

In a patient with such a fracture, the first sign of this complication is often pain in the forearm, increased on passive extension of the fingers. Then the radial pulse ceases. If this is lost after fracture at the elbow, and does not return when the patient is warmed, the artery should be exposed and painted with papaverine (Kinmonth 1952). For the established condition a muscle-sliding operation is required.

CHAPTER 13

# THE WRIST AND HAND

## LOWER RADIO-ULNAR JOINT

Lesions of the radio-ulnar joint are rare, and cause pain felt at the wrist only. Hence it is easy to forget the existence of this joint and to look only at the wrist. It is part of the routine examination of the wrist to perform full passive supination and pronation at the lower radio-ulnar joint, before examining the passive and resisted movements at the wrist itself. The lower forearm must be grasped when testing these two movements, to prevent any strain falling on the carpal joints.

Rotation through 180° is present at a normal radio-ulnar joint, the ulna remaining stationary as the radius revolves round it.

### Capsular Pattern

If both passive extremes are painful, arthritis is present. A mal-united fracture just above the wrist leads to osteoarthrosis later. If there has been no injury, non-specific arthritis must be present. Its nature is not at all evident; the only clear facts are: (*a*) all endeavours to stretch the joint out aggravate the condition, whereas (*b*) one injection of triamcinolone into the joint affords full, and nearly always permanent, relief.

In a patient who already has rheumatoid arthritis this joint may become affected too, often bilaterally. If so, triamcinolone is again effective, but may have to be repeated at six- to twelve-monthly intervals.

The patient's forearm is fully pronated; the prominence of the lower end of the ulna is now clearly visible. The joint line is identified by palpation, the examiner pushing the radius and ulna backwards and forwards on each other and feeling for the plane at which this occurs. A point is chosen on this line not more than 5 mm above the upper edge of the lunate bone, since the joint extends for only 1 cm upwards from that edge. A syringe containing 1 ml of triamcinolone suspension is fitted with a fine needle 2.5 cm long. It is thrust in vertically and strikes bone; it must then be withdrawn a short distance and a number of tiny adjustments made until it is felt to pass between the radius and ulna. The injection is then given.

### Non-capsular Pattern

Pronation is of full range and painless; supination is limited by painless bony block. This results from mal-union of a Colles's fracture and consequent shortening of the radius. The limitation of movement is of course permanent.

If this phenomenon is accompanied by pain at one or both extremes, osteoarthrosis has supervened. The symptoms are not severe, and a bandage about the wrist may ease discomfort. Triamcinolone intra-articularly is well worth a trial.

When tenosynovitis of the extensor carpi ulnaris muscle exists at the groove at the base of the ulna, full passive supination is apt to hurt for no very obvious reason.

#### Resisted Movements

When these hurt, the fault does not lie locally. The examiner must resist the movement by grasping the lower forearm, to avoid stress on the wrist. Resisted pronation causes pain felt at the upper forearm in golfer's elbow, very rarely as the result of an actual lesion of the pronator teres muscle. In my experience, the pronator quadratus is never affected. Resisted supination hurts at the elbow and upper forearm in lesions of the biceps and supinator muscles; again no local lesion is responsible.

# THE WRIST JOINT

Lesions at the wrist result from injury, overuse or arthritis, usually rheumatoid. The history is seldom distinctive, and examination, clinical and radiological must be relied on for diagnosis. Since pain is not referred appreciably from tissues lying at the distal extent of a limb, patients with wrist trouble know quite well that their symptoms originate there.

## Inspection

This may reveal swelling. If there is a history of trauma, fracture should be suspected; if not, rheumatoid arthritis, which is usually bilateral. A ganglion is visible and palpable, and can often be burst and can always be punctured, disappearance confirming the diagnosis. Multiple large ganglia occur in longstanding rheumatoid arthritis.

## Examination of Movement

Examination comprises 21 movements:

1. The radio-ulnar joint—two passive rotations.
2. The wrist—four passive movements; flexion, extension, ulnar and radial deviation.
3. The wrist—the same movements carried out against resistance.
4. The thumb—passive movement at the trapezio-first-metacarpal joint and the resisted thumb movements.
5. The fingers—resisted abduction and adduction. These movements must be included, since patients with a strained interosseous muscle at its proximal extent usually complain of pain at the wrist.

In tenosynovitis the evidence obtained when the passive movements of the wrist are tested is sometimes misleading. A movement that might be regarded as merely relaxing a tendon often, in fact, pushes it painfully down its sheath; hence the discomfort elicited in this way may be misinterpreted.

## Crepitus

One of the classical signs of tenosynovitis is crepitus. Fine creaking when the tendon moves inside its sheath indicates roughening of gliding surfaces such as follows overuse, and is common only at the abductor and extensor tendons where they curl round the lower radius. In hyperacute cases, the crepitus on movement may be felt even at the bellies in the upper forearm—myosynovitis. A much coarser creaking is palpable in tuberculosis and advanced rheumatoid disease. Crepitus does not have to be sought; it obtrudes itself. However, in slight or chronic tenosynovitis or in tenovaginitis, crepitus is often absent, and it must not be thought that the absence of crepitus shows the tendons to be normal or excludes a diagnosis of tenosynovitis.

## Passive Movements at the Wrist

Flexion, extension and ulnar and radial deviation must be tested. Limitation of movement in each direction indicates arthritis; limitation in two directions only suggests a disorder localized to one joint or persistent carpal subluxation. In these conditions the resisted movements are painless. The following disorders occur.

### Capsular Pattern

The capsular pattern is about the same amount of limitation of flexion as of extension at first. In long-standing severe arthritis, fixation in the mid-position supervenes.

### Traumatic Arthritis

In my experience, this does not occur in the absence of a carpal fracture. I have never known a case of simple traumatic arthritis last more than a day or two.

The clinical diagnosis of carpal fracture is usually simple, whereas the radiograph taken soon after the injury may reveal no lesion. There is a history of trauma, not necessarily severe. The whole wrist is swollen. Passive flexion and extension movements are limited by muscular spasm, coming on with a vibrant twang. The patient should be asked on which side of the wrist he feels his pain. If a passive deviation movement towards the painful side hurts more than that away from this side, it is clear that squeezing the carpal bones together causes pain: further evidence of fracture. Palpation of the site of tenderness shows which of the bones has been damaged. The bone most often fractured is the scaphoid, since it spans the joint between the proximal and distal rows of carpal bones. The above signs are constantly present and are more reliable in pointing to the diagnosis than the radiograph taken immediately after the accident. One taken two weeks later reveals the damage to bone. Fractures of the scaphoid bone require treatment by immobilization at once; hence, when the above signs are elicited, a plaster cast should be applied immediately, holding the joint in mid-position but in radial deviation; this posture ensures that the fractured surfaces are pressed together. A second radiograph is taken a fortnight later. So long as the diagnosis remains uncertain, physiotherapy, active exercises, etc., are contraindicated, since they predispose to non-union. In un-united fracture, Russe's (1960) bone grafting by the anterior approach avoids damage to the blood supply which enters the scaphoid bone from the dorsal aspect. Successful operation has been described 22 years after the fracture (McDonald & Petrie 1975).

## Rheumatoid Arthritis

This is common. In addition to the limitation of movement, the joint is visibly swollen, warm to the touch and the joint capsule is the site of much soft thickening. The chronic stage may progress to virtual ankylosis in slight flexion; the swelling then diminishes but seldom disappears and the local warmth ceases. The disorder usually affects both wrists, often after the fingers have been affected. Gout, dermatomyositis, Reiter's and gonococcal arthritis must be excluded.

In the acute stage, if pain is severe, immobilization of the wrist for some weeks by an Elastoplast bandage or a cock-up splint is indicated. In the subacute or chronic stage, triamcinolone is usually very successful. No attempt is made at intra-articular injection, but the areas of capsular thickening and tenderness are identified and infiltrated each in turn until the whole affected region has been treated. The actual injection is very painful, but the result, especially in the chronic case, excellent.

## Osteoarthrosis

Generalized osteoarthrosis of the wrist may follow severe injury, or the use of vibrating tools; in the elderly no cause is usually apparent. Limitation of movement without appreciable capsular thickening is accompanied by crepitus when the wrist is moved within the possible range.

The radiograph shows osteophytes and one or more diminished joint spaces with sclerosis of the bony margins. Diffuse cystic change may be noted. By contrast, minor osteoarthrotic change seen on the X-ray photograph is compatible with perfect function.

No treatment has appreciable effect; the symptoms seldom warrant arthrodesis.

## Non-capsular Pattern

*Persistent Subluxation of a Carpal Bone.* The sign that draws immediate attention to internal derangement at the wrist joint is limitation of movement in one direction only. This is found when carpal subluxation occurs at the wrist, muscle spasm limiting extension of the wrist while the other movements remain of full range, though not necessarily painless. The site of the subluxation is easily found by looking at the wrist when held in flexion (see Plate XI); the projection can be seen and felt with ease, and the ligaments about the capitate bone are tender, especially at the lunate-capitate and capitate-third-metacarpal joint lines. Clinically, the capitate bone has subluxated. However, radiography reveals no displacement. It is easy to argue that postulated osseous subluxations which do not show radiologically are imaginary; but the edge of the capitate bone merges with the others and cannot be visualized separately on the radiograph, nor can its position be measured against the superimposed margins of the other bones. Moreover (*a*) the clinical signs of an intra-articular displacement are clear; (*b*) the undue projection is visible on full flexion; (*c*) manipulative reduction is accompanied by a click and the immediate restoration of full range; and (*d*) there is a liability to recurrence. It has been argued that the manipulation ruptures an adhesion; but what adhesion placed at the dorsum of the joint can limit extension, and why should a ligamentous adhesion, once ruptured, lead to recurrence?

Manipulative reduction is easy to perform during traction and consists in separating the proximal from the distal row of bones and then gliding them anteroposteriorly (see Volume II). If the subluxation has been present for several months, some of the ligaments about the capitate bone remain strained and, though a full range of movement is restored at once, the extremes of movement remain painful. One or two sessions of adequate deep massage then afford full relief. A recurrence is treated by immediate reduction.

*Disorder at an Isolated Joint.* Three conditions give rise to solitary limitation of extension at the wrist, but all show clearly radiologically. They are Keinboch's disease (aseptic necrosis of the lunate bone), un-united fracture and isolated osteoarthrosis. In the first case, sclerosis and deformity of the lunate bone are shown by X-rays; at the lunate-capitate joint, localized disappearance of articular cartilage (seldom with osteophytes) is seen. Localized osteoarthrosis comes on some years after an un-united fracture, especially of the scaphoid bone. The projecting osteophytes can be seen and felt; marked limitation, more particularly of extension resulting. Sometimes there is little or no pain.

## Ligamentous Sprain

There are several different sites.

*Ulnar Collateral Ligament.* This follows imperfect reduction of a Colles's fracture, or fracture of the styloid process of the ulna. Inspection reveals the radius united with deformity, and examination of the passive movements at the wrist shows that only radial deviation hurts. Spontaneous cure takes a year; but an injection of triamcinolone is rapidly curative.

*Radial Collateral Ligament.* Sprain here is very rare and is characterized by pain felt only on the extreme of passive ulnar deviation. In fact, the condition usually present when a sprain here is suspected is tenovaginitis of the thumb tendons at their carpal extent. Trial of the resisted movements prevents error. An injection of triamcinolone affords lasting relief. Massage is also effective but several sessions are required.

*Lunate-capitate Ligament.* This is common, and may occur without subluxation at the joint; alternatively, it may persist after a subluxation of some months' standing has been reduced. There is pain felt at the dorsum of the wrist at the extreme of flexion, all the other passive movements proving of full range and painless. Search for tenderness reveals the exact site of the sprain. Deep massage is always curative in a few weeks, even if the condition has persisted (as it often has) for several years.

Differential diagnosis is difficult between a severe sprain of this ligament and a minor degree of bony subluxation at the lunate-capitate joint. In a doubtful case, no harm is done by an attempt at reduction, followed at once, if it is found that there is nothing to reduce, by deep massage.

Occasionally other ligaments are sprained; perhaps the radiolunate, the capitate-third metacarpal (see Fig. 56), or the ulnar-triquetral (cuneiform). The site of tenderness is always carefully sought, remembering that these sprains are often multiple, the search continues even after the most obvious spot has been found.

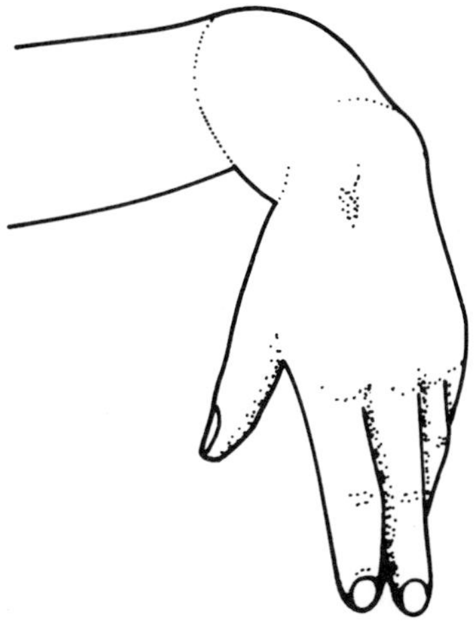

**Fig. 56.** Rupture of the capitate-third-metacarpal ligment.

Unless *all* the sprained ligaments are given adequate massage, the patient is condemned to a permanently troublesome wrist; for there is little or no tendency to spontaneous recovery and steroids are not effective at these ligaments.

Chronic ligamentous sprain at the wrist differs from that at all other joints (except the coronary ligaments at the knee and the deltoid ligament at the ankle) in that forced movements, with or without anaesthesia, afford no benefit. Indeed, they further overstretch the painful ligament and tend towards aggravation. By contrast, the scar can easily be mobilized by deep massage with recovery; all other methods are of no avail, including manipulation, steroid injections, many months' immobilization in plaster, or operation. Indeed, permanent minor disability will be avoided only when deep massage is recognized as the only effective treatment for these ligamentous strains at the wrist.

*Ligamentous Rupture.* This follows a severe flexion injury and leads to permanent instability of the wrist. The ligament that usually ruptures is the capitate-third-metacarpal; a depression can be palpated at this point on full wrist flexion, and the bone can be seen not to flex with the rest of the wrist. After a month, the symptoms cease, but recur if the patient exerts the wrist much. Care and a wrist strap are called for, but the joint remains unstable permanently; for the ligament does not unite and cannot be reconstituted by surgery.

A physiotherapist ruptured this ligament and kept subluxating her capitate bone. She was treated by three injections of the same sclerosing agent as used for the lumbar ligaments, with considerable increase in stability. Subluxation had occurred every month or two, but by being somewhat careful, there had been no attack for the year after treatment. The injection itself was very painful and each time the wrist remained sore for ten days. A second patient also proved a success. Subluxation had occurred almost daily for four years, but after two infiltrations he had remained symptom-free for six months. In a third case the injections proved a failure.

## Resisted Movements at Wrist

Extension, flexion, radial deviation and ulnar deviation at the wrist are all tested against resistance, with the elbow held in extension. If this condition is not observed, false negative responses may be elicited in cases of golfer's or tennis elbow. The resisted thumb and finger movements follow since the thumb tendons also move the wrist, and the interosseous muscles, if damaged proximally, cause pain felt at the wrist.

Pain elicited by the resisted carpal movements may be felt in two places—at the elbow or at the wrist. This differential localization by the patient indicates correctly where the lesion lies. If the pain is felt in the upper forearm or lower arm, a golfer's or a tennis elbow is present. If one (or two congruous) movements cause pain near the wrist, a tendinous lesion is present.

### Pain on Resisted Extension

If the pain is felt at the wrist, the extensor tendons of the wrist, seldom of the fingers, are affected. Crepitus is occasionally felt when the carpal extent of the extensor indicis muscle is involved. If the fingers are kept flexed voluntarily, the extensor digitorum longus muscle is thrown out of action; now, should the resisted movements towards extension still hurt, the carpal extensors are involved. Whether resisted radial or ulnar deviation hurts indicates whether the extensor carpi radialis or the extensor carpi ulnaris is involved. In the former case, the lesion is sought with the wrist held in full flexion and will be found at the insertion of the tendons into the bases of the second and third metacarpal bones (sometimes one, sometimes both). This is a pure tenoperiosteal strain, therefore incurable by any operation slitting up the tendon sheath; there is no tenovaginitis or tenosynovitis. If the extensor carpi ulnaris tendon is at fault, the lesion has by contrast three possible sites, identified by discovery of the site of tenderness while the wrist is held in full radial deviation: at the base of the fifth metacarpal bone (tenoperiosteal); at the extent of tendon between the triquetral (cuneiform) bone and the ulna; at the groove in the lower extremity of the ulna. It is when the tendon is affected in this groove that the puzzling phenomenon occurs of pain elicited at the extreme of passive supination of the forearm.

If the disorder is due to strain or overuse, both deep massage (Paton 1978), and triamcinolone injection are successful. If the tendon is warm to the touch, swollen or nodular, the inflammation is probably rheumatoid; if so, massage is harmful but the steroid succeeds. Tuberculous and gonorrhoeal tenosynovitis have virtually disappeared but an occasional gouty case is encountered.

### Weakness on Resisted Extension

When testing resisted extension at the wrist reveals painless weakness, full neurological examination is required.

*Bilateral Weakness.* If this is confined to the extensor muscles at both wrists, lead poisoning is suggested. If this is not a factor, carcinoma of the bronchus should be suspected.

*Unilateral Weakness.* This occurs in: (*a*) Radial pressure palsy from, for example, a crutch or the edge of a chair impinging on this nerve in the arm or fracture of the humerus at mid-shaft. (*b*) Sixth or (seldom) seventh cervical root palsy. In the former, the flexors of the elbow also lose power; in the latter, the triceps and wrist flexor muscles are much weakened. (*c*) Eighth cervical root palsy. The extensor and flexor carpi ulnaris become weak and, when the resisted extension movement at the wrist is tested, the hand deviates radialwards. If so, the extensors and adductor of the thumb are also weak.

### Pain on Resisted Flexion

If the pain is felt in the lower forearm, the flexor tendons of the wrist or fingers are at fault. Resisted flexion of each finger and resisted radial and ulnar deviation are tested, and the affected tendon defined. When the flexor digitorum profundus is affected, the tender extent is usually about 4 cm long at the lower forearm. When the flexor carpi radialis is affected, the whole distal extent of the tendon is usually tender, sometimes including the tenoperiosteal junction at the base of the second metacarpal bone. When the flexor carpi ulnaris is affected, tenderness must be sought at two sites: proximal and distal to the pisiform bone. In the latter instance, deep palpation through the thickness of the hypothenar muscles is required. Both triamcinolone injection and adequate deep massage quickly afford full relief at all these sites.

*Rheumatoid Tenovaginitis.* This disorder is apt to involve one flexor tendon near the carpus. During the first few weeks the distinguishing feature is diffuse swelling and local heat palpable at the front of the forearm, combined with tenderness over an extent of tendon greater than is expected in cases due to overuse. Usually within a month, the swelling resolves into a series of nodules on the tendon; local heat persists. Treatment by one or two infiltrations with triamcinolone gives lasting quiescence. Rheumatoid arthritis does not supervene, at any rate for the next 15 years.

A swelling, similar to that causing trigger-finger, sometimes forms at a flexor digitorum tendon at the wrist. This sets up pressure on the median nerve where it passes under the transverse carpal ligament and is one of the causes of the carpal tunnel syndrome.

*Tuberculous Tenosynovitis.* This is a disease of the past in Britain. A swelling forms that can be made to fluctuate from palm to lower forearm—'compound palmar ganglion'.

*Foreign Body Tenosynovitis.* An uncommon cause of tendinous trouble at the wrist is movement of a foreign body embedded in the forearm. Even after many years—the longest period that I have so far encountered was 32 years—a small fragment of metal, e.g. lead shot or shrapnel, may suddenly work its way out of the fleshy mass of muscle in which it has lain and, in the course of some hours or a day, move down and lodge at the wrist. Crepitating tenosynovitis results. This condition should be suspected if the forearm is scarred and the patient believes that fragments of metal remain. The position of the foreign body should be identified by palpation. It is then pushed downwards by the fingers. When it has reached the middle of the palm, it disappears; it can no longer be felt and it ceases permanently to trouble the patient.

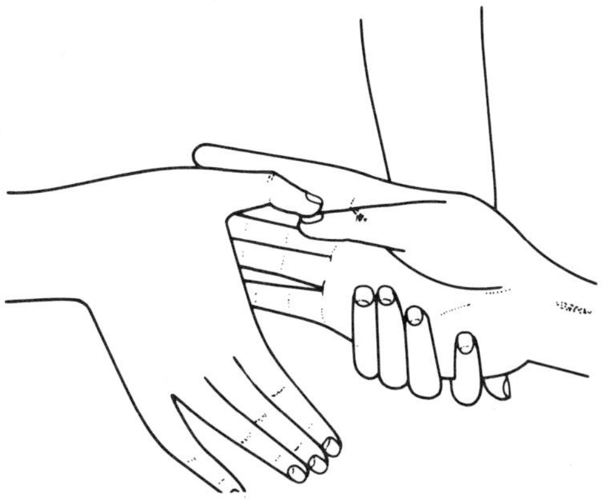

**Fig. 57.** Resisted extension of the thumb. While the patient's hand is held, he presses his thumb upwards against the examiner's thumb.

### Weakness on Resisted Flexion

This finding indicates a seventh cervical root lesion and is associated with marked loss of power in the triceps muscle. The triceps jerk is seldom sluggish.

An eighth cervical root palsy leads to weakness of both the ulnar deviators of the wrist. In such a case during the resisted flexion movement, the hand is seen to deviate radialwards. Corroboration is found in associated weakness of the extensor and adductor muscles of the thumb.

## THE THUMB

Since both arthritis and tenovaginitis at the thumb give rise to pain felt at the wrist, no examination of the wrist is complete without a study of the passive and resisted movements at the first carpometacarpal joint.

A small thumb since birth may indicate a congenital deformity at the lower cervical spine of the Klippel-Feil variety. Widening and shortening of the distal phalanx of the thumb occurs in the distal absorption of bone that may complicate psoriasis.

In arthritis at the trapezio-metacarpal joint, the thumb is often visibly fixed in adduction; the osteophytes can be seen and felt.

## Passive Movement

### Trapezio-first-metacarpal Joint

Only one passive movement need be tested at the trapezio-first-metacarpal joint: backward movement during extension. Since the anterior aspect of the capsule of the joint is that most affected, this is the movement that always hurts in arthritis even when the others do not; limitation of movement is largely confined to abduction. Tenderness is most obvious at the front of the joint. In osteoarthrosis, crepitus can usually be elicited by pressing the bones together and sliding the first metacarpal bone to and fro over the trapezium. The radiograph shows the condition clearly. It is often bilateral, sometimes in association with osteoarthrosis of the fingers. In traumatic arthritis, the X-ray photograph reveals no abnormality; pain may go on for months.

Deep massage to the capsule of the joint on alternate days relieves traumatic arthritis within about a fortnight; in osteoarthrosis, silicone oil injected into the joint often eases the pain for many months. In severe osteoarthrosis, arthrodesis provides a strong and painless thumb with some limitation of movement, whereas excision of the trapezium gives more mobility but a weaker though painless joint.

For injection a short needle of large bore is used and 2 ml of silicone oil (12 000 centistoke) is required. The physiotherapist opens the joint space by grasping the patient's thumb and pulling hard, applying countertraction with her other hand at the elbow. The distraction enables the grooves between the bones to be felt easily (except in gross rheumatoid swelling) and the needle is inserted at right angles to the first-metacarpal shaft. The point of the needle becomes intra-articular at about 1 cm.

## Resisted Movements

Arthritis at the carpo-first-metacarpal joint may be simulated by tenovaginitis at the base of the thumb (de Quervain); for the passive movements slide the tendon up and down within its sheath, thus setting up painful friction. Hence there is often pain on some of the passive wrist and thumb movements; but, when the resisted movements are tested, extension and abduction are found to hurt, thus incriminating the tendons.

### Pain on Resisted Extension

This is always associated with pain on resisted abduction. Resisted flexion and adduction do not hurt (Fig. 57). The pain may be felt only in the lower forearm; if so, the abductor longus and extensores pollicis tendons are affected where they curl round the shaft of the radius just above the wrist.

Crepitus is present in recent cases; the tendons are tender over an extent of 4 cm. When the tendons are affected where they curl round the radius, a few sessions of deep massage prove curative. This was confirmed by Paton (1978) who had used this treatment since 1947 without failure. A month's immobilization had been tried in 544 cases (Thompson et al. 1951) but they found that 44% of factory workers relapsed and had to be splinted again. So cumbersome and uncertain a measure seems hardly worth considering, yet it was advocated in a leading article in the *British Medical Journal* in 1972 (1528). If the pain is felt diffusely, radiating down to the thumb and up the forearm, the tendons of the extensor brevis and abductor longus are probably affected at their carpal extent. If so, crepitus is absent, but a localized thickening can be seen at the radial side of the wrist and there is a small area of great tenderness at the radial styloid process. This is an example of the phenomenon I named 'associated tenderness'. The bone is more tender than the tendon itself, though this area of bone has no connection with the tendons. When the tenovaginitis ceases, the bony tenderness ceases too; so they must be related.

Tenderness of the abductor longus and extensor brevis tendons in their common sheath occurs in three places: (1) at the level of the carpus; (2) at the insertion of the abductor longus into the base of the first metacarpal bone; (3) at the groove on the base of the radius. The tenderness of the styloid process of the radius must be ignored, since no lesion exists at this point. The condition is quite disabling since it hurts considerably whenever the patient grasps anything.

The extensor longus pollicis is very seldom affected at the wrist. Cure by massage takes about a fortnight.

*'Styloiditis Radii'.* Sometimes the pain at the styloid process is so noticeable that the patient says his wrist is painful and tender at that point, but does not mention pain on moving the thumb. This is very puzzling unless the relationship of an abductor and extensor tenovaginitis of the thumb to tenderness of the styloid process is kept in mind. When associated with pain on resisted extension and abduction movements of the thumb, tenderness at the styloid process merely indicates that the carpal extent of the tendons is at fault; no lesion at the actual process is present. The condition has been described under the misnomer 'styloiditis radii'; this is putting the cart before the horse, because the tenovaginitis is

the primary lesion and the bony tenderness continues until the tendons recover.

Before steroid treatment existed, this condition caused much trouble. Now one, at most two, injections of triamcinolone cure. The only difficulty is to place the injection correctly, along the gliding surfaces between tendon and tendon sheath.

The patient sits with the radial side of his wrist uppermost, the hand held in ulnar deviation with the thumb well flexed. A small syringe with a very fine needle 2 cm long is filled with 0.5 ml of triamcinolone suspension. The tendons are now identified and the needle thrust in almost horizontally, parallel to them, just above the base of the first metacarpal bone. The needle is guided to the free surface between sheath and tendon, and as the fluid is injected a little sausage forms along the tendons as far as the styloid process. The patient is seen ten days later and, if not fully recovered a second injection is given.

Operation is effective, but obsolete. The tendon sheath is exposed at its carpal extent and slit open longitudinally over a 3 cm length. Since the tendon now runs in a sheath that no longer fits, the patient is cured; but he has had an anaesthetic, two days in hospital and a scar 5 cm long for a disorder easily put right by conservative means. There is also the waste of hospital facilities and needless expense to the National Health Service to be considered.

Massage is effective in three months, but also out of date, except at a hospital where steroids are not used and the cold orthopaedic surgical waiting-list is over two months long. Immobilization is useless, even when persevered with for months.

Awaiting spontaneous cure is certainly not worth while since the disorder takes three to four years to resolve, with considerable disablement during all that time.

*Rheumatoid Tenovaginitis.* This may occur at the carpal extent of the abductor longus and extensor brevis pollicis tendons. Marked soft swelling of the tendon sheath provides the first sign. The gross thickening contrasts with the slightness of the symptoms, thus distinguishing the disorder from that described above, where the pain and disability are far greater than might be expected from the minor degree of swelling. Treatment by one or two injections of triamcinolone is successful; recurrence is unlikely, and there is no particular tendency to later rheumatoid arthritis.

## Pain on Resisted Flexion

Pain felt when this movement is tested by resistance exerted at the distal phalanx shows the flexor pollicis longus tendon to be at fault. If it is affected at its metacarpal extent, an injection of triamcinolone is effective, but deep massage useless. If it is affected at the wrist, crepitus is sometimes palpable and steroid injection or deep friction equally successful.

*Trigger-thumb.* During active flexion of the thumb a swelling on the flexor pollicis longus tendon may become engaged in the tendon sheath. The patient then cannot voluntarily extend the thumb again, since it is fixed in flexion at the interphalangeal joint. He straightens the thumb by using the other hand, there is a snap and movement is restored. The swelling can be felt moving up and down as the patient flexes and extends the thumb; it lies just proximal to the head of the first metacarpal bone.

An injection of triamcinolone is often effective symptomatically although the node remains. If the symptoms recur, a small plastic operation slitting up the tendon sheath longitudinally in the region of the swelling affords immediate and lasting relief.

## Weakness of the Thumb Muscles

Weakness of adduction and extension of the thumb characterizes a disc herniation at the seventh cervical level with consequent eighth root palsy. It is associated with weakness of ulnar deviation at the wrist.

Weakness of abduction is scarcely perceptible even when the abductor pollicis brevis muscle is markedly wasted as the result of a cervical rib compressing the lower trunk of the brachial plexus. Wasting with some weakness of the thenar muscles occurs with severe pressure within the carpal tunnel.

Weakness of extension of the fingers as well as of abduction of the thumb can result from pressure on the posterior interosseous nerve at the elbow (Guillain & Courtellemont 1905). Spinner (1968) showed that this nerve passes over the surface of the humeral epicondyle, under an arch formed by the origin of the supinator muscle. This is attached at the tip and at the base of the epicondyle, leaving an aperture for the nerve. If this free edge is tendinous—the arcade of Frohse (1908)—it may compress the nerve. Capener (1966) drew attention to the possibility of the edge of the supinator muscle compressing the posterior interosseous nerve, but unaccountably regarded this event as a cause of tennis elbow.

Weakness results, of course, when a tendon ruptures; this is usually obvious. Rupture of the extensor longus pollicis is an uncommon complication of fracture at the lower end of the radius. After a Colles's fracture, the tendon may become frayed by the bony irregularity at the fracture line, finally parting during, as a rule, the second month. The treatment is surgical. Tendons may also rupture in advanced rheumatoid arthritis.

Ischaemic contracture may affect the belly of the flexor longus pollicis muscle; if so, the metacarpophalangeal and the interphalangeal joint can each be extended singly, but not simultaneously—an example of the constant length phenomenon.

## CARPAL TUNNEL SYNDROME

Irritation of the outer aspect of the median nerve near the wrist was briefly discussed by me (Cyriax 1942) under the heading 'median perineuritis'. One case was recorded in which such severe twinges were felt in the thumb that two fruitless operations had been performed for a suspected foreign body in the pulp; cure (which lasted 12 years before I lost sight of the patient) followed two local anaesthetic injections about the median nerve at the wrist. However, the condition remained rather a nebulous entity until the appearance of the paper by Brain et al. (1947). Previous accounts had appeared attributing the condition to a median neuritis, i.e. a primary affection of the parenchyma. The only exception was Marie and Foix (1913) who described 'neuritic thenar atrophy' due to pressure on the exterior of the nerve from the anterior carpal ligament. This was revealed post-mortem in a woman of 80 who had much thenar wasting.

The first symptom is pins and needles felt at the front of the outer three-and-a-half digits of, usually, the right hand. The fact that the radial, but not the ulnar border of the ring finger is paraesthetic, combined with the fact that only the palmar surface (except at the distal phalanges, where the median nerve supplies also the dorsal aspect of the digits) of the fingers is affected, strongly suggests pressure, exerted at the distal part of the limb, on the median nerve. In, for example, sixth cervical root palsy due to a disc lesion or in cervical rib of median development, such accuracy is not attained. The patient notices that using the hand increases the symptoms and rest gives temporary relief. Advantage can be taken of this fact in diagnosis. If splinting the patient's wrist for a few days abolishes the paraesthesia, pressure on the median nerve at the wrist is confirmed. If the other hand becomes affected too, as happens in about a third of all cases, the complaint of pins and needles in both hands is very reminiscent of the thoracic outlet syndrome. After the condition has been present

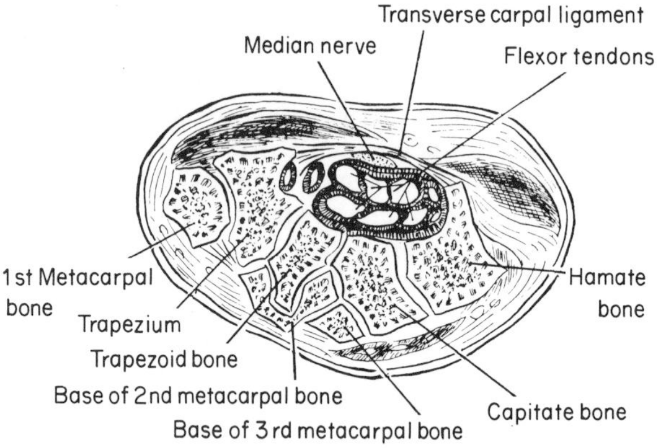


**Fig. 58.** Transverse section of the carpus.

for many months, pain may come on in the palm and forearm, but the pins and needles remain in the hand only.

### Diagnosis

The problem is to differentiate a cervical disc lesion, the thoracic outlet syndrome and pressure on the median nerve in the carpal tunnel. The history is the most informative and the radiograph the least, since this is a disorder of middle age—when X-ray changes in the cervical spine are to be expected in normal individuals.

In the carpal tunnel syndrome, the pins and needles are increased by use of the hand and appear at the anterior aspect of three-and-a-half digits. There is no paraesthesia above the wrist, though there may be aching.

In cervical disc lesion, the pins and needles come and go, day or night, in an erratic fashion, and do not actually last more than an hour at a time. Nothing in particular brings them on and they are felt within the hand and all fingers, not at any aspect.

In the thoracic outlet syndrome, at least for the first few years, the pins and needles are strictly nocturnal, waking the patient after some hours' sleep. Usually all the digits are affected, not on any aspect.

When the carpal tunnel is at fault, examination of the neck for articular signs or of the thoracic outlet for the release phenomenon is negative. By contrast, when the wrist is held extended and the patient flexes and extends his fingers while the physician presses at the front of his wrist, the pins and needles may be evoked and recognized by the patient as his familiar sensation. The physician may feel a swelling on a digital flexor tendon (analogous to that causing the trigger phenomenon) which, as it moves under the transverse carpal ligament, sends a shower of pins and needles down the digits. So does keeping the wrist flexed for a minute and suddenly extending it.

Wasting and weakness of the thenar muscles are not to be expected in the early case; however, it is occasionally encountered. In Stevenson's (1966) series of 120 patients, two-thirds of whom had symptoms of six months to several years, wasting was noted in 29%.

Any diagnosis based largely on negative findings is tentative. Hence, therapeutic confirmation is always required. Triamcinolone is injected into the carpal tunnel and the patient seen ten days later. Though the relief may not be permanent, cessation for some weeks is diagnostic.

### Treatment

The patient sits, with wrist fully extended. A syringe containing 2 ml of triamcinolone suspension is fitted with a needle 4 cm long. A spot on the palmar aspect, 3 cm above the wrist, is chosen and the needle thrust in almost horizontally, so that it travels in the tunnel parallel to the tendons and nerve. It thus passes along them and does not penetrate the nerve. The needle is advanced to almost its full length and the injection given with its point under the ligament.

## Varieties of Compression

### Subluxation of the Lunate Bone

As the result of injury, not necessarily very severe, the patient's wrist becomes suddenly fixed. Extension is impossible; a few degrees of flexion can be obtained. Median paraesthesia comes on at once, leading to numbness within a few days and obvious muscular weakness within a week or two.

Radiography does not reveal the subluxation at all clearly, since the lesion is a fixed rotation of the lunate bone.

Surgery is required at once.

### Rheumatoid Arthritis, Gout, Myxoedema, Sepsis, Rubella, Acromegaly and Pregnancy

Thickening of the transverse carpal ligament and of all the tendons in the tunnel, may result from the general disease of fibrous tissue occurring in rheumatoid arthritis. Division of the transverse carpal ligament is required.

In an acute gouty attack affecting the flexor tendons, such swelling may result that the median nerve is severely compressed. Even if the attack is quickly controlled by indomethacin, butazolidine or colchicum, conduction may take six months to recover. In these cases, cutaneous analgesia is more marked than muscle weakness.

Murray and Simpson (1958) put forward evidence that the paraesthesia in the hands that often accompanies hypothyroidism results from an accumulation of myxomatous deposits within the carpal tunnel; they found thyroid extract was usually effective. The same occurs in acromegaly (Woltman 1940), and in pyogenic infection of the hand. It has also been described in pregnancy.

Ellis (1973) has reported a case of gross swelling within the carpal tunnel during an attack of rubellar polyarthritis. Hydrocortisone had no effect; hence after three days' severe pain the transverse carpal ligament was divided with immediate relief. Microscopy showed infiltration with polymorphonuclear leucocytes which he attributed to a viral synovitis.

### Swelling on a Digital Flexor Tendon

If the swelling is large, a characteristic symptom is mentioned. The patient complains that he cannot flex his fingers actively on waking in the morning but has to work them up and down with the other hand at first. This loss of active movement coming on after a period of immobility is accompanied by median numbness. Search for the swelling must not be confined strictly to the territory of the carpal tunnel; for it may lie several centimetres up the forearm. If the swelling lies close to the palm and in connection with the tendon running to the fourth or fifth finger, the thenar branch of the median nerve escapes pressure and the pins and needles occupy the index, long and ring fingers only.

Treatment consists in acupuncture. About half of all such cases are relieved, at any rate for some years, by careful location of the swelling and the passage of a needle right through it. Presumably, a small fluid core is liberated by the needle. If acupuncture fails, division of the transverse carpal ligament is indicated.

### Colles's Fracture

When immobilization of the wrist ceases, say six weeks after the break occurred, and the patient begins to move his wrist again, the median nerve may catch against the callus.

### No Palpable Abnormality

These are the cases favourable to treatment by triamcinolone and account for about half the total. One injection, perhaps another a fortnight later, suffices to afford lasting relief. It is uncertain whether the sheath of the nerve is lastingly desensitized or inflammation of the tendons leading to local swelling is abated. If injections fail, the transverse carpal ligament should be divided.

Electromyography is helpful in prognosis; for Stevenson (1966) found that a motor latent period exceeding seven milliseconds from wrist to thumb showed that the effect of conservative treatment would be temporary only.

### Occupational Causes

Repeated use of the hand while it is held in extension at the wrist grinds the median nerve against the carpal bones. Hence scrubbing on hands-and-knees or using clippers is often the aetiological factor. After the harmful exertion, the nerve stays tender, being apt to produce pins and needles on very little provocation for some weeks afterwards.

Avoidance of the causative work, aided by local triamcinolone, is indicated. Division of the transverse carpal ligament is without avail.

## Partial Syndromes

### Direct Trauma

A fall on the outstretched hand may bruise the branch of the median nerve to the thumb, at the point where it crosses the medial aspect of the trapezio-first-metacarpal joint. For many months afterwards the patient suffers pain and paraesthesia in the thumb alone. The symptoms are usually thought to be psychogenic.

Although it is not easy to find the exact spot with the point of a needle, one injection of 2 ml of 0.5% procaine solution is lastingly curative, but it may take two or three attempts to infiltrate about the nerve correctly.

### Stick Palsy

A patient, perhaps with chronic nervous disease or osteoarthrosis in both hips, may habitually squeeze that part of the median nerve running to the index and long fingers by holding his walking-stick the wrong way. Instead of gripping the curved handle of his stick across his palm, he may grasp it longitudinally in line with his forearm. All the pressure is then borne at the exact point of emergence of the median nerve from under the distal edge of the transverse carpal ligament. Persistent paraesthesia in the index and long fingers results, which division of the ligament does not alter.

### Palmar Flexor Tendon Swelling

Pins and needles in the long and ring fingers result from a largish swelling on a digital flexor tendon at its emergence just beyond the distal edge of the transverse carpal ligament. The trigger phenomenon is absent and the swelling easy to miss. It should be trimmed surgically; division of the ligament is of no avail.

## PRESSURE ON THE RADIAL NERVE

This is rare. A minor subluxation of the scaphoid bone may lead to stiffness of the wrist and paraesthesia at the dorsum of the three-and-a-half radial fingers owing to pressure on the nerve in the anatomical snuff-box. Examination of the wrist shows the pattern characteristic of internal derangement—limitation of extension only. Manipulative reduction restores movement at the wrist and abolishes the pins and needles simultaneously.

An osteoma projecting dorsally at the base of the third metacarpal bone (sometimes the result of an accessory centre of ossification there) may engage against the branch of the radial nerve to the index and long fingers. When the hand is then moved from side to side during wrist flexion, a sharp twinge is felt as the nerve engages against the projection and rides over it; the dorsum of these fingers then tingles for several minutes. The exostosis can be removed if the symptoms warrant.

If the sensory branch of the radial nerve catches against the lower edge of the radius, the patient describes a characteristic action as bringing on the paraesthesia. This movement consists in bringing the arm backwards from the dependent position and then twisting it into full medial rotation with the elbow straight; he then flicks the forearm into full pronation and the wrist and fingers into flexion. This position stretches the radial nerve to the maximum and a sharp tingle results. An injection of triamcinolone suspension is given where the nerve crosses the edge of the radius.

## THE HAND

Pain in the hand usually results from local trauma or overuse. Much weight should be given to the history and the site of pain, which is usually felt exactly at the site of the lesion. Conversely, when pain in the hand is referred from above, the patient knows it. Inquiry is made for changes in colour such as suggest a circulatory disorder, e.g. Raynaud's disease or a cervical rib pressing on the subclavian artery or vein. Pain persisting in hands and feet since early childhood occurs in boys with angiokeratoma corporis. The hands are normal but the skin of the lower trunk is covered with tiny dark spots. The cause is a deficiency of the enzyme α-galactosidase.

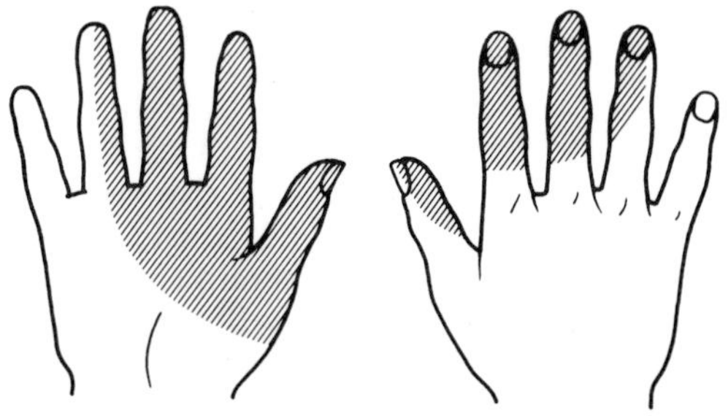

**Fig. 59.** The paraesthetic area in median nerve compression at the wrist.

### Paraesthesia

Numbness and pins and needles in the fingers are a common symptom which has been named 'acroparaesthesia'. They are felt in the hand irrespective of the level at which the causative pressure is exerted, hence the relevant nerve trunk—identified by which fingers and which aspect are affected—must be examined from neck to hand. Pins and needles in all four limbs

| | |
|---|---|
| Thumb alone | Numbness only—occupational pressure on the digital nerve at the outer side of the thumb<br>Pins and needles—contusion of the thenar branch of the median nerve |
| Thumb and index finger | Fifth cervical disc lesion |
| Thumb, index and long finger | Fifth cervical disc lesion or cervical rib |
| Thumb, index, long and adjacent side of ring finger | Palmar surface—median nerve in carpal tunnel<br>Dorsum—radial nerve |
| Thumb and fifth finger | Tumour of humerus |
| All five digits of one or both hands | Thoracic outlet syndrome |
| All five digits of both hands | Cervical central disc protrusion |
| Index and long fingers | Palmar surface—trigger-finger or stick-palsy<br>Indeterminate—sixth cervical disc lesion<br>Dorsal surface—carpal exostosis or subluxation |
| Index, long and ring fingers | Sixth cervical disc lesion or carpal tunnel syndrome |
| All four fingers | Sixth cervical disc lesion |
| Long finger alone | Sixth cervical disc lesion |
| Long and ring fingers | Sixth cervical disc lesion, stick-palsy |
| Long, ring and little fingers | Seventh cervical disc lesion |
| Ring and fifth fingers | Seventh cervical disc lesion or thoracic outlet syndrome |
| Ulnar side of ring and whole fifth finger | Pressure on ulnar nerve at elbow or palm |

characterize disorders such as peripheral neuritis, diabetes, pernicious anaemia, and central cervical disc lesions.

*Localized Paraesthesia.* The main diagnostic points are—Which fingers? Which aspect? (See above.)

As always, when a nerve twig, trunk or root is pressed on, even if the paraesthetic area appears to identify the one affected, the whole nerve must be examined from spine to digit; the above indications are probabilities, not certainties. When an area that does not correspond to any one nerve is described, the lesion must lie above the differentiation of the brachial plexus.

## Muscles of Hand

The muscles most often strained are the interosseous bellies. They may receive a direct injury and are in any case bound to be damaged when a metacarpal shaft is fractured. Musicians, especially violinists and pianists, sprain these muscles by an over-vigorous movement during fingering, and, unless treated, may be permanently unable to play perfectly again.

When, as is commoner, a dorsal interosseous muscle is strained, the pain in the hand is elicited by a resisted abduction movement of the extended fingers. The tender spot in the muscle must be found—the patient's sensations are a good guide—and deep massage given there. Even after months of disablement that has resisted every conceivable treatment, a musician can be confidently assured that he will be able to play again tomorrow night. Two or three sessions of massage are curative.

Tendinitis of an interosseous muscle at the base of one of the first phalanges may be difficult to distinguish from a strain of the joint itself. Though the tender spot is level with the joint and that side of the joint is slightly swollen, some of the passive movements at that joint hurt, others do not, i.e. the non-capsular pattern. It is then that pain elicited by a resisted movement clarifies the diagnosis.

Differentiation is important, for three to six sessions of adequate deep massage cure a tendinitis, however long-standing, but have no effect on traumatic arthritis.

Occasionally an abduction sprain of the thumb overstretches a thenar muscle, most often the origin of the oblique abductor muscle at the base of the second or third metacarpal bone.

Considerable ingenuity is required in testing the small muscles of the hand and in finding the tender spot in the structure thus identified. The physiotherapist too must take considerable trouble to find the position that allows her finger the best access to the tissue at fault, perhaps by pressing one metacarpal bone forwards and the adjacent one backwards.

All the intrinsic muscles and their short tendons respond immediately to adequate massage, but not to steroids. On the long flexor tendons in the palm, by contrast, massage has no effect, but triamcinolone is successful.

*Weakness* of the interosseous muscles of the hand characterizes a first thoracic root lesion. If one interosseous muscle is weak and wasted in isolation, localized pressure (usually occupational) on the deep palmar branch of the ulnar nerve in the palm should be suspected. In cervical rib with extensive weakness, the ulnar half of the flexor profundus digitorum and the flexor carpi ulnaris are usually affected too.

## Joints of the Hand

Arthritis occurs at any of the hand joints and gives rise to limitation of movement. The pattern for the joint is an equal degree of limitation of flexion and extension; except in severe arthritis rotation is painful at extremes rather than limited in range. The history, combined with the appearance of the joint, provides the clearest pointer to the type of arthritis present. The relevant points are: whether the onset is apparently causeless, traumatic, or the result of immobilization because of neighbouring sepsis; whether the affection is multiple or single; whether the distal or the proximal joints were affected first; whether the capsule of the joint is swollen or not; whether the joint changes colour or not; whether there is a family history of gout or Heberden's nodes.

### Rheumatoid Arthritis

This never begins at the distal interphalangeal joints, whereas osteoarthrosis usually does. Rheumatoid arthritis often begins as stiffness of the fingers on waking in the morning; at this stage no clinical signs may be perceptible, but the sedimentation rate is markedly raised. Sooner or later one or more metacarpophalangeal or proximal interphalangeal joints of one or both hands develop the familiar spindle-shaped swelling. Later on, ulnar deviation of the fingers is characteristic. The mechanism is as follows: during gripping, as the fingers flex they also deviate ulnarwards in the normal individual, partly owing to the slight tilt on the metacarpal heads, partly because the tendons of the interosseous muscles lie at the medial side of the joint. By dint of much gripping, the ulnar deviators become stronger than the radial deviators. The deviation in rheumatoid arthritis is initiated by these two factors, and the effect is then enhanced by the extensor tendon gradually shifting towards the ulnar side of the joint and pulling the phalanx over each time the muscle contracts.

An identical picture is presented by multiple subacute arthritis complicating Reiter's disease, gonorrhoea, chronic gout, psoriasis and the early stage of scleroderma. In psoriasis the nails are ridged.

Care should be taken not to assume too readily that the symptoms in a patient with rheumatoid arthritis are due to articular disease. A trigger finger is a common complication, since the tendons are also very apt to be affected. Sometimes the swelling becomes large enough to prevent active, but not passive, flexion of a finger. Since movement is easily restored by a small plastic operation on the tendon sheath, correct diagnosis is important. A ganglion lying between the head of the second and third metacarpal bones must not be mistaken for rheumatoid arthritis.

Intra-articular triamcinolone is the treatment of choice when only a few joints are affected and the patient not in an acute flare. Fenoprofen, ibuprofen, ketoprofen and naproxen should be tried in turn until the most effective is found and the dose ascertained. However, Kleinkort and Wood (1975) advocate phonophoresis using 10% hydrocortisone ointment. Ultrasonic waves possess obvious advantages over repeated multiple injections when the disease involves many digital joints. Recently, surgery has been advocated in the early stage, in order to obviate the invasion of bone, cartilage and ligament by the inflamed synovial tissue, so as to avoid irreversible change. Once the rheumatoid synovium has been removed surgically or by radio-isotope injected intra-articularly, it seldom grows again; hence distension of the joint and stretching of the ligaments ceases. Invasion of subchondral bone with formation of cysts and destruction of articular cartilage is also postponed by this means. A good case can therefore be made out for early surgery, the difficulty being that some half of all cases do well without. It is thus a question of selecting the cases that will do badly.

Vaino (1967) considers that the indications for operation are: (*a*) patients under 40 years old, specially women; (*b*) raised ESR at the onset; (*c*) abnormality of the albumin/globulin ratio at the onset; (*d*) rapid development of bony erosion visible radiographically. Moberg (1967) states that two areas of synovial hypertrophy appear early in rheumatoid arthritis, the larger on the dorsum of the joint, the smaller lying anteriorly. Each develops close to the nutrient foramen, causing obstruction, and cells appear to be released from these areas of hypertrophy which degenerate with the release of an enzyme that attacks cartilage. Early synovectomy may postpone this damage.

## Osteoarthrosis

This may result from a severe injury; if so, only one joint is affected. In the apparently causeless cases of multiple involvement that occur in elderly patients, usually women, a strong familial trend is evident. The distal joints are affected first; after many years the disorder spreads to the proximal interphalangeal joints, very seldom to the metacarpophalangeal joints. The knobbly appearance of the joint is quite different from rheumatoid arthritis, for the base of the distal phalanx can be seen projecting abruptly as two small rounded bosses at the dorsum of the joint. A varus deformity, usually at the index, may develop at a distal joint. Both hands are usually affected more or less symmetrically. The radiograph shows the osteophytes and erosion of cartilage clearly. From time to time, a new node forms at an affected joint; while it is growing there is pain for a month or two and occasionally the fingertip goes pink. This mottled pink is different from the shiny red of gout. After a month or two the discoloration passes off and the node stops hurting.

Heberden's (1802) nodes and osteoarthrosis cause little in the way of symptoms. They are unsightly and cause aching and clumsiness. Since the distal finger joints fix in 45° flexion in the end, arthrodesis seldom brings much improvement unless an intractable painful traumatic arthritis supervenes after injury. Some patients are pleased to have the exostoses removed surgically for cosmetic reasons.

## Traumatic Arthritis

This is common, and results from direct contusion, indirect sprain, chip fracture or reduced dislocation. The history is characteristic; the joint itself is swollen in the spindle shape resembling rheumatoid arthritis. After severe trauma, the joint is often warm to the touch for about a month. Movement is limited; the active, passive and resisted movements must all be tested in case a tendinous lesion coexists.

All treatment is futile. The joint recovers, whether treated or not, in six to eighteen months, depending on the severity of the original trauma and the age of the patient. Whether the patient uses the joint enough to make it ache or not has no effect on the ultimate result. Steroids, so useful in traumatic arthritis at the toe joints, afford no corresponding benefit in traumatic arthritis at the fingers. Immobilization, of course, strongly contraindicated.

### Unreduced Dislocation

At the interphalangeal joint of the thumb, dislocation is sometimes mistaken for traumatic arthritis; it is extraordinary how the local swelling obscures the deformity. Examination shows the joint to be fixed in full extension, quite different from arthritis in which flexion and extension are equally limited.

In late cases, reduction is impossible and arthrodesis in 45° of flexion gives a good result.

### Immobilizational Stiffness

Before the days of antibiotics this was the common result of splintage for sepsis. The fingers must not be splinted for a day longer than is absolutely necessary, and never in full extension.

### Gout

Involvement of the hands is usually a late manifestation of the disease. The familial predisposition and the history of recurrent attacks, clearing up completely, beginning at the big toe and later spreading to other joints, is diagnostic. The shiny red appearance of the joint is characteristic.

When chronic gout comes on gradually in an old man, the onset and the clinical appearance of the joints may perfectly mimic rheumatoid arthritis. Tophi in the ears and a raised blood uric acid level finally appear, but are of little diagnostic aid in the early, doubtful case. Therapeutic testing with butazolidine is the quickest way to a clear answer.

Indomethacin 25 mg four times a day or phenylbutazone 200 mg three times a day have displaced colchicum. They cause subsidence of the acute attack within a day or two.

### Clicking Finger Joint

Traction on the finger of up to 5 kg has no effect, but when this is increased by 2 or 3 kg more the phalanges spring apart and radiography shows an intra-articular bubble of air, suddenly coming out of solution from the synovial fluid (Roston & Haines 1947). This is the same phenomenon as in caisson disease. The gas takes 20 minutes to dissolve again; until then the pop cannot be repeated. Fisk (personal communication, 1973) has made the interesting suggestion that the clicks felt and heard on spinal manipulation possess the same mechanism—a bubble of air forming within a facet joint.

## Tendons of the Hand

### Tenosynovitis

The flexor tendons in the palm may develop much coarse grating in advanced rheumatoid arthritis. Such chronic tenosynovitis causes little or no symptoms. If the discomfort warrants, triamcinolone injected into the affected tendon sheath is effective.

### Trigger Finger

A swelling on any of the digital flexor tendons may form just proximal to the metacarpophalangeal joint. When big enough, this gives rise to trigger finger or trigger thumb. When the digit has been fully flexed actively, the swelling engages within its sheath and becomes fixed in this position. The affected finger, usually the third or fourth, can then no longer be extended by muscular action; the patient has to free it by pulling at it with his other hand, whereupon it disengages with a snap. The swelling on the tendon is easy to feel in the palm or thenar eminence, just proximal to the head of the metacarpal bone. Some cases are apparently causeless; others due to multiple minor trauma (e.g. using a pair of clippers); yet others complicate rheumatoid arthritis. If necessary a small operation enlarging the relevant part of the tendon sheath by slitting it up affords permanent cure, but many patients are hardly disabled enough to wish this done. In minor cases an injection of triamcinolone usually abolishes symptoms for months or years.

Rarely, the swelling may become so large that active flexion of the finger stops at half-range. The fact that passive flexion is not limited draws immediate attention to the digital flexor tendon. Equally rarely, the swelling may form on the proximal part of the tendon in the palm and interfere with the branch of the median nerve running to the index and long fingers, causing pins and needles at the adjacent surfaces of these two digits.

A small tender swelling may form on the flexor tendon level with the proximal crease of the finger. It causes no symptoms unless the patient carries a suitcase; the local pressure then hurts.

## Ruptured Tendon

*Mallet Finger.* Any injury that forcibly flexes the distal finger joint while it is actively held in extension may cause rupture of the extensor insertion at the base of the distal phalanx. A cricket ball is often the culprit. The distal joint can be fully flexed voluntarily; the elastic rebound of the tissue takes it back to 45°, the last 45° cannot be actively performed, although the passive movement remains full. The dorsal aspect of the base of the phalanx is tender and swollen.

Treatment should be instituted at once. In young persons the affected finger should be fixed in full flexion on the palm of the hand by one piece of strapping running along from the dorsum of the finger to the front of the wrist covered by another piece of strapping encircling the hand (Fig. 60). This position ensures full relaxation of the distal part of the tendon (since the distal joint is held in full extension) while the tendon is held taut proximally by fully flexing the proximal interphalangeal joint. The strapping is kept on for four weeks; union between tendon and bone is then firm. In elderly patients, keeping the metacarpophalangeal joint fully flexed may lead to undesirable stiffness; hence it is best to fix the distal joint in full extension and the proximal joint in full flexion by a small plaster gutter, leaving the metacarpophalangeal joint free. This is kept on for a month, but union is less sure. Attempts to suture the tendon to the bone operatively are so seldom successful that the late case is best left untreated.

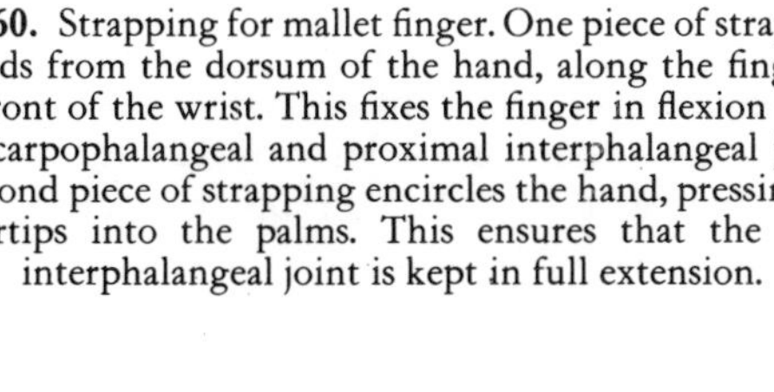

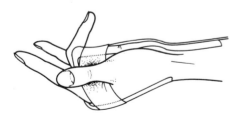

**Fig. 60.** Strapping for mallet finger. One piece of strapping extends from the dorsum of the hand, along the finger to the front of the wrist. This fixes the finger in flexion at the metacarpophalangeal and proximal interphalangeal joints. A second piece of strapping encircles the hand, pressing the fingertips into the palms. This ensures that the distal interphalangeal joint is kept in full extension.

*Ruptured Flexor Tendon.* Rupture of the flexor digitorum longus at its insertion into the base of the distal phalanx is a rarity. The whole tendon recoils into the palm where it lies bunched up, giving rise to a swelling superficially resembling Dupuytren's contracture. The distal finger joint cannot be actively flexed, although the passive movement is retained. Arthrodesis is called for if the patient's work is interfered with.

## Ganglion

A ganglion sometimes forms between the heads of the second and third metacarpal bones, and is nearly always mistaken for rheumatoid arthritis. It gives rise to vague local aching. Inspection of the hand shows the swelling to project between the bones; movement at the two adjacent metacarpophalangeal joints is of full range and painless; the radial side of the second and the ulnar side of the third metacarpophalangeal joint are clearly not swollen, and palpation reveals a fluctuant swelling. Acupuncture affords permanent relief; I have yet to meet a recurrence.

A ganglion may form on the front of the palm just distal to the hamate bone. It lies hidden under the hypothenar muscle bellies and causes no symptoms until it becomes large enough to compress the ulnar nerve. Ulnar paraesthesiae and weakness result, for which no cause can be found as the nerve is followed down from the base of the neck, until this swelling is detected in the proximal part of the palm. If the sensory branch to the ulnar fingers and to the hypothenar muscles has already been given off, weakness without cutaneous analgesia results, affecting the adductor pollicis, the interosseous and the two medial lumbrical muscles. Up to 5 ml of mucus may be obtained on aspiration. If the ganglion fills up again quickly, as it is apt to do, it should be removed before the palsy becomes too severe. I have encountered only one instance of a swelling on the flexor digitorum tendon running to the fifth finger, prominent enough to compress the ulnar nerve. The condition was bilateral and the enlargement lay 4 cm above the wrist joint.

An ulnar palsy of similar nature comes on in workmen who repeatedly hit a lever with the front rather than the side of the ulnar border of the hand. Thrombosis of the ulnar artery has also been recorded, after similar repeated local minor trauma.

### Multiple Xanthomas

These occur in the extensor tendons of the fingers at the dorsum of each hand and along each proximal phalanx. The tendons present a number of closely spaced, discrete nodules, causing visible projections that can be seen to move up and down with the tendons. No symptoms result and no tendency to rupture. Coincident bilateral involvement of the tendo Achillis is almost a certainty. Finally, large nodes form on the extensor tendons at the dorsum of the foot and on the front of each upper tibia and the back of the upper ulna. The blood cholesterol level is usually greatly raised, to twice or three times the normal level (200 mg).

A corn-oil diet has been shown (Jepson 1961) to diminish the cholesterol level in the blood, and, if the patient regards treatment as worth while, should be continued indefinitely. Mason and Perry (1965) treated four patients with large xanthomas on knees and elbows with clofibrate (2 g daily for two years) with disappearance of the swellings and the serum cholesterol fell from 1100, 500, 460 and 325 to under 250 in each case. Bengal grain is now under trial.

If the projections on the long bones annoy, they can be excised.

## Bones of the Hand

Clubbing of the distal phalanges occurs in pulmonary disease. Since clubbing occurs mainly in disease of the lungs and upper colon, especially ulcerative colitis—both tissues innervated by the vagus—the suggestion has been made that, in some obscure way, the disorder is mediated via the vagus nerve. This was given considerable confirmation by Flavell (1956) who reported that the clubbing disappeared after section of the nerve, later confirmed by Holling et al. (1961). Doyle (1970), however, regards hypertrophic osteoarthropathy as a result of disturbance of the hormonal control of sodium absorption in the proximal renal tubules.

Swelling of the terminal phalanges with radiographic evidence of erosion at the tip of each bone occurs in psoriasis; the nails are ridged. The whole skeleton of the hand enlarges greatly in acromegaly. In sclerodactyly the bones of the fingers are narrow and tapering, with the skin stretched tightly over them; the joints are contrastingly prominent. In scleroderma the thickening lies at the phalanges, between the joints. Congenital absence of the thumb nails occurs in the patella-nail syndrome, characterized by a diminutive patella, subluxation of the head of the radius, and a bony projection (visible radiologically) arising from the blade of each ilium above the acetabulum.

Fractures are common.

### Post-traumatic Osteoporosis

This is a curious and rare sequel to injury, first described by Sudeck in 1900. It nearly always follows a fracture of the forearm near the wrist (e.g. Colles's) or of the leg near the ankle. Cases have been described, however, after an otherwise unexceptional sprained ankle, not even treated by splintage.

A week or two after the accident the wrist and fingers swell and there is considerable pain on movement. The distal part of the limb becomes cyanotic and cold; the lower leg becoming almost black when left dependent for a few minutes. The range of movement at carpus (or tarsus) and fingers (or toes) diminishes rapidly. Trophic changes supervene and the nails stop growing. The radiograph, which showed no such change just after the injury, reveals severe osteoporosis involving the distal part of the broken bone and the entire hand or foot, far more than can be accounted for by immobilization. Union of the fracture proceeds normally.

The cause is unknown. Spontaneous recovery (which may never be complete, some stiffness remaining permanently) takes one to two years. Active use of the injured hand or foot should be enjoined. The radiograph shows a degree of atrophy so extreme as to suggest that the bones of the foot might easily give way under the stress of weight-bearing; moreover, softening, such that the affected bones can easily be cut with a knife post-mortem, has been described. Nevertheless, no harm results from ordinary weight-bearing activities and I have seen no case of subsequent deformity.

There appeared to be no effective counter to Sudeck's atrophy until McKay et al. (1977) treated a case of five months' standing with guanethidine. This drug displaces noradrenaline from storage at the sympathetic nerve endings, thus causing prolonged sympathetic block. They employed Hannington-Kiff's method (1974) of regional intravenous infusion on two occasions five weeks apart and describe lasting benefit. Hannington-Kiff (1979) reported relief from causalgia in 10 patients.

## Palmar Fascia

A painless contracture of the palmar fascia, named after Dupuytren (1832), but first described by Astley Cooper in 1822, may develop slowly, usually towards middle age, and lead to fixed flexion deformity of the fingers. It affects the ring finger most often, but sooner or later the third and fifth fingers also become involved. It is usually bilateral, but considerably more advanced on one side than the other. The palmar fascia thickens, becomes adherent to the skin and the cause of the deformity is obvious. The disorder is familiar; four-fifths of the patients are men. Rarely the plantar fascia is also affected.

In the early stage, the patient should himself be taught to stretch out his finger daily so as to elongate the palmar fascia as fast as it contracts. Later, a plastic operation using a Z-shaped incision is indicated, followed by splintage in extension of the fingers.

## Digital Nerves

Occupational pressure on the radial side of the thumb leads to numbness rather than pins and needles at the outer border of the distal phalanx. The workman is found to steady his hand against the edge of his bench. Recovery usually takes six months. Rarely the ulnar side of the little finger suffers in the same way.

Swelling on a digital tendon in the palm may squeeze a digital nerve and set up paraesthesia felt at the contiguous sides of two fingers.

Direct trauma may bruise the thenar branch of the median nerve where it crosses the trapezio-first-metacarpal joint leading to pins and needles in the thumb.

A ganglion adjacent to the hamate-fifth-metacarpal joint may lead to an ulnar palsy.

Many nervous diseases begin by setting up symptoms referable to the hand, e.g. cervical rib, cervical disc lesion, neuroma, syringomyelia, paralysis agitans and chorea.

# OEDEMA OF THE HAND AND FOREARM

### Angioneurotic Oedema

When oedema of the dorsum of the hand occurs without apparent cause, it is termed 'angioneurotic'. It may be allergic, but in some cases the chief underlying factors are psychological. The oedema is usually most marked on waking, disappearing as the day goes on. Pitting is easily produced. No treatment appears to make any lasting difference, unless an allergic sensitivity is discovered until Thompson and Felix-Davis (1978)'s discovery that tranexamic acid, 1 g three times a day could abort attacks.

### Interference with Lymph or Venous Return

Cervical rib, thrombosis of the axillary vein, or interference with the drainage of lymph as the result of operation (usually for cancer of the breast), or carcinomatosis of the axillary glands should be considered. When caused by idiopathic thrombosis of the axillary vein, spontaneous recovery seldom takes longer than a month.

### Post-traumatic Oedema

The cause of this uncommon sequel to injury to the hand is obscure. The distinguishing feature is that the oedema stops abruptly at the wrist or elbow instead of gradually fading away. The ridge formed by the upper extremity of the oedema is clearly palpable. The patient may allege much pain and disablement, and may add that the grip is weak and the hand numb. The oedema is clearly real, but there is a full range of movement at every joint, and no weakness or wasting of the muscles is discernible. Radiography reveals at the most some disuse atrophy. The supposition that the condition is an hysterical manifestation has received support from the work of Scott and Mallinson (1944), who cured a number of patients by psychotherapy, some in a few weeks.

In some (possibly all) cases the oedema is an artefact, produced by the application of a tight band. It was much commoner during the war years of 1939–45 than it is now.

CHAPTER 14

# THE THORAX AND ABDOMEN

Symptoms referable to the thorax arise from a wide variety of disorders, not all of them visceral. Preoccupation with visceral disease leads to neglect of the somatic causes of thoracic pain. Thoracic disease may give rise to symptoms felt wholly outside the thorax, in the abdomen perhaps, or in a limb only. If the patient's symptoms depend on activity and posture rather than on visceral function, their provenance from the moving parts should be particularly considered.

Clinically, *the thoracic spine begins at the third vertebra*, the upper two thoracic joints and nerve roots being best examined as part of the neck. The upper two thoracic segments form the inner aspect of the upper limb, thus being most easily examined with the cervical segments that make up the rest of the limb.

## SOURCES OF THORACIC PAIN

### The Neck

Displacement of part of the third or fourth cervical intervertebral disc sets up pain felt to radiate as far as the root of the neck; at the fifth and sixth levels, pain felt as far as the mid- or interscapular area is commonplace; at the seventh level the pain is often wholly mid-thoracic, sometimes at its most intense at the lower angle of one scapula. Great opportunities for mistaken diagnosis thus exist; for extrasegmental reference of pain from the dura mater still puzzles clinicians.

Even more misleading reference occurs at times. Instead of a cervical disc lesion setting up scapular pain it may give rise to pectoral pain only. This is no greater a transgression of the rules of segmental reference than the pain being felt in the third or fourth thoracic dermatome posteriorly. Being a rare site of reference, however, the true diagnosis may not even be considered.

### The Thoracic Joints and Dura Mater

Internal derangement at a thoracic joint gives rise to pain felt centrally or to one side of the posterior thorax. If the intercostal nerve root is compressed, pain is usually felt posteriorly first, then spreading anteriorly. Deep breathing may hurt. In disc lesions of primary posterolateral evolution, the pain may be unilateral and anterior only, in the thorax or, less often, the abdomen. Occasionally, a thoracic disc lesion sets up sternal pain only. In first and second thoracic disc lesions the ache is felt at the lower scapular area radiating to the ulnar side of the palm or the inner arm respectively.

Compression phenomena occur at the intervertebral joints, causing central posterior or bilateral pain, sometimes referred round to the side of the lower thorax, usually unilaterally.

Ligamentous pain occurs in ankylosing spondylitis and vertebral hyperostosis, felt at the interscapular or sternal area. Rarely, sternal pain may arise from the manubriosternal joint.

### The Ribs

Fracture is common and results in localized pain lasting six weeks at most. Disease is rare and is usually due to bacterial invasion or secondary malignant deposits. Tietze's painful swelling of a costochondral junction is uncommon.

### The Muscles

The intercostal muscles are, of course, slightly torn when a rib breaks; they may also be bruised or strained by direct contusion. Bruising of the digitations of the serratus anterior occurs. In these cases, the pain is very localized.

A more diffuse thoracic pain, often referred to the arm as far as the elbow, results from strains involving the pectoralis major or latissimus dorsi muscles. Athletes may strain the posterior inferior serratus muscle.

## The Bones

An angular kyphos is often very difficult to palpate at the thoracic spine. Wedge fracture of a vertebral body, if uncomplicated, causes symptoms for not longer than three months. For the first week there is often girdle pain. Kyphotic compression of the anterior aspects of the vertebral bodies gives rise to a posterocentral bone-to-bone ache that can go on unchanged for decades. Senile osteoporosis causes no symptoms unless, as may happen, pathological wedge fracture occurs.

Osteitis deformans, aortic aneurysm, tuberculous caries and secondary malignant deposits in the spine or sternum naturally set up pain arising from diseased bone. One case of aspergillosis acquired in England has been encountered.

## The Nerves

Neuritis of the spinal accessory, long thoracic or suprascapular nerve gives rise to a constant unilateral scapular pain lasting three weeks. In herpes zoster, the vesicles appear after three or four days. Early in the course of neuralgic amyotrophy, bilateral upper thoracic pain is felt, but it spreads to one or both arms within a few days. In the early stages of a thoracic intraspinal neuroma, the symptoms may be posterior thoracic only. Brown (1828) described a case of a girl of 17 who felt pain running to the front of the chest on manual pressure at the 7–8th thoracic vertebrae.

## The Diaphragm, Pleura and Lung

Diaphragmatic pain (C3, 4, 5) is often felt at the shoulder at each breath, i.e. at the fourth cervical dermatome, in correspondence with the main embryological derivation of the diaphragm. Pain arising from that part of the pleura not in contact with the diaphragm is also brought on by respiration but is felt in the chest. The lung is insensitive, but large tumours invade the chest wall, setting up local pain and causing spasm of the pectoralis major muscle, with consequent limitation of elevation of the arm. They may also cause limitation of thoracic side flexion away from the affected side.

'Pleurodynia' is the name given at one time to pain felt along a thoracic dermatome increased by breathing or coughing, i.e. almost always a thoracic disc protrusion with root pain.

### Epidemic Myalgia

The onset is sudden and, if fever is absent, diagnosis may be difficult. The pain is felt all over both sides of the thorax from the costal margins to the upper arms. A deep breath hurts. All sorts of movements may be found vaguely uncomfortable, but when repeated a few minutes later, they do not hurt. The illness behaves like a diffuse bilateral pleurisy and recovery takes 10 to 14 days.

## The Myocardium

The heart is developed from the first, second and third thoracic segments. Hence pain originating here may be felt spreading from the thorax to the root of the neck and to the upper limb as far as the ulnar border of the hand on the left or on both sides. Alternatively, there may be thoracic pain; or, less often, pain confined to the left or both upper limbs.

## The Aorta

Thrombosis of the lower aorta leads in due course to intermittent claudication in the legs and absence of the femoral pulses. An occasional case is encountered of posterior lower thoracic pain only, before blood flow in the iliac arteries is much diminished. Such cases are very puzzling and the diagnosis remains in doubt until femoral pulsation becomes impaired later.

Haematoma formation after intra-aortic injection of contrast material sets up left-sided lower thoracic pain.

## Venous Thrombosis (Mondor's Disease)

Unilateral pain at the front of the thorax may coincide with the appearance of a tender cord running from the pectoral area to the umbilicus, rendering full elevation of the arm painful. The cause is thrombosis of the thoraco-epigastric vein. Spontaneous recovery takes a month or two.

# THORACIC DISC LESIONS

Since most cervical and lumbar symptoms are nowadays generally regarded as having an articular origin, the question naturally arises: are thoracic symptoms also caused by disc lesions? In my view, they are (Cyriax 1950*a*). The marked signs that eventually serve to clarify the diagnosis in cervicolumbar protrusions seldom appear at the thorax, however long a patient is kept under observation; hence this theory is correspondingly difficult to prove. Moreover, operation, which has established the pathology of disc lesions in the lumbar and cervical regions so firmly, is very seldom necessary at the thoracic spinal joints. For this reason, an editorial article in the *British Medical Journal* as lately as February 1976 gave an exhaustive list of causes of pain felt along a rib, without mentioning a thoracic disc lesion.

At the cervical and lumbar joints an alternation exists that simplifies diagnosis. A minor degree of protrusion interferes with the joint, not yet with the nerve root; hence local pain and articular signs are at their most obvious when neurological signs are lacking. By contrast, when the protrusion has passed posterolaterally and interferes little with joint movement, it exerts its maximum pressure on the nerve root; hence root pain and clear neurological signs supervene as the articular symptoms and signs fade.

Disc lesions occurring at the thoracic joints by no means show this characteristic sequence. There is an extraordinary variation in the mode of onset; moreover, the articular signs are seldom obvious, and neurological signs are conspicuous only by their absence. Clinicians therefore properly hesitate to inculpate a thoracic joint as the source of what used to be called 'fibrositis', 'pleurodynia', 'intercostal neuritis', or intercostal neuralgia (Nicod 1818). It should be noted that pain deep breathing occurs just as readily when a disc lesion compresses the dura mater via the posterior ligament as in pleurisy; connection with respiration has then no differentiating significance, though doubtless this fact is responsible for the invention of 'pleurodynia'.

Diagnosis is always difficult, confusion with visceral disease being excusably very frequent. Indeed it is always safest to approach diagnosis from two aspects, the absence of signs of visceral disease balancing and confirming those of an articular plus nerve root disorder.

### Spontaneous Cure

Though scapular and lumbar pain can go on indefinitely when caused by a cervical or low lumbar disc lesion, unilateral root pain has a set period and seldom lasts more than four and twelve months respectively. No such tendency exists at the third to twelfth thoracic levels and root pain, usually at one costal margin, with or without a posterior component, can continue unchanged for many years. The length of time that root pain has continued determines reducibility at cervical and lumbar levels; by contrast it presents no such criterion at the thorax; a disc lesion, even in a young person, may well prove reducible after constant root pain for ten years.

## Symptoms

### Thoracic Lumbago

The patient bends or twists and is suddenly fixed in flexion by severe posterior lower thoracic pain, central or unilateral. A deep breath usually hurts more than coughing; the reverse is true in lumbar lumbago, when a cough hurts but a deep breath is seldom uncomfortable. A few days in bed ensure recovery but recurrence is to be expected, brought on by bending or twisting the trunk, especially during compression of the joint, i.e. when carrying a weight.

The pain may be at one side of the posterior thorax on one occasion, on the other the next time; movement of the loose fragment across the midline is common. The same phenomenon may be noted during manipulative reduction; a click may be felt that makes the pain change sides. (This is one of the phenomena that made me realize 30 years ago that thoracic pain was caused by disc lesions.)

The pain often radiates along the relevant dermatome, as in cervical and lumbar disc lesions, i.e. round to the front of the chest, usually at about the level of the lower costal margin, but also to the side of the sternum or to the abdomen in high and low lesions respectively. Central disc protrusion may cause radiation round both sides of the anterior thorax.

### Sternal Pain

Occasionally, upper- or mid-thoracic lumbago causes pain felt anteriorly only, at the sternum or epigastrium. Since the onset is sudden, during say lifting, the symptoms suggest coronary thrombosis and differential diagnosis may not prove easy at first, especially as this type of onset is apt to occur in middle age. A quick test is to ask the patient to take a deep breath, which aggravates the pain in disc protrusion but not when the myocardium is at fault.

## Thoracic Backache

Slow protrusion causes posterior thoracic backache, often coming on after sitting for some while in flexion, and is commoner in patients who already have an excessive thoracic kyphosis. The pain may be central or unilateral, most often at the lower part of the thorax, and the history discloses a clear relation to posture and exertion. The pain is often intermittent, according to what the patient does, and often absent for months on end.

The nuclear self-reducing lesion is common in those who sit for long periods each day, e.g. typists. The patient wakes comfortable and for the first few hours up feels nothing. Then sitting brings on the posterior thoracic ache which increases as the day wears on. Standing and lying abolish the ache in a few minutes. There is no pain on Sundays. The cause is a posterior bulging of the joint contents, which recede as soon as excessive flexion is no longer maintained.

Symptoms of pleural, intercostal muscular, costal and dural provenance are all increased on coughing or deep inspiration; hence respiratory exacerbation serves to rule out cardiac pain only. Pressure on the dura mater at any thoracic level does not, as at the lower levels, give rise to limitation of straight-leg raising, but the pain caused by a lower thoracic protrusion may be increased, or the pain on neck flexion aggravated, during *full* straight-leg raising.

## Root Pain

*Primary Posterolateral Protrusion.* This occurs at the thoracic joints no less than at the cervical and lumbar. In these cases, the posterior component is absent and the unilateral pain confined to the front of the chest or to the abdomen (Brown 1828). There is no correlation with visceral function but clear correspondence with posture and activity. These cases give rise to much diagnostic difficulty (Player 1821) and are responsible for the idea that manipulators can cure angina, gastritis, cholecystitis and the like, by doing something unspecified to the spinal joints that they declare alters autonomic tone.

If the eleventh or twelfth thoracic nerve root is compressed, there is pain in the iliac fossa perhaps radiating to the testicle. Occasionally, the abdominal component is absent and pins and needles in groin or testicle may be the only symptom leading to a diagnosis of 'testicular neuralgia'.

In upper thoracic disc protrusion the symptom may be merely a band of unpleasant tingling as the patient runs his hand down the front of his chest. Another unusual symptom is impingement against the nerve root, only when the dura mater is drawn upwards. The patient states that he feels nothing unless he bends his head right forward, when he notices a sharp stab of pain at one side of the sternum, sometimes accompanied by pins and needles in the mid-pectoral area.

*Secondary Posterolateral Protrusion.* This is the commoner type of onset, but now the history of posterior unilateral pain, later radiating to the costal margin, naturally draws attention to the back of the trunk. Even so, the fact that a deep breath and sometimes, a cough aggravate the pain often misdirects attention to the pleura.

In general, the likelihood of anterior thoracic and abdominal symptoms stemming from pressure on an intercostal nerve root is forgotten. Obviously, most thoraco–abdominal pain has a visceral source, but when symptoms at the front of the trunk are independent of visceral function, and alter with posture and exertion, the possibility of thoracic root pain should be considered more often than is the present habit. Manipulative reduction can then be performed within the medical sphere.

## Spinal Cord Symptoms

Pins and needles come on in both feet, gradually spreading to include the legs and thighs. Then weakness and some numbness of the legs sets in. There is no backache to speak of, but vague girdle pains are usually mentioned. Pressure from a central protrusion on the thoracic cord clearly accounts for some cases of what used to be called transverse myelitis (Key 1838). Osteophytes compressing the spinal cord have been described (Bailey & Casamajor 1911; Damany 1914).

# Physical Signs

## Inspection

The patient stands with light falling evenly on his back, its general shape being noted. The angular kyphos characteristic of a collapsed vertebral body is quickly seen and can later be palpated; a flat lower lumbar spine and excessive upper lumbar-lower thoracic kyphosis suggests a past adolescent osteochondrosis. Absence of the lumbar lordosis with a marked thoracic kyphosis suggests ankylosing spondylitis. Scoliosis and kypholordosis dating since adolescence are immediately visible, of course, but neither has any significance; for disc lesions are not more common in patients with these postural deformities than in others. Scoliosis confined to the upper thorax and lower neck suggests unilateral cervical rib or congenital vertebral deformity of the Klippel–Feil type.

## Active Movements

*Upper Thoracic Pain.* Since the common cause of upper thoracic pain, especially posterior, is a *cervical* disc lesion, examination must begin at the neck, and only if this is negative need a local origin be considered at all. Moreover, scapular pain can result from a scapular lesion or from disorders like long thoracic or suprascapular neuritis, the signs of all of which are revealed only on examination of the upper limb. Lesions at the apex of the lung may affect the first thoracic root, and are identified only when the strength of the small muscles of the hand is tested. Hence, not only the neck movements but the whole routine testing of the upper limb must be completed before the thorax is examined.

Neck flexion has two results; movement at the cervical joints and stretching of the dura mater. The fact, therefore, that neck flexion provokes a thoracic pain is no evidence that it has a cervical origin, whereas if any other movements of the neck hurt, a cervical lesion is highly probable.

Scapular movement also has two results. In a local lesion this may be uncomfortable, but scapular approximation pulls on the first and second thoracic nerves, and tends to stretch the dura mater upwards just as does neck flexion. Hence in a thoracic disc lesion at any level, this movement is apt to hurt via this unexpected mechanism and must not be thought to incriminate a scapular muscle.

*Lower Thoracic Pain.* Pain arising from the neck or upper two thoracic joints does not reach below the sixth thoracic dermatome (see Figs 14–16). Pain felt below this level, particularly if it lies fairly close to the spine, has a thoracic source, and the thoracic joints are examined. The movements tested are flexion, extension, both side flexions and both rotations. Range is tested; the normal range of active rotation of the thorax on the pelvis is 70° in each direction. If pain is provoked, its site must be noted. Care is taken to inquire for pain occurring at half-range; for a painful arc, especially on rotation, is common and pathognomonic of a disc lesion.

## Passive Movements

The patient sits, his hands on his abdomen. The examiner stands, grasping his shoulders, holding his knees between his own. The pelvis is thus fixed while the passive rotation is carried out. Rotation to 90° in each direction exists at the thoracic joints in all but the elderly—more than can be performed actively. It follows that in thoracic articular lesions much more discomfort can be elicited by passive than by active movement.

Passive extension is tested with the patient prone. Each joint is pressed towards extension with a slight jerk in the hope that it will hurt at one level more than another, or that greater resistance will be encountered, thus identifying the exact level of the lesion. Unfortunately, the same amount of discomfort or stiffness is apt to be elicited at several adjacent levels.

## Stretching the Dura Mater and Nerve Roots

*Neck Flexion.* This stretches the dura mater upwards, since the neck is 3 cm longer in full flexion than in full extension. In consequence, this movement is apt to tauten the dura mater against an intraspinal projection or to lift up a nerve root until it impinges. Hence, the symptoms of any intraspinal space-occupying lesion at a thoracic level may be exacerbated by neck flexion. The sign is common to disc lesions, small benign tumours and disseminated sclerosis (in which connection it was described by Lhermitte in 1929).

Sometimes, although neck flexion has not caused or increased symptoms, it aggravates the pain after it has already been elicited by passive rotation, when the thorax is held twisted to the extreme of range. It can then be deduced that an articular lesion exists, interfering with dural mobility. This can be only a posterior projection, i.e. a disc lesion.

Rarely neck flexion may bring on or aggravate interscapular or sternal pain in ankylosing spondylitis. Just as an occasional case of lumbar spondylitis shows bilateral limitation of straight-leg raising, so can this dural sign be elicited when the thoracic joints are affected. Presumably the spondylytic inflammation has reached the dura mater.

*Scapular Approximation.* For a long time it was obscure to me why scapular approximation is apt to increase the pain caused by a disc lesion at any thoracic level. In the past, this finding had been repeatedly misinterpreted, and led to disc lesions being attributed to trouble in the trapezius or in a rhomboid muscle. Such attribution to either muscle is easily disproved, for passive approximation of the scapulae (which relaxes these muscles) hurts just as much.

Scapular approximation pulls on the first and second thoracic nerve roots and sets up scapular pain, of course, in first and second thoracic nerve root pressure. But it thereby lifts also the whole thoracic extent of the dura mater upwards. This movement is apt to elicit pain when even a lower thoracic disc lesion is present. Indeed, as manipulative reduction proceeds, it may be the last sign to disappear.

*The First Thoracic Stretch.* Another sign exists, positive only when the mobility of the first thoracic root is impaired.

The patient is asked to bring his arm out horizontally in the coronal plane, and to bend his elbow until his forearm points vertically upwards. This should not alter the symptoms. He is then asked to flex his elbow fully, putting his hand behind his neck. This stretches the ulnar nerve, which pulls on the first thoracic nerve root, setting up the pain in the scapular area or arm.

## Parenchymatous Involvement

Conduction along an intercostal nerve is seldom appreciably affected in thoracic root pressure caused by a protruded disc; hence, articular signs with root pain without signs of impaired conduction are the usual combination. A small area of cutaneous hypersensitiveness or analgesia is occasionally demonstrable anteriorly; alternatively, a wide band is found with borders so ill-defined as to afford no real help towards indicating the level of the protrusion. Occasionally a small patch of analgesia in the groin characterizes pressure at the twelfth thoracic level. Paralysis of one intercostal muscle would, on the contrary, be highly significant, but I have yet to detect this phenomenon. Electromyography might help here.

Disc protrusion at the first thoracic level should provide a welcome exception, since clear signs of a first thoracic root palsy would obtrude as soon as the strength of the small muscles of the patient's hand is tested. However, I have not yet encountered a case of unilateral first thoracic root pressure severly enough to weaken the muscles. Cases with neurological signs were all found to suffer from other conditions, e.g. malignant deposits in this vertebra, pulmonary sulcus tumour, neuroma, pressure by a cervical or first rib, or on the ulnar nerve at the elbow or wrist.

## Root Palsy

I have encountered only two such cases. Each patient had a band of analgesia parallel to and just above the inguinal ligament, and weakness of the muscle there was manifested by marked bulging on resisted flexion and rotation of the trunk (T11).

The numbness took six months to go; strength returned to the oblique muscle in six and twelve months respectively.

## Spinal Cord Signs

Pressure on the spinal cord is rare, but in all cases of suspected thoracic disc protrusion the signs of an upper motor neurone lesion should be sought, whether articular and nerve root signs are present or not. If the posterior displacement lies strictly centrally and has come on slowly, articular and nerve root signs are absent, but in large postero-lateral protrusions, the signs of both disorders may be combined.

Pins and needles felt in both lower limbs on neck flexion may prove the only symptom or sign, occurring equally with a central cervical, as with a central thoracic (but not lumbar) protrusion. In a recent minor case, not severe enough to warrant immediate laminectomy, much anxiety is naturally aroused. Some progress and require operation, but there are cases of slight spastic uni- or diplegia, caused by a thoracic disc lesion, with symptoms and signs that remained unaltered for up to 20 years. Even osteopathy has in some cases proved harmless, though it has also precipitated catastrophe requiring immediate laminectomy.

## Resisted Movements

At the thorax, the resisted movements have particular importance. Unlike the cervical and lumbar regions where muscle lesions scarcely occur, the muscles of the thorax and abdomen can suffer strain leading to post-traumatic scarring and persistent symptoms. A pectoral or intercostal muscle may be affected in this way, as may the latissimus dorsi, the inferior posterior serratus, the rectus or the oblique abdominal muscles.

Resisted rotation is best tested sitting as for passive rotation, and the result compared with the response to active and passive rotation. Side flexion is best tested with the patient standing, the examiner resisting the movement by applying his hip to the patient's, grasping his far shoulder, and asking him to bend away from the side where the examiner stands (Fig. 61).

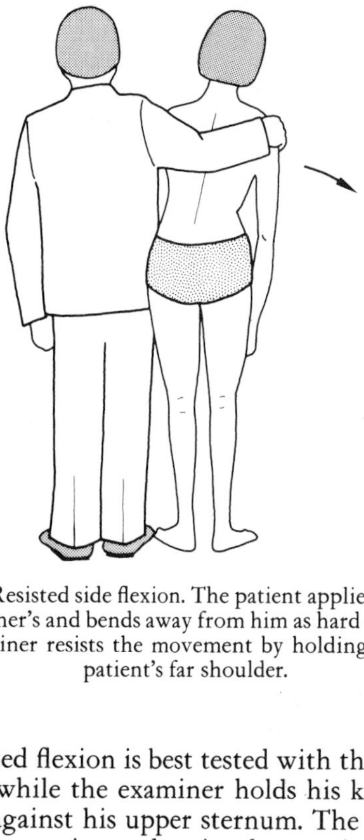

**Fig. 61.** Resisted side flexion. The patient applies his hip to the examiner's and bends away from him as hard as possible. The examiner resists the movement by holding on to the patient's far shoulder.

Resisted flexion is best tested with the patient sitting, while the examiner holds his knees and presses against his upper sternum. The response to active, passive and resisted extension can be simply contrasted by asking the prone patient to: (*a*) lift his chest off the couch with his arms behind his back; (*b*) push himself up with his arms letting the back sag (press up); and (*c*) attempt extension against the examiner's pressure at the base of the neck and at the knees.

Psychogenic symptoms at the thorax are not uncommon. By the time the neck has been examined, then the arm down to the hand, then the active, passive and resisted thoracic movements, followed by the lumbar spine, sacroiliac joints and lower limbs, the patient is hopelessly confused and has put forward a self-contradictory pattern. Pain provoked by resisted thoracic movement is a particularly likely allegation in such cases; for the patient is apt to equate effort with pain. Hence, a pattern indicating an inconceivable series of lesions emerges.

## Radiology

This seldom affords any help in disc lesions. The physical signs show that a protrusion is causing symptoms, but I am unable to reach greater clinical accuracy than to estimate the level as upper, mid- or lower thoracic. Should an isolated joint within the requisite bounds chance to show a markedly diminished joint space or much larger osteophytes than the others, this provides little guide to the joint affected. Calcification of one or more discs has no significance.

Myelography is urgently indicated when signs of pressure on the spinal cord are present; it reveals the level of the obstruction. Posterolateral protrusions are difficult to demonstrate unless Jirout's technique of dynamic pneumomyelography is employed (see p. 278). In any case, myelography is called for only preparatory to laminectomy; an operation that the degree of these patients' disablements seldom warrants. Surgery is apt to prove dangerous and should be advocated with reserve.

# INTERPRETATION

The pattern that emerges when a thoracic disc lesion is present is, as elsewhere, the partial articular pattern characteristic of internal derangement. Pain, therefore, is to be expected, and perhaps limitation, on some but not other of the thoracic active movements; more pain when these movements are carried out passively; no pain when the same movements are attempted against so great a resistance that the joint stays motionless.

As always in internal derangement, the partial capsular pattern emerges. One side flexion or rotation movement is limited, the other not. As a rule two, three or four of the active movements of the thorax hurt; correspondingly four, three or two do not. Often the articular movements elicit the posterior ache only, not affecting the anterior component which is apt to be increased on neck flexion alone. In difficult cases comparing the results of passive and resisted extension may prove helpful. A combination of articular with dural signs is common, but either may exist alone. Not only neck flexion but approximation of the scapulae often brings on the pain, because this movement pulls on the dura mater via the upper two thoracic nerve roots.

One rotation, often both, especially when carried out passively, nearly always hurts in a lower or mid-thoracic disc lesion. In a minor case, this may be the only painful movement. Even so, if passive rotation hurts and resisted rotation does not, a clear articular sign has emerged. If neck flexion now increases the ache present on full rotation, the diagnosis is clear.

So little movement is possible at the upper two thoracic joints owing to rigidity of the first and second ribs and sternum that, in lesions at these two levels, the articular signs may be wholly absent, only the movements stretching the nerve root increasing the pain.

Muscle lesions do not radiate pain from the posterior thorax to the anterior; this fact taken alone exculpates the muscles. If a resisted movement hurts and the passive movements—other than the one that fully stretches the muscle—do not, a muscle lesion is present. If no movement hurts, the pain is unconnected with the moving parts, and renewed search for a visceral origin must be undertaken.

*Caution.* There is one pattern of which the examiner must beware. Active side flexion away from the painful side is *limited* and painful; both passive rotations are full and painless. Since the movement most likely to hurt in a thoracic disc lesion is rotation, such marked restriction of side flexion without corresponding interference with rotation suggests an extra-articular lesion. Neoplasm of the lung or even in the upper abdomen may be present, alternatively, there is an intraspinal neuroma at a lower thoracic level. The last three cases I saw with this sign had, respectively, carcinoma of the hepatic flexure of the colon, neoplasm of the lower lung and a dumb-bell neuroma at the tenth level, lying partly inside and partly outside the spine.

## Treatment

### Postural Prophylaxis

In kyphosis, the posterior aspect of each of the joints between the vertebral bodies gapes and the anterior aspect is narrowed. This is, of course, the position of the joint most favourable to retropulsion of the intra-articular contents. The cervical and lumbar lordoses have the welcome effect of reversing this inclination of the joint surfaces: they thus serve to prevent displacements at the upper and lower extent of the vertebral column. These lordoses happily placed at the more mobile spinal joints necessitate the existence of an intermediate compensatory kyphosis; otherwise the centre of gravity of the body would lie too far anteriorly. In consequence, kyphosis has developed at the thoracic part of the spine, where movement and, by corollary, the likelihood of displacement of a fragment of disc, is fortunately greatly restricted by the rigidity of the thoracic cage.

It should be realized that even in individuals so supple that they can bend backwards and put their head between their thighs, the thoracic spine, owing to the inextensibility of the sternum, has been shown by radiography never to extend beyond a straight line. Hence, it is quite hopeless to expect a patient to maintain a thoracic lordosis; no such achievement is possible. Any patient with a lower thoracic disc lesion should avoid flexing his back and, more important, should not rotate it during flexion, especially if lifting a weight; he must avoid prolonged compression of the joints, i.e. carrying, and should maintain as great a degree of extension as possible during weight-lifting.

Those who sit all day and develop the—usually lower—thoracic ache due to posterior nuclear bulging must have their work rearranged so that the maintenance of kyphosis is no longer necessary. To this end, papers should be placed higher on an inclined plane so that the office worker has to lean away from them, i.e. backwards. A music stand supporting paper above the typewriter forces a typist to look upwards. A drawing-board may be held almost vertically.

Swimming is the only advantageous sport in thoracic (or lumbar) disc lesions. When the body floats, all compression strain on the joint ceases, and keeping the head out of water involves some degree of trunk extension: the beneficial posture. This does not apply to diving, since this involves a sudden impact during trunk flexion.

*Childbirth.* Lying in bed during the puerperium is a common cause of backache in young women. It has nothing to do with pregnancy, relaxed ligaments or sacroiliac strain. It is the result of lying in bed in 'the nursing mother's position', i.e. pillows behind the thorax while the back sags into kyphosis all day. The pillows should support the lumbar spine and she should lie face downwards at intervals during the day.

## Manipulative Reduction

This is attempted in all cases, unless a contraindication exists. Success is almost invariable. It is the tendency to recurrence that provides the problem.

*Contraindications.* Pressure on the spinal cord precludes any attempt at manipulation, i.e. a spastic gait, incoordination of the lower limbs, extensor plantar responses. Such patients should be left alone and laminectomy considered.

Paraesthetic feet show that the lesion has begun to touch the spinal cord. In such cases manipulation is contraindicated but traction is well worth trying, and, in cases of not too long standing, may well succeed. Manipulation during anticoagulant therapy may lead to intraspinal haemorrhage, as reported in one case after chiropractice (Dabbet et al, 1970).

*Indication for Manipulation.* The articular signs are of the expected type, some hurt, some not, usually unilaterally. One or both rotations prove painful. Limitation, if present, is usually of one rotation only. Dural signs are elicited but spinal cord symptoms and signs are absent. No signs of interference with an intercostal nerve root are detected.

All the findings that, at cervical or lumbar levels, show that manipulation will fail, have no bearing on lesions lying between the third and twelfth thoracic vertebrae. Whether the root pain came first or followed posterior aching, how long the root pain has been present, whether the history suggests a nuclear or a cartilaginous protrusion—none of these considerations is material. Nuclear protrusions are most uncommon and come to light only when the attempt at manipulative reduction fails; if so, the protrusion is usually centrally placed in a patient with considerable thoracic kyphosis.

*Technique.* Manipulative reduction should be carried out (*a*) without general anaesthesia and (*b*) during traction. The actual manipulations are described in Volume II, and only general principles require mention here.

Traction is applied by two assistants—one pulling on the patient's arms or head (depending on the level of the lesion), the other at his feet. If two physiotherapists trained in this work are employed, they can help the manipulator a great deal by altering their line of pull at the same moment as he forces the requisite movement.

After each manipulation, the patient stands up and states what difference (if any) he notices; the manipulator notes any objective alteration in the range of movement at the affected joint. This precaution prevents patients being made worse, as is sometimes unavoidable during general anaesthsia. As long as any particular manipulation does good, it is repeated. When it ceases to help, the manipulator passes on to the next one. This goes on until full reduction has been secured, or the patient has clearly had enough for one day, or it becomes evident that the protrusion is irreducible.

Once well, the patient should attend again quickly if he suffers a recurrence, indeed, it is an exceptional patient with a thoracic disc lesion who attends less often than once every year or two. It is only the upper four thoracic levels, where disc lesions are uncommon, where so little joint movement is possible that reduction is normally permanent. However, many patients can be kept continuously comfortable by having their protrusion reduced by manipulation at once whenever it recurs.

*Oscillatory Technique.* The to-and-fro movements popularized by Maitland are particularly useful in two sets of circumstances. (*a*) A thoracic disc lesion may cause considerable aching, but very minor articular signs; this is particularly apt to happen secondary to wedge-fracture. (*b*) The patient has such severe thoracic lumbago that the ordinary manipulations are difficult to tolerate. Oscillatory manoeuvres continued for five to fifteen minutes often reduce the displacement to the point where the ordinary manoeuvres become possible.

*Sustained Traction.* Thoracic disc lesions seldom protrude centrally and remain fixed in that position. If they do, especially if the patient has a postural kyphosis or an old crush fracture, manipulation may be dangerous or unlikely to succeed, or both. Alternatively, a history of gradual onset may suggest a pulpy protrusion. Or, manipulative reduction, when tentatively begun, may aggravate the symptoms. When pins and needles are felt in the feet, manipulation is always avoided and traction is indicated. In such cases, reduction by sustained traction should be attempted at once (see Volume II); it seldom fails. The traction lasts 30 to 45 minutes daily; a small woman may need 35 kg, a large man 70 kg.

## Prevention of Recurrence

The same precautions must be taken as are set out under postural prophylaxis (p. 207).

*Corsetry*. Whereas a corset is a great protection against recurrence in lumbar disc lesions, there is no corresponding benefit from wearing a corset with steels extending from the lower buttock to the upper thorax. This is so often prescribed, but is the reverse of what is required. If the thorax is to be immobilized, the more the lumbar spine is free to move, the better. Hence the cloth part of the corset can enclose the pelvis or not, as the patient and corset-fitter prefer, but the steels must start at the mid-lumbar region only (for a lower thoracic disc lesion) or at the lowest thoracic level (for a mid-thoracic lesion). Even so, a corset is seldom effective, and is very cumbersome.

*Ligamentous Sclerosis*. Since the thoracic spine is devoid of lordosis, the patient, though he must do his best, cannot always keep his intervertebral joint so tilted that it is open wider in front than behind. This is particularly so after fracture of a vertebral body or in osteochondrosis or Schmorl's nodes; for consequent kyphosis at the joints either side of the wedging is considerable, and the supra- and interspinous ligaments on each side become overstretched.

In all cases in which a marked tendency to recurrence becomes manifest, sclerosing injections into the ligaments joining the spinous processes should be given. The result may not become apparent until a couple of months after the third infiltration, but there is a good chance of enhanced stability.

Francis (1973) reported on 14 cases of thoracic disc lesion on which he had carried out Rees's neurofasciotomy with success in each case.

## Recumbency

This is the traditional treatment for all pain of spinal origin felt at the posterior aspect of the trunk. If manipulation and traction both fail, prolonged rest in bed is the only alternative. Happily, this wearisome treatment is very seldom required but, when it is, the outlook is indeed poor; for each recurrence then has to be dealt with by renewed recumbency.

In elderly patients, the capsular contracture of osteoarthrosis prevents the bones from coming apart when weight-bearing ceases. If so, recumbency is fruitless.

## Operation

Laminectomy is feasible only when contrast myelography reveals the site of the protrusion. In early cases of spinal cord compression, laminectomy must be considered and, if the lesion is progressive, carried out. The spinal cord has little space about it within the thoracic neural canal; moreover its blood supply only just suffices. About half of all patients are not improved afterwards, though further aggravation may cease. Others find the paralysis increased after operation, even when the safer anterolateral approach is employed. Hence intervention should be undertaken with reluctance. The alternative is an intradiscal injection of chymopapain (Ford 1969); he reports on two cases, one at the ninth, the other at the eleventh level. The cases of recurrent thoracic pain with increasing pins and needles in the lower limbs that render the patient more and more unable to carry on are best treated by arthrodesis. The myelogram is usually negative, since the protrusion is not yet large enough to indent the dura mater sufficiently to interfere with the flow of contrast material, but clinical examination can determine the level within two or three joints. Arthrodesis carried out over four or five joints has been conspicuously successful in several cases of this kind.

In a survey of operations for disc lesions in Switzerland (Brügger 1960) of 2948 laminectomies, 7 were carried out at thoracic levels, 2 at the eighth, 1 at the ninth and 4 at the eleventh intervertebral joints.

# Osteopathy and Chiropractice

The difficulty in distinguishing between visceral disease and root pressure set up by a thoracic disc lesion is responsible for many diagnostic errors. This has served to strengthen laymen's claims that visceral disease results from vertebral displacements and is curable by their reduction. The osteopath or chiropractor is himself misled when the patient, after his spine has been manipulated, declares that his, say, 'cholecystitis' or 'angina' has ceased. A doctor has diagnosed visceral disease. Finding that his spinal treatment has relieved it, the manipulator naturally imagines that he has really cured a visceral disorder; so does the patient. In consequence, all sorts of theories exist on the effect of vertebral manipulation on the autonomic system.

The many vocal and satisfied patients of lay manipulators—most of them by no means the neurotics so often supposed—combine to show how often a thoracic disc lesion remains unsuspected.

However, there is another aspect to this picture. In 1962 Strohmeyer told me that, of 40 cases of paraplegia admitted to his neurosurgical clinic in Bremen, 28 followed a chiropractic manipulation. Livingstone (1971) reported that in 172 patients receiving chiropraxy, injury resulted in 12. Several patients had a spinal neoplasm, which gives an idea of the care exercised by chiropractors in Germany and Canada in the selection of cases.

## COMPRESSION PHENOMENA

Since some degree of kyphosis is universal at the mid- and upper-thoracic joints, symptoms due to gradual retropulsion are common, especially in individuals with a marked thoracic kyphosis.

### Posterior Bulging at the Thoracic Spinal Joints

Mid- or upper-thoracic central aching is apt to come on in those who sit bent forward for long periods on end. The discomfort is probably caused not so much by an actual disc lesion as by a gradual and slight movement backwards of the entire intra-articular contents at several adjacent joints. After some years this pressure stretches the posterior longitudinal ligament, bulging it backwards against the dura mater. The greater the patient's thoracic kyphosis, the longer he sits bent, and the more he compresses the spinal joints, the greater the likelihood of this occurrence.

Diagnosis is made largely on the characteristic symptoms. The patient wakes comfortable; as the day goes on, the posterior thorax begins to ache centrally, except on Sundays, when he does not sit poring over a desk. The ache gets slowly worse, spreading bilaterally until most of the back of the chest is painful. Carrying anything heavy or sitting for some time increases the symptoms; lying down for a few minutes, later for some hours, brings relief. While the pain is bad, a deep breath usually hurts. This pain goes on appearing by day and ceasing at night, coming on earlier in the morning as the years go by, and taking longer to abate with recumbency. Improvement follows change in the patient's circumstances, e.g. leaving a kyphotic occupation (such as sewing) or acquiring domestic help.

Examination shows minimal articular signs and an absence of all other signs. The patient who describes a complaint that gives rise to practically no signs, and then is found to have practically no signs, must be believed. He is not suffering from psychoneurosis; for hypersensitive patients have multiple symptoms and display exaggeration and incongruity in their signs, not a consistent negative.

For the first 10 to 30 years, the radiograph reveals no abnormality. Finally, anterior erosion takes place, as described below.

In the early stages treatment should be to change the patient's occupation to one more suitable, combined with explanation on how the pain is produced and, by corollary, avoided. Later, as the condition develops, lying down for an hour in the late morning and again in the afternoon may keep the pain within bounds. If this does not suffice, traction is indicated and is best given daily for, say, a fortnight, then at weekly, finally monthly, intervals. Ligamentous sclerosis after reduction is strongly indicated, but may have to be carried out at several adjacent levels. Francis (1973) reports excellent results with neurofasciotomy. Manipulation is contraindicated, for no reducible fragment is present.

### Anterior Erosion

A thoracic kyphosis, in the end, leads to such continued pressure on the anterior aspect of each disc that the front of the bodies of two adjacent vertebrae wear it through and meet. Where bone touches bone, a localized anterior osteophyte appears on each vertebral body, with bone sclerosis at the point of contact. Though this outcrop can be called an osteophyte, its existence does not mean that the whole joint is osteoarthrotic in the sense that a patient may be said to be suffering from osteoarthrosis of the hip or ankle. It is localized pressure phenomenon. Bone contains nerves and is a sentient structure. Hence bone pressing against bone can well cause pain. The osteophyte is not the cause of pain, but the result of the disc erosion that has enabled the bones finally to grind together painfully, and the pain would have appeared had no osteophytes formed. Anterior erosion is the cause of pain in patients who developed Scheurmann's deformity in adolescence.

Anterior erosion of the disc takes years to develop; hence, patients with this condition are nearly always middle-aged or elderly, possess a rounded thoracic kyphosis and give a past history of posterior articular bulging (see above). The intermittent thoracic ache finally becomes constant, and analgesic drugs become necessary. The radiograph shows the typical changes. Not all patients with this radiological appearance suffer much discomfort; the degree of pain caused is extremely variable and more attention should be paid to the patient's statements than to the X-ray appearances.

Clinical examination shows very little. The characteristic kyphosis is noted; the limitation of movement is obvious but the joints are often so stiff that the active movements prove painless and only the passive movements elicit the articular pain.

A conservative treatment sometimes effective is traction, repeated at such intervals (if it succeeds for the time being) as the symptoms warrant. Daily neck suspension provides an alternative.

## Lateral Erosion

Exactly the same mechanism occurs in long-standing severe scoliosis. At the concave side, the intra-articular disc becomes worn through and bone touches bone painfully with the same local sclerosis but less pronounced osteophytes (Brown 1828). Unilateral pain felt in the erector muscles of, usually, the lower thorax is the first symptom. Since the bulge is lateral, not posterior, and thus cannot press on the dura mater or a nerve root, no symptoms arise until bone touches bone. The ache is purely local and unilateral, without radiation to the front of the trunk. A deep breath is painless and dural signs are absent. Finally, the pain becomes constant by day and is aggravated by any exertion tending to press the joint surfaces together, e.g. carrying. For many years a night's rest brings relief, but ultimately the ache may persist round the clock.

The passive movements at the relevant spinal joints hurt; the stiffness is such that the active movements are grossly limited but more or less painless. The resisted movements do not hurt. Sustained traction is the only conservative treatment worth attempting, but often fails. If the symptoms warrant, extensive operative fusion is indicated.

## Thoracic Mushroom Phenomenon

This results from complete attrition of one disc in an elderly patient. Erosion has to be complete, for the thoracic nerve root fills only one-third to one-tenth of the foramen (Svanberg 1915). It may result in central posterior thoracic aching; root pain is also encountered usually unilateral. The patient suffers constant pain except while lying down, whereupon it ceases in a minute or two. In contrast to a lumbar compression phenomenon, sitting and bending forwards do not abolish the pain.

The articular signs are inconspicuous, for the joints are so stiff that no change is felt in the symptoms as the patient moves. In root pain, side flexion towards the painful side is apt to hurt, by further compression at the foramen. Some hyper-aesthesia may develop along the posterior extent of the relevant dermatome. Cord signs are absent. The diagnosis is established by the characteristic history—pain when upright, comfort lying—and the negative clinical findings.

When the pain on keeping the trunk erect is felt centrally, the best hope of lasting relief is arthrodesis. Before this is advised, it is worth while, especially after wedge-fracture, trying the effect of traction. One session may afford some days' relief. If so, this treatment is repeated on, say, alternate days for some years. The local carpenter makes a frame with a pulley, installed at the patient's home.

If the pain is unilateral, extending obliquely downwards along the dermatome, it can often be abolished, at any rate for a year or two, by infiltration about the nerve root. First the correct root has to be identified with a procaine block, the patient standing up afterwards and stating whether or not the pain comes on after keeping upright for the usual length of time. At his next attendance, he may report lasting benefit; if so, the anaesthetic block is repeated. If the relief proves ephemeral, triamcinolone is substituted. This treatment apparently desensitizes the nerve root enough to make compression no longer painful; it is remarkably successful and the relief lasts six months or two years. Thereupon the same treatment is once more effective.

In the mid-thoracic region the intervertebral foramen lies halfway between each pair of ribs. Their adjacent edges are identified and a spot chosen midway between them and 5 cm from the midline. A 2 ml syringe is filled with 2% procaine solution and fitted with a thin needle 5 cm long. This is thrust in almost horizontally, parallel to the ribs. The tip should hit the edge of the lamina and then, by being manoeuvred along a little more deeply, lose touch with bone and enter the foramen. It is passed in another 5 mm and the injection given here.

No anaesthesia at the dermatome results; the effect appears to be on the surface of the nerve root only together with a block of the sinuvertebral nerve.

## Thoracic Neuroma

Though neurologists' statistics show that thoracic neuromas outnumber cervical and lumbar, this has not proved so in cases sent to the orthopaedic physician.

At first nothing distinguishes a neuroma from a simple thoracic disc protrusion, for the cessation of root pain with the passage of time applies only to disc lesions at cervical and lumbar levels. In either case, root pain, with or without central discomfort, is experienced, aggravated by a deep breath, cough, laughing, neck flexion and scapular approximation. The articular signs, however, may prove unusual, side flexion away from the painful side proving limited and painful, whereas neither rotation hurts.

Disc pressure seldom causes any cutaneous analgesia. Hence a patch of numbness along the dermatome, especially if it increases in size as time goes on, arouses suspicion. Pins and needles in one or both feet show that the spinal cord is menaced and call for myelography without waiting for objective signs of impaired pyramidal function.

Thoracic disc lesions very seldom prove irreducible by manipulation during traction. Failure should therefore bring to mind the possibility of a neuroma.

# PATHOLOGICAL WEDGING

The bodies of the thoracic vertebrae become wedged as the result of a number of different pathological processes.

## Adolescent Osteochondrosis

This occurs mainly at the lower half of the thoracic spine (and in the upper lumbar region). Between the ages of 14 and 18, an osteochondrosis may appear at the end-plate of one or two adjacent vertebrae. Osteochondrosis is merely a descriptive label; the cause is nuclear material forcing its way between the end-plate anteriorly and the now unprotected bone, with consequent erosion. Marked wedging results. This concept of anterior nuclear protrusion was first put forward by Beadle (1931). He pointed out that the wedging of the vertebral body was due to prolapse of the nucleus through the end-plate, where it invaded cancellous bone—a phenomenon already described by Schmorl (1927). After a few years, further progress is halted by the formation of a layer of compact bone round the herniation. This permanent barrier accounts for the sclerotic edge seen radiologically. By the age of 19 the lesion has become static and further pressure on bone ceases. The shelf of hard bone shows up well on Beadle's illustrations of microscopic appearances. These facts have recently been confirmed by Swischuck (1970). The process is painless and in itself insignificant, but it leads to a permanent increase in the degree of kyphosis at the affected joints. This posture tends to eventual retropulsion of disc substance, with posterior bulging occurring in patients still quite young.

The lateral radiograph (Plate XVII) shows the condition clearly, but since the disorder often causes no symptoms, X-ray evidence of vertebral osteochondrosis, past or present, must not be regarded as significant, unless the symptoms and clinical signs point to an articular lesion at the affected level.

When adolescent osteochondrosis occurs to a rather lesser degree but over many vertebrae, the disorder is named Scheuermann's disease.

I have never seen a case of Calve's osteochondrosis of the vertebral body itself with consequent wedging.

## Adult Osteochondrosis

In adult life a visible localized rounded kyphosis, involving four to six adjacent vertebrae, is often left over from a past lower thoracic osteochondrosis. Active movement towards extension is considerably limited but painless, whereas flexion, side flexion and rotation are of full range. Passive extension at the kyphosis with the patient prone is felt to be stiff and provokes minor discomfort. Usually, the disorder causes no symptoms, merely a visible convexity. However, as it shows up radiologically and possesses a name, it causes much irrelevant medicolegal argument and may also be used to bolster psychoneurotic symptoms.

## Fracture

Flexion injuries may cause fracture of a vertebral body. The immediate pain usually encircles the trunk at the appropriate level; this girdle pain lasts a week or two. At the end of three months symptoms have ceased; no treatment is necessary unless the patient is seen during the first few days, when a week in bed may be required. If the bone has been damaged, no further trouble need be feared. If the disc has also suffered, endless trouble is to be expected. Permanent kyphosis exists at the joint on each side of the fracture, and manipulative reduction is apt to prove very temporary. Such patients, when involved in lawsuits, are apt to be described as suffering from compensation neurasthenia; some are, it is true, but many others are not. They are suffering from a lesion that the radiograph cannot reveal, and force sufficient to break bone may well injure adjacent cartilage as well. It is unfair to maintain that, because the bone has united, the patient cannot have pain. He may or may not; that is an assessment that cannot be reached by radiography, which is merely evidence that the accident was severe enough to damage bone. The problem cannot be resolved except by clinical examination. Moreover, the flexion deformity may give rise to considerable ligamentous aching in the overstretched supra- and interspinous ligaments and to a feeling of insecurity on bending forwards. In either case, sclerosing injections are indicated. If fixed flexion deformity eventually leads to a compression phenomenon, pain is apt to return, perhaps years later. Occasionally, post-traumatic ossification in the ligaments leads to fixation of the joint and permanent cure.

The convulsion of ECT may, by hyperflexing the spine, drive the nucleus pulposus into the body of the vertebra. No wedging results and slight and transitory pain in the bone from the minor fracture is the only symptom. The radiograph is diagnostic.

## Senile Osteoporosis

This disorder affects the whole thoracolumbar spine and pelvis of elderly persons, more often women (see Plate XXIV); the neck and the bones of the limbs are not appreciably affected.

The bodies of the vertebrae soften; hence the first radiological sign is a marked biconcavity of the vertebral body, caused by disc substance pushing its way evenly towards the spongiosum. At this stage, *there are no symptoms*, and it is a common mistake to suppose that, if a patient has a backache and the radiograph shows senile osteoporosis, this disease accounts for the backache. The same appearance is seen in young patients who once suffered from severe rickets, and in tropical osteomalacia. Later on pathological wedging may occur. If this takes place suddenly, fracture with girdle pain results, leading after a week or two to localized bone pain. After three months, the fracture has united and symptoms have ceased unless the flexion deformity gives rise to retropulsion of the articular contents as a compression phenomenon. If the wedging takes place gradually, it may cause no symptoms, but in due course the compression phenomenon may ensue. Palpation for the kyphos should be followed by radiography.

Nordin (1959), working with the radioisotope $^{47}Ca$, showed that the rate at which bone was laid down was not reduced and that osteoporosis was caused by enhanced resorption of bone, the result and not the cause of a negative calcium balance. Steroid therapy is well known to induce such a negative balance, with increased loss, mainly faecal, of both calcium and phosphorus. Rose (1965) states that fluoride and calcium therapy is without avail. In my experience, 1 g of calcium gluconate three times daily together with an anabolic steroid often prevents further deformity and should be continued indefinitely. Testosterone appears to have no such effect. Calcitonin may prove useful for it lowers the plasma calcium level.

## Pathological Fracture

The angular kyphos is palpable and radiography shows the cause. When this is due to isolated myeloma of the vertebral body X-ray therapy may be permanently effective. Tuberculosis caries has been regarded as calling for immobilization and arthrodesis but Konstam and Blesovsky (1962), working on unpromising clinical material in Ibadan, published a review of 207 cases of spinal tuberculosis treated with isoniazid and *para*-aminosalicylic acid without plaster, the patients remaining ambulant. Even the 56 with paraplegia were allowed to get about as much as they were able. Complete recovery was obtained in 178 cases of the 207, and in 51 of the 56 paraplegics.

## Schmorl's Nodes

These appear for the first time about the age of 16 at the lower thoracic and upper lumbar levels and represent small invasions of the vertebral body by nuclear disc material protruding vertically. They never cause any symptoms, at the time of their occurrence or later. By fixing the nucleus in the centre of the joint and thus preventing a tendency to pressure directed posteriorly they may well protect the patient against posterior protrusion.

# THORACIC SCOLIOSIS

## Congenital Scoliosis

The mother notes that the baby lies always on one side, but the rotation deformity often remains unnoticed and is regarded, when it is perceived later, as an infantile scoliosis.

## Adolescent Scoliosis

This starts at about the age of 10, when the rate of bone growth increases. Owing to the tilt on the articular surfaces of each facet joint, the lower articular process, as it rides upwards during side flexion, is also drawn forwards. As a result, a thoracic scioliosis is prominent on the concave side, the opposite of a lumbar scoliosis where the facet surfaces tilt the other way and the vertebrae are rotated towards the convex side. It is commoner in girls, and the prominent convex side is more often the right. The deformity increases until vertebral bone growth ceases at 16 to 18 years of age. The easiest way to know is radiography of the apophyses at the iliac crest; they fuse at the same time as those of the vertebrae. It then remains static till middle age, when the discs begin to wear away on the concave side; the deformity then increases again. When they are completely eroded and bone touches bone, pain appears for the first time. It is remarkable how seldom the ordinary type of thoracic disc lesion with attacks of intermittent displacement of a loose fragment complicates thoracic scoliosis.

Orthopaedic surgeons disagree on whether treatment makes an appreciable difference to the outcome of scoliosis. Early arthrodesis can obviously stop an increasing deformity from getting worse, and a Milwaukee brace from pelvis to chin and occiput prevents aggravation, but has to be worn for some years, i.e. until bone growth ceases. It is very doubtful if exercises and ordinary corsetry do much for the child; their chief virtue appears to me to be giving the parents the feeling that 'something is being done'. In 1941 the American Orthopaedic Research Committee reported that not one of 425 patients with idiopathic scoliosis derived any benefit from exercises. After the age of 16, nothing further is required, since growth of the vertebrae ceases then. If the angle of deformity between the thoracic spine and the lumbar is less than 60°, a normal life span is to be expected (Zorab 1969).

In Russia, adolescent scoliosis is treated by chemonucleolysis. The nucleus bulges towards the convex side. Reduction of the nucleus by the injection allows correction, but the now normal disc space keeps it within its proper limits (Sampson 1978).

## Secondary Scoliosis

Hemivertebra, neurofibromatosis, thoracoplasty and anterior poliomyelitis affecting the trunk muscles asymmetrically are the likely causes.

It had always been thought that, in scoliosis complicating neurological disorders, the deformity resulted from the unequal muscle pull, the stronger muscle naturally lying on the concave side of the curve. Kleinberg (1951) pointed out that this was not necessarily so. The contrary can happen; moreover, the degree of deformity is not necessarily proportional to the severity of the muscle weakness. Martin (1965) described 14 patients with post-encephalitic Parkinsonism who had developed a scoliosis. Some patients deviated towards, others away from, the more rigid side. In two cases, the curvature was corrected when the operation on the globus pallidus relieved the rigidity. He therefore suggests that the scoliosis is the result of positive neuromuscular action.

# THORACIC ANKYLOSING SPONDYLITIS

In ankylosing spondylitis, the distinctive feature is pain coming and going irrespective of what the patient does. During a good period, no degree of exertion has any effect; during a bad period, the back may ache without provocation. When the thoracic spine is affected, the pain is posterior and central, but when the anterior longitudinal ligament becomes involved, it may be epigastric or sternal and worst on waking. A deep breath does not hurt, but there may be a feeling of tightness, owing to the onset of rigidity at the costovertebral joints.

Realization that the symptoms stem from thoracic spondylitis depends on examination of the whole spine.

A flat lumbar spine associated with an upper thoracic kyphosis is suggestive, and marked limitation of side flexion in each direction at all the lumbar and thoracic spinal joints is pathognomonic. Sacroiliac and lumbar involvement sometimes proceed painlessly; even so, with rare exceptions, the lumbar spine becomes rigid before the thoracic joints stiffen. Since spondylitis in the sacroiliac joints never begins after the age of 40 and usually begins during the twenties, the restriction of lumbothoracic movements is detected long before the age when limitation from advanced osteophyte formation can have set in. When spondylitis has omitted the lumbar spine and has jumped from the sacroiliac to the thoracic joints, diagnosis is very difficult; for thoracic aching due to the spondylitic process begins while a full range of movement remains at the lumbar spine; moreover, there has not been any gluteal or lumbar discomfort. The hint is given by the complaint of an ache worse on waking, coming and going for years without apparent cause or connection with exertion. Clinical examination shows that the range of passive thoracic rotation is limited to 45 or 60° (normal 90°), and that at the extreme of the possible range the movement stops with a hard end-feel and a great deal more pain than would be provoked if merely a minor long-standing disc lesion were present. Repeated radiographs have revealed no abnormality at the thoracic joints, but these clinical findings naturally call for X-ray examination of the sacroiliac joints, at which the telltale sclerosis is nearly always seen. If the sacroiliac joints happen to be radiologically normal, only the immediate and lasting response to phenylbutazone confirms the diagnosis.

Treatment consists of relief from pain and stiffness by means of either butazolidine or indomethacin, and surprisingly small doses often suffice. If there is pain only in the mornings, 100 mg of butazolidine taken last thing at night may enable the patient to wake comfortable. Other patients prefer indomethacin and 25 mg three times a day are often prescribed, but except during an exacerbation, one or two tablets a day are often enough. During a remission, all drugs are avoided.

Surprisingly, fixation of the chest, with consequent reliance purely on the diaphragm for breathing, does not lead to increased incidence of pneumonia, etc. Zorab (1966) states that in a Ministry of Pensions analysis of the cause of death in 70 cases of advanced spondylitis only five were from an acute respiratory disorder.

## LESIONS OF THE THORACIC CAGE

The intrinsic thoracic muscles, notably the intercostal muscles, are liable to direct bruising. The muscles connecting scapula and humerus to the thorax may be painfully strained, especially in athletes. Hence an essential part of the examination of the thorax is to test the resisted movements of the neck, scapula, arm, thorax and abdominal wall.

It should be remembered that diaphragmatic, intercostal or abdominal muscular symptoms and signs, when accompanied by fever, may result from epidemic myalgia, less often from infestation with *Trichinella spiralis.*

### Intercostal Muscles and Ribs

Damage to one or more intercostal muscles follows direct bruising, nearly always at the front of the chest. The ribs may or may not remain intact. Fracture of a rib must involve some muscle fibres tearing close to the break. When there is no displacement of the fractured ends, the surfaces fit and movement here is not a cause of appreciable symptoms. Nevertheless, breathing and other active movements set up pain, clearly of muscular origin. The patient points to the spot in a characteristic way; he places one finger on the exact place. In other painful affections at the thorax the pain is diffuse and he indicates the site of symptoms with the palm of his hand.

Referred pain does not arise from an intercostal muscle, for it is developed at the distal end of one short segment; moreover, it lies superficially.

The main diagnostic difficulty is the primary posterolateral disc protrusion causing anterior pain only; in the other types the pain is posterior as well as anterior and no confusion can arise. Full active trunk extension stretches the affected intercostal muscle and resisted flexion and rotation of the trunk also usually hurt. Luckily these are the very movements that do not hurt a patient with a thoracic disc lesion. Springing the chest wall by pressure on the rib at a distance from the injured point hurts in fracture but not in a disc lesion. Palpation has no diagnostic value, since a referred tender area can always be found at the front of the chest wall in any case of disc lesion with anterior pain. If, however, a fractured rib or a strained intercostal muscle is present, local tenderness defines its exact site.

Medicolegal considerations apart, when the

intercostal muscles are damaged by direct bruising, it makes no difference whether an uncomplicated fracture of one or more ribs is present or not. The cause of pain and the treatment are the same.

Clicking of a costal cartilage is painless. Momentary discomfort, however, is felt when the point of one of the lower ribs hits the iliac crest, as may happen on side flexion of the trunk in patients with exceptionally long floating ribs or with marked scoliosis. Quite severe pain lasting as long as a minute occurs when the point of a rib becomes loose anteriorly and is forced into the substance of the abdominal muscles on trunk flexion. The attacks are recurrent and the patient often supplies the diagnosis himself. Painful swelling of a costochondral junction (Tietze 1921) is visible and palpable. Fibrositis with the same coarse crepitus as may accompany scapulothoracic movement seldom affects the intercostal membrane at a sternochondral junction.

### Treatment

*Muscles.* The intercostal muscles respond very quickly to massage. Especially if he is elderly, the patient cannot mobilize the muscle himself however deeply he breathes; hence pain persists indefinitely, but the scarring is broken down by transverse massage in a very few sessions (see Volume II).

*Fractured Rib.* As already pointed out, it is tearing of the intercostal muscle, not the broken rib itself that sets up pain in uncomplicated fracture. In recent cases the best immediate treatment is local anaesthesia induced at the affected muscle. The pain on breathing may be such as to cause shock, which the anaesthesia immediately abates. The severe pain very seldom returns. Further relief from pain can be achieved by strapping the affected side of the chest. The criterion for its application is the degree of pain, not the fact of fracture; hence, strapping is equally indicated in recent intercostal lesions, whether or not associated with fracture.

Non-elastic strapping is applied horizontally; it must cross the midline at the sternum and at the spine, and must be applied very tightly at the extreme of a full expiratory movement. Fractured ribs unite enough to become painless in four to six weeks and union is invariable; thus, pain persisting after this period has elapsed must arise in the intercostal muscles. Should pain persist longer than a month, deep massage is indicated.

*Loose Rib.* If a loose rib or long floating rib causes sufficient symptoms, its anterior extent can be removed.

## Muscle Lesions

### Minor Trauma to the Diaphragm

These cases are uncommon. They result from blows on the chest with transmitted stress. The pain is on respiration only; no pain is elicited when trunk movements are performed while the patient holds his breath. It is my impression that the central fibres of the diaphragm give rise to pain felt at the point of the shoulder whereas the fibres near the ribs give rise to local pain only.

I have encountered one case only of a painful scar occurring at the attachment of the diaphragm to the back of the xiphisternum. The spot was just within finger's reach. The symptoms had been taken for indigestion for ten years and treated by drugs and finally cholecystectomy. Deep massage at this point gave lasting relief.

### Stitch

This is supposed to arise from the diaphragm and may be an ishaemic phenomenon akin to claudication. The alternative theory is tugging on the diaphragmatic origin of the peritoneal ligaments suspending stomach and liver. Running soon after a meal predisposes to stitch which may be a recurrent phenomenon, coming on at the same moment race after race.

Examination of the patient between attacks reveals no abnormality; after a race deep breathing hurts for a few minutes—nothing else. Lying down stops the pain.

It is alleged that keeping the arms into the sides during exertion postpones or avoids pain. As a rule, nothing avails.

### Lesion of the Pectoralis Major and Latissimus Dorsi Muscles

These are dealt with in Chapter 11 since they are muscles controlling the arm. In the former case, the pain comes on gradually and is felt in the pectoral area, usually spreading down the inner side of the arm to the elbow. Full passive elevation of the arm stretches the muscle and hurts; it hurts also when a rib is fractured close to the pectoral origin and in Mondor's phlebitis. Resisted adduction of the arm also hurts but resisted medial rotation usually does not. The best way to elicit pain in lesions of the pectoralis major is to ask the patient to bring both arms horizontally forward and then press his hands together as hard as he can (see Fig. 45). The two areas most often affected are the inner fibres just below the clavicle or the lowest part of the outer edge close to the ribs. When the differentiation between an intercostal and a pectoral pain is required, and pain on a resisted adduction movement of the arm is not clearly elicited, the following test is useful. The patient places his hand on his hip and tenderness is compared while the pectoralis major is in contraction and in relaxation. In the case of a pectoral lesion, the tenderness is greater on contraction. The pectoralis minor muscle appears never to suffer comparable strain, though it may be involved in contracture of the costocoracoid fascia.

Treatment consists of local anaesthesia or deep massage (see Volume II).

When the thoracic extent of the latissimus dorsi muscle is affected, the pain is localized. Resisted adduction and full passive elevation of the arm both hurt; the thoracic movements are painless. Local anaesthesia often has some lasting effect, and deep massage is quickly curative.

## COSTOVERTEBRAL JOINTS

Movement at these joints lessens as age advances; in consequence, the respiratory excursion of the chest wall diminishes. A thoracic kyphosis, emphysema or a liability to asthma increases the tendency to early stiffness. In such cases, the joints should be kept as mobile as possible by passive forcing, whereupon the patient practises deep breathing exercises that maintain the added range. To this end the physiotherapist places her hands on the lower ribs and increases the respiratory movement of the chest wall by manual pressure (Fig. 62).

In ankylosing spondylitis, the costovertebral joints eventually become fixed as part of the ligamentous ossifying process. During the involvement, which may take years, pain may be felt at one or both sides of the sternum or of the thoracic region posteriorly. It is apt to be most troublesome after some hours' sleep or on waking in the morning, i.e. after relative immobility. Breathing is uncomfortable and the patient feels the respiratory excursion of his chest to be

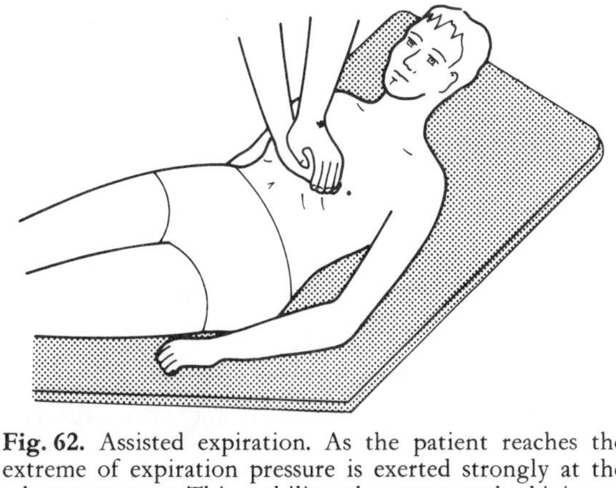

**Fig. 62.** Assisted expiration. As the patient reaches the extreme of expiration pressure is exerted strongly at the lower sternum. This mobilizes the costovertebral joints.

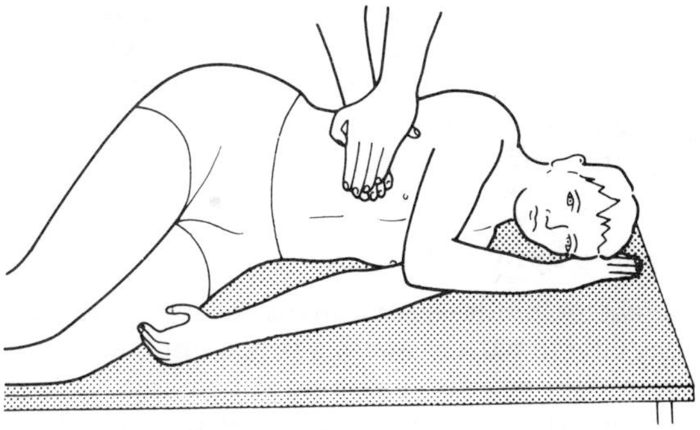

**Fig. 63.** Assisted inspiration. As the extreme of inspiration is reached, pressure is exerted on the lower ribs. This mobilizes the costovertebral joints in the opposite direction to that shown in Fig. 62.

restricted—as indeed it is. The trunk movements do not alter the pain, but make the diagnosis clear, for side flexion of the lumbar spine is largely or fully lost by the time the costovertebral joints are affected. Pressure on the sternum while the patient lies supine reproduces the pain. If one costovertebral joint only is affected, an endeavour should be made to inject triamcinolone into it. Certainly, when the injection is correctly placed, relief is secured within 24 hours and usually lasts many months. If many are affected, indomethacin 25 mg twice daily or butazolidine 100 mg twice daily stops the feeling, but not the fact, of stiffness.

*Postoperative posture and respiration* provide an important field for the physiotherapist. The patient's position in bed is most important, e.g. after thoracoplasty. After operations of any severity on the chest and abdomen, the vital capacity is much diminished. Breathing exercises, postural drainage and manual shaking greatly diminish the incidence of postoperative pulmonary complications.

## THE STERNUM

Most sternal pain has a visceral origin, but there are other sources.

### Lesion of Bone

The sternum may be fractured; if so, an upper thoracic vertebra is often wedged as well. It may also be painfully invaded by metastases. In either case, the bone itself is tender and the radiograph diagnostic.

### Manubriosternal Joint

The cause of trouble at this joint is seldom an injury; monarticular rheumatoid arthritis or ankylosing spondylitis is more commonly responsible. The patient knows exactly where the pain is and the manubriosternal ligaments are swollen and tender. Triamcinolone injected at the joint is most successful.

### Tietze's Syndrome

The costochondral junction may become strained, especially in patients with a persistent cough, e.g. chronic bronchitis. The pain is brought on by a deep breath and cough and is felt to one side of the sternum, about 4 cm from its edge. A small swelling is palpable at the affected junction, and the tenderness at the junction, whereas if the lesion is of the intercostal membrane, it lies between the two bones. If the pain has lasted longer than a month, fracture of a rib cannot be responsible.

Pressure on the sternum or at the lateral aspect of the thorax usually reproduces the unilateral pain, and the site of tenderness is diagnostic. One infiltration with triamcinolone is curative.

### Pain Referred to the Sternum

An upper thoracic disc lesion protruding centrally may give rise to sternal pain only. If so, diagnosis is often difficult, since the upper thoracic joints possess little mobility, confined as they are by ribs and sternum. Hence the active thoracic articular movements may be misleadingly painless, only passive forcing reproducing the sternal ache. But the dural signs are usually clear, neck flexion and scapular approximation reproducing the symptom well.

When the anterior longitudinal ligament is affected in ankylosing spondylitis, the pain may be purely sternal or epigastric.

## LESIONS OF THE ABDOMINAL WALL

An accurate, detailed history is essential in differentiating visceral disorder and thoracic disc lesions from anterior muscular pain. Except in athletes or after an operation for inguinal hernia, anterior abdominal pain seldom results from a muscular lesion; hence this ascription should be made unwillingly.

## Examination of Abdominal Movements

When the abdominal muscles are affected, little information is supplied by the trunk movements of the standing patient; for only extension hurts in lesions of the abdominal musculature. The resisted abdominal movements are tested as follows.

The patient lies supine; then, resting his hands on his lap he sits up. The examiner places one hand on his feet and the other against his sternum, and a strong trunk flexion movement is resisted (Fig. 64). Pain on such resisted movement may be felt in the abdomen, in which case it arises from the rectus abdominis, or in one groin, in which case it arises from the flexor muscles of the hip. The sitting patient is next asked to twist his trunk against the examiner's resistance

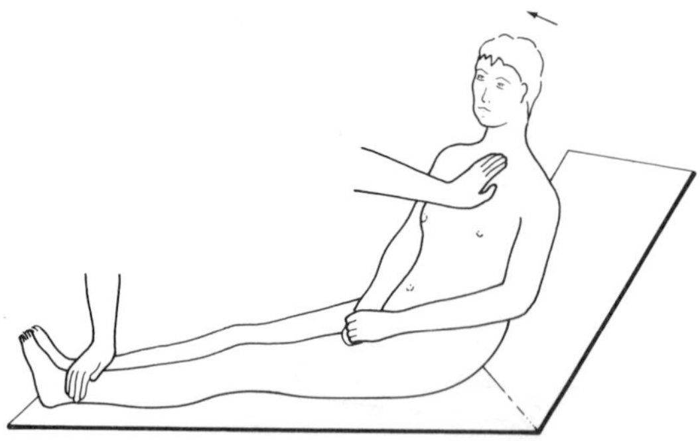

**Fig. 64.** Resisted flexion of the trunk. The examiner supports the patient's legs with one hand, while resisting the patient's attempt to sit up by pressure on the chest. Test for the rectus abdominis muscle.

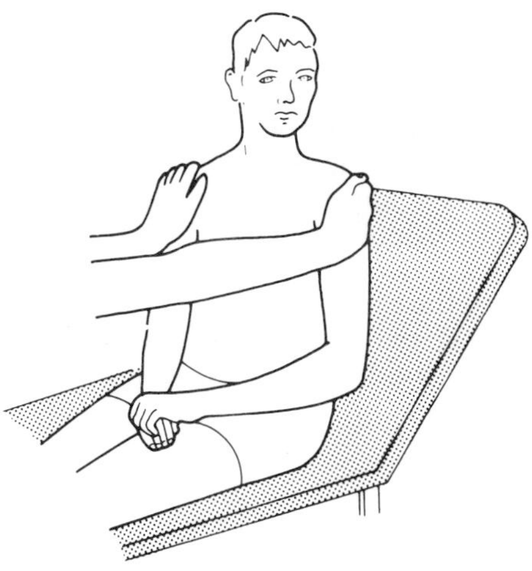

**Fig. 65.** Resisted rotation of the trunk. The patient tries to twist his trunk against resistance applied at his shoulders. Test for the oblique abdominal and serratus posterior inferior muscles.

applied at both shoulders (Fig. 65). Pain on such a movement away from the painful side suggests a lesion of the external oblique muscle; towards the painful side, of the internal oblique muscle. If this sign is positive in a youngster of 14 to 16, the radiography may show avulsion of the iliac epiphysis along the crest, just behind the anterior superior spine.

The structure defined by which movement proved painful should be examined for tenderness near the area where the pain is felt.

If the rectus abdominis muscle is at fault the lesion is most frequently above the umbilicus. Then, full active elevation of the ipsilateral arm, when the patient stands or lies flat, often stretches the muscle and causes the abdominal pain. A small haematoma can often be felt. Tenderness at the pubic insertion suggests fracture or puerperal subluxation of the symphyis pubis rather than a muscular lesion.

When the origin of either oblique muscle from the ribs is affected, tenderness is best elicited by bringing the finger under the costal edge and pressing upwards and forwards. As some tenderness here is normal, the two sides must be carefully compared. The belly of an oblique muscle is involved as a rule at one or other iliac fossa. Chronic appendicitis may then be closely simulated. The following test serves to determine whether the source of pain is in the muscle or viscera.

The semirecumbent patient is asked to raise his head and shoulders from the couch, i.e. to contract his abdominal muscles—and pressure is applied at the spot which has already been found to be tender. The patient is then asked to lie back and relax, and the pressure of the same degree is applied again. If the pain is accentuated in the former event—namely, when the pressure is exerted against taut muscles which protect the underlying viscera— its source must be in the muscles or fasciae of the abdominal wall. If, on the other hand, it is greater when the patient relaxes, the source must lie inside the abdomen.

Gross weakness of the abdominal muscles results from advanced myopathy or anterior poliomyelitis.

The treatment of muscle lesions of the anterior abdominal wall is deep massage (see Volume II).

## SYMPHYSIS PUBIS

Puerperal subluxation results in pain and tenderness felt exactly at the symphysis as soon as the patient gets up after the confinement. Resisted trunk flexion sets up local pain (Fig. 64). Radiography while the patient stands first on one leg, then the other, demonstrates the laxity, which allows up to 1 cm of movement between the bone ends. Obstetricians report that, after division of the symphysis pubis in difficult labour, fibrous union is complete in two months.

The patient should wear a corrugator belt (see Fig. 100, p. 373) for as long as is necessary, usually six weeks. If that does not suffice, intraligamentous sclerosis is required. On one occasion, arthrodesis was called for.

In men, pain arising from the joint is a rarity and responds well to an infiltration with triamcinolone suspension.

The symphysis may be seen radiologically widened in the pubic osteitis that may come on one to two months after prostatectomy. A line of calcification at the centre of the symphysis due to deposition of calcium pyrophosphate occurs in pseudo-gout.

# THE FEMALE BREAST

## Retraction of the Nipple

Weller pointed out that stimulation of the back of the newborn baby's palate by the tip of the nipple initiates the wish to suck and swallow. The nipple must, therefore, pass the 2 cm gap formed by the gums and reach 2.5 to 3 cm beyond, as a result of the length of the nipple itself and the amount of stretch in the areola. This is the minimum elastic yield that must exist for the establishment of the baby's eagerness to suck. Primiparas' nipples should be examined and treatment should be undertaken during the seventh month of pregnancy. The nipple should be everted until it is more prominent than the areola and the expanded tip grasped between the thumb and two fingers. The physiotherapist shows the mother how to apply continued traction.

CHAPTER 15

# THE LUMBAR REGION: APPLIED ANATOMY

Speaking of the disc, Eyring (1969) stated that 'its tendency to break itself apart and crush adjacent vertebrae, to compress nerve roots or cord and to cause untold amounts of suffering have made it one of the most important medical, legal and socio-economic entities.' I agree; for in my experience lumbar disc lesions are responsible for more continuing—yet avoidable—annoyance, frustration, semi-invalidism, general misery and bad temper than any other tissue of the body. In my view, lumbar disc lesions are responsible for well over 90% of all organic symptoms attributable to the lower back. This is a very different belief from 30 years ago. It was then taught, and believed, that affections of the muscles and fasciae of the lumbar area were the usual source of pain. This idea arose from Sir William Gower's lecture in 1904 when he postulated the existence of a disease called 'fibrositis', which, attacking the fibrous tissues of the lower back, caused lumbago. This notion was unchallenged for 41 years until a fresh approach to lumbago was proposed (Cyriax 1945; Key 1945). The new view is now widely accepted and it is largely agreed that a disc lesion causing internal derangement is the cause of lumbago. Indeed, Mixter and Barr stated in 1946 that disc lesions could cause backache only. Schiotz (1958) pointed out, however, that my father, Edgar Cyriax, wrote in *The Practitioner* in 1919 that 'the pathology of the vertebral cartilages has received but little attention. ... As regards the intra-articular cartilages, I can find no mention of any investigations on their morbid anatomy. Presumably the laws that govern the general pathology of fibro-cartilage are applicable to the vertebral cartilages as well. ... In the vertebral column, symptoms are sometimes found that so exactly resemble those induced by cartilaginous displacement elsewhere that it can with safety be assumed that these occur in the spine.' He regards him as the first to consider the possibility that disc lesions cause painful internal derangement.

'Fibrositis' has proved a much more stubborn belief, though it was discredited 30 years ago (Cyriax 1948). The concepts set out in these two papers have now been enthusiastically adopted. But, the pendulum has swung too far and the diagnosis of a disc lesion is now made too readily at the lower part of the vertebral column. There are a number of causes of pain in the back and lower limb other than disc lesions. They are all uncommon and form a small group dealt with in Chapter 17.

'Osteoarthrosis' of the lumbar spine has been challenged for the last 25 years in successive editions of this book, yet even now remains a common ascription. It was still considered the commonest cause of backache at the symposium held at the Mayo Clinic in 1951, although Beneke (1897) and Kahlmeter (1918) had already pointed out that vertebral osteophytosis was secondary to disc degeneration.

## Nomenclature

In this book, the undermentioned terms are used as follows:

*Backache:* Discomfort in the lower back.

*Lumbago:* A sudden access of pain in the lower back causing some degree of fixation and twinges on attempted movement. During recovery from lumbago, a moment is reached when the patient has merely backache. There is no exact point at which this change takes place; hence the differentiation is clear enough at extremes but merges indefinitely at the centre. The distinction between backache and lumbago is important, since the prognosis is so different. Backache may go on for years, continuously, or in spells lasting months. A sharp attack of lumbago nearly always recovers spontaneously in 1 to 3 weeks, even if the patient does not rest in bed. He then remains completely comfortable until his next attack, say, a year later.

*Sciatica:* Pain felt radiating from the buttock to the posterior thigh and calf. There is no name for pain felt only in the buttock, nor for pain of third lumbar provenance felt along the anterior aspect of the limb. Many cases of such radiation are labelled 'sciatica', but I regard such an extension as unhelpful. It would be more apt to revive the obsolete name 'boneshaw' (Arderne 1350) to cover all root pains felt in the lower limb.

## THE ERECT POSTURE

Why are disc lesions so common? Dillane et al. (1966) found in their practice that every year 2.4% of their patients suffered from a lumbago severe enough to request medical help. On the third of June 1967, the latest date for which the Department of Health has issued figures, the number of individuals off work with disc lesions, lumbago and sciatica was 24 400 men and 3160 women, a total of 27 560: roughly one insured person per family doctor in the country. Of these 2360 men and 680 women had been off work for one to four years and 460 men and 540 women for four to eighteen years. Another table gives the incidence as 1.5% of all workers each year. Schultz in Chicago (1975) has stated that one-third of all workmen's compensation is paid for injury to the back. Why does ordinary use of the joints of the spine cause pain so readily, when the other joints of the body can so often withstand lifelong exertion without causing trouble?

The answer is man's acquisition of the erect posture, evolution having entailed reversal of the function of the lumbar spine. Recent discoveries in Africa suggest that men walked upright there between 3 and 5 million years ago (Davis 1973), long enough, one might have thought, to allow better adaptation. But the cerebellum has caught the vertebral column unprepared. Originally it needed to be strong in resisting extension strains; now it must resist repeated flexion. In quadrupeds, there was no appreciable compression; now that man can stand upright, unwonted compression aggravates the stress. As this stance evolved, the whole column should have been redesigned.

In the long evolutionary period from fish to quadruped, the spine had served to maintain the distance apart of the front and hinder parts of the living creature. It never had to bear any compression strain. Moreover, a quadruped has no occasion to bend forwards since his forefeet are already on the ground; in consequence, little reason existed for the development of a structure able to withstand flexion strains. In consequence, the anterior longitudinal ligament is wider (2 cm as opposed to 1.4 cm), thicker (2 mm as opposed to 1.3 mm) and stronger, fibre for fibre, than the posterior longitudinal ligament (Tkaczuk 1968). By contrast, sagging of the spine as it hung between its anterior and posterior supports was undesirable, hence the column became a mechanism strong against extension stress. As soon as the erect posture was assumed the strains of compression and of flexion were imposed on a structure not designed to withstand either. Worse still, the spinal nerves emerged opposite the weakest part of the column—namely, the joints—instead of the exit for each pair lying (as might just as easily have happened) opposite the vertebral body. Worst of all, each spinal joint (except the two uppermost) contained a disc; a ring of fibrocartilage with a pulpy centre. This arrangement stopped the cervical spine from being driven up into the brain when an individual fell on to his head or, seated, on to his buttocks; for the downward momentum of the skull and the upward impetus of the body were cushioned by 22 elastic washers. The likelihood of a vertebral fracture at any level was also much diminished. This buffer was quite satisfactory so long as the spine was kept horizontal and suffered only extension strains, since movement in this direction tended to push the articular contents ventralwards, away from the nerve roots, but as soon as the maintenance of the erect posture forced the joints to bear weight and to accept flexion strain, the system broke down.

Though the discs protected the central nervous system from vertical impact, they are clearly not required by the joints as such. Indeed, the two joints that bear the greatest weight are the ankle and the talocalcanean. As the patient walks, these joints support alternately more than twice the compression applied to any lumbar joint; yet they hold up perfectly for a lifetime, in spite of the absence of any buffer. Again, no symptoms necessarily result from such complete erosion of disc substance that the lumbar vertebrae lie in virtual apposition, bone to bone. Hence it is most arguable that the existence of the intervertebral discs causes more trouble than it prevents.

## THE LUMBAR LORDOSIS

It is puzzling that the spinal column, though a weight-bearing structure, has been designed in a series of curves rather than as a vertical pillar. There are individuals who possess a perfectly straight spinal column from sacrum to neck; they have a graceful carriage and move well. A straight vertebral column is therefore not impossible to construct; indeed, general mechanical principles would suggest that at the spine as at the limbs, a vertical line is ideal for weight-bearing. Aesthetic considerations strengthen this view; for a straight back leads to an agreeable posture, whereas exaggerated lordosis leads to prominence of the belly and buttocks. For years the view has therefore been held, on apparently logical grounds, that the lumbar lordosis should be as slight in degree as possible.

It is my belief that the lumbar and cervical lordoses were developed to protect—albeit not with great success—the posterior longitudinal ligament from excessive strain and to exert an anteriorly directed pressure on the contents of the intervertebral joint. Biologically speaking, the development of the lordosis must be recent and subsequent to the emergence of the capacity to maintain the erect posture; for the spinal curves are absent at birth and during the first year of extrauterine life. The spinal joints most subject to internal derangement are the fifth and sixth cervical and the fourth and fifth lumbar—the areas of the spine where the normal lordosis is most marked. The primary thoracic kyphosis present at birth is thus retained as a compensatory mechanism whereby the erect position can be maintained in spite of lordosis above and below. The existence of the cervical and lumbar lordoses means that the joint-space is wider in front than behind. In this way a slight pressure, directed forward, is constantly exerted on the intervertebral disc during weight-bearing. Figs 66 and 67 show the difference in the tilt on the joint, when a normal subject holds his lumbar spine, first extended, then flexed. The other advantage of the spinal curves is that they act as shock absorbers, a sudden vertical stress being in part converted into movement increasing the curves. In patients with a flat spinal column, the intervertebral disc has no such protection, and it is noticeable that patients with a lumbar spine devoid of anterior convexity are more apt to suffer from backache than those with a normal degree of lordosis. Clearly, if the joint surfaces lie parallel when the patient stands erect, a slight degree of trunk flexion begins at once to squeeze the disc backwards; whereas the existence of a lordosis ensures that the trunk has to be well flexed before the obliquity is reversed and the back of the joint becomes wider than the front.

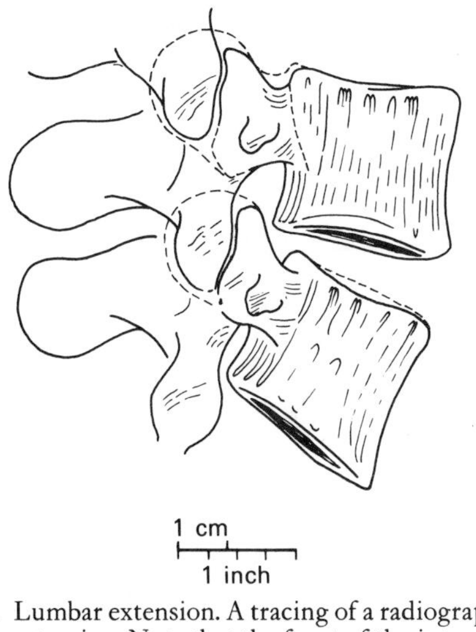


**Fig. 66.** Lumbar extension. A tracing of a radiograph taken in trunk extension. Note that the front of the intervertebral joint gapes widely (12 mm) whereas the posterior aspect is narrowed (5 mm). When the articular surfaces are thus tilted the pressure of the body weight forces the contents of the joint forwards.

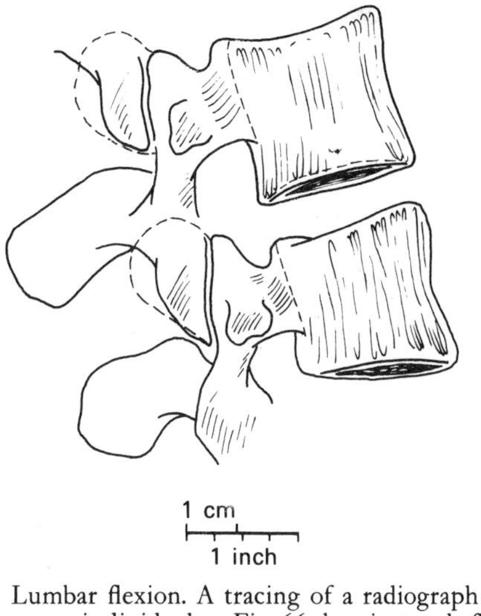


**Fig. 67.** Lumbar flexion. A tracing of a radiograph taken from the same individual as Fig. 66, but in trunk flexion. Note that the inclination of the joint surfaces is now reversed. The anterior aspect of the joint space (6 mm) has become less than the posterior (7 mm). The intra-articular contents tend to be forced backwards. This is the dangerous tilt.

Already, Brackett (1924), had worked out that lifting with the lower back flexed was the cause of pain there.

The phenomenon of a painful arc (Fig. 68) on trunk flexion throws light on intra-articular mechanics. Discography with contrast material injected into a lumbar intervertebral joint shows how the nucleus tends to move backwards during trunk flexion, both in normal and in abnormal joints. When patients with a normal lumbar curve stand erect, the disc is pushed anteriorly. As trunk flexion proceeds the moment comes at the half-flexed position when the surfaces have moved enough to reverse the tilt. At this point a mobile fragment of disc moves sharply backwards, jarring the dura by pressure transmitted through the posterior longitudinal ligament. Further trunk flexion may not alter the position of the disc again; the remainder of flexion is then painless. Alternatively, the pain may reappear at the extreme of trunk flexion, if the loose part is squeezed yet farther backwards. Hence a painful arc is pathognomonic of hypermobility of a fragment of the intra-articular disc in a spinal joint.

It is well to remember that most people develop backache more readily when standing half-bent forwards than fully flexed. The reason is that, once the trunk has passed below the horizontal position, body-weight exerts traction on the lumbar joints. This is not offset by muscle contraction, since in full flexion the muscles are inevitably relaxed. Such negative pressure within the joint is not exerted if the individual bends forwards only a short distance. It is also for this reason that it is seldom when bending to lift that lumbago comes on but when the trunk is coming up again, the muscles contracting strongly while the articular surfaces still retain their kyphotic obliquity. This fact also serves to discount osteopaths' idea of lumbago being caused by sprain of a facet joint when it is taken beyond its normal range of movement. At half-flexion no articular structure is on the stretch.

## Practical Bearing

In the past, the prescription and technique of postural exercises have been too much guided by aesthetic considerations. In fact, the prevention of future backache has the prior claim; it is such a universal symptom that prophylaxis is worth while from a child's early days. It is to the gymnasts who teach at schools that we must look first for a reversal of policy. No endeavour must be made to persuade children to bend down and touch the floor. Those who can, well and good; those who cannot must not force their trunks, nor have them forced, towards flexion. Lessons on how to sit and lift maintaining the lordosis should become part of gymnastic school training everywhere. Once such postures become second nature, they can be carried on into working life indefinitely.

The control, therefore, that aesthetic considerations used to exercise over the child's posture should be tempered by knowledge of the frequency and mechanism of disc protrusion. Once growth has ceased, postural exercises are powerless to alter the shape of the bones. However, they may well be harmful if they include movement towards flexion, for they are still

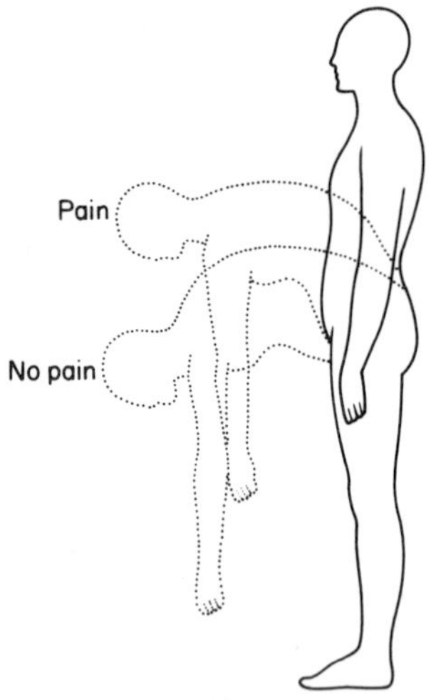


**Fig. 68.** A painful arc on trunk flexion.

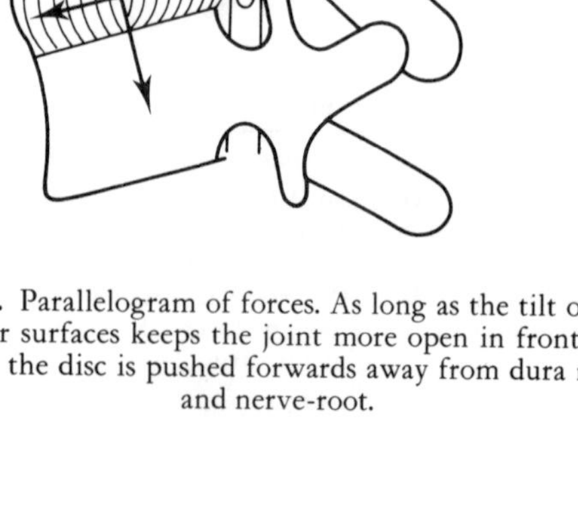

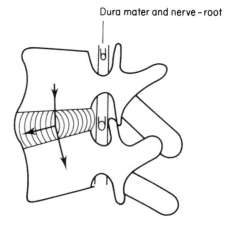

**Fig. 69.** Parallelogram of forces. As long as the tilt on the articular surfaces keeps the joint more open in front than behind, the disc is pushed forwards away from dura mater and nerve-root.

capable of stretching ligaments and moving a loose fragment of disc to an unfavourable position. There is a sort of fetish that no one is healthy unless he bends to touch his toes a number of times every morning. Many disc lesions are the result of acting on this extraordinary idea. Hospitals still exist in England where flexion exercises are ordered for back trouble under the physiotherapist's supervision, and in Canada and the USA exercises are prescribed towards flexion as a matter of course. This is the result of Dandy's misconception. Writing in 1929, he took the view that 'the normal anterior curvature of the lumbar spine would be expected to throw greater localized effects of trauma on the posterior side of the disc ... Then the relatively thin and incomplete posterior ligaments would more readily permit protrusion of a tumour in the intervertebral disc.' This is a most reasonable opinion, but ignores the parallelogram of forces, as does Paul Williams's reasoning. Even sitting with the back convex is advised and car manufacturers who ask for authoritative medical advice on seating are sadly misled although proper seating had in fact been described by Taylor in New York in 1864. When the sufferer from backache finds that flexion exercises increase his discomfort, alas he congratulates himself on affecting the right spot. The potential harm inherent in postural exercises based only on 'health and beauty' concepts should be explained to all.

### 'Postural Pain'

Posture is a concept, a shape, not a disease. Hence the phrase 'postural pain' adds nothing to what is already said when a patient complains of backache. In all lesions of the moving parts, the posture adopted by the part at fault influences symptoms. When standing with the knee fully extended hurts a patient with arthritis in his knee, he is not regarded as suffering from postural knee-ache; if this posture hurts, it is agreed by all that a lesion exists at the knee. Backache arising from the moving parts varies according to posture; in other words, the pain alters as the stress on some lumbar structure is altered. A change in symptoms corresponding to the stresses acting on the lesion is common to all disorders of the moving parts. If the pain is then called 'postural', the most that this adjective has implied is that the pain due to the unnamed lesion alters with the position of the affected part. Brown (1828) pointed out that in scoliosis the intervertebral cartilage becomes atrophied by pressure absorption on the concave side. Nevertheless, the idea is widespread that, if an individual with backache has a 'bad' posture, the two are connected. This popular notion is an obvious misconception; for not only do many people with 'good' posture suffer from backache but an equal number with a 'bad' posture do not. There is only one posture that enhances the likelihood of backache—namely, a flat back—and this is the one long regarded as 'good'. This view has been confirmed by Hult (1954). He studied 1200 workers and found that the incidence of back trouble and of radiographic signs of disc degeneration was the same in those with scoliosis or kypholordosis as in other individuals.

Backache arises, whatever the posture, as the result of some lesion. The diagnosis must state the nature of this lesion, and name the tissue responsible for the pain. 'Postural' does neither. Indeed, the many different ideas about backache are mostly dependent on uncertainties about the mechanics of the lumbar region. The application of simple anatomical fact to the problem of backache is set out later in this chapter.

## PREVENTION OF RECURRENCE

Once the displacement is reduced, or the protrusion has been removed at laminectomy, the question of preventing recurrence arises.

### Postural Advice to the Patient

It is not so much what the individual does as the posture he adopts to do it that matters. This was brought out very clearly by Magora (1972). His statistics, based on a study of 3316 individuals, showed that back troubles were caused by prolonged standing, lifting and bending in 29.9% of workers and by prolonged sitting in 12.6%. Of those who alternately sat and stood only 1.5% developed backache. Like many other structures, the disc can stand short-lived strains well, but not prolonged stress maintained in the same direction, as Lindblom (1952) showed in rats' tails.

The mechanics of lumbar disc protrusion must be explained to the patient. He must be told that, so long as his lumbar spine is held in lordosis, movement backwards of the loose part of the disc is virtually impossible. He must be shown how to stand, sit (not crossing his legs), bend, and lift, using his knees rather than his back. His car-seat and his chair at home and at the office must be corrected so that the hollow in his back is maintained while he is seated. He must go on all fours if he wants to do things on the ground, e.g. weeding. Neurosis is prevented by explaining that the disorder is purely mechanical, and not the precursor of crippling disease. With the exception of digging, he can go on doing whatever he did before; it is merely the way of doing it that has to be changed. Tennis and similar games must be avoided by patients with a fragment of cartilage loose in the joint; but in patients with a tendency to nuclear protrusion, the quick up and down of tennis does not matter.

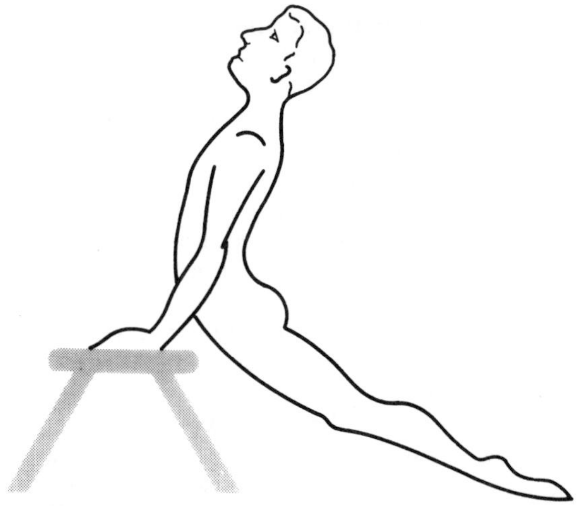

**Fig. 70.** Hypertension exercises. The weight of the lower limbs provides traction. Engagement of the low lumbar spinous processes shifts posteriorly the axis about which the intervertebral joint moves. Now the hinge lies behind the joint and hyperextension draws apart the whole extent of the two articular surfaces. This represents the only useful exercise in lumbar disc lesions.

## Avoidance of Exercises

Exercises that maintain or enhance lumbar mobility are contraindicated after a disc lesion. It is by keeping the joint still, not by moving it, that further intra-articular displacement is best prevented. Patients should be taught how to use their sacrospinalis muscles to keep the lumbar joints motionless in extension and to flex the trunk at hips and thorax. The inculcation of a permanent postural tone in the sacrospinalis muscles is taught as soon as the patient is seen. He must grasp the idea of how preventing movement at a joint, when forces act on it, itself involves muscular exertion. Yoga exercises should be avoided since they demand trunk flexion with the legs held straight. Hamstring pull then flexes the pelvis on the lumbar spine. Crouching with the legs fully flexed, knees on thorax, also flexes the pelvis on the sacrum, but this is not so if the hips are fully abducted and the knees fully flexed in the Indian manner.

For patients who insist on performing exercises, one exists that is logically defensible. In full extension of the lumbar spine, either the spinous processes engage—only ligament buffering—or the apex of each facet impinges against the lamina of the vertebra below. The axis about which further extension takes place must now shift posteriorly to these three points of bony contact. Hence the patient puts his hands on a stool and straightens his arms, bringing his trunk almost vertical but letting his legs stretch out backwards. He lets his trunk sag; passive lumbar extension results (see Fig. 70). During this exercise (active for the arms, passive for the lumbar joints) each intervertebral joint surface is drawn away from its fellow by movement about this posterior hinge during the traction afforded by the weight of the buttocks and thighs. This has the opposite effect of prone-lying trunk extension exercises, whereby contraction of the sacrospinalis muscles squeezes the vertebrae together. Moreover, the fullest extension is not attained, hence the hinge-effect is lost.

## Avoidance of Compression

If a heavy object has to be carried, compression on the lumbar spine can be avoided by making the object bear directly on the iliac crest or on the sacrum. The strain then passes from pelvis to limbs, sparing the lumbar joints.

# THE INTERVERTEBRAL DISC*

The disc serves six purposes:

1. To increase height by adding to the length of the spine.
2. To join the vertebrae together and yet allow movement between them.
3. To distribute the load equally over the surface of the vertebral body. The semifluid consist-

*Interested readers should apply to Winthrop Laboratories for their Medi-cassette entitled *Backache and Lumbar Disc Lesions*, by G. Symonds (1976).

ency of the nucleus ensures that the whole disc bears the same stress, however the joint is tilted (Nachemson 1960).

4. To act as a buffer when an individual falls on his head or, seated, on to his sacrum. Part of the impact is cushioned by the elastic structure of cartilage.
5. To keep the lateral facets the correct distance apart.
6. To maintain the size of each intervertebral foramen. This is not often important since the aperture is three to ten times larger than the root (Svanberg 1915).

## Historical Note

When a syndrome has become widely recognized, it is always found to have been described before in papers that attracted no attention at the time. In the Museo Nacional de Antropologia in Mexico City stands a pottery vase 50 cm high dating from the Monte Alban II period, 200 BC. It is an accurate representation of the lumbar spine, body, pedicle, lamina and processes. Between each vertebral body is a wide space indicating the disc (see Plate II/2).

Vesalius was the first to describe the appearance of the intervertebral disc in 1543. Weitbrecht (1742) described a tissue intermediate between cartilage and ligament joining each two vertebrae together. The fibres formed lamellae crossing each other. Cotugno wrote a book on sciatica in 1764 (*De Ischide Nervosa Commentarius*), ascribing it to dropsy of the dural funnel enclosing the nerve. In his later book (1775) he ascribes sciatica to 'abundant or acrid fluid abiding in the outer vaginae of the ischiadic nerve'. This correct attribution to dropsy of the dural sheath of the nerve root was forgotten. He pointed out that semiparalysis with wasting was commonplace. Lassègue had already noted wasting of the muscles in the affected limb by 1864. In 1838, Key reported two cases of paraplegia caused by protrusion of disc. Riadore (1843) ascribed root pain to compression at the intervertebral foramen and recognized degeneration of the intervertebral disc. Virchow (1857) reported a herniated disc post-mortem; he regarded it as caused by trauma.

In 1888, Charcot described the characteristic spinal deformity in sciatica and Ribbert (1895) produced protrusion in rabbits by puncturing the intervertebral disc. Kocher (1896) described a case of rupture of the second lumbar disc after a fall on the heels, and in 1910 Krause removed a tumour at the third lumbar level which microscopy showed consisted of fibrocartilage. In 1916 Elsberg drew attention to 'spinal chondromata', and in 1911 Goldthwaite described one case, and Middleton and Teacher two cases, of flaccid paraplegia with paralysed sphincters resulting from 'exaggerated prominence of the fifth lumbar disc' of traumatic origin. The latter put a segment of spine into a vice and reproduced the expulsion of the disc experimentally. Dandy (1929) described two cases of paraplegia caused by extrusion of disc substance but the first operative results to be published were those of Alajouanine and Dutaillis (1928). Little notice was taken of these papers until Mixter and Barr's article in 1934 on sciatica cured by removal of protruded disc material. The first two books on disc lesions were by Mauric (1933) in Paris and Glorieux (1937) of Bruges. The latter's myelographic plates are particularly clear.

### Cartilage and Pulp

Between the bodies of each two lumbar vertebrae lies the disc. It is the largest avascular structure in the whole body. The structures here are:

*The End-Plate.* This consists of hyaline cartilage covering the articular surfaces of each vertebral body, with many little perforations centrally. Vernon-Roberts (1975) dissected 300 elderly people's spines and found that, however gross the degeneration of the disc, the end-plate was never fully worn through.

*The Annulus Fibrosus.* This consists of layers of fibrocartilage attached to the end-plate, the vertebral bodies and the anterior and posterior longitudinal ligaments; it surrounds the nucleus. There are about a dozen of these concentric lamellae posteriorly (Weitbrecht 1742; Joplin 1935). They have been compared to the layers of an onion, but run in different directions, crossing each other; this arrangement (like a Japanese fingerstall) gives the annulus great strength. Round the circumference, the fibrocartilage sinks into the vertebral body forming a strong band. The spongy structure of cartilage provides hydrostatic lubrication (McCutchen 1964). Were the liquid contained within cartilage not retained by viscous resistance, it would be squeezed out as soon as the disc bore weight. The disc would then be reduced to an inelastic solid, half its original thickness. Cartilage contains neither blood vessels nor nerves, hence all damage is permanent, union and regeneration being impossible; yet Mathews (1977) still speaks of 'healing'. Being devoid of nerves (Jung &

Braunschwig 1932), the lesion of itself cannot cause pain; fracture or degeneration of the disc cannot cause symptoms unless some other tissue is secondarily affected.

*The Nucleus Pulposus.* At birth the nucleus occupies the centre of the intervertebral joint. But during growth the anterior aspect of the vertebral body grows faster than the posterior. Hence in adult life the nucleus has come to lie slightly behind the centre. It consists of a softish, gelatinous polysaccharide and forms the cushion between the vertebrae, during compression exerting hydrostatic pressure, uniformly distributed. Harrison (1821) had noted that when the spine adopted a position of strain 'the intervertebral substance is compressed in one part and spread out in the opposite direction'. On return to a neutral posture, it was 'entirely restored by its inherent elasticity'. It bulges when cut (Goldthwaite 1911). In the young it is quite distinct from the annulus, less so in adults, and by late middle age has disappeared completely. The disc has then become uniform throughout its substance and consists of the familiar 'crab-meat' removed at laminectomy. For this reason, nuclear disc protrusion is rare in the elderly. If the nucleus erodes the spongiosa of a vertebral body, the prolapse is known as a Schmorl's node. If this is caused by injury, Joplin (1935) has noted that the sclerotic edge does not appear for three to four months.

The function of the nucleus is partly to act as shock-absorber, and partly to change shape when the vertebrae tilt on each other, thus maintaining a uniform distribution of stress throughout the joint. The water of which the nucleus is largely composed is retained by the innate affinity protein–polysaccharide combinations possess for tissue fluid. It can therefore be punctured with impunity at discography or when a needle is introduced too far during lumbar puncture or sinuvertebral block.

*Nerves within the Disc.* It is a well-established fact that cartilage, in addition to being avascular, is also insensitive, containing no nerves. Much search has gone on for nervous filaments within the disc. This has disclosed that the connective tissue at the surface of the disc is innervated and that tiny fibrils penetrate its outermost lamella for a fraction of a millimetre only (see Plate XXXIX). The rest of the disc is devoid of nerves.

## Bearing on Treatment

Cartilage is hard and its displacement, in whatever joint of the body it occurs, is often susceptible to manipulative reduction. This should be done at once in all suitable cases, so as to minimize ligamentous overstretching at the back of the joint.

Nuclear material is soft and usually cannot be successfully manipulated back into place. If a manipulation is attempted, the technique is different; sustained pressure replaces the sharp jerk, since it is now the intention to squeeze rather than to click the displacement back into position; but the endeavour is apt to fail. Most pulpy protrusions are reducible only by traction or by rest in bed.

# THE AGEING OF CARTILAGE

Cartilage is an avascular structure; hence it cannot unite or regenerate after it has been damaged. This applies to the intervertebral disc no less than to the meniscus at the knee, where it is admitted on all sides that a tear never heals. Even in articular (as opposed to intra-articular) cartilage, Davies et al. (1962) showed by electron microscopy in young adult rabbits that no evidence of cell division is discernible. Tonna and Cronkite's radioisotopic studies show cartilage to be a static tissue. They found that in rats no detectable multiplication of cells took place after the first month of life. Nine months after injection of tritated thymidine, cartilage cells were still loaded with it, whereas it disappeared in a month from rapidly dividing tissues. Burnett's (1965) research with the electron microscope in Tasmania has led him to state: 'Articular cartilage turns out to be a remarkably static tissue.' Mauric (1933) stated that the disc contained no blood vessels in adult life, and in Portugal, Miniero (1965) devoted a book to a detailed description of the vertebral arterial and venous supply. His photographs of injected specimens from fetal life to 80 years old show consistently that the disc itself is entirely devoid of blood vessels. This lack of blood in the intervertebral disc was confirmed once more by Hassler (1970) though his micro-angiographic studies showed some vascularization at the vertebral margin of the fibrocartilage in babies. These vessels had atrophied by the age of 12 and all trace of them was absent in adults. Yet one of the arguments put forward for the treatment of lumbago by rest in bed is 'to allow the disc to heal'. This impossibility is important medicolegally, since there is (*a*) no certain relation in time between damage to a disc and the first attack of internal derangement and (*b*) a permanent liability to recurrence. Once a loose fragment of fibrocartilage has moved, the crack cannot unite so as to prevent another displacement.

The nutrition of articular cartilage appears to begin from the surface and penetrate towards the bone, not the reverse. The permeability of cartilage lessens with age, and Stockwell showed that in a three-month-old rabbit silver proteinate passes quite readily into articular cartilage from its free surface, but penetrates much less at 2 years old. Lowered cell nutrition and reduced elasticity lead to damage to the gliding surfaces which are then no longer adequately covered by the film of synovial fluid on which virtually friction-free movement depends. This is how Stockwell considers that osteoarthrosis is caused, and certainly the scanning electron microscope (magnification 100 000) has shown marked surface alterations in arthritis. However, Lenoch (1970) has pointed out that in alkaptonuria granules of pigment appear first in the deepest layers of cartilage, gradually working their way to the surface. These granules cannot stem from the synovial fluid, which is pigment-free. He considers that the primary lesion in osteoarthrosis lies in the subchondral bone, degeneration of which interrupts the channels of cartilaginous nourishment. Brodin (1973) has pointed out that nutrition suffers if synovial fluid is no longer sucked in and out of cartilage. This happens equally if (*a*) no pressure or (*b*) constant pressure is applied to an area of cartilage. It is thus intermittent loading and unloading that prevents degeneration.

Backache and disc degeneration are not synonymous. This was first pointed out by Hirsch (1959) when he said that full degeneration of the disc resulted in no movement and therefore no pain. The fact that back troubles are a disease of middle-age was shown by Herndon (1927) who analysed 941 cases of injury and found the incidence to be: 16 to 19 years: 20 cases; 20 to 29: 82; 30 to 39: 110; 40 to 49: 97; 50 to 59: 47; and 60 to 69: 12. After the age of 20, the time off work averaged 1 month, but it was only 2 weeks in the youngest group. Many patients with multiple degeneration suffer no discomfort. This was proved by Unander-Scharin in 1950, when he investigated 116 767 cases of sickness, 4.5% of which were due to lumbosciatic pain. He found the frequency of such symptoms to diminish markedly after the age of 60. Were backache due to disc degeneration—the widespread belief today—the incidence would rise as age advanced. That degeneration of the discs is a universal phenomenon not necessarily causing any trouble was confirmed afresh by Gresham and Miller (1969). They dissected out the third, fourth and fifth lumbar discs post-mortem in people who had had no back troubles. Between the ages of 14 and 34 years 90% of the discs were found normal. At 35 to 45, degeneration had set in in 75%. After the age of 46 ever single fifth lumbar disc was degenerate, and only a quarter of the fourth lumbar discs were normal. This was confirmed again by Ritchie and Fahrni (1970) who found that degeneration of a lumbar disc began during individuals' twenties. They tested various parts of the disc for hardness and reported consistent softening of the posterior part alone by the age of 45. At 80, all the annular lamellae had become totally disorganized.

Many patients are distressed at being told that they are suffering from one or more 'degenerate discs'. This suggests an irreversible and crippling phenomenon. The term should be discarded, for disc degeneration is universal as age advances and causes no symptoms. Disc protrusion is painful whether degeneration has set in or not. Degeneration without displacement compresses nothing and so cannot cause symptoms. The phrase is therefore pathologically inaccurate and psychologically undesirable. This fact was confirmed by statistics issued by the Department of Health in 1971. During 1967, the frequency of lumbago at different ages was 1% under 20 years of age; it reached 10% in the 35 to 39 age group and then rose by 1% each 5 years, reaching a maximum of 15% at 60 to 64 years. It fell to 3% (the same as in the 20 to 24 age group) at 65 years and over. Sciatica behaved in roughly the same way: 0.3% under 20, 10% aged 30 to 34 years, 15% at 50 to 54 years, 24% at 60 to 64 years and 4% over 65 years. If degeneration of the disc was the cause of symptoms, the incidence would not decrease with advancing years.

## Calcification of the Disc

This occurs after haemorrhage and in chondrocalcinosis. It may well be asked how calcium salts could reach the disc. Beadle (1931) showed that blood could suffuse from the adjacent part of the vertebral body via the many small holes in the end-plate. He illustrated replacement of part of the disc by vascular granulation tissue. Using a dye, Nachemson et al. (1970) showed that, though the perimeter of the end-plate was impermeable, vascular buds connected the marrow of the vertebral body with the centre of the end-plate. Thence diffusion occurred to the annulus fibrosus. Clearly this situation makes nuclear calcification possible. Such diffusion was shown by Maroudas et al. (1973) to be just adequate to maintain nutrition only if the lowest value of glycolysis (drawn from the literature) was accepted.

Calcification of the nucleus indicates past haemorrhage, but has no bearing on the patient's present symptoms.

In chondrocalcinosis it is the annulus not the nucleus which calcifies.

## THE PRESSURE WITHIN THE DISC

Many calculations had been made, some leading to impossibly large theoretical loads on the joint. Nachemson carried out valuable research by in vivo discometry, and published a book and four further papers setting out the results (Nachemson 1962, 1972; Nachemson & Morris 1963; Nachemson & Lind 1969). He measured the intradiscal pressure by means of a needle thrust into the nucleus, thus directly assessing the pressure when the individual adopted different postures. Initially, he found that in an excised lumbar spine the ligaments about the joint exerted a pressure of 0.7 kg. Jayson et al. (1973) subjected 78 discs excised from cadavers together with the adjacent vertebral bodies to increasing pressure. They found that a damaged disc might burst with as little as 50 lb/in$^2$ but ten of the normal discs withstood 1000 lb without damage.

The intradiscal pressure is dependent on the load. Movement of part of a disc depends on the state of the disc, the inclination of the joint surfaces and the centrifugal force acting on the disc. Strong muscles tend further to squeeze the joint and to enable heavier loads, i.e. more centrifugal force, to act on the disc. This situation, i.e. that however strong they are, the lumbar muscles contribute nothing to the prevention of lumbar disc lesions, is not yet appreciated, and the generalization that the stronger the muscles the more stable the joint is erroneously accepted. In probably every hospital in the country exercises are blithely ordered in both prophylaxis and treatment.

### Nachemson's Findings

Striking confirmation of the accuracy of the facts deduced from clinical observation and set out in successive editions of this book has emerged from Nachemson's work. He has led the experimental approach to the mechanics of the lumbar spine for 20 years and published a summary of his findings in 1975. He has established the following.

If the pressure within the disc while an individual is standing is taken to be 100, then on lying supine it is 25, while lying on the side 75 and while sitting 150. Standing bent slightly forwards is also 150; sitting bent slightly forwards is 180. Standing bent well forwards is 210 and sitting bent well forwards is 270. Here indeed is the mathematical confirmation of the dangers of sitting and of flexing the trunk, even when standing.

When an individual weighing 70 kg lay supine, the load on the third lumbar disc was 30 kg. This was reduced to 10 kg when 30 kg traction was applied. Standing set up a pressure of 70 kg, which rose to 100 kg while sitting. Bilateral full straight-leg raising brought the recumbent pressure to 120 kg. Active trunk extension while lying prone raised the pressure to 150 kg, again a clear indication that such exercises should be avoided. Lifting a 20 kg weight by straightening the knees with the back hollow increased the pressure to 210 kg, whereas it mounted to 340 kg if the lifting was carried out with the back bent and the legs straight. When different portions of the unsupported back were tested with the individual sitting, the least pressure was in lordosis; the more the lumbar spine was extended the less the intradiscal pressure. If the seated patient lifted his trunk upwards by pressing with his hands on his thighs, the stress was further diminished. Indeed, this is the only way in which a patient with severe lumbago can sit.

Nachemson also emphasizes that the decade when back troubles are most frequent is between 40 and 50 years; clear evidence that degeneration of any lumbar tissue cannot be the reason for back symptoms. He goes on to say that it remains to be proved that strong muscles avoid painful episodes and that it has never been shown that patients liable to backache have weak muscles. He advises the use of a chair with a lumbar support, as was advocated by Taylor in 1864. When weights are lifted, lumbar flexion must be avoided. It is clear that Nachemson, the foremost authority on the mechanics of the lumbar joints, has confirmed what had already been determined, albeit less exactly, by clinical methods.

## Damage to the Disc

If it is entire, the disc cannot protrude unless the posterior ligament ruptures. When time and the multiple minor traumata of ordinary active life have initiated damage, the cartilage becomes slightly, then more, cracked, but being devoid of nerves there is no warning discomfort. In the end, a fragment forms that is either completely detached within the joint or lies hinged. The stage is now set for the first attack of internal derangement, i.e. lumbago if the loose piece lies centrally or root pain if the fragment lies posterolaterally within the joint.

Since the two end-plates lie nearly parallel a displaced fragment of disc can occupy an indefinite number of positions. The situation is not the same as at the knee where the semi-detached fragment of meniscus can lie only at one or other side of the dome of the femoral condyle, i.e. either 'in' or 'out'. At the knee, therefore, displacement and reduction are both sudden phenomena, heralded by a click. At a lumbar joint, by contrast, although the onset of lumbago is often instantaneous, spontaneous reduction during rest in bed is usually a slow process. The displacement recedes a little day by day, the symptoms and signs waning correspondingly. Manipulative reduction is often as sudden as the onset, and the click may be heard and felt.

The nucleus sometimes pushes past the annulus; if so, pure herniation of pulp with an intact annulus results (Fig. 72). If the annulus is cracked and part of it moves, the centrifugal force always acting on the nucleus may push pulpy material into the breach. As a result, any cartilaginous displacement of sufficient size and standing becomes aggravated by secondary herniation of pulp into the gap. This may take the shape of a collar-stud, the narrow track at the annulus forming the stem of the stud, if so, manipulative reduction becomes impossible.

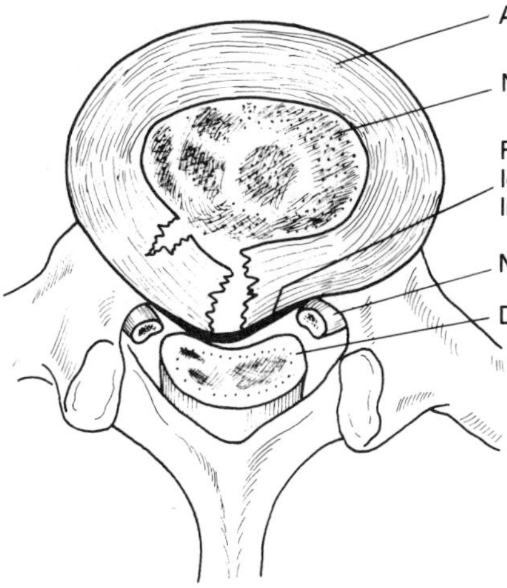


**Fig. 71.** A cartilaginous disc lesion. An annular crack has led to posterior displacement by hinging. The posterior longitudinal ligament is bulged out backwards and pressure exerted on the dura mater: lumbago results. No nuclear material has extruded, hence reduction by manipulation is simple.

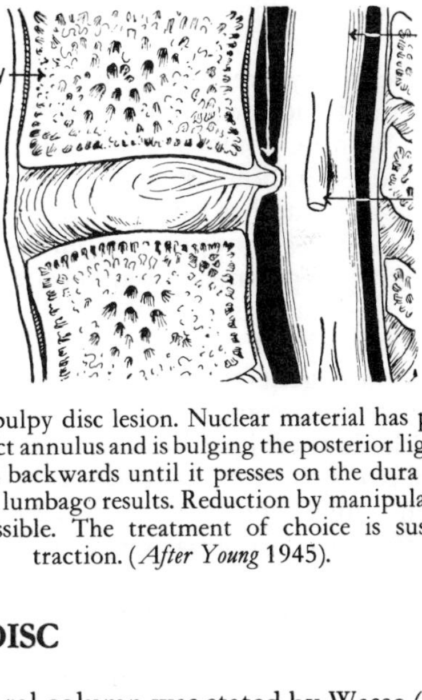


**Fig. 72.** A pulpy disc lesion. Nuclear material has pushed past the intact annulus and is bulging the posterior ligament longitudinal backwards until it presses on the dura mater. Bachache or lumbago results. Reduction by manipulation is often impossible. The treatment of choice is sustained traction. (*After Young* 1945).

# HYDROPS OF THE DISC

The water content of the disc was calculated by Püschel in 1930, and found to diminish steadily with age. At 18 years old the fifth lumbar annulus consisted of 72% water, the nucleus 81%. By the age of 35, these figures had decreased to 65 and 78%. In fact Beckett (1724) had already pointed out that elderly people grow shorter as the result of the 'intervening cartilages' becoming harder. The loss of height due to a day's compression of the vertebral column was stated by Wasse (1724) to be 1.5 to 2.4 cm, less in the elderly. It was worked out again in Hungary on 1000 individuals (de Puky 1935) and was attributed to decreased water content of the discs. It turned out to be 17.1 mm for men and 14.2 mm for women, an average of 0.68 mm per disc.

There is a theory that lumbago is caused by sudden swelling of the disc as the result of its rapidly absorbing fluid. This ignores several obvious facts.

1. If the disc were to swell, it would force the vertebral bodies apart. Since two-thirds of the intervertebral joint lies anterior to the axis about which flexion and extension take place, the spine would be fixed in extension, whereas in lumbago the spine is fixed in flexion.
2. Radiography in recumbency, i.e. without compression strain on the joint, does not show an increased width of the joint space during lumbago. Moreover, some patients deviate *towards* the painful side.
3. Intra-articular cartilage is avascular, hence it cannot suddenly change its nature and become absorbent. The meniscus at the knee is not found swollen when removed during an effusion into the joint. In any case, where would this fluid suddenly appear from? A more reasonable hypothesis would be haemarthrosis, which can, after all, come on in a few moments. But evidence of past haemorrhage is a rare finding at laminectomy, though Beadle (1931) did show that vascular granulomas could form within the disc by extravasation of blood through the multiple small apertures at the central part of the end-plate. Hence calcification must have this aetiology. Vernon-Roberts (personal communication, 1975) dissected 300 lumbar spines and detected no evidence of past haemarthrosis in any of the 500 intervertebral discs he examined. He found red degeneration not to be uncommon, but this was not altered blood, since the pigment contained no iron.
4. Fluid suddenly permeating the disc would not come on with a click during trunk flexion. Still less would it disappear with another click during manipulative reduction.

The evidence therefore strongly opposes this hypothesis.

## RADIOLOGY

The real use of a lumbar radiograph is negative, to show that no other disorder is present. But X-rays are today frequently studied in a vain endeavour to decide whether or not a disc lesion exists. Nothing could be more fallacious. What the radiograph shows is whether the disc is thick or thin and whether osteophytes are present or not. But a disc can atrophy without displacement; alternatively, protrusion can occur at a joint where the space is of full width. Osteophyte formation is itself symptomless; it merely indicates some degeneration, as is almost universal in elderly people, some of whom have never had backache in their lives. What matters is whether or not a displacement is present—and this the straight radiograph cannot show. Another error is to aver that a normal radiograph excludes a disc lesion. No one would, after inspecting the X-ray photograph of a young man's knee, say whether his meniscus was torn or not, nor would radiographic evidence of displacement be expected. Similarly, the X-ray appearances of the bones of the back cannot be expected to exclude damage to cartilage—a radiotranslucent tissue.

Osteophytosis with or without a diminished joint space is secondary to disc degeneration and results from ligamentous traction lifting up periosteum. Bone then grows out to meet its limiting membrane. Most osteophytosis is directed laterally or anteriorly and does not matter. Rarely an osteophyte projects posteriorly, compressing the dura mater or a nerve root. This finding is often significant and connected with symptoms.

Degeneration of a disc, once it becomes considerable, appears as a diminished joint space with osteophytosis on the radiograph. When a disc is ground to pieces entirely, the joint space disappears and bone all but touches bone, only the end-plates intervening (Plate XVII/1); in many such cases the mushroom phenomenon supervenes. If the disc is reduced to rubble and passes anteriorly, its remnants can often be seen lying enclosed by two bony peaks (Plate XXI). The nucleus can herniate into the body of a vertebra; this phenomenon causes adolescent osteochondrosis, alternatively Schmorl's nodes. Complete absence of the joint space is compatible with painless function, but not with a full range of movement. The fact that the joint space is of normal or diminished width does not indicate where the posterior—the important—part of the disc happens to be lying. Hence the appearance of the disc space on the radiograph adds nothing for or against a clinical diagnosis of displacement of a disc fragment. This view has since been confirmed by Soderburg and Andren (1956). They began with the idea that a diminished disc space with osteophytosis reduced the risk of protrusion, but finally found no correlation between the clinical and radiological findings. Roberts et al. (1978) found that neither static nor moving radiographs of the lumbar spine were of any value in predicting the response to manipulation.

The first time a disc has been made visible by radiography was by Worthington (1980) at Nottingham University. He was able to visualize normal discs by nuclear magnetic resonance. A strong magnetic field makes the nuclei of atoms briefly emit radio signals. These are picked up and processed through a computer, thus affording a view of the human body at one plane at a time.

When a firm diagnosis of disc lesion has been made, the fact that this or that joint space is diminished does not even prove that the lesion lies at the narrowed level. For example, at laminectomy for sciatica, it sometimes happens that a patient's symptoms are the result of protrusion at, say, the fourth level (where the joint space is of normal width) and the contents of the fifth joint (where the space is much diminished) are not responsible for any symptoms, degeneration with thinning having gone on silently for years. Moreover, some 20% of patients subjected to laminectomy are found to have two protrusions (Young 1952), not necessarily at the levels the X-rays appeared to indicate.

Markedly diminished joint spaces at the upper lumbar levels are often seen in elderly patients, but disc lesions causing symptoms at the first or second lumbar level are a great rarity. Semmes (1964), at laminectomy on 1500 cases, found one first and two second lumbar protrusions; Collis's (1963) discograms detected one at the second lumbar level and none at the first in 1014 cases. It is clear, therefore, that mere thinning of the disc affords no evidence of protrusion past or present.

Multiple erosion of disc substance leads to considerable loss of height as age advances. Each lumbar disc may well have been 1 cm thick originally. If all five are reduced to a thin wafer the patient becomes 5 cm shorter.

Calcification of a ligament shows that it has probably suffered damage some years before (Plate XXII); bleeding into an intervertebral joint may be followed by intra-articular calcification. Calcification of the disc itself occurs in chondrocalcinosis (pseudo-gout).

## SPONTANEOUS RECOVERY

Pain in the neck, posterior thorax or lumbogluteal area caused by a disc protrusion in the midline can continue indefinitely. This does not apply to acute torticollis or to sudden thoracic pain or to lumbago; in these disorders the tendency to spontaneous recovery in a week or two is considerable. But neckache, scapular aching, posterior thoracic aching and lower backache can go on for many years. The same applies to cases of bilateral root pain. However, the moment the protrusion moves to one side, compressing a nerve root, with easing of the pressure exerted via the posterior ligament against dura mater, a mechanism leading to spontaneous recovery is set in motion. This takes six to twelve months at the three lower lumbar levels; three to four months at cervical levels; an indeterminate time at the first and second thoracic level. Spontaneous recovery from root pain may not occur at all at the third to twelfth thoracic levels.

In sciatica, the more marked the neurological weakness, the sooner the patient loses his pain in the limb. Time must be counted from the first appearance of strong unilateral root pain coupled with cessation of central pain in the trunk; mere lumbar aching radiating slightly to one limb does not suffice, and the time that has elapsed since the pain in the trunk or gluteal area began is wholly immaterial. It is important to realize that the central backache must cease before one can begin counting. If it is not lost, or the symptoms are projected to *both* limbs, there is no limit to how long root pain can last.

There are four ways in which spontaneous recovery is secured; the anatomical result in each case is different.

### Reduction

The displaced part of the disc may return to its bed spontaneously, either during rest in bed or merely because the patient maintains his lordosis, since he finds that trunk flexion is painful. Reduction can also be secured by manipulation or traction. Once back in place, the loose fragment is neither more nor less firmly in place because it shifted slowly during rest in bed or quickly during manipulation, and recurrence is not avoided more by one method than the other. Reduction implies that the damaged tissue no longer protrudes, but what has displaced itself once can do so again. Recurrences are thus to be expected.

Some believe that the click which often signals reduction at a lumbar joint indicates that the loose fragment has been shifted away from the dura mater or the nerve root by becoming even further displaced. Were this so, recurrence would be obviated, for what is not restored to its original position cannot displace itself again and, when a patient who had had 20 attacks of lumbago in his life came to laminectomy, 20 small fragments of disc would be found lying free in the intervertebral canal. This is not so.

## Erosion

A large posterolateral protrusion (Fig. 73) pressing against a nerve root lies in close contact with the dura mater. This pulsates, and jolts the protrusion against the back of the vertebral body at each heart beat. The bone is therefore eroded (as occurs on a larger scale in an aortic aneurysm) painlessly and the protrusion is finally accommodated (Fig. 74). I am indebted to my colleague R. H. Young for explanation of this important phenomenon. The protrusion now ceases to compress the nerve root and the patient recovers fully. What is more, the protrusion now lies in a position from which it cannot become dislodged, and I regard patients in whom recovery has been awaited as the result of this mechanism as no more subject to further attacks than a normal individual. Hence they can resume heavy work and need not wear a corset.

## Root Atrophy

Root pressure from a protruded disc goes on hurting so long as the sheath of the root remains sensitive. Extreme pressure so deprives the compressed extent of root sheath of its blood supply that it loses sensitivity.

As ischaemic root atrophy becomes complete, the pain abates, the appropriate cutaneous area goes numb, stretching the root returns to full range and the root palsy, sensory and motor, reaches a maximum. In other words, the patient has become subjectively better by getting anatomically worse.

Good recovery from the palsy is to be expected when only one root is paretic, but when two adjacent roots atrophy, some lasting loss of power of the weakest muscle, i.e. that common to both roots, may persist. There is very little tendency to recurrence. Hence the patient can exert himself normally and need not wear a corset.

## Disc Shrinkage

Surgeons report that at laminectomy on patients who had severe sciatica years ago, inspection of the disc shows a normal hard cartilaginous surface, level with the bones. The protrusion has receded. It would seem that its extra-articular position deprives the fragment of its nutrient synovial fluid; hence the protrusion slowly shrivels. This must be the mechanism operating in those cases of posterolateral protrusion which recover spontaneously in a year without the supervention of any neurological deficit. This mechanism is not brought into play when the displacement lies centrally, causing pain felt chiefly in the back, presumably because the protrusion still lies intra-articularly, confined by the posterior longitudinal ligament.

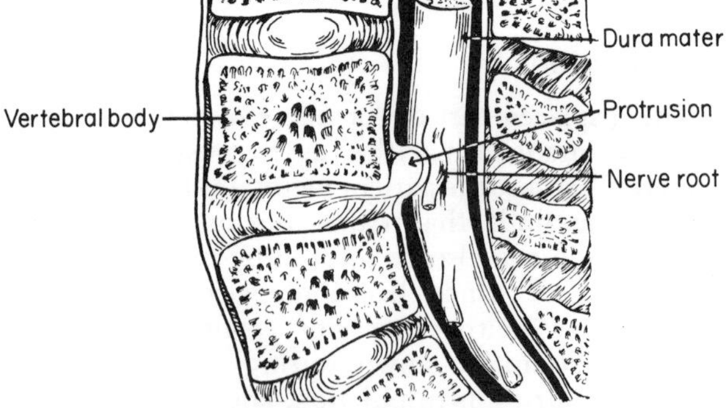


**Fig. 73.** Sciatica caused by herniation of nuclear material at the fourth lumbar level. The protrusion has passed posterolaterally and now impinges on the nerve root. It no longer presses on the dura mater, hence the backache ceases when the pain in the limb comes on. (*After Young 1945*).

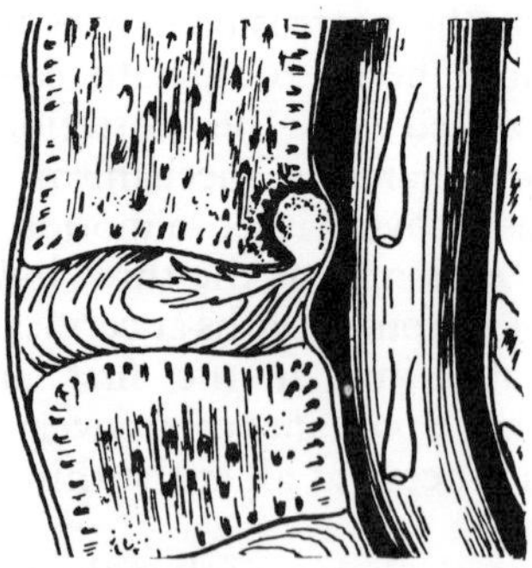

**Fig. 74.** Spontaneous recovery. The postero-inferior aspect of the vertebral body is eroded and the protrusion accommodated. When this process becomes complete dura mater and nerve root are no longer subjected to pressure. Symptomatic recovery is now established. (*After Young 1945*).

## THE MUSCLES

It is an accepted orthopaedic principle that the stronger the muscles about a joint, the more stable it is. This is a sound generalization, but there are exceptions.

This principle does not apply to internal derangement. Who puts the cartilage out in his knee? The professional footballer, whose exceptionally strong muscles and vigorous movements strain the joint in a way unlikely in a weaker man. Strong muscles protect the bones they join against displacement; they do not protect against intra-articular subluxation. Indeed, it can be argued that a man whose muscles enable him to put a 100 kg compression strain on his lumbar joint, is more apt to damage his disc than a weaker individual who can lift only 50 kg. Strong muscles do not prevent internal derangement at a lumbar joint, rather the contrary. Stability here is determined only by the interlocking of the lateral facets and the strength of the many ligaments. This view was confirmed by Nachemson and Lind (1969) who found that the strength of the abdominal and lumbar muscles was 'of doubtful importance' in the prevention of backache. The sacrospinalis muscles lie along the posterolateral aspects of the vertebrae; hence the first effect of their contraction is to squeeze these bones together, thus compressing the intervertebral joints. Only when all the play in these joints has been taken up is the spine moved towards extension. Thus the stronger the sacrospinalis muscles, the more the joint is compressed. It is thus the strong man who puts the greater compression stress on his lumbar joint during lifting. Retropulsion of disc material may ensue, rendered more probable by his muscular prowess. This view is confirmed by the fact that dockers, who have extremely strong sacrospinalis muscles and can thus lift loads beyond the compass of an ordinary individual, suffer ten times the national average for back troubles. As a corollary, patients whose lumbar muscles have been weakened by poliomyelitis seldom develop lumbar disc lesions.

An extension movement from the standing position is initiated by the sacrospinalis muscles. As soon as the thorax passes behind the vertical line, the movement continues by the force of gravity. The abdominal muscles pay out to allow the movement to be carried to its extreme. Pain elicited at the extreme of range is not derived from the muscle by active contraction. For this reason, standing trunk extension, being a passive movement, must be regarded as a test of articular function. If pain of muscular origin is suspected, the spinal movements must be tested against resistance. In fact, myofascial lesions are very uncommon at lumbar levels and result from direct trauma only. In young men, early disc lesions are often called 'sprained muscle', but not by those who test muscles by resisted contraction.

When an individual bends forward to pick up a heavy object, the sacrospinalis muscles pay out and at the extreme of range are fully stretched. When he strains upwards to lift, three forces act on the lumbar joint while it is held in flexion. First, as soon as the lumbar spine on its journey upwards passes the horizontal line, the weight of the trunk begins to compress the joint; secondly, the weight of the object lifted compresses the joint further; thirdly, both sacrospinalis muscles contract and compress the joint further still. Hence the stronger these muscles are, the greater the compression stress on the joint—in other words, the greater the liability to a disc lesion. Although flexion exercises have fallen out of favour, there is hardly a hospital department in the country where back exercises of some sort are not carried out in the 'treatment' of disc lesions, in the mistaken belief either that extension exercises encourage reduction, or that strong muscles beneficially support the joint. Though patients do recover in spite of such exercises, convalescence is delayed, and renewed protrusion during their performance—even if they are merely prone-lying trunk extension exercises—is by no means unknown.

The iliopsoas and the abdominal muscles are the flexors of the lumbar spine; the former flexes the spine when the femur is fixed; the latter flex it when the pelvis is fixed. In the standing patient, once the movement has been initiated by these muscles, flexion proceeds from the force of gravity, the hamstring and sacrospinalis muscles paying out smoothly to let the trunk down.

In acute lumbago, the flexed position of the lumbar spine is maintained by simultaneous contraction of the psoas and sacrospinalis muscles fixing the joint from both aspects in the neutral position. As a result of this flexed posture, the sacrospinalis muscles have to work hard against gravity to prevent the trunk toppling further forwards; since the patient is no longer poised vertically in line with his centre of gravity. This fact accounts for the mistaken idea that lumbago results from spasm or 'fibrositis' of the sacrospinalis muscles. One has only to remember that the muscles extend the joint to realize that spasm of the sacrospinalis muscles is neither the cause nor the result of lumbago. Were these muscles really in spasm, the joints would be held in extension, as happens in the opisthotonos of tetanus. Moreover, if the patient lies prone and the examiner presses on his back, thus extending the joint and relaxing the muscles, the pain increases.

When 'fibrositis' was discredited (Cyriax 1948), more plausible lesions of the non-articular structures were proposed. Fatty lobules are present in the sacrospinalis muscles and their herniation through the lumbar fasciae with strangulation was postulated as a cause of symptoms. Their existence in most normal persons is not denied. Alternatively, the word 'fibrositis' has been changed to 'fasciitis', 'myogelosis' or 'non-articular rheumatism'. That the muscles, fascia and fatty lobules are not affected in lumbago is proved again by the patient's posture; were any of these soft tissue disorders really present, he would instantly relieve his pain by bending backwards and relaxing tension. Indeed, the mere fact that a pain in the back or buttock is increased on bending backwards shows that it arises from a joint and not from the now-relaxed extensor muscles of the lumbar spine and hip joint.

Strange (1966) has put forward quite a different reason for avoiding the word 'disc' and going back to the muscular theory of lumbago. He states that this diagnosis, 'imperfectly made, has been responsible for making tens of thousands of perfectly fit men and women into life-long invalids'. In his address he went on to decry 'thousands of unnecessary operations', 'hundreds of thousands of physiotherapists' hours wasted', 'millions of pounds won in totally improper compensation', 'millions of man-hours of work lost'. Every word of this arraignment earns approval except the plea for a return to a false pathology. If a rational attitude to disc lesions ('displacement of a piece of cartilage' frightens nobody) were promoted, if logical treatment were carried out at once as a matter of course, the word would soon lose the dire significance that it possesses for patients today.

## THE BONES

The lower half of one vertebra and the upper half of the one below share the same embryological derivation and form one segment. When the fetus is 4–5 cm long, the notocord expands centrifugally forming a fissure extending across the segment. This is the disc, which during the whole of fetal life consists of nuclear material only, derived from the notocord. In adult life, the nucleus of the disc provides the only notocordal remnant.

The anteroposterior stability of the lumbar spine depends largely on engagement at the two lateral joints of the articular facets of one vertebra against the corresponding pair above and below (Fig. 75). If the pedicle is lengthened (Plate XXII) or a fibrous defect replaces bone at each isthmus between the superior and inferior articular process, this stability is endangered. Plate XXIII shows the considerable displacement that can occur after excessive removal of bone at laminectomy. Bony defect at the pars intermedia of the articular process may not lead to untoward stretching; if so, the condition is known as spondylolysis (Plate XX/2). However, the fibrous tissue at the defect in the bone may lengthen; spondylolisthesis results (Plate XXII). Since the stretching takes place anterosuperiorly to the lateral articulations of the affected vertebra, the spinous process of the spondylolisthetic vertebra is held in its normal relationship to that of the vertebra below. The body of the vertebra above, however, follows the body of the affected vertebra, and its spinous process therefore lies displaced anteriorly. For this reason, the irregularity of the spinous processes visible and palpable

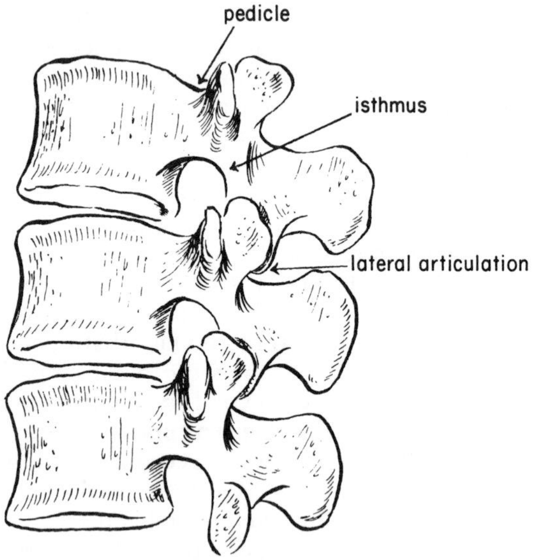


**Fig. 75.** Anteroposterior stability of the lumbar spine. This depends on the integrity of the pedicle and the isthmus and the engagement of facets at each lateral articulation.

in spondylolisthesis appears at the vertebra above that shown on the radiograph to be at fault.

## Congenital Abnormalities

Those who regard any congenital abnormality visible on the radiograph as sufficient explanation for backache are diminishing. Different observers have noted between 15 and 60% incidence of congenital abnormality in the lumbosacral region of patients not subject to backache. Sacralization of the fifth lumbar vertebra has no local significance, but it shows this joint to be fixed and suggests that excessive strain has fallen on the fourth lumbar joint which has had to do the work of two. It occurs in some 10% of ordinary individuals and is usually accompanied by a very narrow disc space, congenitally so. In sacralization, the likelihood of a disc lesion is enhanced at the joint above; recurrence is also more difficult to avoid. A lumbarized first sacral segment has no significance. Spina bifida occulta is a defect of the neural arch and thus unconnected with any joint; it has no significance, except in so far as it may denote poor development of the sacral facets—a factor in spondylolisthesis. Sutow and Pryde (1956) found it present in 28.5% of normal adults, whereas Southworth and Bersack's (1950) figure is 18.6, and Crow and Brogden's 35.7%. These authors examined 936 young men and found only 40.2% devoid of all radiological abnormality. 'Osteoarthrosis' of an abnormal joint between the upper surface of the sacrum and the fifth lumbar transverse process is also symptomless. It is perfectly logical, however, to regard any congenital abnormality, though irrelevant in any single case, as weakening the joint at that level, not by its mere presence, but by causing asymmetry. If, for example, the plane of the two facet joints is not identical, the vertebra must skew as it moves, thus straining the intervertebral joint and predisposing to disc trouble. This has been pointed out by Putti (1927) who described and illustrated the variability of angle at the lumbosacral facets—regarded by him as contributing towards sciatica. Gillespie's investigations (1949) confirmed this hypothesis. He found that any congenital abnormality, however distant from the surfaces at which a vertebra moves (e.g. spina bifida), predisposes to lumbar trouble. In 500 cases of laminectomy, spina bifida was present in 18.2%, whereas in patients attending for non-lumbar disorders, it was only 4.8%. The figure for any bony abnormality (excluding spondylolisthesis) in patients requiring laminectomy was 18.2% as opposed to 8.8% in patients whose back had never troubled them. This eminently probable conclusion was unquestioned until 1971 when Redfield reported on a radiological survey of 2201 heavy workers. Of these 209 were placed in a high-risk category on account of congenital abnormality, 1992 in a low-risk group. The surprising fact emerged that the likelihood of back injury in the alleged high-risk workers was half of that in the low-risk. Tini et al. (1977) came to the same conclusion in Switzerland. They found a fifth lumbar transitional vertebra present in 5% of ordinary people and 6.7% of 4000 patients with lumbar symptoms—a difference that the authors do not consider significant. It may well be, therefore, that radiography has as little value in providing an index of future liability to backache as it has when a disc lesion is actually present.

In contrast, spondylolysis and spondylolisthesis (Plate XX/2 and XXII) are significant, since they may result in painful stretching of ligament or nerve root, but much more often in a disc lesion at the unstable joint (Key 1945). Spondylolisthesis can exist for a lifetime without causing any symptoms.

Hemivertebra itself causes no symptoms. Spontaneous correction above and below the angulation often leads to minimal postural deformity, although the radiographic appearances are most asymmetrical. Hemivertebra may lead to a secondary disc lesion at the oblique joint. Alternatively, it can eventually result in the same painful bony contact of the vertebral bodies as complicates longstanding scoliosis from any other cause.

## Spinal Stenosis

This phenomenon was described and illustrated by Krause in 1910 (Plate LIV*a*, p. 1072) at the fourth lumbar level, and put forward as a contributory cause in compression of the cauda equina by Verbiest in 1954. His patients suffered from spinal claudication and at laminectomy he found a shallow canal with visible dural compression. A spinal canal with an anteroposterior diameter of less than 15 mm was considered abnormally narrow. In Jones and Thomson's series (1968), some of the patients suffered from claudication, others from backache and root pain. Their myelograms suggested that the pressure arose posteriorly, as the result of bulging of the ligamentum flavum secondary to undue approximation of two vertebrae. Porter (1979) found the breadth of the canal 1.4 cm or less in spinal claudication (normal 1.6 cm).

Clearly, individuals with too small a spinal canal are apt to suffer more from encroachment on its space than those whose dura mater can avoid compression by shifting backwards. Heavy workers with spinal stenosis are more at risk than ordinary individuals. Since the size of the neural canal sac can be measured by ultrasound scanning, it is a reasonable precaution for employers to have the canal measured and to warn anyone with a narrow canal to avoid labouring. The technique is merely to record echoes from the posterior and anterior surface of each lamina, and then from the posterior surface of the vertebral body. The time-interval between the echoes from the bones is measured and is proportional to the distance between the reflecting surfaces. The causes of a straitened spinal canal are numerous; Osborne (1974) gives the following list: developmental stenosis, osteophytosis, spondylolisthesis, achondroplasia, spina bifida, osteitis deformans and over-growth of bone after arthrodesis.

Jayson and Nelson (1979) state that the most troublesome is the trefoil-shaped vertebra. In this type the nerve roots fit the shallow lateral recesses with the result that any encroachment inevitably squeezes them. Since the space is increased on trunk-flexion, leaning forwards relieves the pain and paraesthesia on walking. Extension aggravates these sensations. Only surgical treatment avails; the affected vertebrae having to be decompressed even as high as the second lumbar level.

## THE JOINTS

The axis about which anteroposterior movement takes place lies at the junction of the anterior two-thirds and the posterior third of each lumbar vertebral body.

The primary movements at the lumbar joints are flexion, extension and side flexion. Flexion is brought to a stop by the supra- and interspinous ligaments, the ligamentum flavum and the capsule of the lateral articulations, which prevent the facets sliding any farther apart. Bouillet (personal communication, 1961) noted at laminectomy that, at the level of the disc lesion, the interspinous ligament is often torn, sometimes to shreds. He had found a reliable guide to the level of the protrusion. Clinically, palpation may reveal a gap between two spinous processes if the supraspinous ligament has parted. In wedge-fracture, the supraspinous ligament is always overstretched. The posterior longitudinal ligament scarcely limits flexion; for it lies so close behind the pivotal point of the movement. Extension is limited by the abdominal muscles, the anterior longitudinal ligament, bone meeting bone at the lateral joints, and the engagement posteriorly (cushioned by the interspinous ligaments) of the spinous processes. Side flexion is limited by the deep lumbar fascia, the lateral spinal ligaments, the ligaments of one lateral facet preventing further movement apart, and the point of one lateral process meeting the lamina on the concave side.

Very little rotation takes place at the upper four lumbar joints. Engagement of the inferior and superior articular processes largely prevents rotation. At the lumbosacral joint the angle of the facet surfaces is tilted usually to about 45°, but the variation (0 to 80°) is considerable. Hence, a little rotation is possible, limited by the iliolumbar ligaments. A little ligamentous play and a slight shearing play also exist at the facet joints; it is thus an exaggeration to say that rotation is wholly absent at the lumbar spine. Nevertheless, the range is very small and in Sollmann's cineradiographic film of a young woman dancing the twist, the lumbar spinous processes can be seen to remain vertically above each other, rotating with the pelvis but not on each other.

At the spinal joints, increasing limitation of movement is to be expected as age advances, unlike the joints of the limbs, where range alters little from childhood to senescence. Osteophyte formation and ligamentous contracture come to limit the range of movement at the spinal joints so much, that what would be gross limitation in a man of 25 is full range at 70. This absence of an absolute criterion causes much difficulty in diagnosis.

A patient with a small but painless range of lumbar movement is unaware of any rigidity, whereas a patient with ample range but discomfort at extremes states that his back feels stiff. Stiffness at the lumbar spine is thus a subjective phenomenon, unrelated to the amplitude of movement present. This is fortunate, for the spinal joints are the only ones in the body at which a diminished range of movement is advantageous and unperceived by the patient. At all joints other than the spinal, the endeavour is to abolish symptoms by the restoration of as full movement as is possible; the reverse applies to those spinal joints that contain damaged discs.

## The 'Facet Syndrome'

Schiötz's research (1958) has revealed that the first published ascription of back troubles to a disordered facet joint was by Dane—a chiropractor—in 1921. Putti (1927) incriminated the facet joint in sciatica. Since it is the osteopaths who are now promoting this joint, it is regarded as an osteopathic idea by the many doctors who come to hear of their view. Some have accepted this pathology, but there are many reasons for scepticism.

These joints have come into prominence, not because of any scientific research connecting them with backache, but by involvement in osteopaths' prestige. Disc lesions were a medical discovery and these laymen need to be 'one up' on doctors; they therefore invented the 'facet syndrome', inculpating joints that had not been previously considered as a common source of symptoms. They aver that the facet joints 'bind', but neglect to explain how two parallel cartilaginous surfaces can suddenly become fixed, a phenomenon unknown at any other joint. Wyke (1973) has stated that the facet joints do not lock. Inquiry by myself from two medical men practising osteopathy, both of whom had published work on the 'facet syndrome' elicited the response that its existence was mere supposition.

Apart from 'binding', the theories that I have heard propounded are that an intra-articular meniscus becomes displaced or that a synovial tag is nipped. Since synovium contains no nerves, such nipping would be painless, which disposes of the second alternative. Another postulate is the production of a traumatic arthritis at the facet joint, with swelling of the joint and muscle spasm about it.

### Anatomy

The two little facet (zygo-apophyseal) joints maintain stability; they do not bear weight. Nachemson (1962) stated that for loads of less than 200 kg they were subjected to no compression strain. They serve to keep the vertebrae in line and at the lumbar spine prevent rotation (except sometimes at the lumbosacral joint) while allowing flexion, extension and side flexion. At cervical and thoracic levels their surfaces lie obliquely and thus allow rotation as well as the other four movements. Since the articular excursion is 5–7 mm, the capsule is very lax in full extension. Hence, to prevent it becoming pinched between the bones, some of the fibres of the multifidius muscle, as they pass from the superior articular process to the spinous process below, blend with the posterior capsular fibres, keeping them taut (Lewin et al. 1961). At the upper and lower extremities of the joint lie small pads of fat, provided with a synovial fringe. These cushions act as buffers and undergo fibrosis as age advances. Vernon-Roberts (1975) illustrated pseudarthrosis between the apex of each inferior facet and the point where it impinged on the lamina below, in elderly individuals. McCall et al. (1978) found that when the facet joint capsule was injected with an irritant solution no pain was provoked beyond mid-thigh, there was no limitation of straight-leg raising nor discomfort on coughing.

The joints contain small intra-articular menisci (Töndury 1940) extending from the edges of the joint towards the joint cavity. They are present at birth. Dörr (1958) illustrates a small intra-articular meniscus lying towards the base of the facet; this would be pinched on extension and released on flexion of the joint.

Innervation stems from the medial branch of the posterior ramus, which crosses the joint capsule, giving off fibres to it. The nerve then continues downwards to supply also the joint below.

### Arthrography

Glover's arthrograms of the facet joints, displayed during a lecture in 1972, show a dumb-bell shadow. The oil injected within the joint flows up and down to where the joint surfaces are not in contact. Where they are in apposition, no room for the oil seems to exist. The interesting point is the large size of the upper shadow, occupying a large part of the intervertebral foramen. This sphere indicates the considerable length of ligament necessary to allow the bones to move apart when an individual bends forwards. The upper shadows shows a circular defect which he attributes to the nerve root. Clearly, an effusion into the synovial joint could exert pressure on a nerve root and set up a sciatica ceasing when the patient bent forwards. In fact, one such case has been described (Kendall 1972). The myelographic shadow showed no disorder when the spine was straight, but, on full lumbar extension, complete occlusion of the foramen was visible. At laminectomy the capsule of both facet joints was found hypertrophied.

## Evidence Against the Facet Hypothesis

There are two different sets of facts that militate against the idea of backache resulting from facet joint lesions. The first is that gross disorders there seldom cause backache. The second is the conflict between the physical signs found present and the existence of a lesion in that position.

*Known Lesions of the Facet Joints.* In many instances of the disorders detailed below, there is no backache. Strong reasons therefore exist for not ascribing lumbar symptoms to a disorder of the lateral facet joints.

Six disorders are recognized, in addition to the capsular hypertrophy described above:

1. *Incongruence.* When a disc has become completely eroded, as often happens to elderly people, the vertebral bodies lie about 1 cm closer together than originally. Such approximation clearly causes gross incongruence of the articulating surfaces at the facet joints, which slide down to adopt permanently the position of full extension. Yet these old people are conspicuously free from backache.
2. *Angulation.* After a wedge fracture of a vertebral body has united with deformity, marked tilting of the fractured bone on that above is inevitable. A much increased gap can be felt between the spinous processes; indeed, the supraspinous ligament has often ruptured. Lack of parallel between the articulating facet surfaces must supervene, but these patients seldom suffer any inconvenience.
3. *Distraction.* Posterior spondylolisthesis is possible only if the upper facets shift backwards on the superior articular processes of the vertebra below. This can be seen clearly on a lateral or oblique radiograph. Yet such gross overstretching of the capsule of the two joints is usually painless.
4. *Osteoarthrosis.* Lewin's (1966) radiological studies of people *without backache* showed osteoarthrosis of the facet joints in 15% of individuals aged 26–45, rising to 60% above that age.
5. *Spondylitic arthritis.* Bywaters (1968) described pannus at the facet joints in spondylitis ankylopoetica, with marginal erosion of cartilage.
6. *Adult spondylolisthesis.* This is a disorder in which the facet joints really do 'bind'. Cartilaginous, then bony, attrition with large osteophytes can reach such an advanced stage that the joints become wholly disorganized. This allows one vertebra to slip forwards about 1 cm. This might well be regarded as painful, yet many such patients have no backache.

*Conflict with Clinical Factors.* The history may contain facts that exclude ascription to a facet joint. It is not a central structure. Hence, it cannot give rise to central pain, or pain that starts centrally and then shifts to one side, or pain that starts to one side and then becomes central. Only a fragment of cartilage loose inside the intervertebral joint can move in this way. Sitting for some time is a common cause of backache, yet keeping the spine motionless in a posture close to the mid-position cannot conceivably strain the facet joint. A cough may be stated to hurt, and the facet joint does not lie in contact with the dura mater. Moreover, when root pain follows on backache, the lumbar symptoms often cease when the pain in the lower limb becomes established. This could not happen if the facet joint were at fault. Since it is common knowledge that lifting a heavy object is more likely to cause lumbago than just trunk flexion, the lesion ought to lie in a tissue that is compressed during weight-bearing. There is only one such: the disc. Moreover, during trunk flexion the facets move apart; hence, even if they were weight-bearing, they could not do so in that position.

Inspection may show the lumbar spine to be held deviating from the vertical. Should the list be away from the painful side, as often happens, muscle spasm about an irritated joint is excluded. The same applies to an alternating scoliosis. If a displaced meniscus were present, mere side flexion away from the painful side or trunk flexion would disengage the lesion at once, whereas very few backaches abate on full trunk flexion. Were a facet joint to develop a traumatic synovitis so that the swelling of the joint encroached on the intervertebral foramen enough to pinch the nerve root, full trunk flexion would immediately tauten the facet joint capsule and enlarge the foramen. Yet few sciaticas indeed obtain relief by bending fully forwards.

There exists one set of clinical signs that would do well for a facet disorder: the patient who is forced by sciatica to hold himself bent forwards and deviated. Trunk extension is impossible owing to the provocation of severe root pain which often ceases on full flexion. These patients' signs correspond with what could well be expected from a deranged facet joint. However, this is the very syndrome that nearly always calls for laminectomy. At operation, a disc protrusion is found and removed. The patient recovers without anything being done to his facet joint.

Neck flexion stretches the dura mater and lumbar pain thus set up can result only from a central prominence. In cases of real doubt, epidural local anaesthesia can be induced. Since the fluid injected cannot enter the facet joint, and procaine of 1:200 strength causes surface anaesthesia only (no root palsy results), relief following the induction shows that the lesion was capable of compressing the surface of the dura mater.

### Conclusion

The history or clinical signs are nearly always inconsistent with ascription of lumbar trouble to a facet joint. Since gross lesions of the facet joints cause neither backache nor disease elsewhere, it is most unlikely that the postulated minor transient lesion—whatever it is—'without irreversible change' could have any effect. Since fixation of the facet joints from senile obliteration of the disc or of the whole segment from tuberculosis or septic infection or ankylosing spondylitis causes no disease elsewhere either, it is not at all probable that the minor degree of derangement that the osteopaths allege could be dangerous to health. Moreover it is up to them, the advocates of this hypothesis, to put forward some evidence that their notion is correct, or at least based on some clinical findings that interested medical men can investigate.

### Facet Locking

Lay manipulators are proud of their capacity to 'lock' the facet joints. By this they mean pushing them to the extreme of range, whereupon they will not move any further. Side flexion of the neck one way accompanied by rotation in the opposite direction crowds the facet joints together until they are fixed. The neck is then rigid, since all the slack has been taken up. But this cannot be termed 'locking' for the joint is not locked at all in the sense that a displaced meniscus locks the knee. It is merely held at the extreme of range, whereupon no more movement is possible, as happens whenever bone meets bone at any joint, e.g. impingement of the olecranon against the humerus on full extension at the elbow.

In this extreme position of the neck, so laymen aver, any further strain now affects only the joint they propose to treat. This involves the supposition that each vertebral joint moves to full range before the adjacent joint moves at all. To me it is remarkable that, in spite of their compression of the joints and fixation at the extreme of range in this way, osteopaths' manipulations can still prove effective. Even if their ideas were correct—a bone out of place or limited movement at a joint—it is obvious that the last way to attempt reversal of either phenomenon would be manipulation during compression. Their ideas about the advantages of 'locking' the facets result in the best adjuvant to manipulation at the cervicothoracic joints, i.e. adequate traction, being denied to osteopaths and chiropractors. In fact, Bihaug (personal communication, 1974), experimenting with a cadaveric spine from which the muscles but not the ligaments had been removed, found that it was anatomically impossible to lock the facet joints.

## THE LUMBAR LIGAMENTS

The lumbar ligaments are often regarded as liable to strain, but ligaments become sprained when a joint is forced beyond its normal range. However, the pain of lumbago comes on when the patient, having bent fully to lift, is halfway up again—a moment when the joint is near mid-range and, in consequence, no ligament is tense. Hence, 'lumbosacral strain' is a misnomer.

### The Posterior Longitudinal Ligament

This ligament plays an important part in disc protrusion. It occupies the midline but is deficient on each side (Weitbrecht 1742); hence a protrusion initially presenting centrally meets the barrier of a tough ligament. The resistance of the ligament (Dandy 1929) tends to push the protrusion back again anteriorly and accounts for the regular occurrence of spontaneous reduction in lumbago. After repeated attacks, the protrusion is apt to shift towards a zone of lesser resistance, i.e. to one or other side of the ligament. As a protrusion enlarges, therefore, it usually becomes unilateral. As a result, central pain in the back is replaced by root pain in the lower limb.

Should the posterior longitudinal ligament rupture, it is then possible for the entire contents of the intervertebral joint to extrude backwards.

If so, the cauda equina is subjected to strong pressure and severe bilateral sciatica results. In addition, the third and fourth sacral roots may be compressed and paralysis of the bladder ensues. This may become permanent unless early laminectomy relieves the pressure quickly.

Cases have been described of lumbar puncture being followed by a lumbar disc lesion. It is very doubtful whether the introduction of the needle bears any relevance to the disorder; for, were it a question of extrusion of nuclear material via the puncture in the posterior longitudinal ligament, manipulative reduction would prove impossible. In fact, manipulative reduction usually succeeds, and it is clearly the flexed position in which the patient has been maintained, not the needle itself, that has caused the displacement.

## Supraspinous Ligaments

These join the tips of the spinous processes and limit the amount of flexion possible at each intervertebral joint. When a vertebral body is fractured, the ligament is overstretched and may rupture, leaving a palpable interspinous gap. At laminectomy the ligament may be seen to be torn at the level of the protrusion.

In disc protrusion at the third, fourth or fifth level, the fifth lumbar supraspinous ligament is found tender. Hence this finding is not a reliable guide to the level of the lesion.

The interspinous ligaments lie more deeply. Being closer to the fulcrum they have little effect in stopping flexion. In any case, they are made of much weaker tissue than the supraspinous ligaments. It takes some strength to force sclerosant fluid into the latter, but the less dense interspinous ligament offers hardly any resistance. In 21% of normal adults one lower lumbar interspinous ligament is deficient (Rissanen 1960).

## Iliolumbar Ligaments

These have an important bearing on patient's symptoms and signs. These ligaments anchor the transverse processes of the fifth lumbar vertebra to each iliac crest and to the sacrum. They therefore restrict side flexion, which has a much smaller range at the lumbosacral joint than at the other lumbar joints. The fourth lumbar joint is capable of great side flexion; hence, in a patient with a protrusion at this level, the joint can gape so much that the displacement is accommodated. In other words, he presents marked deformity and thus avoids most of the pain. The same degree of accommodation is not possible at the lumbosacral joint; in consequence, the deformity is slight but the pain correspondingly severe.

## Alleged Ligamentous Laxity

The first edition of Hackett's book attributing back troubles to ligamentous laxity appeared in 1956. Harrison (1821) had already stated that the spinal ligaments could become stretched, thus allowing a single vertebra to become displaced. He advocated 'restoring the displaced bones to their natural situation' more than fifty years before osteopathy based itself on the same idea. Riadore (1843) had made the same suggestion. Ever since, the notion has been gaining ground that excessive movement at an intervertebral joint is a cause of pain. It is true, of course, that diminished mobility at an intervertebral joint is a commonplace; by comparison, adjacent normal joints may appear hypermobile. Excessive movement does occur in anterior and posterior spondylolisthesis, and is then visible radiologically.

Advanced degeneration of a disc or osteophytosis (often both together) naturally limit joint movement. A sacralized fifth lumbar vertebra is fixed by bridges of bone. After adolescent osteochondrosis, several adjacent joints may move very little. Some elderly patients without osteophytosis or disc degeneration may have gross symptomless stiffness due to diffuse ligamentous contracture. When cineradiography shows two vertebrae scarcely to move on each other at all, the joint is rightly regarded as very stiff. These partly fixed joints may further hypermobility at the joints above and below (Bosman 1972) and it is here, not at the stiff joint, where he considers the trouble to lie.

The undisputed fact of different degrees of mobility has been fostered by osteopaths. They feel for variations in the range of movement at each spinal joint in turn. They quite correctly perceive differences, but incorrectly attribute diagnostic significance to them. The fact that these findings do not provide an accurate guide to the level of the lesion is shown at laminectomy, when a large disc protrusion may be disclosed at a joint with a good range of movement and radiologically normal, whereas the adjacent joint had been found very stiff and X-rays had shown osteophytes and a narrow joint space. Naturally, the real test is to find out at which level passive movement best elicits the patients' symptoms.

The most obvious cause of ligamentous overstretching is a wedge-fracture, which greatly elongates the ligaments between two spinous processes, sometimes to the point of rupture. Gross laxity follows advanced attrition of a disc, such that the two vertebral bodies lie in virtual apposition. This event renders the intervertebral ligaments up to 1 cm too long. In neither case does this ligamentous laxity cause symptoms. Quite apart from the fact that it is the interdigitation of the lateral articular processes that holds the vertebrae in line, ligamentous laxity elsewhere is known to cause instability, not pain. For example, permanent lengthening of a collateral or a cruciate ligament at the knee, or of the acromioclavicular ligaments makes subluxation possible, but does not hurt. Though differences in mobility between one spinal joint and another are a real entity, they have no bearing on symptoms.

Pain arises not from instability of the intervertebral joint itself but from instability of a fragment of disc lying within it. If this shifts to and fro for little cause, recurrent pain is to be expected. Manipulative reduction succeeds easily, but does not last long. The fact that sclerosing injections have helped affords no proof that ligamentous strain has been abolished but rather that the ligamentous contracture provoked has limited movement to the point of preventing attacks of internal derangement.

The bogy of the 'hypermobile segment'—dangerous to manipulate—is put forward by lay manipulators in order to scare off physiotherapists. What happens when such joints are manipulated in the osteopathic manner I do not know. Nothing special, I feel sure; for osteopathy had existed for decades before this caution was invented. All I can say is that my physiotherapists and I have, using our methods, repeatedly manipulated patients with good result in whom the lateral radiographs showed a clear shift of one vertebra on the next at the extremes of flexion and extension.

### 'Kissing Spinous Processes'

The space between the spinous processes is subject to great individual variation. Some authorities consider that trunk extension can pinch the interspinous ligaments enough to cause pain—this notion is easily disproved by local anaesthesia of the allegedly affected ligaments, since the pain when they are pinched remains and clearly has another source. Vernon-Roberts (1975) has illustrated pseudarthrosis at the points of bony contact. Congenital approximation occurs when the processes are unusually large, and causes some limitation of extension without discomfort.

## PAIN ARISING FROM THE LUMBAR LIGAMENTS

I do not myself believe that pain arises from the spinal ligaments, except at the atlanto-occipital and the atlanto-axial joints. Not because of insensitivity (as anyone who has had intraligamentous sclerosant injections can vouch) but because bony engagement and stress on the disc takes the strain first. There appears to me to exist a considerable body of evidence that neither overstretching nor laxity causes symptoms arising from the ligament itself. Indeed, Rolander (1966) found that removal of the intervertebral joints and posterior ligaments led to no increase in the mobility of one vertebral segment on another. Division of the ligamentum flavum had a small effect only. He found that the disc was the main stabilizing tissue. However, it must seem most improbable to most readers that the spinal ligaments should be the only ones in the whole body from which pain does not ordinarily emanate at all. Nearly all observers in this field share views directly contrary to my own. For example, the title of the book of one of my colleagues, O. Troisier (1974*a*), is *Sémiologie et Traitment des Algies Discales et Ligamentaires du Rachis*. This aetiology for backache has already been put forward by Harrison in 1821 who wrote 'Ligaments become relaxed and suffer a single vertebra to become displaced'. His remedy was to restore the displaced bone to its natural position. Riadore (1843) shared this view.

My reasons are as follows.

### Stretched Ligaments

*Fracture.* When a vertebral body suffers a wedge-fracture, the posterior ligaments inevitably are suddenly and severely elongated. The bone pain lasts three months, but the permanent overstretching of the ligaments hardly ever causes any symptoms.

*Spondylolisthesis.* In these cases, the elongation is even more extensive, amounting to 1–2 cm of both anterior and posterior longitudinal ligament. It takes place gradually during growth, but while it is going on the adolescent seldom suffers any discomfort.

*Traction.* This causes considerable tension on the ligaments of the spine. Yet, during traction, the backache nearly always ceases.

*Painful Arc.* Many patients with backache possess a painful arc on trunk flexion. Yet at half-flexion no ligament is on the stretch.

*Ligamentous Stress.* Ligaments are strained when the joint is forced beyond the extreme of the normal range. However, in lumbago, the pain starts when the muscles contract and the joint is squeezed while still in some kyphosis on coming up from full flexion. (This is why 'lumbosacral strain' is so misleading a term, suggesting as it does an overstretched ligament.) Moreover a common way to develop increasing backache is sitting a while with the lumbar spine scarcely flexed at all. Clearly no ligament is responsible for backache so caused, for none is on the stretch.

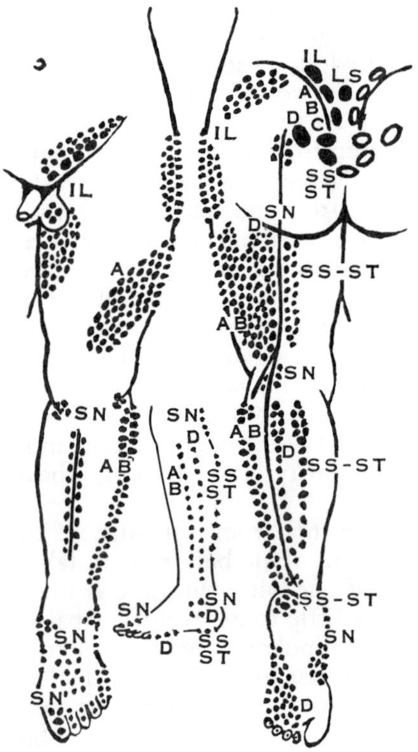


**Fig. 76.** The diagram for Hackett's book, indicating where the injection is made, depending on the area to which pain is referred. (*By kind permission of the author and Blackwell Scientific Publications*).

## Lax Ligaments

No greater ligamentous laxity exists than when complete erosion of the disc has occurred, whether from spontaneous attrition as age advances, destruction by chymopapain or removal at laminectomy. In the elderly, ligaments originally spanning a joint 10 mm wide may now need to be only 1 mm long. Yet these are the very patients conspicuously immune to backache.

None of these facts alters my full agreement with Hackett and Ongley that ligamentous injections are a potent method for abolishing backache. The method devised by Ongley and the solution of dextrose and phenol that he advocates are described in Volume II.

# LUMBAR 'OSTEOARTHROSIS'

*'Osteoarthrosis' of the lumbar spine is an imaginary disease.* Not only does osteophyte formation at the intervertebral joint cause no symptoms, but it is beneficial, and is the mechanism whereby pain in later life is prevented. It is particularly apt to appear at the lateral side of each intervertebral joint, where the disc is weakest.

## Articular Insensitivity

For the proper comprehension of backache, the most vital point to grasp is that the lumbar joints are insensitive to osteophytosis and internal derangement. The analogy with the knee does not hold. Internal derangement of the knee hurts the sensitive knee joint, which becomes the site of a painful traumatic arthritis. At the lumbar joints internal derangement is of itself painless, the ligaments of the joint being insensitive to the pressure exerted by the displacement. *Pain in lumbar protrusions is wholly dependent on whether or not the displacement presses on neighbouring sensitive structures.* The most obvious proof of this surprising state of affairs is the typical history given by patients suffering from primary posterolateral protrusion of disc material. Though they have suffered internal derangement at a low lumbar level from the first, they have not had, and will not have during the whole evolution of their disorder, one moment's backache, since the protrusion has, from the onset, missed the dura mater and compressed the nerve root only. Hence symptoms are felt only in the lower limb throughout the whole course of the disease. The patient with the largest protrusion of all, that causing root atrophy, has no backache. Another proof is afforded by the induction of epidural local anaesthesia. None of the solution gets inside any joint; only the dura mater and its investment of the nerve roots is rendered anaesthetic, yet the pain disappears, although the protrusion is still present as an articular phenomenon. It has been argued that the pain in lumbago is caused by pressure on the posterior longitudinal ligament. This is not so; for, quite apart from the prominent signs of interference with dural mobility, epidural local anaesthesia destroys the pain for the time being and, though it might be thought to render the posterior surface of the ligament anaesthetic, it cannot reach the anterior surface against which the disc protrusion is pressing. It is the anaesthesia of the dural tube that secures relief. Moreover, when the posterior ligament ruptures and massive extrusion of the disc results, the backache does not cease.

*It follows that the lumbar joints are insensitive. Hence, osteophyte formation cannot be expected to set up symptoms.* If it did, nearly all elderly people would suffer intractable backache.

*Osteophyte Formation.* Weight-bearing exerts a centrifugal force on the contents of each lumbar joint. When in middle-age degeneration of the disc becomes considerable, the bulging in each direction during weight-bearing pulls on the ligaments, especially laterally and anteriorly. Ligamentous traction now lifts the periosteum off the edge of the bone. Periosteum is the limiting membrane of bone and just as traction on the plantar fascia at its calcanean origin lifts up periosteum, whereupon new bone grows in to fill the gap, so does this familiar process affect the edge of the vertebral body. New bone gradually forms in the space between vertebra and periosteum, and in due course an osteophyte appears. The lumbar joint being insensitive, this is a painless process. Osteophyte formation brings three benefits. First, it replaces soft ligament with hard bone and the disc becomes cupped in bone—a strong hindrance to further protrusion. Secondly, the osteophytes limit mobility, thus preventing the very movements that might otherwise have resulted in an attack of internal derangement. Thirdly, the weight-bearing area is increased, so that the pressure per unit area diminishes.

Radiological surveys have shown that, by the age of 50, lumbar osteophytosis is present in 90% of normal men and, at 65, in 80% of normal women. Yet, these are the very ages when the incidence of backache and sciatica has begun to decline. Really elderly people rarely suffer backache, though this is the moment when degeneration of the disc is at its maximum (Office of Health Economics 1973). Moreover statistics from California (Leavitt et al. 1972) show the highest incidence of back troubles in the decade 40 to 49, dropping by a third between 50 and 59 years of age, and by two-thirds beyond 60. It must therefore be abundantly clear that degeneration of any tissue in the spine cannot provide the explanation for back troubles.

Anyone who still imagines that lumbar osteophyte formation causes a painful condition known as 'osteoarthrosis' should visit a clinic where middle-aged heavy workers, e.g. dockers, are see on account of a disorder unconnected with backache—say, renal calculus. He will see, on radiograph after radiograph of the urinary tract, gross osteophyte formation at all the lumbar vertebrae. Questioned, the patient insists that his back has never troubled him. The fact is that, sooner or later, heavy work results in lumbar trouble unless osteophyte formation comes into play as a protective mechanism. Those who carry heavy weights for a living and whose vertebrae adapt themselves by throwing out osteophytes are able to go on with such work until late middle age, whereas those who do not develop 'osteoarthrosis' develop disc lesions instead and turn to other jobs. Admittedly, these osteophytes are not a perfect protection, and cases of discogenic pain are encountered notwithstanding marked osteophyte formation, largely because osteophytes have formed anteriorly and laterally but not posteriorly. When, as rarely happens, a posterior osteophyte enlarges enough to compress the dura mater or a nerve root, symptoms do of course result (Plate XXVI/1). The lumbothoracic spinal joints are not the only ones where osteophyte formation is symptomless, e.g. the cuneo-first-metatarsal joint.

## Schmorl's Nodes

Another protective mechanism is the development of Schmorl's nodes. Unfortunately they are rarely seen where they are most needed, i.e. at the fourth and fifth lumbar levels, being common only at the lower thoracic and upper three lumbar joints. This radiographic appearance indicates that the nucleus pulposus has protruded vertically into the body of the vertebra. The herniation into bone is continuous with the nucleus, as was shown by Beadle's (1931) microscopic sections and Collis's (1963) discogram (Fig. 77). Erosion proceeds slowly and painlessly, greatly diminishing the centrifugal force exerted by the nucleus

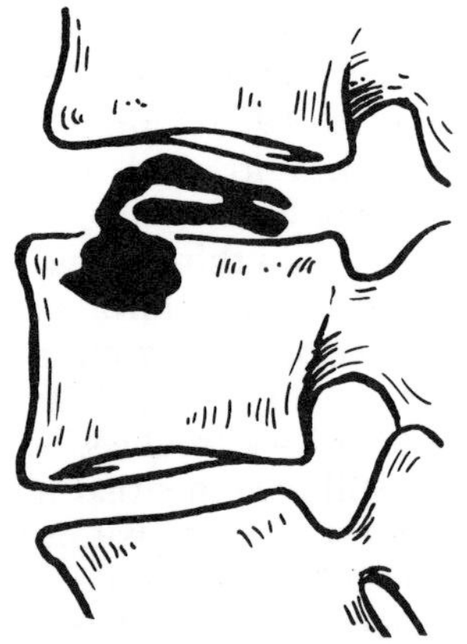

**Fig. 77** Schmorl's node. The normal biocular pattern of the disc is shown. The contrast material outlines the node, demonstrating the connection. (*Reproduced from Collis 1963*).

on the annulus and preventing it from tending to shift backwards. Hence it helps to fix the nucleus, but unhappily not at the joints where such protection is most desirable. Vernon-Roberts (1975) examined 300 spines of elderly people post mortem and found 40% to have one or more Schmorl's nodes.

## THE DURA MATER

This tough membranous tube runs from the foramen magnum of the skull to the caudal edge of the first or second sacral vertebra. The lower level varies a good deal and once in a hundred cases the theca ends below this point and is then apt to be pierced by the needle when epidural local anaesthesia is attempted via the sacral hiatus. It keeps the spinal cord, as far as the first lumbar level, then the cauda equina, buffered in a fluid medium. This liquid is continuous from ventricles to sacrum. A vascular jolt, e.g. coughing, momentarily enlarges the intradural veins and starts an impulse transmitted throughout cerebrospinal fluid. From it emerge 30 pairs of nerve roots covered by the dural sheath which ends at the distal edge of the intervertebral foramen. Cotugno likened this sleeve to a funnel (1775).

### Dural Mobility

The dura mater moves slightly in relation to the vertebrae it traverses. This has been unwittingly noted in two classical signs of meningeal irritation—neck retraction and Kernig's sign. Extension at the neck relaxes the dura mater as much as possible, and has its minor counterpart in local pain brought on by neck flexion in a thoracic or a lumbar disc lesion. Occasionally a large mid-thoracic protrusion actually limits the range of neck flexion. Kernig's sign is merely another way of demonstrating limitation of straight-leg raising, and has its counterpart in the patient with sciatica who cannot sit up in the bath without bending the knee of the affected leg. Whether the dura mater is immobilized by inflammation within or compression from without, the movement is limited because it stretches the dura mater from below, via the sciatic nerve. These signs have been accepted for decades, but their mechanism has not been elucidated, because hitherto the dura mater has not been regarded as possessing a mobility of its own, independent of movement at the joints it spans.

Dural stretching from above and below is painful in some patients but not in others with apparently identical lesions. The cause for this discrepancy was elucidated by Reid's (1958) anatomical studies in New Zealand. In the course of 38 autopsies, he found that, in patients over 25, no less than 31 had developed localized shortening of the dura mater. As a result, the dura mater had been drawn downwards so far that the thoracic roots could be seen running upwards to their respective foramina. Breig (1960) attributes this shortening to shearing forces between the dura mater and the wall of the neural canal damaging epidural tissue with consequent scarring. Clearly, the presence or not of dural signs in any one case of lumbago will depend not only on the size of the protrusion but on whether or not the theca has undergone contracture.

### Dural Sensitivity

The dura mater is often regarded as insensitive, chiefly because pricking the membrane during lumbar puncture is not felt by the patient. This is not an effective stimulus, any more than is acupuncture of the bowel. When laparotomy is performed under local anaesthesia of the abdominal wall, the intestine can even be divided without any pain. Yet no one denies the tension pain of colic. The dura mater behaves in the same partly sensitive way; it does not feel a prick but, when its mobility is impaired, resents stretching.

Edgar and Nundy (1966) made an important contribution to the study of pain arising from the dura mater. They investigated its nerve supply and found that it was innervated from the sinuvertebral nerve by three separate routes. However, these fibres all ran to the ventral aspect of the dura mater, no nerves being traced to, or discovered at, the dorsal surface of the membrane. This partial innervation confined to the anterior aspect of the dura mater explains why no pain is felt at lumbar puncture when the needle pierces the membrane. By contrast, a central disc protrusion bulges out the posterior ligament enough to compress the sensitive anterior aspect of the theca. Myeloscopy (MacNab 1980) has shown that the dura mater is very sensitive to touch. He says 'we had not realized before how sensitive the dura mater is. Even touching the surface with the tip of the myeloscope produces backache'. Here is experimental proof that the dura is the sentient membrane responsible for backache (Cyriax 1945). In arachnoiditis the nerve roots no longer lie surrounded by cerebrospinal fluid but can be seen to lie matted together by a curdlike substance.

*The Main Dural Symptom.* This is felt in the posterior aspect of the trunk on coughing; curiously enough, in the thoracic region, a deep breath evokes the pain better than a cough. Occasionally a patient avers that constipation increases his lumbar or root pain, defaecation bringing relief. This is an example of pelvic venous congestion transmitting increased pressure to the intradural veins. It would not be surprising if the severe backache that sometimes heralds anterior poliomyelitis arises from the dura mater.

*The Dural Signs.* These are: (*a*) pain in the back brought on by neck flexion and (*b*) pain in the back set up by straight-leg raising. This pain may then be further increased by neck flexion. O'Connell (1956) made radiographic measurements in full flexion and full extension of the neck and his findings confirmed these views. He showed that in full flexion the length of the front and back of the cervical spinal canal increased by 1.5 cm and 5 cm respectively, compared with full extension. Neck flexion thus moves the dural tube upwards an average of 3 cm, and draws the thoracic extent of the dura mater with it. Breig (personal communication, 1972) has shown that the dura mater stretches transversely but not longitudinally.

## Comment

In lumbar disc lesions, the most remarkable feature is that the symptoms, although caused by displacement within a joint, arise from pressure transmitted indirectly to the dura mater and not from any pressure exerted on the articular structures themselves. For years, if the lumbar movements hurt, the common cause of backache was sought in the bones, joints, ligaments, muscles, fasciae—in other words, in the moving parts of the back. Unexpectedly, the intra-articular disc, invisible on the radiograph, provides the prime cause of backache, and the dura mater, formerly thought to lie inert and insensitive within the spinal canal, is the sentient structure whereby derangements of the spinal joints make themselves felt. The experimental findings of Smith and Wright (1958) substantiate these views. By passing nylon loops round different structures in the back at laminectomy and pulling gently on these threads later, they found: (*a*) the nerve root very sensitive, mere touch sufficing to provoke pain and limitation of straight-leg raising; (*b*) the dura mater only slightly sensitive, an ache appearing in three cases out of five; (*c*) the interspinous ligaments and the ligamentum flavum insensitive; (*d*) the posterior longitudinal ligament (tested in one case) sensitive. Unless this dual mechanism is understood, it is not possible to make sense of the signs presented by patients with, for example, lumbago. The articular protrusion is the primary cause of pressure; it bulges out the back of the intervertebral joint. The ligaments are insensitive and nothing is felt until the bulge is large enough to compress the dura mater.

Since the mechanism is dual, the physical signs would be expected to be dual too. They are: dural and articular. It is possible painfully to stretch the dura mater by traction exerted from a distance—dural signs—and painfully to force the protrusion against the dura mater by movement at the affected joint—articular signs. For this reason, the subtitle of my paper on lumbago in 1945 was 'the mechanism of dural pain'. Though the suggestion made then that lumbago is caused by internal derangement of a low lumbar joint is now widely accepted, the concept of dural pain has not filtered through appreciably.

## Dural Reference

The mechanism of the production of pain in disc lesions is not merely academic; for readers of Chapter 3 will remember that the manner of reference of pain from the dura mater defies the rules of segmentation that all other tissues observe. False localizing symptoms are, therefore, commonplace, and deceptive. Indeed, there is no pain felt between the waist and the feet that could not originate from a lumbar disc lesion. The pain in acute central lumbago at a low lumbar level may spread to any of the following sites: the whole abdomen below the umbilicus; one or both groins; up the trunk posteriorly to the lower thorax; down the front, outer side or back of both thighs; to the coccyx. This clinical finding was experimentally confirmed by Fernström (1957) who found that abdominal pain could be provoked at lumbar discography. Later, in 1960, he reported pain in head, shoulders or chest in 1.3% of patients undergoing discography. None of these symptoms has the slightest localizing value, and it must be remembered that, in lesions affecting the dura mater, ordinary anatomical tenets are regularly transgressed. Difficulty arises when pain in one buttock (first lumbar dermatome), one groin (twelfth thoracic dermatome) or the iliac fossa (lowest three thoracic dermatomes) is set up by a low lumbar disc lesion causing little or no concomitant backache. Renal pain, chronic appendicitis or a lower thoracic disc lesion is then closely simulated and differential diagnosis becomes extremely difficult at times. The removal of the appendix for lumbago is no rarity, and by no means an easily avoidable error. Luckily, in those hospitals where it is carried out, epidural local anaesthesia provides a simple answer in all cases of doubt.

By contrast, the area occupied by the root pain in the lower limb is highly significant; for the affected dermatome is clearly outlined.

## LUMBAR INNERVATION

The classic complete account of the spinal nerves is contained in Hovelacque's (1927) book. Further studies were carried out on monkeys by Stilwell in 1956. By means of intravital staining he was able to demonstrate even very delicate nerves in carefully prepared sections. He found the anterior and posterior longitudinal ligaments to be well supplied with nerves entering both from above and below and overlapping. In contrast to Edgar and Nundy, he found the dorsal aspect of the dura mater to be supplied with nerves exclusively from the autonomic plexus, whereas the ventral half was supplied by a recurrent branch from the sinuvertebral nerve containing both autonomic and somatic fibres (Fig. 78). This nerve travels back through the intervertebral foramen, composed of elements derived from two adjacent roots.

The annulus fibrosus has nerves confined to a thin layer of connective tissue on its surface; no nerves penetrate the annulus. This is plainly shown in Bradley's microphotograph (Plate XXXIX). The interspinous and flaval ligaments possess nerves along their surfaces only; no fibres are detectable entering their substance.

The facet joints are innervated by the medial branch of the posterior ramus.

Each sinuvertebral nerve emerges from the posterior ramus 2 mm distal to the posterior ganglion, receives a branch from the sympathetic chain and then loops back into the spinal canal curving upwards round the base of the pedicle (Luschka 1850). Thence it runs towards the

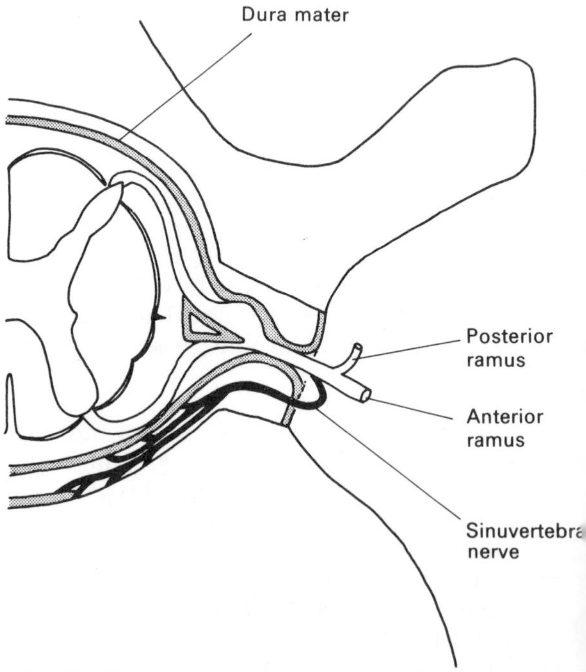


**Fig. 78.** The sinuvertebral nerve emerges from the intervertebral forearm and then doubles back to supply the posterior longitudinal ligament and the anterior aspect of the dura mater. (*After Hovelacque 1927*).

midline, reaching as far as the posterior longitudinal ligament (Pedersen et al. 1956). Filaments supply the ligaments, periosteum and dura mater, but neither of these authors could detect nerve fibres within the annulus fibrosus itself.

The posterior rami pass downwards obliquely each dividing into medial and lateral branches. The medial branch crosses the posterior aspect of the base of the transverse process, where it lies in a ligamento-osseous tunnel at the junction of the transverse and the superior articular process (Fig. 79). It crosses the facet joint, giving off twigs to it. The terminal fibres now pass along the lamina, anastomosing with their neighbours and ending in the interspinous ligament. Each nerve sends fibres to the facet joint above and the one below, which are thus supplied by nerves from two segments (Lazorthes & Gaubert, 1957). Microscopy showed the nerves to contain both sensory and sympathetic elements. No lumbar nerve reaches the skin of the lumbar region, which is supplied entirely via the thoracic roots.

In 1973 Bradley, Professor of Anatomy at Melbourne University, kindly showed me his recent dissection of the anterior and posterior lumbar rami. As Plate XLI shows, the posterior ramus divides into two branches, medial and lateral. The medial twig divides into two just beyond the edge of the transverse process, one running to the adjacent facet joint capsule; the other, longer, extends to the corresponding joint below. The lateral branch innervates adjacent periosteum and nearby fibres of the sacrospinalis muscle.

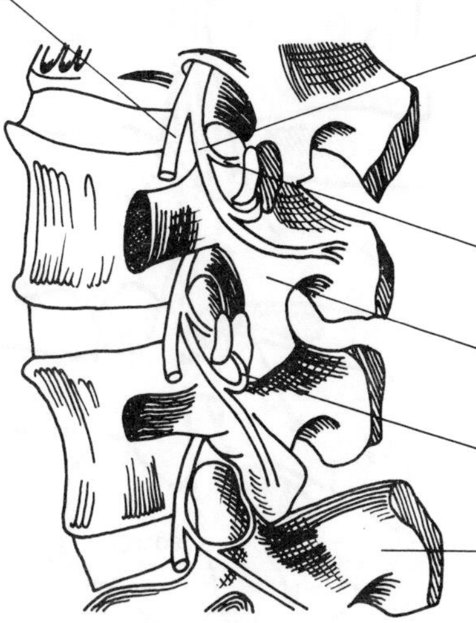


**Fig. 79.** The posterior rami at the second, third and fourth lumbar levels. (*After Pederson et al. 1956*).

The first to attribute a pathological significance to the sinuvertebral nerve was Leriche (1924). During laminectomy for painful amputation stumps, he noted excessive congestion of many small arteries and veins within the spinal canal. He considered abnormal stimuli conducted by the sinuvertebral nerve as responsible for the congestion and, probably, the pain.

# THE LUMBAR NERVE ROOTS

## Obliquity

The lumbar roots emerge in pairs from the dura mater and reach the foramen of exit by passing downwards and outwards across the body of the vertebra and the posterolateral aspect of the intervertebral joint. At the third, fourth and fifth foramina, disc protrusion can result in root compression, whereas at the first and second lumbar levels the root emerges high up in the intervertebral foramen, above the intervertebral joint, thus escaping impact.

The downward slope of the lower nerve roots has an important practical application. It is possible for a protrusion lying almost centrally at the fourth level to pinch the fifth root, whereas by presenting a little more to one side, it can compress only the fourth root (Fig. 81). A larger

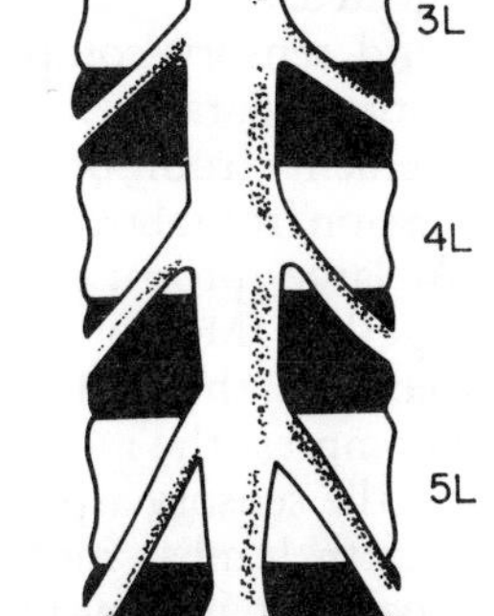

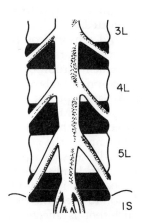

**Fig. 80.** The relation of the lumbar nerve roots to the intervertebral discs (black). From a photograph of a dissection. (*Reproduced from Burns and Young 1945*).

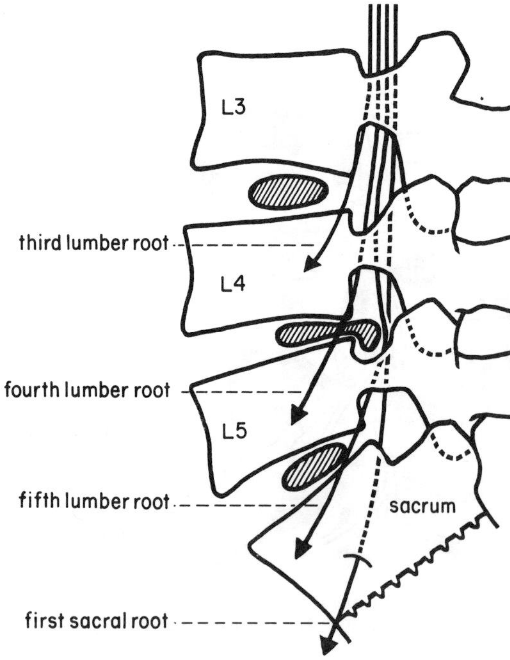


**Fig. 81.** Compression of the fifth lumbar nerve root by a protrusion at the fourth level. This diagram shows clearly that a herniation appearing just to one side of the posterior ligament misses its own nerve root, since this has already passed too far laterally. It is apt to impinge against the root emerging one level below. (*After Laurence 1955*).

protrusion can, of course, squeeze both roots. Similarly, a protrusion at the fifth level may affect the first sacral or the fifth lumbar or both roots. A fourth lumbar palsy indicates that the lesion lies at the fourth level; a first sacral palsy, at the fifth lumbar level; but a fifth lumbar palsy leaves the issue indeterminate. Hence, it is always best to confine the diagnosis to a statement on which root is affected.

The motor and sensory components of the nerve root emerge separately; hence a purely motor (impingement from below) or purely sensory (compression from above the root) paresis is common. A large protrusion affects both components together. Moreover, a protrusion emerging between, say, the fifth lumbar and first sacral root can compress the motor aspect of the lumbar root and the sensory aspect of the sacral root, causing a fifth lumbar motor, and a first sacral sensory, palsy. It is very rare for a third lumbar disc lesion to affect the two roots; at this level, the third root is affected alone. At the fourth and fifth levels, the third and fourth sacral roots may be compressed alone or in combination with the lower lumbar or upper sacral roots.

## Dural Investment of Nerve Roots

The nerve root draws out with it an investment of dura mater that extends, judging by clinical data, for at least 2 cm. The existence of this short sleeve derived from the dura mater was deduced on clinical grounds (Cyriax 1949*b*). The anatomical studies of Frykholm (1951) confirmed its presence and post-mortem specimens were illustrated (Brain 1954) delineating the extent of the dural pouch. Many observers must have been puzzled to note that the fourth and fifth lumbar dermatomes start in the lower thigh; yet the pain of sciatica usually includes the upper thigh and buttock. The pain occupies not only the whole extent of the relevant dermatome, but also a proximal area where, until Sicard and Leca's report (1954), the dermatome was thought to be absent.

Over 200 years ago, Cotugno (1764, 1775) distinguished between pain radiating to the front of the thigh from the hip joint and posterior crural pain stemming from the 'ishiadic' nerve. He pointed out that in posterior nervous sciatica many cases developed semiparalysis and muscle wasting. He viewed the cause of sciatica as 'abundant or acrid fluid in the outer vaginae of the sciatic nerve'. This correct attribution of the root pain to oedema of the dural sheath lacks only the reason for the dropsy. Root compression with consequent paresis was described again by Fontana in 1797.

The sciatic nerve trunk beyond the dural sleeve is insensitive locally, and compression here merely gives rise to distal paraesthesia. It withstands pressure well since only one-tenth of its cross-section consists of conducting fibres; the rest is epineurium.

The fact that the dural sleeve does not extend beyond the vertebral foramen is confirmed by experience during the performance of sinuvertebral block. The needle, just before reaching the posterior aspect of the vertebral body, may brush against the nerve root. This event causes an odd feeling like water trickling down the patient's limb, but no pain. It is thus clear that the dural investment terminates at the edge of the foramen.

This fact elucidates an unusual phenomenon. Rarely, pins and needles with numbness come on without discomfort. In most of these cases, painful sciatica soon supervenes. Such an onset indicates that the protrusion has passed laterally rather than posteriorly and is impinging against the nerve root just beyond the distal extremity of the dural sleeve. If the protrusion enlarges and moves in a posterior direction it reaches the sensitive investment and the expected root pain comes on. Exceptionally, this does not happen, and a painless root palsy appears. This event may be mistaken for 'sciatic neuritis'.

## Sheath and Parenchyma

The nerve roots consist of two parts, sheath and parenchyma, each with a different function.

### Mobility of the Sheath

Each root has an external aspect—the dural sheath—which moves in relation to neighbouring structures. Experiments during laminectomy have shown that the lower two lumbar roots undergo an excursion of about 0.5 cm during straight-leg raising. Restriction of mobility at these two roots limits the range of straight-leg raising, since the sciatic nerve lies behind the hip and knee joints. Restriction of mobility at the third lumbar root limits the range of prone-lying knee flexion, since the femoral nerve lies in front of the hip joint. Moreover, the occurrence of a painful arc on straight-leg raising (Fig. 82) shows that the nerve root moves in relation to the posterior aspect of the joint. A bulge here may form a projection against which the nerve catches; if it is small, the root slips over it, causing momentary pain, after which the rest of the movement further stretching the nerve is painless.

Pain, whether in the back or lower limb, caused by straight-leg raising, is often increased by neck flexion. Now, if a pain brought on by straight-leg raising is aggravated by neck flexion, the tissue whose mobility is impaired must run in a continuous line from the neck to below the knee, passing behind the hip and knee joints. There is only one such structure—the dura mater and its continuation, the sciatic nerve.

In sciatica, the lumbar spine may deviate in a manner calculated to minimize pressure on the sensitive sheath of the nerve root. If a protrusion lies at the axilla of the root, the patient deviates towards the painful side, more so on trunk flexion, thereby avoiding dragging the root against the projection. This deviation is involuntary; the patient is unaware of the way he moves on bending forwards and cannot prevent himself doing so. If the protrusion lies lateral to the nerve root, he preserves the root by deviating away from the painful side. These two antalgic postures were noted by Brissaud in 1890.

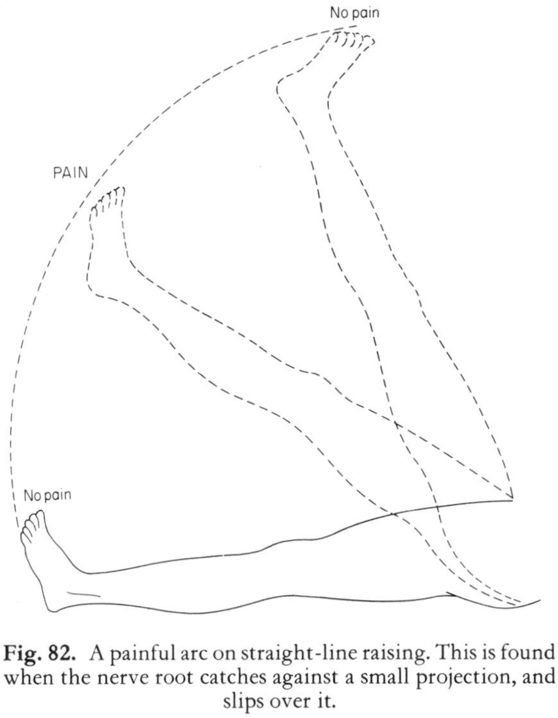


**Fig. 82.** A painful arc on straight-line raising. This is found when the nerve root catches against a small projection, and slips over it.

### Conduction

Each root has an internal aspect—the parenchyma—which serves conduction only; it is not concerned with mobility. Hence, interference with the parenchyma leads to a lower motor neurone lesion. Pressure on the sheath of the root, though painful, may not be great enough to affect conduction as well as mobility; if so, the tests for mobility show interference and for conduction, no interference. Greater pressure impairs both mobility and conduction. Pressure greater still may cause ischaemic root atrophy, whereupon the sheath loses its sensitivity and the protective reflex limiting straight-leg raising ceases. Then the hamstrings no longer contract to protect the nerve root; in consequence, the range of the movement of stretching the nerve becomes of full range at the same time as the palsy becomes complete.

I have never met a case of an isolated sciatic neuritis (apart from neuralgic amyotrophy) at the lower limb, and doubt its existence. Were such a disorder to occur, only the parenchyma would be affected; hence mobility could not be restricted, only conduction.

The fourth sacral root lies centrally in the lumbar region, protected by the posterior longitudinal ligament. It is very seldom compressed by a protruding disc, for this tends to be turned off to one or other side by the strong central resistance. Interference with this root leads to perineal and lower sacral pain, weakness of the bladder and anus, and analgesia and weakness, together with numbness in the saddle area. This root is not stretched during straight-leg raising, and in isolated compression dural and nerve sheath signs are both absent. More often, massive extrusion of disc material compresses the entire cauda equina and severe bilateral sciatica accompanies the fourth sacral root palsy.

## PRACTICAL BEARING

It follows from the matter set out in this chapter that a patient suspected of a lumbar disc lesion must be logically examined on the principles dictated by applied anatomy. Fortunately this is quick and simple. The routine is:

*The Bones*
- Inspection
- Palpation
- Radiography

*The Joints*
- Visible deformity standing still
- Lateral deviation on movement
- Range of movement
- Pain elicited at one or more extremes of movement; where is this felt?
- Painful arc

*Dura Mater*
- Neck flexion alone
- Straight-leg raising
- Neck flexion during stretching of nerve root

*The Nerve Roots*
- Sheath: estimating mobility
- Parenchyma: testing conduction

This examination suffices for the identification of a disc lesion. It does not take account of differential diagnosis, which is dealt with in Chapter 17.

CHAPTER 16

# THE LUMBAR REGION: EXAMINATION

The examination of a patient complaining of backache follows a logical sequence as given below.

## The Patient Walks In

1. Inspection of gait and general appearance as he enters.

## The Patient Sits

2. History.

## The Patient Stands

3. Inspection of the posterior aspect of the trunk and lower limbs. Spinal deformity, pelvic tilt. The position of the thigh and wasting are noted.
4. Asking the patient to point to the level and extent of his pain.
5. Noting the range achieved on each active movement at the lumbar joints.
6. Noting change in range or pain when the examiner aids the lumbar movement.
7. Noting if any movement alters a lumbar deformity.
8. Noting if any movement causes pain and if so where.
9. Noting the presence or absence of a painful arc.
10. Testing the muscles while the joints are held motionless, i.e. the resisted lumbar movements.
11. If any question of a weak calf muscle has arisen, asking the patient to rise on tiptoe first on the good, then on the bad, leg only.

## The Patient Lies Supine

12. Testing the mobility of the dura mater by neck flexion, straight-leg raising and neck flexion during straight-leg raising.
13. Testing the mobility of the dural investment of the fourth lumbar to second sacral nerve roots.
14. Testing conduction along the second to fifth lumbar nerve roots.

## The Patient Lies Prone

15. Testing conduction along the first and second sacral nerve roots.
16. Testing the mobility of the dural sleeve of the third lumbar nerve root.
17. Palpation for lumbar deformity.
18. Carrying out a series of small extension thrusts at each lumbar joint in turn, in order to determine at which level the symptoms are best reproduced. In addition, muscle guarding may be felt at the level of the lesion. Palpation for tenderness yields no useful information except when a fractured transverse process is suspected.
19. Sinuvertebral nerve block. If arthrodesis or a steroid injection is necessary, it is essential to determine at which level the lesion lies. For example, the radiograph may show spondylolisthesis at one level and a very narrowed joint space at the next level. The effect of a sinuvertebral block is then decisive.

## Further Measures

20. Radiography.
21. Sometimes, electromyography.
22. Sometimes, lumbar puncture.
23. Sometimes, myelography or epidurography.
24. Sometimes, discography.
25. Sometimes, exploratory laminectomy.

When the function of every low lumbar structure has been fully tested, the hip joints with the muscles that control them, and the sacroiliac joints, are examined. Occasionally, too, arterial examination is relevant.

Since backache is a common psychogenic symptom, the question of neurosis arises. Interspersed between the relevant observations, therefore, some tests are included to which ordinary patients' responses are uniformly negative. In this way, the examination singles out those who put forward the self-contradictory patterns characterizing pain partly or wholly of emotional origin. It also prevents the reverse error—namely, a mistaken diagnosis of psychogenic pain in an obviously neurotic patient who, nevertheless, happens to have a genuine lesion.

## Preliminary Inspection

Before the history is taken, a glance is given at the overall picture presented by the patient. Does he walk in aided or unaided? How did he travel from his home to hospital? These findings may or may not tally with his account later of the degree of disablement. What is his posture and his gait? As he seats himself, does he do so easily or with the caution that denotes the need to avoid severe twinges? If his seated posture is unexceptional, he must possess 90° range of flexion at hip and knee. A glance at his face gives an idea of how he has been sleeping and how badly the pain is affecting him; how does this compare with his account, perhaps, of severe pain and sleepless nights?

Patients brought in on a stretcher may well be suffering from severe lumbago or chronic osteomyelitis; for sitting is nearly always the most painful position in fourth and fifth lumbar disc lesions (but not at the third level, when the articular signs are often reversed). Arrival in a wheelchair should inspire caution.

# HISTORY

## Lumbar Symptoms

Doctors have a tendency to become impatient with diseases that pass on neither to death nor to recovery. Many are uninterested in disorders that seldom lead to appreciable crippledom and yet run a variable chronic course over which it is difficult to achieve control. Most physicians and nearly all surgeons become bored by the backaches that are daily described to them. In fact, backache is a symptom hard to evaluate, and *all* cases of backache are in essence 'difficult'. Hence, every possible assistance is needed, and a detailed history in chronological sequence is the first stand-by. No effort should be spared to find out what the symptoms have been, and are now; when they started, and what vicissitudes the back has suffered during the years. Where was the pain originally; has it ever spread elsewhere; how did it begin; was it constant or intermittent; has it altered lately; what brings it on; is it affected by posture or rest or exertion? How severe is the pain and what is the degree of disablement? All this must be ascertained.

When the symptom is backache, the following questions are kept in mind:

1. Is this a disc lesion or one of the uncommon causes of backache?
2. If it sounds like a disc lesion, is the protrusion hard or soft, large or small, central or unilateral, stable or unstable? The behaviour of symptoms, as from their first appearance, is highly indicative. Is there any pointer to the level? If a posterolateral protrusion is suggested, is it primary or secondary?

   It must be realized that it is only the history that can suggest the mushroom phenomenon or a nuclear self-reducing herniation.
3. What sort of a person is the patient? Does his account of his pain follow one of the well-known sequences? Do the activities that make the pain better or worse tally with the rest of the story? Do the described degree of pain and his daily activities fit in with his appearance and with the disablement that he outlines?

However simple the case seems, the patient should always be induced to talk about his reaction to his symptoms.

*Time.* This has both diagnostic and medicolegal bearing.

If a patient has had backache for years, progressive, serious disease is ruled out. Only a few disorders give rise to episodic pain, and only intermittent internal derangement repeatedly fixes a joint within its range of movement. Constant displacement of a part of the disc may get neither greater nor smaller for years; there is no limit to how long such a backache may last without recovery or aggravation. By contrast, a month or two of increasing backache, often in an elderly patient, may well signal lumbar metastases. In spondylitis, the pain spreads up the trunk.

A disc is damaged by prolonged wear and tear; it may also suffer in an accident. Should an annular crack be caused by an injury, it may not become complete for a year or two. Once it is complete, many months may elapse before the patient makes the movement that brings about displacement; now, for the first time he becomes aware of his lesion. Hence a gap of weeks, months or years may separate the accident from its eventual, nevertheless direct, result. This long interval between cause and effect involves great medicolegal difficulties and distresses counsel and judge who, naturally, expect guidance on the relevance of injury to a symptom beginning later. In fact, in disc trouble, no theoretical limit exists to the interval between an accident and the onset of pain. Moreover, it is always arguable that the trouble is due to an antecedent injury. Alternatively, years of wear and tear on the disc can cause a fragmentation that becomes clinically noticeable owing to internal derangement at any time during a patient's lifetime. This is *not* the same thing as the suggestion—often put forward by defending counsel—that, since the radiograph shows osteoarthrosis, the plaintiff was bound to get pain sooner or later anyhow.

There is no time limit for backache caused by a disc lesion and histories dating for 20 years are commonplace; 50 years is not unknown. The reason appears to be that, as long as the protrusion remains small and central, it is kept intraarticular by the posterior longitudinal ligament. It thus preserves its synovial nutrition and does not shrink with the passage of time. By contrast, in sciatica, the protrusion passes beyond the edge of the vertebra, outside the joint, and the patient recovers by the protrusion shrivelling.

*Similarity.* When patients relate symptoms caused by a low lumbar disc lesion, the outstanding feature is the similarity of the accounts. Each is describing the effects on himself of events taking place in a closed cavity lying in the midline of the lumbar area. Since pain arises only from pressure exerted alternatively on the dura mater or on a nerve root, there is a limit to the number of different events which can take place. 'All discs are alike, and all other disorders are different' is a sound working rule.

In general, the ache due to disc trouble is increased by exertion, especially lifting, i.e. flexion during increased compression. The patient, even when free from all symptoms, can, if he chooses, bring his pain on by, for example, digging for some time. Merely keeping the lumbar spine in kyphosis by sitting, driving a car or in an armchair, brings on backache relieved by standing up. Turning in bed often occasions a twinge. Avoidance of activity, recumbency, and maintaining the lordosis lessen the backache.

By contrast, the way pain is referred from the back when a lumbar disc lesion is present is very variable, since the dura mater does not obey the rules of segmental reference, and pain spreading up to the scapulae, forward to the lower abdomen and down to the coccyx is as common as the proper segmental reference to the lower limbs.

## Characteristic Histories

By lumbago is meant severe backache coming on suddenly and temporarily fixing the patient.

### Annular Lumbago

The story is typical of internal derangement. The patient states that he bent down; as he came up again he felt a click and was seized with severe lumbar pain, locking him in flexion, less often in side flexion. Heberden (1802) describes the attack as 'sudden cramp in the muscles lasting two or three days making all motion intolerable'. The pain is more often bilateral than unilateral. After some seconds or minutes, he could straighten up but agonizing twinges prevented any but the most cautious movement, and coughing and sneezing were very painful. A rare symptom is a momentary, painless giving-way of both legs, as if all postural sense had ceased in both lower limbs (neurologists describe this phenomenon in other disorders as the 'drop attack'). He retired to bed and the pain gradually eased, until, after some days or weeks, he was symptom-free. He remained so until a year or two later when a similar movement brought on the same train of events. The patient's account is the exact counterpart of internal derangement at the knee; a strain is followed by severe local pain and locking in flexion. A displacement lying at the back of his lumbar joint forces the patient to bend forwards, holding the joint in kyphosis so as to accommodate the protrusion; for, while erect, he squeezes the protrusion still further backwards, increasing the already painful pressure on the dura mater. Gradual reduction during rest in bed, i.e. during relief from the compression inherent in the erect position, follows the attack, but recurrence is very probable. Cartilage, having no blood supply, cannot unite once fractured, and a fragment that has moved once can always move again.

### Nuclear Lumbago

The history in cases of nuclear herniation is equally characteristic. The patient did some heavy work involving much stooping and lifting, e.g. laying a concrete path. After some hours he felt a slight backache but thought little of it.

That evening after sitting for an hour or two in his armchair, the back felt stiff and ached. He slept comfortably, but woke next morning unable to get out of bed because of severe lumbar pain. He stayed in bed for a week or two and recovered. A pain that appears to be brought on by rest in bed and yet abated on further recumbency is puzzling. Sooner or later, he had another attack. This account describes the onset of a displacement slowly increasing in size and first giving rise to symptoms many hours after the maintenance of the causative posture, i.e. a nuclear protrusion. Pulp oozes; cartilage subluxates in an instant. The distinction has an important bearing both on treatment and on the maintenance of reduction. A hard fragment can be manipulated; a soft protrusion recedes most quickly with traction. A patient with a pulpy lesion can safely play tennis again; for, though he bends down, he comes up again instantly and the prolonged flexion that sets up nuclear movement does not come into operation. On the other hand, a patient with a cracked annulus has to be constantly on his guard.

## Combined Lesion

This is no new concept. In 1934 Mixter and Barr found at laminectomy that in 18 consecutive cases the protrusion was of annular material only in 7, nuclear only in 4 and both in 7.

## Backache

A patient who declares that his lumbar pain was central or bilateral at first, but is now unilateral, must have a disc lesion. His statement indicates that the lesion has moved from the centre of the back to one side. In order to move in this way, the lesion must occupy a central cavity; and there is only one such, the intervertebral joint, and the only tissue it contains is the disc itself. The converse does not hold, for a patient with either a disc lesion or ankylosing spondylitis may describe unilateral pain in the buttock later becoming central and lumbar.

Backache which changes sides is more often caused by a fourth than a fifth lumbar disc lesion; an ache in the buttock that alternates suggests sacroiliac arthritis. Rather a similar story is recounted by patients with two low lumbar disc lesions, i.e. at both the fourth and fifth levels.

In very early disc lesions, or in those that remain minor, the characteristic feature is aching dependent on how much the patient exerts his back. This is the cause of the ordinary backache to which almost everyone is subject. Any work involving stooping is followed by pain or occasions sudden twinges; if he takes things quietly, he feels little or nothing. He may experience difficulty in straightening up after bending or in getting up out of an armchair or car (i.e., after the maintenance of kyphosis has allowed some posterior shift of part of the disc). Turning in bed is often mentioned as occasioning a twinge awakening him.

A curious alternation sometimes takes place in long-standing backache caused by a disc lesion. For some or many years the patient wakes comfortable and then gets backache varying in intensity according to what he does: the expected pattern. Eventually, the situation reverses itself and he gets pain waking him in the early hours and easing when he gets up; an occasional patient is encountered who has had to leave his bed for half an hour before dawn for years. He may be able to do quite heavy work by day without discomfort. The second half of this history does not suggest a disc lesion at all, but the first half of the history is characteristic, and the fact remains that the only effective treatment is epidural local anaesthesia. Rarely, a small chronic disc lesion sets up matutinal pain only, but the common cause of backache worst on waking is spondylitis ankylopoetica.

## Compression Phenomena

A different account designates a self-reducing disc lesion. The patient, often in his twenties or thirties, wakes comfortable. After he has been up for some hours, the back begins to ache. This continues, often getting slowly worse as the day wears on. When he goes to bed the pain ceases after an hour or so. Again he wakes comfortable, and it is an essential part of the diagnosis that for the first hour or two up, the patient can bend in every direction and feel nothing, whereas the same movements performed in the afternoon are painful. The mere fact that a backache ceases when the patient is in bed is not evidence of a nuclear self-reducing type of lesion; he must be able to move his back fully and painlessly in every direction for the first hour each morning. The treatment of a nuclear self-reducing disc lesion is restricted; it does not include manipulation, traction, corsetry or recumbency. Sclerosing injections provide the first approach, posterior ramus blocks the second and arthrodesis the third.

The mushroom phenomenon is also the result of compression. The patient is an elderly man, who after standing for 10 or 15 minutes gets backache. Further standing makes it severe, and if circumstances force him to stay upright for longer, bilateral sciatica may be added to the backache. The moment he sits or lies down the pain ceases, never in longer than a minute. This sequence is also described in spondylolisthesis, both with and without a secondary disc lesion, but the patient is then usually much younger. No treatment avails appreciably for the mushroom phenomenon when it causes backache except the prevention of compression by arthrodesis. However, if the main symptom is root pain, this can usually be abolished, certainly for many months on end, by an injection of triamcinolone about the nerve root, using the same technique as for a sinuvertebral block.

## Pain on Coughing and Sneezing

This suggests interference with the dura mater, but is not pathognomic of a disc lesion. A neuroma is very apt to result in pain worse on coughing or sneezing usually felt in the lower limb rather than the back. In active sacroiliac arthritis, a cough raises the intra-abdominal pressure, thus momentarily distracting the sacroiliac joints; hence, a cough hurts in one buttock.

## Consistency

The following facts help to differentiate a nuclear from a cartilaginous displacement. Backache brought on *after* (some hours later or even next day) rather than *during* exertion, suggests slow nuclear oozing. Pain in the back, buttock or lower limb increasingly evoked by sitting and relieved by restoration of the lordosis has the same significance. By contrast, backache coming on as soon as exertion starts suggests an annular lesion. If a click initiates or abolishes symptoms, the fragment is clearly cartilaginous.

## Position

The patient is asked to indicate at what level he felt his pain at the onset, and to state whether it began centrally or to one side of the midline. He must describe any subsequent change in position of his pain and say whether it radiated elsewhere or shifted. Upper lumbar pain—'the forbidden area'—is very seldom the result of a disc lesion, whereas this is the common cause of purely low lumbar symptoms.

If a central pain becomes unilateral, a central lesion has shifted to one side: a possibility only if a loose body occupies a central cavity in which it is free to move to one side. This is just what happens in disc trouble.

Central pain cannot arise from a muscle or a facet joint, in which pain would be unilateral from the first.

Pain at one or other side of the sacrum, later leading to central backache, coming and going irrespective of what the patient does, characterizes spondylitis ankylopoetica. The same significance attaches to diffuse lumbar pain, often worst on waking, that spreads up to thoracic levels in the course of some years.

## Stability

If a heavy worker gets an attack of pain in the back less than once a year, it is clear that the loose fragment of disc is pretty stable. In contrast, pain occurring each few months without any particular exertion implies great instability. Easily successful manipulative reduction also suggests instability and the probability of early recurrence.

Central backache coming and going independent of exertion is most unlikely to be caused by disc trouble, but more probably indicates flare and subsidence in spondylitis ankylopoetica. Recent central backache slowly getting worse suggests spinal neoplasm or tuberculous caries.

## Reducibility

If several weeks' rest in bed are needed before the patient can return to work, he suffers real economic hardship. If a couple of days suffice, his attacks hardly matter. If one manipulation puts him right each time, all he needs is a capable manipulator. However, a displacement insusceptible to manipulation that, untreated, lasts for months or is relieved only after some weeks' traction must be taken seriously and every endeavour made to prevent recurrence.

## Size

Marked articular signs suggest a large protrusion. Fixation of the joint in deformity noticeable to the patient implies a considerable blocking of the joint. If he is fixed flexed by central pain, he is clearly indicating a posterior displacement. If he states that one hip projects, he is describing deviation of the lumbar spine away from the prominent side. Tilt to one side suggests trouble at the fourth, rather than the fifth lumbar level; a fourth lumbar disc lesion is almost a certainty if the deviation varies in direction from one attack to another, or if it alternates from moment to moment. A lateral list implies that the dura mater has to be held to one side or the other of a central projection.

Statement that the foot feels numb, or that it flops when the patient walks or that he finds that he cannot rise on tiptoe, naturally suggests a root palsy; this too is evidence of a large protrusion.

## Neurosis

The patient with emotional trouble which he centres on his back does not really know what he ought to feel; he therefore describes not his symptoms but his degree of suffering. When asked to describe his trouble, he talks of 'it' or of feeling 'so bad', and can give no clear account of where his pain was at first, and is now, how long ago it began, and how it has altered since. Such a patient, if not interrupted, can talk for 20 minutes without mentioning his symptoms at all. He dilates at length on the circumstantial evidence for its reality: his disablement, and the reaction of his family to it, the number of different doctors consulted, diagnoses made and treatment undergone. When asked what took him to all those doctors in the first place, he rarely answers simply 'my backache' but explains that it was his inability to do things, or because his friends, perceiving his suffering, insisted on it.

When the question arises of how his pain has varied during the years, if it has spread and if so where to, what activities or postures make the pain better or worse, he becomes restive and makes it clear that he finds the physician's questions tiresome, irrelevant and displaying inexperience. This contrasts strongly with the patient with organic backache, who is only too pleased at last to have found a physician displaying an interest in his backache; he is only too delighted to give full details.

A genuine minor lesion in a neurotic patient presents a more difficult problem. He knows what to say; but the discrepancy between his symptoms and the degree of disablement, and then with the physical signs, is too great to pass unnoticed. He may be unable to go out or to work; yet he can travel up to hospital alone, walking into the clinic room with an easy gait. It must be remembered, however, that severe neurosis is no bar to the development of acute lumbago. In such a case, of course, the severe pain is balanced by equally marked physical signs.

## Lumbago without Disc Lesion

There are six rare conditions in which a history of lumbago is described and yet internal derangement is not the cause—fracture, spondylitis ankylopoetica, afebrile osteomyelitis, tuberculosis, and tabes.

*Pathological Fracture.* A patient with malignant disease of the lumbar vertebra, senile osteoporosis or, yet more rarely, no predisposing lumbar disorder, may describe sudden lumbar pain on lifting an object, followed by difficulty in straightening up again. Though the history is similar, inspection of the lumbar spine shows the angular kyphos; the radiograph is diagnostic.

*Ankylosing Spondylitis.* When this disease attacks the lumbar spine, the patient can suddenly and painfully sprain the stiffening lumbar joints by lifting something heavy. The attacks simulate lumbago, but the pain may be *upper* lumbar and in any case, by the time these events are described, the range of both side flexion movements at the lumbar spine is visibly impaired.

*Spondylitic Invasion of the Disc.* In the early stage of lumbar involvement by ankylosing spondylitis, post-mortem studies have demonstrated (Bywaters 1968) granulomatous invasion of the disc. This is weakened and becomes slowly replaced by vascular connective tissue. Such softening of the disc can clearly lead to fissures, fragmentation, and in due course, sudden attacks of internal derangement at a time when no clinical limitation of movement is detectable. These bouts result from a disc lesion, the damage to which is secondary to the spondylitic process, not to ordinary wear and tear.

This disorder must be distinguished from a liability to lumbago in a patient who later on happened to develop spondylitis.

*Tuberculosis of the Disc.* This possibility is most deceptive, since it is caused by sudden central protrusion of a disc weakened, not as is usual by trauma or overuse, but by tuberculous disease. This disorder perfectly mimics the history and physical signs of a first attack of lumbago, caused by an uninfected disc, since, after all, it still is at the moment purely a disc lesion. The infection not yet having eroded bone, the radiograph reveals no abnormality and the sedimentation rate may well be normal. Naturally, such a case is bound to be treated at first for lumbago on standard lines, and it is only the lack of response to treatment that leads to radiography repeated later on. One such patient, treated by me by manipulation for a third lumbar disc lesion, remained pain-free for a year afterwards; the first radiograph to show erosion of bone was taken 18 months after the onset.

Naturally, manipulation of a lesion that later proves tuberculous suggests negligence to the patient and could lead to medicolegal difficulties. But it is doubtful if any real harm accrues to the patient with very early caries, even if manipulation should accelerate the invasion of bone. After all, until this becomes visible radiographically, no patient would accept nor doctor initiate the tedious treatment that tuberculosis necessitates. Hence, nothing effective can be done until the disease has reached the same stage either way.

*Chronic Afebrile Osteomyelitis.* The patient is sent up by ambulance as a case of acute lumbago. The story is of some weeks' increasing pain at the centre of the back coming on for no obvious reason. Severe pain stops the patient standing and nothing arouses suspicion at first except that coughing does not hurt; surprising in such an acute case. Examination, however, shows a complete absence of dural signs and epidural local anaesthesia does not abate the pain.

*Calvé's Disease.* While the vertebral body is flattening out (vertebra plana) several weeks' severe backache result, but the patient is a child.

*Tabes.* Lumbago is occasionally mimicked by tabes. Cases occur of lumbar crises instead of gastric crises. The patient suffers periodic attacks of severe lumbar pain without vomiting, for which, on examination, there is no lumbar lesion to account. Absence of tendon reflexes at the lower limbs naturally leads to examination of the reaction of the eyes to light and to the serological tests for syphilis.

## Root Pain

Pain caused by a lumbar disc lesion may be felt in the lower back only. Root pain may supersede or be added to it. Unilateral root pain often occupies one clear dermatome and is then an aid in diagnosis. Whether the lumbar pain disappears or not when the root pain comes on is important in prognosis and treatment.

*Extrasegmental Reference.* In lumbago, the pain may spread up the back of the trunk to the scapulae, anteriorly to the abdomen and groins, down any aspect of the lower limbs, or to the coccyx. This radiation has no bearing on the level of the articular lesion, and is not as severe as the lumbar pain itself. When, as happens occasionally, referred pain only is present, diagnosis becomes difficult, for pain felt down both lower limbs or in one or both groins does not sound much like lumbago. Indeed, when the right groin only is affected, a diagnosis of 'chronic appendicitis' is often made.

There are two difficulties here. First, pain from a low lumbar disc lesion is often felt at the side of the sacrum or in the upper buttock. Yet the upper buttock is covered by skin of first, second and third lumbar derivation, and the lower buttock by skin formed from the first and second sacral segments. Hence, in theory, compression of the fourth and fifth lumbar nerve roots cannot give rise to pain in the upper buttock—exactly where such pain usually begins. It would seem that the uppermost component of the root pain is due to irritation of the edge of the dura mater and forms part of the extrasegmental reference from that tissue. The compression of the adjacent dural sleeve of the nerve root can then be regarded as responsible for correct segmental reference to the distal part of the lower limb. Secondly, pain in the groin can arise in three separate ways. It may provide merely an example of extrasegmental reference, and thus possess no localizing significance. But it may also represent the proximal part of third sacral root pain. If the pain spreads to the groin and along the inner aspect of the thigh to the knee, the third sacral dermatome is fully outlined, but if the pain is in the groin only, the significance is ambiguous. It may also represent correct segmental reference from a lowest thoracic root involvement. These three possibilities have to be assessed separately.

*Dermatomic Reference.* Unilateral root pain is a considerable help in diagnosis, giving a good pointer to which nerve root is at fault. Pins and needles or numbness afford an even better clue, provided the patient can give a clear account of where they are felt.

Pain in the groin suggests third sacral root compression, not first lumbar root pain. The latter is very rare and more apt to make the groin paraesthetic. Third sacral pain travels along the groin and down the inner side of the thigh to the medial aspect of the knee. Pain at the front of the thigh characterizes a second or third lumbar root lesion; if the front of the leg is included the third lumbar root is singled out. In such a case, if the pain is severe, the patient cannot lie flat in bed at night for the first week, but has to sleep sitting in an armchair, thus relaxing the third nerve root. Pain at the outer thigh and leg, crossing to the dorsum and inner aspect of the foot, occurs with fourth and fifth lumbar root lesions. If the big toe is affected alone, either root may be responsible, but if the second and third toes are also involved, it is the fifth root. Sometimes it is the second, third and fourth toes. Pain reaching the outer two toes along the lateral border of the foot indicates that the first sacral root is affected, and pain from buttock to heel characterizes the second sacral root. Pressure on the third sacral root gives rise to pain in the groin, radiating along the inner thigh to the knee, whereas pressure on the fourth sacral root may give rise to perineal pain and weakness of bladder and rectum.

As a rule, when the root pain comes on, the backache ceases; this is to be expected since a protrusion that moves from the centre to one side naturally stops compressing the dura mater at the same moment as it reaches the nerve root. This does not apply when pressure is applied to the fourth sacral nerve root. The determination of this moment is important in assessing the past and future duration of a root pain, since calculation can begin only from the cessation of the lumbar pain and its transference to the lower limb. Backache continuing when the root pain appears can go on indefinitely, especially when the back aches more severely than the limb. In elderly patients the backache seldom disappears when the sciatica comes on, and after the age of 60 no term can be put to a sciatic pain accompanied by some backache.

Primary posterolateral protrusions usually come on slowly in patients aged 20–35. They never impinge on the dura mater at all, hence premonitory backache is absent. The patient describes pain brought on gradually by sitting, felt at the calf, at the back of the knee, or at the posterior aspect of the thigh. After some weeks or months, the entire posterior aspect of one lower limb aches the whole time except in bed; the pain may extend to the buttock in the end. A cough hurts the limb. This history is important, for such protrusions are always irreducible by manipulation.

Numbness is often described; if so, the distal extent enables the dermatome affected to be identified. Some days' or weeks' severe sciatica suddenly abating within a few hours, with the onset of a numb foot, characterizes root atrophy. Some patients complain that the foot and leg feel cold. This is not a misinterpretation of numbness, for Stary (1956) showed by thermometry that the limb is often actually colder than its fellow, presumably as the result of loss of the circulatory pump in those with a weak calf muscle.

Alternating sciatica suggests the sacroiliac arthritis of ankylosing spondylitis; less often it designates a disc lesion at the fourth lumbar level, changing sides. Rarely a disc may develop two protrusions, one at each side of the posterior longitudinal ligament, bilateral root pain resulting. Another cause is two protrusions, one at the fourth and another at the fifth on the other side. Massive extrusion of the whole disc after rupture of the posterior ligament compresses the whole cauda equina: weakness of the bladder and perineal–anal–rectal–sacral numbness then accompany the bilateral root pain. Bilateral sciatica without alternation characterizes spondylolisthesis, the mushroom phenomenon and malignant disease. Pain of similar distribution is described in bilateral osteoarthrosis of the hip, aortic thrombosis, spinal claudication and the lightning pains of tabes.

## Paraesthesia in the Lower Limb

Paraesthesia without root pain can result from diseases like disseminated sclerosis, diabetes or pernicious anaemia. More often (in cases referred to the orthopaedic physician) the cause is pressure on the spinal cord from space-occupying lesions at any cervical or thoracic level, usually central disc protrusions. It is important to remember that such central protrusions may give rise neither to local pain (then or previously) nor to any interference with the mobility at the relevant joint. For example, a doctor with a spastic paresis of both legs for 17 years never had any neckache. He had a full and painless range of movement at his neck, and yet myelography revealed a very large disc protrusion at the sixth cervical level, which was removed. Sometimes a clear sign emerges; one patient complained of pins and needles in his big toe only on bending his head forwards; this was abolished by manipulative reduction carried out at his neck. In other cases of pressure on the spinal cord, suspicion is aroused by the fact that the paraesthesiae are bilateral, yet neither spondylolisthesis nor the mushroom phenomenon is present. Alternatively, they may occupy an area not corresponding to any root or peripheral nerve area. For example, an elderly man whose cervical disc displacement was reduced (with some difficulty) had had neckache for ten years and one year's paraesthesia extending from both patellae to all the toes of each foot—an impossible anatomical distribution for any one pair of nerve roots or nerve trunks. Another patient whose mid-thoracic disc protrusion responded to traction had had 18 months' pins and needles at the inner three toes of one foot, spreading to the same toes of the other foot for the previous three months.

Hence, pins and needles felt in one or both lower limbs without root pain focuses attention on the spinal cord at cervical and thoracic levels rather than any low lumbar lesion (with the exception of spondylolisthesis).

### Pressure Paraesthesia in One Lower Limb

Pins and needles, often with numbness over a lesser area, are apt to accompany root pain when the protrusion compresses the sensory part of the root, by impingement from above. Accurate dermatomic distribution results. The possibilities are:

| | |
|---|---|
| Front of thigh | Second or third lumbar nerve root; pressure on the middle cutaneous or obturator nerve |
| Outer side of thigh | Pressure on lateral cutaneous nerve or genitofemoral nerve at iliac crest |
| Front of leg | Third lumbar nerve root |
| Outer leg | Fourth or fifth lumbar nerve root |
| Big toe | Fourth or fifth lumbar nerve root; saphenous nerve below knee |
| Big and second toes | Fifth lumbar root, tight tibial fascial compartment, loose body in knee, pressure on second digital nerve |
| Big and two adjacent toes | Fifth lumbar root |
| All toes | Compression of peroneal nerve at fibula; combined pressure on fifth lumbar and first sacral root |
| Second toe and sole | Loose body in knee |
| Second, third and fourth toes | Fifth lumbar root |
| Fourth and fifth toes | First sacral root; Morton's metatarsalgia |
| Heel, calf and posterior thigh | Second sacral root |
| Saddle area, anus and scrotum | Fourth sacral root |

### Pressure Paraesthesia in Both Lower Limbs

Spondylolisthesis
Spinal claudication
The mushroom phenomenon
Cervicothoracic disc lesions protruding centrally
Spinal neoplasms, benign or malignant

## EXAMINATION

Nothing is easier than to decide that the patient has a disc lesion. But it is by no means enough to say 'another disc'. This bare statement lacks all the detail essential to the formulation of an accurate prognosis and the prescription of proper treatment. Many relevant questions must first be answered. Is it large or small? Is it in place or out of place? How long has it been displaced? Is it cartilaginous or nuclear or both? In which direction has it moved? At which level does it lie? Is it movable or fixed, stable or unstable? Is it likely to get larger or to recede? Is it dangerously placed? Is it causing severe pain in the trunk or limb? Is there marked lumbar deformity which may become permanent? Is it interfering with a nerve root enough to cause a palsy? If so, is one root compressed or two? In either case, does the palsy matter, and will it eventually recover by vertebral erosion, cartilaginous shrinkage, pressure atrophy or reduction, and, if so, how much longer will that take? Have adhesions formed about the root? Moreover, how stoical or hypersensitive is the patient?

Although the shift from posterocentral to posterolateral is slight anatomically, patient's signs vary in emphasis according to this change in position of the protrusion. In the former case, articular and dural signs predominate. When pain felt in the limb supervenes, the articular signs diminish and may disappear at the same time as the root signs become obvious.

If a patient is examined for a suspected disc lesion at a time when no displacement is present, nothing is found. He must be seen at a time when the symptoms are present, and the diagnosis must be a disorder from which full recovery is possible—not, for example, osteophytosis.

## Inspection

The patient's gait should be noted as he enters the room, together with the way he moves to sit down and the position which he prefers when seated. These important diagnostic aids are lost if the patient is first seen lying in bed at home or in hospital. The patient's face should be scrutinized to assess how badly the pain is affecting him constitutionally. The peaky facies and sunken eyes of ankylosing spondylitis may be seen. However, occasionally spondylitic patients are fat and cheerful, so too much reliance cannot be placed on appearances in this disease.

The patient stands with the whole posterior aspect of the body bared from head to foot. The light should fall from a source behind him, so that unilateral shadows do not give a false idea of the shape of his trunk. The following are noted:

### The Position of the Pelvis

Is it horizontal or oblique? If it is oblique, the legs are not the same length. Seven per cent of normal people have a difference of 1.2 cm or more in the length of the legs. Alternatively, fixed flexion deformity exists at the hip; if so, the knee on that side is held forwards, compared to its fellow; in more obvious cases, the heel is off the ground.

Boards are placed under the foot of the shorter limb until the pelvis becomes horizontal. If the lumbar tilt ceases when the iliac crests are rendered level, it is the result of the short leg. If it remains, the deviation is intrinsically lumbar. If the list to one side is accompanied by a lower thoracic or lumbar rotation deformity, it is unrelated to recent symptoms, representing merely a scoliosis present since adolescence. If there is no rotation, the deviation signifies a lumbar articular lesion.

If the patient has discomfort while standing, or on lumbar flexion or extension, his short leg is raised by a platform under his foot. If this eases or abolishes his pain, he should wear a raised heel indefinitely. The same applies to patients with shortening greater than 1 cm, to those with recurrent lumbago (when the frequency of attacks may be lessened by abolition of the shearing strain on the affected joint), and in those whose shoulders are markedly out of level.

### The Shape of the Lumbothoracic Spine

Is there an angular kyphos? If so, a vertebral body has become wedge-shaped, as the result of tuberculous caries, neoplasm, fracture, localized osteitis deformans or senile osteoporosis; alternatively, gross thinning of two adjacent discs gives rise to this appearance. Does the patient stand upright or is he bent forwards at lumbar spine and hips? This flexed posture is typical of acute lumbago, but is also seen in bilateral arthritis at the hips.

Does he stand evenly on both legs? In sciatic root pain due to a disc lesion or neoplasm of the ilium, the patient may be unable to put the foot on the painful side flat on the floot, and stand with all his weight on the painless limb, resting the other foot on tiptoe.

Is the back unduly flat? If so, is the thoracic kyphosis greater or less than usual? If it is less (i.e. the lumbothoracic column forms a vertical line), the cause is a failure in development, the infantile flatness of the lumbar spine persisting into adult life. This posture leads to a graceful carriage but an enhanced likelihood of disc protrusion. If the thoracic kyphosis is exaggerated, spondylitis ankylopoetica or adolescent osteochondrosis should be suspected in the young and osteitis deformans or senile osteoporosis in the elderly.

Is there an excessive lordosis? If this is compensated by an equally excessive thoracic kyphosis, the postural deformity dates from adolescence. If there is no such compensation, the whole spine lying at a level anterior to the sacrum as the result of an acute localized lordosis, spondylolisthesis is present.

Is the lumbar spine regular? A mid-lumbar shelf in the spinous processes characterizes spondylolisthesis at the fourth lumbar level. The upper spinous processes lie at one level; then a step is seen, the lower two processes projecting level with it. Concealed spondylolisthesis occurs, visible and palpable when the patient stands, but disappearing when the joint is relieved of weight-bearing. Hence, radiography while the patient lies down does not reveal the displacement (Plate XXXVI).

Is there any lateral deviation of the spine? If

so, is it towards or away from the painful side? If the protrusion lies lateral to the nerve root, this is drawn away from the projection and the trunk deviates away from the painful side; if the displacement lies medially, i.e. at the axilla of the root, the patient deviates towards the painful side. When the nerve root is gripped by a protrusion embracing both sides like a nut-cracker, the root cannot move either way and gross limitation of trunk flexion without appreciable deviation results. Gross deviation results from fourth (Plate XV) but very seldom from fifth lumbar disc lesions, on account of the stabilizing effect of the iliolumbar ligaments. Alternating deviation is diagnostic of protrusion at the fourth lumbar level. It indicates that the dura mater slips from one side to the other of a small midline projection; as he is unable to keep it perched on the apex of the protrusion, the patient cannot maintain a vertical posture. Long-standing lateral deviation without rotation occurs in hemivertebra (Plate XXV). The angulation is sudden and often seen to have its apex at an upper lumbar or lower thoracic level. Though itself not a cause of pain, hemivertebra may lead to a disc lesion at the oblique joint, or to such complete erosion of cartilage that bone grinds against bone (as in scoliosis). In either case, symptoms then begin. Tuberculous caries may affect only one side of a vertebral body; if so, an angular lateral deformity arises without rotation.

Is there any rotation? Adolescent or congenital scoliosis is always accompanied by rotation. Hence, lateral deviation accompanied by rotation prominent on the concave side is long-standing and unconnected with a recent disorder; lateral deviation without rotation is recent and relevant. Antalgic postures were described by Brissaud (1890), Remak (1894), Ehret (1899) and Young (1951), and later in the 1954 edition of this book. They were set out afresh by de Sèze in 1955, who pointed out that deviation away from the painful side commonly indicated a fourth rather than a fifth lumbar displacement. He confirmed the description of these three types of deviation: (*a*) towards the painful side; (*b*) away from the painful side; and (*c*) alternating. There exist, however, three further undescribed postural effects of a protruded disc: (*a*) no deviation when the patient stands erect, but marked deviation, usually towards the painful side, on attempted trunk flexion; (*b*) the reverse: deviation standing which disappears towards the extreme of trunk flexion; and (*c*) a momentary deviation at the arc, i.e. when the trunk is flexed halfway (Plate XIV/I). This clinical finding was confirmed by Newman (1968).

Lastly, does the patient's posture conform to the alleged site of pain? Hysterical patients may allege lumbar pain and hold themselves bent sideways; yet the lumbar spine is held vertically, the tilt occurring at the thoracic and cervical spine. This is the reverse of a genuine deformity; if the lumbar spine deviates, correction is maintained by side flexion in the opposite direction at the thoracic joints so that the shoulders are level and the head erect.

## The Level of Pain

The patient is asked to point with one finger to the centre of pain. Care must be exercised against ascribing pain felt at the second or third lumbar levels to a disc lesion. When a disc lesion results in local pain, this is felt on a level with, or just below, the joint affected. Lower thoracic disc lesions are not uncommon and at the twelfth joint often set up pain felt at the first lumbar level. First and second lumbar disc lesions are extremely rare; third lumbar lesions contribute 5% of the total. There thus exists an upper lumbar region about 10 cm wide—'the forbidden area'—where pain is very seldom the result of a disc lesion. Pain in the forbidden area suggests ankylosing spondylitis, neoplasm, caries, aortic thrombosis or reference from a viscus.

## Muscle Wasting

Apart from myopathy and anterior poliomyelitis, wasting of the muscles of the trunk is a rarity. Visible wasting of the muscles of the buttock and posterior thigh occurs in arthritis at the hip and in first and second sacral root palsies. In arthritis of any severity at the hip, the quadriceps muscles waste too. If the buttock on the painful side is the larger, neoplasm deep to the gluteal muscles is probably present.

## Muscle Spasm

If the sacrospinalis muscles are seen to stand out, spasm holding the lumbar spine in lordosis, serious disease is the likelihood. It is, however, remarkable that Gower's (1904) attribution of lumbago to erector muscle spasm ('fibrositis') went unchallenged for 41 years (Cyriax 1945) in view of the flexed posture of such a patient's lumbar spine. Since he stands in kyphosis the trunk in front of its centre of gravity, the sacrospinalis muscles are merely contracting normally to present his toppling further forwards. Were involuntary muscle spasm present, the spine would be fixed in extension.

## Other Signs

If the foot turns a dusky red on standing but blanches on elevation, advanced arteriosclerosis is present, suggesting intermittent claudication as a possible cause of the patient's painful limb. In Sudeck's osteoporosis the dependent ankle and foot are almost black.

The patient's trunk may look compressed from above downwards, as if it had sunk into itself. This appearance suggests osteitis deformans, senile osteoporosis or advanced degeneration of the discs leading to diminished joint spaces at all the lumbar joints.

The recent development of genu varum in an elderly patient suggests osteitis deformans.

## Spinal Movements

It is well to realize that the lumbar movements carried out voluntarily from the erect position are largely passive, not active, in their diagnostic import. Though the patient initiates the movement by muscular force, gravity then comes into play and does the rest. This statement has been confirmed by MacConaill and Basmajian (1969) whose electromyographic studies showed that muscle activity ceased entirely on full trunk flexion, the ligaments then bearing the entire stress. Only if, having bent as far as is comfortable, he is asked to bend a little farther, do the muscles contract again. If differentiation between a muscular and an articular lesion arises, the examiner should test the joint by gently forcing the required movement before repeating it against resistance.

The two questions that testing the lumbar movements helps to answer are: (*a*) Do the lumbar movements evoke or alter the symptoms? (*b*) What is the state of the lumbar joints?

The patient stands and four movements are investigated: extension, two side flexions and flexion. Range is watched and painfulness ascertained. If pain is evoked, the patient is asked when and where it is felt. Since flexion is the movement that most often hurts, it is performed last, lest a persisting ache after this movement obscure the responses to the other movements.

Since lumbago and sciatica are variants of the same disorder, the signs are interchangeable. Occasionally, patients with sciatica are found who adopt the flexed posture of lumbago (Plate XIV/2); in most of these cases, the pain in the limb is intensified by trunk extension, whereas trunk flexion and, later, straight-leg raising prove painless. By contrast, patients with only lumbar pain may show the lumbar deviation, limitation of trunk flexion and of straight-leg raising on one side that are most typical of sciatica. Painless clicking occurring at the lumbar spine on movement shows that a loose fragment of cartilage alters position but not enough to compress a sensitive structure.

*Caution.* Whether spinal movement is limited or not is most difficult to assess, because there is no absolute criterion. Whereas at most normal joints the range of movement is the same in childhood as in old age, this is not so at the lumbar joints. Thus, a young person may bend his trunk sideways until his upper shoulder lies vertically above his lower; the same individual, 40 years later, may well possess only a few degrees of lumbothoracic movement. Yet he may feel no stiffness or discomfort, or indeed have anything the matter with his back at all. Hence, a range that would have been considered grossly pathological during adolescence may be normal in an elderly man. Any estimate of what is, or is not, likely to be pathological limitation of lumbar movements has to take into account the patient's age and habitus. This difficulty in separating the important from the harmless causes of limited lumbar movement is the reason why some doctors insist on a radiograph in every case. This is justified, up to a point, but factors may appear in the history (e.g. pain of many years' standing) or the examination which clearly indicate that the lesion is not, in fact, osseous.

## Extension

This may be limited or of full range, painful or painless. In acute lumbago, extension is lost altogether on account of the block at the back of the joint. Were it limited by muscle spasm, as many authorities maintain, it would be the abdominal and psoas muscles that were contracting, not the sacrospinalis. In fact, no such spasm can be felt to occur at the abdominal wall and flexing the hip joints does not increase the lumbar extension range.

In minor degrees of backache, extension is often painful at full range. Quite a common pattern in unilateral backache is: extension hurts centrally but full flexion hurts at one side of the back. Painful limitation of extension occurs in serious disease of the spine, including spondylitis ankylopoetica. Painless limitation of extension characterizes osteophyte formation. If a disc lesion and osteophyte formation coexist, the extreme of such movement towards extension as is possible often proves painful.

If trunk extension sets up pain felt in the buttock or the lower limb, its origin must be articular, for in this position the lumbar joints are stretched, the sacroiliac joint subjected to a rotation strain and the hip joint is extended, whereas the lumbar and buttock muscles are relaxed. Trunk extension hurting at the front of the thigh occurs in third lumbar disc lesions and arthritis at the hip. When pain in one buttock is brought on by· trunk extension, the question arises whether it is extension of the lumbar or of the hip joint that is responsible; for osteoarthrosis of the hip joint may set up pain felt only at the gluteal extent of the third lumbar dermatome. A stool is put in front of the patient and he puts his foot on it, flexing the thigh. From this position he can extend his lumbar joints keeping the hip flexed. When trunk extension is severely limited by pain shooting down the back of the limb, the outlook for the success of conservative treatment is poor; many such cases require laminectomy. Rarely, when lumbar extension is attempted, it may cease abruptly long before full range is reached, the trunk bouncing forwards with a sharp twinge to the flexed position again. This is the same springy block as occurs when the meniscus is displaced at the knee and designates a buckled end-plate.

## Side Flexion

*All serious diseases of the lumbar spine result in limitation of the range of both side flexion movements.* A practised eye is required, since the range of this movement diminishes with the patient's age. Hence, knowledge of what range an individual of that age and shape ought to possess must be correlated with that actually found present.

Tuberculosis, malignant and benign neoplasm, chronic osteomyelitis, old fractures and spondylitis ankylopoetica all give rise to marked painful limitation of these two movements. Painless limitation of side flexion in an elderly patient denotes osteophyte formation, osteitis deformans or advanced osteoporosis. Limitation of side flexion in one direction only is usually associated with visible lateral deviation the opposite way when the patient stands; it signifies a block lying at one side only of one joint—in other words, a lumbar disc lesion, usually at the fourth level.

One or both side flexion movements may hurt. If each hurts on the side towards which the patient bends, he is clearly squeezing something painfully. This can result only from a lesion placed intra-articularly; for all the other structures on that side of the lumbar region are relaxed in this position. If it hurts on the side away from which he bends, he is stretching both joint and muscle; then, as elsewhere, it is the discovery later that the resisted movement in the opposite direction is painless that incriminates the joint. Alternatively, if extension and side flexion away from the painful side both hurt, the symptoms must arise from the joint since full extension relaxed the sacrospinalis muscle. In patients under 60 years old, when side flexion hurts on the side towards which the patient bends, an attempt at manipulative reduction is much less likely to succeed than when side flexion away from the painful side hurts. If any lumbar movement other than flexion hurts in the lower limb instead of at the lumbar region or upper buttock, manipulation nearly always fails, especially if the patient is less than 60 years old.

A *painful arc* may be felt on side flexion. It takes two forms. The early part of the movement hurts, but at full range the pain has ceased. Alternatively, the patient may complain of pain as his trunk passes the vertical on swinging from side to side. A painful arc is pathognomonic of a disc lesion, for it shows that the dura mater rides over an articular projection, usually at the fourth level.

## Flexion

Flexion is initiated by contraction of the psoas and abdominal muscles; then gravity takes over, aided by gradual relaxation of the sacrospinalis muscles. This finding was confirmed by Flint (1965) who showed by electromyography that the rectus abdominis muscle is active only at the start of trunk flexion. Inman and Saunders' (1942) post-mortem studies showed that the whole spine is 7 cm longer in full flexion than in full extension and this movement stretches the dura mater upwards.

Patients with any serious disease of the lumbar spine flex from the hips, the lumbar spine being fixed in lordosis by spasm of the sacrospinalis muscles. This sign accompanies limitation of side flexion. In patients with considerable kypholordosis, the lumbar spine may stay extended when the patient flexes in what looks like the limitation of severe disease, but if side flexion is of adequate range, this appearance can be disregarded. An occasional patient with lumbago flexes with a rigid back, but this must not be attributed to a disc lesion until radiography has demonstrated that no other disorder is present. A limited capacity to bend forwards without the intense spasm of vertebral disease, means that the patient is prevented from stretching the dura mater or a sciatic nerve root. Thus in central lumbago, pain limits standing trunk flexion and, as a corollary, straight-leg raising often is later found bilaterally limited. This is by no means invariable, since in subacute lumbago trunk flexion standing is often found limited, whereas straight-leg raising is of full range. The difference lies in the degree of protrusion present when the joint is, and is not, compressed by the body weight. This fact has an important medicolegal bearing, for it is *not* an inconsistency when a patient with lumbago cannot bend forwards but is found to possess a full range of straight-leg raising. What he cannot do is to sit up on the couch with his legs extended in front of him; for the body weight is then once more borne by his affected lumbar joint. Only this discrepancy is evidence of ill-faith. When manipulative reduction is carried out in lumbago, full straight-leg raising is often afforded by the first few manoeuvres, whereas it takes considerably more treatment to restore full trunk flexion from the erect position.

In lumbago, neck flexion often hurts in the lumbar region, as this movement stretches the dura mater from above, just as straight-leg raising stretches it from below. Sometimes a pain created by flexing the trunk is, therefore, increased by neck flexion. It might be argued that neck flexion stretches the sacrospinalis muscles as much as it does the dura mater. This is true, but if resisted extension at the neck is tested, it proves painless, thus exculpating the muscle. If, in a patient with lumbar articular signs, neck flexion increases the pain, the articular lesion must be such as to impair the mobility of the dura mater; in other words, a posterior projection exists at the joint.

In unilateral pain, whether in the lower back or the limb, the patient, though he stands upright symmetrically, may be found on flexion to deviate towards or away from the painful side, according to which side of the nerve root the protrusion has passed. By contrast, other patients, who have a lateral tilt at the lumbar spine while standing upright, lose it at the extreme of flexion. This finding implies that accommodation for the block at the posterior aspect of the joint is no longer necessary owing to the increased distance apart of the articular surfaces. An alternating scoliosis may also be seen, the patient deviating one way as he bends down, but coming up deviating the other way. This means that the dura mater has to be held to one or other side of the projection.

Limitation of trunk flexion because of pain felt in the limb posteriorly shows that the patient cannot stretch his sciatic nerve root beyond a certain point. Usually this is associated with pain felt in the lower lumbar region or upper buttock on one or two of the other movements of the lumbar spine. However, usually in primary posterolateral protrusion, limitation of trunk flexion may prove the only sign, the other three lumbar movements being of full range and painless. In such a case the alternation between articular signs and root signs is seen at its clearest.

Pain appearing when full flexion is reached merely implies that some structure is painfully stretched or moved. It is not a muscle, for the ligaments bear all the tension at the extreme of range. In a disc lesion, the mechanism is twofold. First the dura mater lies stretched against the back of the intervertebral joint on full trunk flexion; hence it will be applied more strongly to the projection at the extreme of range. Secondly, when the intervertebral joint is held in kyphosis, its contents tend to be squeezed backwards; hence the projection may increase in size. For this double reason, full flexion nearly always hurts in lumbar disc lesions. If trunk flexion causes central backache, the trouble must lie at the joint or its posterior ligaments. If trunk flexion sets up unilateral pain felt in the buttock, although reference from the lumbar region is the common source, a torsion strain is applied to the sacroiliac joint and the gluteal structures are stretched. Hence these tissues must be examined subsequently; if they prove normal, the pain has a lumbar origin.

## Painful Arc

The patient feels the transient pain at mid-range, and may be seen momentarily to falter at this point. An arc shows itself in two ways. The patient may state that, as he reaches the halfway-down position, a momentary lumbar pain is felt. If this is not felt on the way down, it should be looked for on the way up from trunk flexion, for this is the best means of eliciting the sign. Alternatively, the patient may be seen suddenly to deviate laterally at half flexion, returning to a symmetrical posture as soon as this point is passed, up or down (Plate XIV/1). He is quite unaware of this momentary deviation. Usually pain is felt at the arc; occasionally it is visibly present but devoid of discomfort. A painful arc is usually associated with pain at the extreme of one or other of the lumbar movements, but it can be an isolated finding. While standing, patients can induce the arc by tilting the pelvis to and fro on the lumbar spine rather than by flexing the spine on the pelvis.

A painful arc means that a fragment of disc lies loose in the joint and alters its position at the moment when the tilt of the articular surfaces reverses itself as the lumbar spine passes from lordosis to kyphosis. The pain, but not the visible deviation as the patient bends, is abolished by epidural local anaesthesia; hence, the mechanism must be a jarring of the dura mater via the posterior ligament as the fragment shifts. A painless momentary deviation at half-range implies that the articular surfaces open to ride over a projection within the joint, but that the loose piece does not project enough to interfere with the dura mater.

A painful arc, whether on flexion or, less often, on side flexion, is extremely helpful in diagnosis. It is pathognomonic of a disc lesion. It is a particularly valuable sign (*a*) in young patients with early disc lesions in whom the other lumbar signs are either not distinctive, or capable of more than one interpretation; (*b*) in medicolegal cases when it may be alleged that symptoms are caused by muscular or ligamentous strain (but at half-range no muscle or ligament is on the stretch); (*c*) when neurosis is suspected, since this is a physical sign which, in my experience, occurs only in organic lesions.

## Interpretation

The distinctive finding in low lumbar disc lesions is the partial articular pattern that identifies internal derangement. Part of the joint is blocked, part is free; hence some movements prove painful at their extreme, some not. If there is limitation of range, its degree is unequal in different directions and the capsular pattern does not emerge. The severity of the signs depends on the size of the displacement, but the pattern has the same quality. The situation is the same as in the neck where acute torticollis (the analogue of lumbago) is characterized by gross partial articular signs, whereas in chronic disc lesions causing pain in one scapular area, they are minor, but still possess the same distinctive asymmetry.

The expected pattern is that of a partial joint lesion, and this usually emerges on examination. The pain may be shown to have a lumbar articular provenance, and yet be felt unilaterally. Of the four lumbar movements, only one, two or three may hurt. If they all hurt, as is common in severe lumbago, the pain on one movement may be much greater than on the others. Limitation of movement may be confined to flexion, or to one side flexion movement and not the other. In short, in minor degrees of displacement some movements are slightly blocked and, therefore, painful, but not limited; others are of full range and painless. In major obstruction, although all four movements may hurt, they hurt unequally and some are grossly limited, others not. Such asymmetry may accompany central or unilateral pain, depending on the position of the displacement. Moreover, a painful arc is often present, especially in minor cases. This occurs at a moment when no ligament is on the stretch and is pathognomonic of an interarticular loose body shifting its position when the tilt on the joint surfaces is reversed.

## No Movement Hurts

If no lumbar movement causes any discomfort, there are four possibilities.

*Pain Referred to the Back.* In times past, almost all backache in women was regarded as arising from the pelvic organs. Doctors forgot that men get backache too, just as often. Indeed, Robertson (1924) stated 'surely no surgeon today can believe that simple retroversion of a normal uterus causes backache.' Now, most gynaecologists regard backache of uterine origin as a rarity (Jeffcoate 1969).

Pain referred to the back suggests serious intra-abdominal disease.

*Quiescent Lumbar Disc Lesion.* If no displacement of annulus or nucleus exists at the time that the patient is examined, there are neither symptoms nor signs. A history of past lumbar pain dependent on posture and exertion makes the diagnosis clear.

*Spondylolisthesis.* When spondylolisthesis causes backache without a disc lesion, the lumbar movements are usually found to be painless.

*Bruised Dura or Nerve Root.* The ache in the back or the limb is usually constant, unaltered by any posture or exertion, except that it is often worse at night in bed. Yet the history leaves no doubt that the trouble started with an attack of lumbago or sciatica.

An epidural injection is required diagnostically, and settles the question at once. It is also the treatment of choice, abolishing the persistent bruising of dura mater or nerve root that has led to the continued ache.

## THE PATIENT LIES SUPINE

How the patient moves to get on to the couch should conform with the degree of disablement reported in the history and indicated by the lumbar movements. In suspected malingering, the patient is asked to sit on the edge of the examination couch, then to swing himself round, still sitting up, until his legs lie outstretched before him on the couch. If he sits in this position comfortably, a full range of straight-leg raising exists *while the lumbar joint is supporting the body weight.* It is fair to contrast this finding with the range of trunk flexion already ascertained, and of straight-leg raising as determined later.

The sacroiliac joints are now tested by pressure downwards and outwards on each anterior superior spine of the ilium. The range and painfulness or not of flexion, rotation and, if necessary, abduction and adduction at the hip joints is determined next; the resisted hip movements may require testing for pain or weakness.

Testing the sacroiliac joints, the hip joint and the muscles about it involves eight manoeuvres, none of which normally hurts a patient with minor lumbar trouble, although in acute lumbago almost any movement of the legs hurts the back; if so, the severe lumbar signs present overshadow these minor findings. It is true that full hip flexion both flexes the lumbar spine and pulls slightly on the sciatic nerve roots; it may therefore hurt a little. Medial rotation at the hip may set up discomfort in the buttock in an occasional case of sciatica, again by pulling on the nerve root. This fact was confirmed by Brieg and Troup (1979) who found that the sciatic nerve trunk was stretched up to 1 cm on full medial rotation of the hip in cadavers. However, the resisted hip movements cannot hurt the back in any circumstances. These eight tests therefore possess a dual purpose, partly to ascertain the integrity or not of the tissues under examination, partly to assess the patient's sincerity. If he alleges that all these movements set up or increase his backache, this is gross exaggeration.

## Straight-leg Raising

### Historical Note

Lassègue wrote his book on sciatica in 1864 without mentioning limitation of straight-leg raising, and it was his pupil Forst who drew attention to this sign in 1881 (Romagnoli & Dalmonte 1965). In 1884, de Beurmann showed on a cadaver that straight-leg raising stretched the sciatic nerve trunk. In 1901, Fajersztajn demonstrated on the cadaver that straight-leg raising on the painless side drew the dural tube downwards, thus exerting tension directly on the nerve roots on the affected side. He suggested this was the reason why lifting the painless leg hurt the affected limb. In 1910, Zizina concluded that when crossed straight-leg raising hurt, the lesion must lie in the spinal canal. Yet for years, limited straight-leg raising was misunderstood and was considered the result of spasm of the piriformis muscle squeezing the sciatic nerve trunk. That this was a fallacy should have been evident because: (*a*) when the muscle does contract fully, straight-leg raising does not become limited; (*b*) in sciatica, the thigh does not fix in abduction and lateral rotation as it would in piriformis muscle spasm. Inman and Saunders (1942) were the first to show that straight-leg raising moved the nerve roots. They found that the third root did not move at all, the fourth root very little, but the fifth lumbar and first and second sacral roots were stretched downwards 2 to 5 mm, starting at 15° and reaching a maximum at about 70° range of straight-leg raising. The piriformis theory was finally refuted by Smith and Wright (1958), who, by later pulling on threads placed round the nerve roots at laminectomy, were able to reproduce root pain and limitation of straight-leg raising on the conscious patient.

### Technique

In normal individuals, the range varies from 60 to 120° and, at the extreme, an uncomfortable stretching is always felt at the back of the knee. Straight-leg raising exemplifies the constant length phenomenon which characterizes extra-articular limitation of movement, for the range of flexion at one hip differs from its fellow only when the knee is held in full extension. This proves that the tissue at fault spans at least two joints and runs behind both the hip and knee joints. If neck flexion now increases the pain in the limb, the structure at fault must run up to the neck, spanning another 24 joints. The cause of limitation of straight-leg raising is spasm of the hamstrings; it is an involuntary protective mechanism preserving the dura mater and the lower spinal roots from painful traction analogous to the muscular spasm set up by appendicitis or arthritis. One has only to realize this useful purpose to shudder at the days (not so far in the past) when straight-leg raising was forced under anaesthesia.

Straight-leg raising is limited in meningeal irritation from any cause and is known as Kernig's sign. This merely elicits limitation of straight-leg raising in a different way, by showing that the knee has to flex when the trunk is flexed on the thigh; the order in which the diagnostic movements are performed has merely become reversed. Again, in meningitis, neck flexion soon does more than just hurt; it becomes impossible and in severe cases the neck is fixed extended to spare all tension on the dura mater.

When straight-leg raising is tested, the patient's pelvis must not be allowed to rise off the couch, nor may the pelvis be allowed to rotate forwards, so that what now looks like straight-leg raising is really abduction at the hip joint. The leg is lifted as far as it will go, until muscle tension prevents further movement. Whether the end-feel is abrupt or gradual is noted; in the latter case, an attempt is made to push the limb a little farther. The patient states if pain is produced and, if so, where it is felt. (Throughout this discussion on straight-leg raising, the assumption is made that full flexion at the hip is possible. If it is not, the question of arthritis at the hip joint or the 'sign of the buttock' arises and the considerations set out in this section do not apply.)

The range of straight-leg raising is first estimated on the painless side. In disc lesions, at the extreme range, pain is sometimes felt in the other thigh or buttock on account of tension transmitted via the dura mater, especially if the protrusion lies between dura mater and nerve root at the fourth level. The range on the painful side is noted next. This is nearly always limited in pressure on those roots whose trunk passes behind the hip joint (i.e. the fourth and fifth lumbar and the first and second sacral). The examiner must not mind gently forcing straight-leg raising, as long as this causes only slight pain and the hamstring muscles do not terminate the movement abruptly. Otherwise he will miss a painful arc or those uncommon cases where pain begins at, say, 45° and the leg then goes on up to 90° without increased discomfort.

When the straight limb has been raised to the point where pain just begins, the patient is asked to flex his neck, keeping his trunk still. This often increases the pain by pulling on the other end of the nerve root via the dura mater. It is a useful test, proving that the tissues whose mobility is painfully impaired runs from above the neck to below the back of the knee, and there is only one such structure: the dura mater continuous with the sciatic nerve trunk. Had this diagnostic manoeuvre been carried out regularly, the disputed question of sacroiliac subluxation or a lesion of the facet joint causing sciatica would have been resolved years ago, for by no stretch of the imagination can neck flexion be regarded as altering tension on the sacroiliac of zygo-apophyseal ligaments.

Some clinicians, when the straight leg has been raised as far as it will go, passively dorsiflex the foot. Whether additional pain is produced or not, this does not appear to yield any further information.

## Significance

Straight-leg raising tests the mobility of the dura mater from the fourth lumbar level downwards. It also tests the mobility of the fourth and fifth lumbar nerve roots, and of the intraspinal extent of the first and second sacral nerve roots. It remains a valid test only so long as the dura mater and its investment of the nerve roots retain sensitivity.

*Straight-leg Raising as a Dural Sign.* Just as neck flexion stretches the dura mater from above, so does straight-leg raising stretch it from below. Hence, any hindrance to the normal mobility of the dura mater leads to a corresponding limitation of straight-leg raising. Since the theca lies centrally, it is pulled on equally whichever leg is raised; hence the limitation is usually bilateral when the symptoms are felt in the back. This is indeed the usual finding in severe lumbago, when a large posterocentral bulge touches the dural tube. It is remarkable how gross a limitation of straight-leg raising may result, considering that the excursion of the membrane is only a couple of millimetres. Unilateral lumbago often gives rise to unilateral restriction of straight-leg raising, or to a greater degree of limitation on that side.

The larger the protrusion, the more straight-leg raising is limited. Indeed, in really acute lumbago it may prove impossible to lift either leg off the mattress at all. When the dura mater is compressed via the posterior longitudinal ligament, the range of straight-leg raising varies inversely with the size of the protrusion, and indicates any change in impact by altering instantly. Though the dura mater may have suffered compression for months or even years, and thus be regarded as likely to remain bruised for some time after release, this is not so and straight-leg raising becomes of full range as soon as the pressure ceases. Hence it provides a most useful and delicate criterion during an attempt at manipulative reduction, showing from moment to moment how the displacement is shifting. However, a full range of straight-leg raising is achieved before reduction is complete. Once a displacement has largely receded, it may still cause pain on lumbar movements, tested standing since the joint is now subjected to pressure again, causing renewed bulging. The range of straight-leg raising is an equally sensitive index when reduction by traction is under way, but is not a reliable guide when tested immediately after the session. It must be estimated each day *before* treatment is begun. When reduction is almost complete, a painful arc on straight-leg raising often appears. When reduction by recumbency is in progress, a full range of straight-leg raising suggests that the patient should now start getting up for increasing periods.

Epidural local anaesthesia abolishes the dural symptom (pain on coughing) and the two dural signs (pain on neck flexion and limited straight-leg raising) of lumbago for the duration of the anaesthesia. The protrusion is left unaltered, but it now impinges on a membrane no longer sensitive. After the injection, visible articular signs do not alter and a lateral list, or a momentary deviation at the arc, can still be seen. However, these phenomena are now unaccompanied by any pain.

The absence of dural signs in an apparent case of acute lumbago should make the clinician pause. If the pain in the back is so severe that the patient cannot move out of bed, yet coughing does not hurt, and it is accompanied by a full range of straight-leg raising, afebrile osteomyelitis should be suspected. In cases of doubt the induction of epidural local anaesthesia proves diagnostic, since anaesthesia confined to the outer aspect of the theca has no effect on a lesion in bone.

Rarely, in ankylosing spondylitis straight-leg raising is severely limited on both sides by pain felt in the back. A cough does not hurt and epidural local anaesthesia does not increase the range. Presumably, the dura mater is involved in the spondylitic process. If this is not confined to the outer aspect of the dural membrane, but affects its whole thickness, anaesthesia of the external surface only would be without effect.

*Straight-leg Raising for testing the Mobility of the Dural Sleeve of a Lumbar Nerve Root.* In 1942 Inman and Saunders put needles into the nerve roots of cadavers and showed by radiography that the sciatic nerve roots begin to be drawn downwards only after 15 to 30° upward movement of the straight-leg. The third lumbar root did not shift. This corresponds exactly with clinical findings which show that only the fourth lumbar to second sacral roots are stretched; hence in pressure on the third lumbar or lower two sacral roots, no interference with this mobility is to be expected. The lumbar nerve roots are mobile, though the excursion is slight when they are watched during straight-leg raising while they are exposed at laminectomy. The range was measured by Goddard and Reid (1965) and found to be 1.5 mm for the fourth lumbar root, 3 mm for the fifth lumbar and 4 mm for the first sacral. This may not seem much; yet gross signs result from any hindrance to mobility at the intervertebral foramen. If the root cannot move freely, straight-leg raising on the affected side is usually markedly restricted, neck flexion often increasing the root pain thus provoked. In fourth lumbar disc lesions, straight-leg raising on the unaffected side often hurts in the painful limb; sometimes the limitation is bilateral. This finding designates an axillary protrusion, straight-leg raising on the good side drawing the dura mater and the affected nerve root towards that side, against the prominence lying to the medial aspect of the root. Rarely, straight-leg raising is limited on the painless side only; again this suggests a fourth lumbar protrusion.

In cases without neurological deficit, the degree of restriction of straight-leg raising is proportional to the pressure exerted on the nerve root. The situation is the same as in lumbago, and reduction of the displaced fragment leads to full painless range at once. However, the situation changes when conduction becomes impaired. Now it is the degree of interference with conduction that affords the true criterion of the size of the protrusion. It is a commonplace to see a patient one day with, say, 60° limitation of straight-leg raising without neurological signs. A week later, the same patient may have developed a root palsy, but without any further restriction of straight-leg raising, though the protrusion has clearly got larger. Finally, there is the patient who has developed an ischaemic root palsy; his pain has ceased and his straight-leg raising has returned to full range, yet his protrusion has become maximal. Now, the degree of straight-leg raising has become most misleading. The clinician must, therefore, be aware of this alteration whereby, in large protrusions against the nerve root, the severity of the palsy takes over from straight-leg raising as the criterion of the degree of interference.

A painful arc may appear on straight-leg raising, usually from 45 to 60°, movement above and below being painless. This sign implies that the nerve root catches against the protrusion and slips over it, i.e. it is of small size and localized.

The sciatic nerve trunk can also be stretched enough to transmit added tension to the sciatic nerve roots by medial rotation at the hip. This shows itself in two ways. When the straight-leg has been raised as far as possible, the root pain thus set up can be increased on rotating the hip medially. The patient with considerable limitation of straight-leg raising soon learns that his stride is less stilted if he laterally rotates his hip. He is thus seen to walk with his foot turned out.

*Full Straight-leg Raising in Disc Lesions.* Straight-leg raising is not necessarily limited even in severe sciatica due to a disc lesion, and it must never be assumed that, because straight-leg raising is of full range, a disc protrusion cannot be present. If it so happens that the nerve root emerges a little higher up in the foramen than is usual at the lower two lumbar levels, stretching the nerve root will not bring it into contact with the emergent protrusion, hence straight-leg raising cannot become painful or limited. Some of the most severe and intractable (apart from laminectomy) cases of low lumbar disc protrusions show gross limitation of extension or of side flexion at the lumbar joints, the attempt at either movement being prevented by an access of severe pain in the lower limb. If so, trunk flexion and straight-leg raising may even relieve the ache.

After unsuccessful laminectomy, straight-leg raising may rise to full range, leaving the root pain unabated. In recurrence after successful laminectomy, straight-leg raising may become limited again, but quite often does not.

Straight-leg raising cannot pull directly on the second or third lumbar nerve roots (as was confirmed by Goddard & Reid in 1965); hence, in protrusion at these two levels, straight-leg raising is always of full range. Indeed, the root pain may even be relieved thus, since hip flexion slackens the femoral nerve, thus diminishing tension on these two roots. By contrast, in other instances, the root pain at the front of the thigh is elicited on *full* straight-leg raising by root traction due to the downward pull on the dura mater from the roots below.

Straight-leg raising does not pull on the fourth sacral root, since this root does not reach the lower limb. It is only when massive extrusion of the whole disc has taken place and the whole cauda equina is trapped that bilateral root pain and marked restriction of straight-leg raising supervene on both sides.

In lower thoracic disc lesions, straight-leg raising is always of full range, and only seldom uncomfortable.

In the elderly, who usually suffer backache as well as the root pain, straight-leg raising is seldom limited, though often painful at its extreme, in the minor disc displacements common at that age.

If there is such a condition as isolated 'sciatic neuritis' (I have never met with a case), straight-leg raising cannot become limited, since this would be a primary parenchymatous lesion, not affecting the dural sleeve and hence leaving mobility unimpaired.

Straight-leg raising is not limited, and often not even painful at its extreme, in the ordinary backache that results from a minor low lumbar disc lesion. In these cases, articular signs only are to be expected.

*Inconsistencies in Neurosis.* If the range of straight-leg raising is limited, the range of trunk flexion, standing and of sitting with the legs outstretched must be restricted in equal degree. Inconsistency in this direction is a common finding in psychoneurosis and malingering. The converse does not hold; for many perfectly genuine disc lesions restrict trunk flexion but not straight-leg raising, since in the former case the protrusion is greater owing to the compression strain on the joint. Unless this difference is appreciated, injustice may be done to patients with medicolegal claims. Similar considerations apply to gross lumbar lateral deviation visible when the patient stands but straightening out when he lies prone, or to limitation of trunk extension standing but not lying. As soon as the joint is relieved of the compression of body weight, the pressure of the protrusion against dura mater or nerve root eases, and the signs correspondingly diminish. These phenomena are thus organically determined and must not be thought inconsistencies and evidence of neurosis. By contrast, when the signs are greater when the body weight is *off* the joint, this suggestion indeed arises.

*Limited Straight-leg Raising Without Disc Lesion.* The causes of limitation of straight-leg raising in other than disc lesions are: any intraspinal lesion, e.g. tumour at or below the fourth level, malignant disease or osteomyelitis of the ilium or upper femur, ankylosing spondylitis, fractured sacrum, ischiorectal abscess and haematoma in the hamstring muscles. In all the above conditions affecting the buttock, hip flexion is limited too, hence the 'sign of the buttock'—slight limitation both of straight-leg raising *and* of hip flexion—emerges, and the physician is thereby warned (see Chapter 23).

### Stages of Straight-leg Raising

*Full Painless Straight-leg Raising.* As set out overleaf, a full and painless range of straight-leg raising by no means excludes a lumbar disc protrusion.

*Pain on Full Straight-leg Raising.* Pain evoked at the extreme of range suggests a small protrusion and is common in elderly patients' sciatica and after laminectomy.

*Painful Arc on Straight-leg Raising.* The protrusion is so small that the nerve root merely catches against it and slips over.

*Limited Straight-leg Raising: No Neurological Signs.* This indicates a not very large protrusion. A minor degree of pressure exists close to the intervertebral foramen, interfering with mobility but not conduction.

*Limited Straight-leg Raising: Neurological Signs.* The range of straight-leg raising is largely independent of the degree of parenchymatous involvement; for it measures only the mobility of the dural sleeve of the nerve root. This double finding indicates a great degree of pressure near the intervertebral foramen, enough to have compressed the parenchyma as well as the root sleeve, i.e. to impair conduction as well as mobility.

*Full Straight-leg Raising: Root Palsy.* It may happen that a patient after some hours' or days' severe sciatica reports that his pain suddenly eased and, at the same time, his foot went numb. This indicates root atrophy. The posterolateral disc protrusion becomes maximal and compresses the root so hard that it becomes insensitive from ischaemia. When stretched, no protective reflex is evoked, since the root sleeve is no longer sentient. Hence straight-leg raising reaches full painless range within a few days, at the same time as conduction along the root ceases; in consequence, the full syndrome of muscle-weakness, absent reflex and cutaneous analgesia appears. The patient has become symptomatically better by becoming anatomically worse.

## Tests for Conduction

Conduction must be carefully tested both for diagnosis and to arrive at a proper choice of treatment. The magnitude of parenchymatous involvement must be assessed. The greater the degree of interference with conduction, the greater is the force compressing the nerve root; in other words, the larger the protrusion. It is a safe rule that signs of interference with conduction, apart from minor paraesthesia, mean that an attempt at reduction by manipulation or traction will fail. By contrast, recent limitation of straight-leg raising without neurological deficit is encouraging.

Often a root palsy is incomplete. If the protrusion compresses the upper aspect of the root, a sensory palsy results; if the pressure comes from below, the palsy is motor. Large protrusions compress the whole root and cause both motor and sensory impairment; a full palsy is always present in root ischaemia.

A disc lesion, in general, affects only one nerve root. A protrusion just to one side of the midline tends to compress the root below itself (see Fig. 81, p. 250), whereas a more lateral protrusion catches the root at the same level as itself. Emergence of a disc material at the interval between the fifth lumbar and first sacral root quite often produces a fifth lumbar motor and a first sacral sensory palsy. Owing to the obliquity of the fourth lumbar to second sacral roots, it is possible for two roots to be compressed by one large protrusion. This happens at both the fourth and fifth lumbar levels; hence fourth–fifth lumbar, or a combined fifth lumbar and first sacral palsy can occur. Triple palsies are extremely rare, and so are combined third–fourth palsies; in either case, neoplasm should be suspected. When it compresses the nerve root, the disc protrusion has moved to one side or the other of the posterior ligament; therefore, bilateral weakness of muscle is scarcely ever caused by a disc lesion, although both ankle jerks occasionally disappear in unilateral sciatica.

### Physiotherapist's Duty

It is the duty of the physiotherapist who treats a lumbar (or, for that matter, cervical) disc lesion by an attempt at reduction, to examine root conduction before beginning manipulation or traction, and at intervals during treatment, especially if the patient is not doing well. A patient may be seen on one day and reduction advised; yet by the time treatment begins a few days later, a palsy may have supervened. The physician has no means of discovering this; it is the physiotherapist who must note and report this event, since the change makes attempted reduction futile. It is not uncommon to see patients in whom a lengthy course of treatment has been continued in the presence of the clearest signs that the endeavour is vain.

## Resisted Movements

Resisted flexion of the hip is weak in second or third root palsy. If contraction of the psoas muscle is both weak *and* painful, the physician must remember that he is testing part of the posterior abdominal wall and that neoplasm here, or at the upper lumbar spine itself, is the usual cause of this sign. If so, the foot is usually hot, owing to interference with the sympathetic chain. Painless weakness of the psoas muscle is hardly ever caused by a disc lesion, except as the lesser part of a third root palsy. If, then, this muscle is weak *alone*, serious disease at the second lumbar level must be suspected, e.g. neuroma; if the paresis is bilateral, secondary neoplasm. Secondary deposits at the upper femur also give rise to pain and weakness on resisted flexion at the one hip, but in that case the passive hip movements are restricted and painful.

The muscles controlling the foot are examined next. The tibialis anterior is tested by asking the patient to dorsiflex his foot strongly. Unless the examiner puts all his power into resisting this movement, minor weakness is not detected, since the normal individual's strength far surpasses the examiner's. The tibialis anterior muscle is derived largely from the fourth lumbar segment and is not appreciably weakened in a third or fifth lumbar palsy. The extensor hallucis is tested next; the examiner is stronger than the patient in this instance. It forms part of the fourth and fifth lumbar myotomes. Thus, although weakness of this muscle shows that the protrusion is big enough to have resulted in muscle weakness, it does not help to indicate whether it is the fourth or the fifth root. Eversion of the foot tests the peroneal muscles; normally, these are stronger than any examiner's resistance. They are supplied by the fifth lumbar and first sacral roots; hence weakness here is common to a lesion of either root. If the extensor hallucis muscle is also weak, the fifth lumbar root is at fault; if the calf muscles are weak, the first sacral root is inculpated.

During this examination, other diseases occasionally come to light, e.g. peroneal atrophy. Since the disorder is painless, minor degrees are scarcely noticed by the patient, and the discovery of long-standing bilateral weakness of the tibialis anterior and peroneal muscles may be thought recent and arouse a justified but mistaken suspicion of spinal metastases.

## Sensory Signs

Search is made for cutaneous analgesia. In second lumbar root palsy the cutaneous analgesia occupies the whole of the front of the thigh from groin to patella. If the third lumbar root is involved, this begins at the patella and continues along the front and inner side of the leg to just above the ankle. In fourth lumbar root palsy, the big toe is often analgesic; in a fifth root palsy, the big and two adjacent toes. When the first sacral root is affected, skin sensitivity may be impaired at the outer border of the foot as far as the two smallest toes. A second sacral root palsy may give rise to a numb heel. Disc lesions very seldom give rise to bilateral neurological signs; hence if the paraesthesia is symmetrical, spondylolisthesis or neoplasm should be considered.

The *knee jerk* is sluggish or absent in third lumbar root lesions.

The *plantar reflex* should be tested in any patient who complains of upper lumbar backache, or that the limb drags or feels weak or heavy, or when muscular weakness of an unusual distribution is encountered, particularly bilaterally.

# Arterial Examination

Pulsation should be felt for at the femoral, dorsalis pedis and posterior tibial arteries if intermittent claudication is suspected. In patients with claudication, pulsation is necessarily absent in the arteries at the ankle, but the converse does not hold, pulsation being absent for years without claudication appearing. When the internal iliac artery is blocked alone, the buttock claudicates but the femoral artery pulsates normally. Pitting oedema of one foot suggests venous thrombosis or angioneurotic oedema unless it is accompanied by gross neurological signs, when it usually indicates pelvic malignant disease. Inflamed varices at the ankle, empty and invisible when the patient lies, may cause local heat; if this is found, the ankle should be examined again while the patient stands and the veins show up. In thrombosis of the external iliac artery, the affected leg and foot are cold for many hours after exertion; after a day or two of rest in bed, this difference on the two sides disappears. The tibia may be warm in osteitis deformans. Secondary deposits at the second lumbar level may affect the sympathetic supply, giving rise to a warm foot and markedly increased arterial pulsation at the ankle.

## THE PATIENT LIES PRONE

The calves are inspected anew. Wasting may be visible in a first or second sacral root palsy. Weakness of the calf muscles due to a disc lesion is never extreme enough to be detectable on plantiflexion against resistance, but can be demonstrated by asking the patient to stand tiptoe first on the painless leg then on the painful one.

The ankle jerk is then tested. It becomes unilaterally sluggish or absent in fifth lumbar and first or second sacral root palsy. Once having disappeared, in about half the cases it never returns even years after complete recovery. Hence in recurrent sciatica, its absence implies that the patient has had a root palsy, but not necessarily that any large protrusion exists now. Bilateral absence of the ankle jerk occurs in an occasional case of unilateral sciatica, and rarely the ankle jerk disappears only on the painless side. Both ankle jerks may disappear in spondylolisthesis, tabes, malignant disease and after some years of the mushroom phenomenon. Slow return of the foot after the tendon has been struck and the muscles have contracted suggests hypothyroidism. Not all individuals possess tendon reflexes; bilateral absence of knee and ankle jerks may or may not indicate some generalized disorder but has no significance in, for example, a probable disc lesion.

Weakness of the quadriceps muscles is best tested with the patient prone; the two sides are compared. The patient should be stronger than the examiner. In a third lumbar root palsy, the quadriceps is weakened, in severe cases in conjunction with the psoas muscle. Bilateral weakness occurs in myositis, localized myopathy and spinal neoplasm. Weakness accompanied by increased pain indicates a partial rupture of the quadriceps or a fractured patella.

The state of the hamstring muscles is best demonstrated by asking the patient to flex his knee against resistance (Fig. 83); this time the examiner is stronger than the patient. Weakness of the hamstrings shows that, if a disc protrusion is responsible, the first or second sacral root is compressed, i.e. that the lesion lies at the fifth lumbar level.

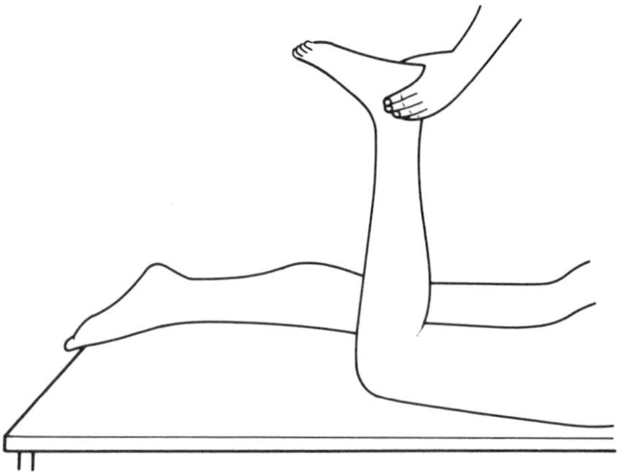

**Fig. 83.** Resisted flexion of the knee. The examiner resists the movement by pressing against the patient's heel.

Weakness of the buttock muscles is seldom demonstrable by testing resisted extension at the hip, but wasting, sometimes gross, is often visible. It is best noted by asking the patient to contract his buttock muscles; the muscles on the normal side stand out prominently; those on the affected side remain flat and can be felt to remain very podgy on palpation. Increase in the size of the affected buttock is found in neoplasm at the ilium or a cold abscess originating from the sacroiliac joint.

### Prone-lying Knee Flexion

This is the test for the sheath of the third lumbar nerve root (Fig. 84; Plate IV/2).

When a patient lies supine, flexion at the knee involves flexing the hip too; hence the quadriceps muscle and femoral nerve are relaxed above in proportion as they are stretched from below. However, when a patient lies prone, the hip remains extended as the knee flexes and the constant-length phenomenon comes into play. In fact, patients with impaired mobility of the third root sleeve can often be seen, while lying prone, to take the tension off the root by raising the pelvis off the couch and flexing the hip. Limitation of prone-lying knee flexion indicates a lesion

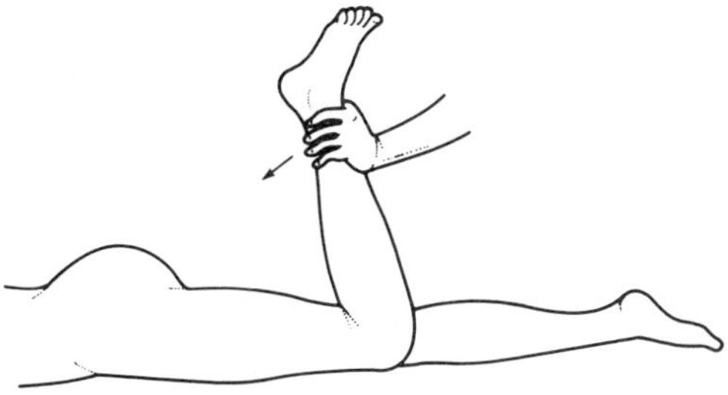

**Fig. 84.** The test for the third lumbar nerve root. The patient lies prone so that the hip remains extended. As the knee is flexed the third lumbar nerve root is stretched via the femoral nerve. In disc protrusion at the third lumbar level, flexion at the knee is unilaterally painful at its extreme, occasionally limited in range. Exceptionally, where a lesion lies at the axilla of the root, full flexion of the knee on the painless side hurts the thigh on the affected side.

connected with the muscles or nerves at the anterior aspect of the thigh. If the quadriceps is neither abnormally adherent to the shaft of the femur (e.g. after fracture of the femoral shaft) nor painful on resisted contraction, the muscle is exculpated and the limiting factor must be the nerve. Prone-lying knee flexion is to the third root what straight-leg raising is to the four roots below. Unfortunately, it is a far less constant sign than straight-leg raising. In most third root lesions, it is painful at full range rather than limited. Since the extreme of this movement is uncomfortable in any individual, the question is the degree of pain: a very much less satisfactory criterion than visible limitation of movement.

If it is limited, the amount of movement obtainable varies according to the size of the protrusion (except in root atrophy) in the same way as does straight-leg raising, and provides the same useful criterion during attempted reduction.

## Palpation

The lumbar spine is palpated for any irregularity of the spinous processes. The physician should run his hand quickly down the central furrow of the spine feeling for any projection that arrests the progress of his fingers. Occasionally, congenital shortening or lengthening of one spinous process leads to unfounded suspicions.

An angular kyphos indicates wedging of a vertebral body or complete loss of two adjacent disc spaces; a shelf indicates spondylolisthesis. In concealed spondylolisthesis the irregularity is visible and palpable as the patient stands, but can no longer be felt when the patient lies down (Plate XXXVI). If an irregularity can be felt erosion of bone in the course of osteoporotic wedging, fracture, tuberculous caries or secondary neoplasm should be suspected. As in all disorders affecting bone, radiography is then essential.

Rupture of a supraspinous ligament causes a palpable gap between the spinous processes, which feel farther apart than their fellows. At operation Bouillet has found this a good criterion for the level of a disc lesion.

Palpation of the tissues overlying the lumbar intervertebral foramina was found by Bihaug (1980) to have prognostic value. He found that pressure there with his thumb, if it provoked pain in the limb, was followed by laminectomy in 51% of 123 patients. If no pain was provoked, 24% needed operation. When the pain was set up in the limb, neurological deficit was more frequent, usually of first sacral provenance.

## The Resisted Lumbar Movements

These should be tested if three possibilities have arisen. (*a*) Was there direct unilateral trauma to the lumbar spine? If so, the last rib or one or more transverse processes may have been injured. These minor fractures show themselves clinically as muscle lesions, giving rise to pain on resisted contraction of the sacrospinalis muscle. (*b*) Is the patient suspected of psychogenic symptoms? If so, comparison of the effect of active, passive and resisted movements may well prove informative. (*c*) Does the examiner believe in sprain of a lumbar muscle? Then the muscles must be tested separately from the joints.

The tests for the sacrospinalis muscles are three: resisted side flexion standing (see p. 206), then prone-lying trunk extension and side-lying trunk side flexion are performed. The patient lies prone and the examiner resists extension by placing one hand at the backs of the knees, the other at the upper thorax posteriorly. The response to this movement may be profitably compared with that to passive extension. To this end, the patient lifts his thorax off the couch by extending his elbows, letting his body sag. Lastly, the patient turns to lie on one side, crosses his arms in front of his chest and, without using his elbow, lifts his thorax off the couch. The physician steadies his thighs during the movement (Fig. 85).

If the resisted movements show that one or more transverse processes have probably been fractured, palpation helps to identify the level. Radiography is clearer still.

One difficulty in interpretation may arise. As was set out in the previous chapter, the first effect

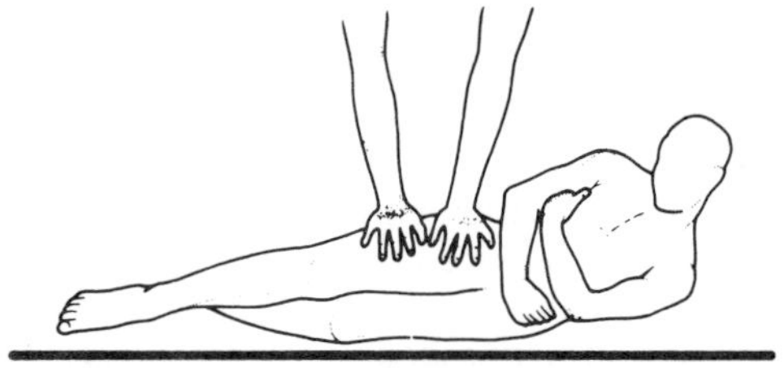

**Fig. 85.** The test for the sacrospinalis muscle. The patient lies on his painless side, his thigh supported by the examiner. He crosses his arms in front of him and lifts his thorax off the couch without using his elbow. This puts a strong strain on one sacrospinalis muscle. This movement is found painful in fracture of a transverse process.

of contraction of the sacrospinalis muscles is to compress the lumbar joints. Hence, resisted extension may hurt even in a disc lesion. However, passive extension relaxes the muscles while straining the joint, hence, it is only the combination of painful resisted extension with painless passive extension that directs attention to the muscle. The sample applies to side flexion.

### Forcing Extension

If examination of the trunk or lower limb fails to show at what level a disc lesion lies, the attempt should be made by oscillatory forcing of extension. As the patient lies prone, a series of pressures towards extension is given, starting at the sacrum and repeated at each lumbar joint. The patient is asked to state at which level the thrusts provoke the greatest discomfort, and the examiner notes at which level muscle guarding is evoked.

Tenderness of a supraspinous ligament is no help, since whatever the level of the disc lesion, the fifth ligament is always the most sensitive. Looking for tenderness of muscle is, of course, quite pointless in an articular lesion.

## DIAGNOSTIC LOCAL ANAESTHESIA

Sometimes the pattern obtained on examination shows merely that the symptoms arise from the moving parts of the back, but whether from a disc lesion or not is uncertain. Alternatively, testing the sacroiliac joint and performing the lumbar movements both hurt, and it is not clear whether the lesion is lumbar or sacroiliac.

In such cases, epidural local anaesthesia should be induced diagnostically. The solution is confined within the neural canal by bone and ligament; it can escape only by the intervertebral foramina (Plate xxxi). Hence it anaesthetizes the dura mater and its investment of each nerve root; it cannot reach the muscles or pass intra-articularly. If the symptoms arise from indirect pressure on the dura mater or a nerve root because of minor diplacement of a fragment of disc, the bulge presses on a surface now rendered insensitive; hence pain ceases for the duration of local anaesthesia. If this simple means of confirming or disproving a diagnosis of an early disc lesion were applied more universally the controversy around the disc *vs* the 'facet syndrome', sacroiliac strain, lumbar muscle or ligament sprain, 'fibrositis' and fatty nodules would be resolved; for this diagnostic infiltration, in a high proportion of cases, causes the pain to disappear for the time being. This implies that the lesion affects the dura mater or nerve root. The facet joints, the muscles and fasciae, together with their fatty denizens, do not lie centrally and cannot in any circumstances compress the dural tube. If the injection does not alter the pain, diagnosis is difficult and the alternative causes of lumbar pain must be considered.

## RADIOGRAPHY

The X-ray photograph has no positive value in disc lesions, since it cannot show the position of cartilage—a radiotranslucent tissue. Its proper use is in differential diagnosis. Since bone disease is rare and nearly all backache arising in the moving parts has an articular origin, it suffices to demonstrate the absence of any bony disorder to draw attention to the joint, in other words, to disc trouble. A diminished joint space shows the disc to be thinned but many discs atrophy as age advances without becoming displaced, and a normal disc space by no means excludes gross displacement of disc material. Even when a disc lesion is clearly present and the radiograph shows a narrow space, laminectomy may reveal that no protrusion exists at the level of the degenerate disc but that the lesion is recent and at an interspace of normal width radiologically. Middle-aged or elderly patients with psychogenic trouble often possess a symptomless diminished joint space, and excessive reliance on radiography then gives unwarranted credence to their allegations. By discography, Collis (1963) showed that 56% of herniations arose at intervertebral spaces of normal thickness, 34% at a narrow space, and 2.7% at a space where posterior spondylolisthesis was visible.

Osteophytes also show, and indicate that the bulging disc has exerted enough ligamentous pull to lift up periosteum. The disc is now cupped in bone. The loose fragment of fibrocartilage is therefore less likely to shift than before, but, as the osteophytes form chiefly laterally and anteriorly, they are not very usefully placed.

Posterior osteophytosis is of course important, if the bony projection becomes large enough to impinge on the dura mater. In fact, such a prominence is rare, and causes intractable backache, though seldom bad enough for the patient to accept laminectomy. Spondylolisthesis is a relevant X-ray finding in bilateral sciatica or paraesthesia in both feet; for the nerve roots may catch against the shelf below. Much more often a disc lesion forms early in the unstable joint and backache or unilateral sciatica in an adolescent often has this cause. Sacralization of the fifth lumbar vertebra is also significant, for immobility of the fifth lumbar joint leaves the fourth with double work to do; hence a disc lesion there is apt to begin in adolescence.

Calcification of the disc has been described in pseudo-gout and can follow haemorrhage into the joint; it is not painful.

## Myelography

When a neuroma is suspected, contrast myelography is obviously indicated, and the investigation is also useful in patients with atypical signs in whom the alternative diagnosis is hysteria. Apart from that, a myelogram is seldom required and need be considered at all only if laminectomy is contemplated. In a straightforward disc lesion causing sciatica, it is unnecessary, since the surgeon will look at both the fourth and fifth lumbar levels in any case. Moreover, if the protrusion has passed well laterally, the dural tube is not indented and it does not show; this happens in about a quarter of all cases. Gurdjian and Thomas's (1970) figures for invisibility are 11.9% at the fourth lumbar level, 23.8% at the fifth. Hence a negative finding does not exclude herniation. Nor for that matter is a positive finding necessarily relevant. Both cervical and lumbar filling defects may be entirely symptomless. Lindblom and Rexed's post-mortem studies (1948) showed large disc protrusions in 17 cases but in only 6 had there been any pain in the back or lower limb. Trowbridge and French (1954) found lumbar myelographic defects in 14 out of 25 patients without symptoms. Hitselberger and Whitten (1968), investigating patients with suspected acoustic tumour, extended their observations to the spinal canal. Even when they excluded all patients with a past history of back troubles, they detected myelographic defects indicating disc abnormality in no less than 37%. This fits in well with McRae's (1956) post-mortem finding of seven symptomless posterior protrusions in 18 individuals. In 109 patients aged over 30 he found 93 with myelographic abnormalities; however, in 46 controls there were 23 with visible deficits. In 20 people aged over 60, all had protrusions, 14 causing symptoms, 6 not. Myelography has a further disadvantage. A defect may be seen at, say, the fourth level, nothing at the fifth. This does not prove that there is no disc protrusion at the fifth level. The surgeon, wrongly reassured by seeing only one defect, removes only the visible protrusion. Reliance on myelography is thus one cause of failed laminectomy.

An important reason for avoiding myelography wherever possible is the irritative effect of all contrast media on the arachnoid membrane. More and more cases are coming to light of intractable pain caused by repeated investigations, especially with pantopaque. The others followed unsuccessful laminectomy. At the symposium held by the International Society for the Study of the Lumbar Spine at Utrecht in 1977, no less than 327 such iatrogenic cases were assembled in five papers. Arachnoiditis is a serious complication, the frequency of which has only lately become recognized. As early as 1973, Shealy warned against repeated myelograms. He reviewed 400 patients, admittedly sent to his Pain Rehabilitation Centre in Wisconsin and thus a selected group, and found 30 with evidence of arachnoiditis. This figure included six who had contrast radiography without subsequent operation. Nowadays some radiologists put a steroid suspension into the theca after a myelogram as a routine precaution against arachnoiditis. Metrizamide is water soluble and is stated to be much less liable to produce arachnoiditis.

A tendency is becoming increasingly manifest to treat the myelogram rather than the patient. Once laminectomy has been decided on on clinical grounds, it is perfectly reasonable, but seldom helpful, to carry out myelography first. If no deficit is seen, the operation is carried out just the same. If a protrusion is seen at, say, the fourth level, this finding does not exclude another at the fifth level, more laterally placed and thus invisible.

It is a major error to let the myelographic appearances dictate whether or not to operate. Laminectomy is called for in severe pain refractory to conservative treatment. It is impossible to see pain on an X-ray photograph, and the degree of patients' symptoms bears no relation to the size of a discogenic defect.

In order to retain a just perspective, the physician must remind himself of the many identical cases judged clinically, that he treated successfully in the era before myelography was so overprescribed and overrated. Certainly, the contrast shadow—positive or negative—has no bearing on the decision to operate or not. But it does exert strong pressure, both for and against, which must be wholly resisted.

## Epidurography

This way of introducing the contrast medium is much to be preferred to intrathecal injection in the diagnosis of disc lesions. For a start it has none of the unpleasant sequelae occurring after myelography. Since it does not call for rest in bed afterwards, it can be used on an out-patient basis. Indeed, Plate XXXI shows an epidurogram carried out by me on a colleague in 1961. He had the injection and immediately walked down to the radiography department to be photographed. In 1962 Luyendijk compared the surgical findings with the reports of myelography and canalography in 35 cases when the two differed. Myelography turned out misleading in every case, canalography in only four cases. Ellis came to the same conclusion (1976), comparing the accuracy in 48 cases. Again, in 35 the interpretations conflicted and operation showed the myelogram to be incorrect in 31 instances, the epidurogram in only four. Indeed, Luyendijk stated (1962) that out of 241 cases canalography afforded insufficient information in only seven. This is very understandable, since the latter outlines the tissues across the entire width of the spinal canal, the contrast medium oozing down the nerve roots (Plate XXXIV). Myelography visualizes merely the central intraspinal area.

## Venography

This can be carried out either via puncture of a vertebral spinous process or by catheterization of the femoral vein. Little additional information is gained and the method has been largely abandoned. The anterior internal iliac veins run symmetrically from the medial aspect of one pedicle to the next, crossing the disc just lateral to each edge of the posterior longitudinal ligament. A protrusion thus compresses this vein and a unilateral defect in the flow is seen on the contrast venogram. The paper by Rettig et al. (1977) contains clear illustrations.

## Jirout's Dynamic Pneumoradiography

Succeeding editions of this book have emphasized that compression of the intervertebral joint increases the signs of interference with joint and with dural mobility. This is most obvious in subacute lumbago when the standing patient is found unable to bend forwards appreciably, but straight-leg raising (though often causing lumbar pain) is of full range. Again, a cough may hurt with the patient standing but not lying. A marked lumbar deviation to one side may cease when the patient lies down. Such findings imply that the displacement—and with it the severity of the signs—protrudes farther during weight-bearing, and somewhat recedes when the joint is relieved of compression strain. My views since 1945, that the symptoms and signs of lumbago result from impingement upon the dura mater, have met resistance, because a myelogram taken during lumbago usually shows no indentation of the dural shadow. Others have maintained that a protruded disc cannot reduce itself.

My deductions from clinical data have been confirmed by Jirout's work in Prague.

*Spinal Compression.* He noted that, at laminectomy, muscle relaxation and relief from weight-bearing sometimes combined to allow a disc protrusion, already demonstrated by myelography, to disappear. He therefore applied a 40 kg longitudinal compression to the patient's spine by means of straps about shoulders and buttocks. After some ten minutes of such compression he was able to see the bulge reappear.

*Pneumo-myelography.* Jirout's method is a highly original piece of research and depends on the fact, first demonstrated by him, that the dura mater has an anteroposterior mobility. He appositely calls the method 'dynamic pneumoradiography'.

With the patient in horizontal position lumbar puncture is performed and 40 ml of spinal fluid withdrawn. The table is then tilted to 30° Trendelenburg position and only 20 ml of air are injected. While the tube is flaccid under such reduced pressure the anterior contour of the air column, i.e. the anterior wall of the dural sac at the level of L4 to S1 vertebrae shifts slightly backwards, so that the width of the anterior epidural space increases. A further injection of 60 ml of air is now given, strongly distending the theca and, in normal individuals, the second radiograph shows that the anterior contour of the air column has shifted anteriorly, the width of the anterior epidural space decreasing by an average of 3 mm. The dural membrane is now strongly applied to the posterior aspect of each vertebral body, outlining each bony concavity and the posterior margin of each disc. In disc protrusion, especially when it projects centrally, this dural movement is present above and below, but absent at the site of the obstacle. Such localized restriction of dural mobility is diagnostic of a space-occupying lesion, nearly always a protruded disc. Furthermore, on the second radiograph, since the projection has pushed the dura mater backwards, this can be seen to have lost its normal curve for several segments above and below. The air shadow shows the tube to run in two straight lines to the apex of the protrusion, where a dural angular kyphos is seen. Since the theca is already under such strong tension, it is not surprising that further stretching is resented—in other words, that in lumbago neck flexion and straight-leg raising cause added pain. Pneumoradiography has thus enabled many disc displacements to be visualized which ordinary contrast myelography failed to reveal. Moreover, he has been able to show the protrusion to be mobile; for longitudinal compression of the lumbar spine increased the bulge; this was demonstrable in half of his 240 cases.

In Jirout's book (1969) radiographs clearly illustrate the increased protrusion caused by compression and the recession when this strain ceases. They also show the dura mater tightly stretched over posterocentral displacements. Since so many regard protruded discs as irreducible, and many others do not consider the dura mater implicated in lumbago, the importance of this objective confirmation of deduction from clinical findings is manifest.

Mathews' (1968) research at St Thomas's Hospital has confirmed this mobility by an alternative method. Using epidural contrast radiography, he has shown the changes before, during and after both traction and manipulation (Plates XXXII and XXXV).

## Discography

*O. Troisier**

This diagnostic method involves introducing radio-opaque oil into the nucleus pulposus. The posterolateral approach avoiding the dura mater is to be preferred; 1 ml of dimer oil suffices and, indeed, an intact disc will not take a larger volume.

When the disc is normal the liquid stays central as a round or bilocular shadow (Plate XXXIII, third disc). Invasion of the annulus via small cracks in its substance demonstrates degeneration. A protrusion can be visualized, usually emerging posteriorly or posterolaterally. At the moment of injection at any one level, lumbar pain is often brought on, but has little localizing significance. By contrast, if the root pain is provoked, the correct level has almost certainly been singled out.

When the results of discography are correlated by the findings at laminectomy later, the correspondence in my cases has proved 80–85%. Sometimes the contrast shadow was not appreciably altered in patients who, at laminectomy, were found to have large protrusions consisting wholly of annulus. Annulograms confirm this fact, thus confirming that disc lesion can be annular, nuclear or mixed.

A review of 197 patients with pain, the back or limb in whom discography was carried out at the third, fourth and fifth lumbar levels yielded the following results:

| | |
|---|---|
| 5 patients all three discs normal | 2.54% |
| 48 patients single disc lesion | 24.36% |
| 97 patients double disc lesion | 49.24% |
| 47 patients triple disc lesion | 23.86% |

In other words, just about half of all patients had two abnormal discs and only one in forty had wholly normal discograms.

In a few instances, the fluid escaped from the intervertebral joint into the epidural space. This indicates a complete annular crack but not necessarily any protrusion. Plate XXXIII shows such an unintended epidurogram, and is of particular interest in outlining the fifth lumbar nerve root. It is easy to see how a protrusion either at the fourth level (at the edge of the posterior ligament) or at the fifth level (impinging more laterally) can compress the fifth root.

Hudgins (1977) found that discography yielded 17% false negative and 22% false positive shadows.

---

*Chef du Service de Médicine Orthopédique, Hôpital Foch. Paris.

CHAPTER 17

# THE LUMBAR REGION: DIFFERENTIAL DIAGNOSIS

An account follows first of the varieties and levels of disc lesions; then of the other conditions that predispose to disc lesions; finally, of disorders causing backache or pain referred to the lower limb unconnected with the intervertebral discs.

## DISC LESIONS

A damaged disc can move in eight different ways at each joint and in each case the displaced material may consist of nucleus, fibrocartilage or both. Protrusion takes place at each of the five levels (though it is rare at the upper two). This amounts to more than a hundred possibilities in lumbar disc lesions alone.

The symptoms and signs that result are summarized below.

### The Eight Ways

#### Gradual Small Posterior Displacement

The symptom is backache, brought on by stooping or lifting, relieved by staying erect or resting, such as almost everyone suffers from occasionally. If the protrusion compresses the dura mater centrally, the pain is central or bilateral. If it lies a little to one side of the midline, the symptoms are felt at one side of the lower back or in the upper buttock.

The signs are *articular* only. There is a full range of movement at the lumbar spine, some extremes hurting, some not; often, a painful arc. Straight-leg raising is of full range and painless. Examination of the lower limbs reveals no abnormality.

#### Swift Large Posterior Displacement

This results in lumbago. The patient is seized with severe pain in the lower back, coming on instantaneously during bending in the case of a cartilaginous displacement, often with a click; alternatively, coming on gradually hours after a period of stooping, and increasing for perhaps a day, when part of the nucleus pulposus protrudes.

There is a constant ache, punctuated by severe twinges on any unguarded movement. The pain may radiate to any part of the lower half of the body, including the abdomen (dural reference). The patient is immobilized in flexion or lateral deviation; he hobbles to bed. A cough and sneeze are agonizing; the dural symptom. The signs are (*a*) *articular* and (*b*) *dural*. The articular signs are fixed deformity at the joint and painful limitation of movement in the asymmetrical manner indicating an intra-articular block. The dural signs are bilateral limitation of straight-leg raising and lumbar pain on full neck flexion.

#### Massive Posterior Protrusion

If the posterior longitudinal ligament ruptures, the whole disc is extruded posteriorly, compressing the entire cauda equina against the anterior aspect of the two laminae. The sciatic nerve roots are then squeezed on each side; in addition, the central component exerts such pressure on the third and fourth sacral roots in the preganglionic position that the bladder may become permanently paralysed. The symptoms are bilateral sciatica and severe lower sacral and perineal pain together with urinary incontinence. The signs are: bilateral limitation of straight-leg raising often with a root palsy on each side; analgesia at the saddle area, perineum and anus; weakness of the bladder and anal sphincter. Dandy's paper depicts the central protrusion very clearly (1929).

## Posterolateral Protrusion

This may be secondary or primary; the former is the commoner.

*Secondary.* The patient suffers a number of attacks of backache or lumbago. This time, just as the pain in the back is passing off, it transfers itself to one aspect of the lower limb, front, outer side, or back, according to the level of the protrusion. In addition to the root pain, pins and needles, numbness and aggravation on coughing may be mentioned.

The signs are now fourfold, relating to the joint, the dura mater, the dural sleeve (mobility) and the parenchyma (conduction). At the fourth and fifth levels they are: limitation of trunk flexion because of pain in the lower limb; one or two of the other lumbar movements may hurt in the lumbogluteal region; nearly always limitation of straight-leg raising; the root pain often increased by neck flexion; sometimes a root palsy. In the elderly, the signs are less obvious. There is then often unilateral backache together with sciatica; the pain does not necessarily leave the back when it appears in the limb, as occurs in the young or middle-aged. Trunk flexion may hurt in the lower limb, but is often of full range; the other lumbar movements hurt in the lumbar region; straight-leg raising is seldom limited, merely painful at full range; evidence of impaired conduction is uncommon.

In third lumbar disc lesions the movements are often reversed, since it is now bending backwards that stretches the nerve root; hence trunk flexion may even relieve the root pain.

*Primary.* A young adult (18–35) develops an ache in the calf or posterior thigh on sitting. This gets slowly worse over a period of weeks or months, eventually spreading to the buttock and foot. There is no backache, and the root pain is seldom really severe. Examination shows limitation of trunk flexion, often with lateral deviation; the other three lumbar movements do not hurt; marked unilateral limitation of straight-leg raising, often with added pain on neck flexion; seldom appreciable signs of impaired conduction at the affected root.

## Anterior Protrusion in the Elderly

*Mushroom Phenomenon.* This compression phenomenon shows itself in two ways: (*a*) as backache with, after a while, discomfort also in both lower limbs and (*b*) as unilateral root pain without backache.

The patient is elderly. Though my youngest to date was 40 at the onset, most are in their sixties, and in unilateral root pain, often over 70. In the end, numbness and pins and needles in the feet may come on if circumstances compel the patient to stand for too long. Since walking includes standing, the patient may complain of pain in the back or limb on walking in a manner resembling intermittent claudication. Alternatively, spinal claudication may be mimicked, especially if the feet readily become paraesthetic. Since the pulses at the ankles are often absent in elderly patients, colour may be lent to a vascular attribution. It suffices to ask if the pain continues if he stands still; if it does, claudication is excluded.

The symptom is pain in the back or in one limb, present only after he has kept upright for, say ten minutes (i.e. standing or walking). If he continues erect, the pain increases and after about 20 minutes he has to sit or lie down. Within two minutes of becoming seated, or a few seconds of lying, all discomfort ceases. This compression phenomenon continues indefinitely, getting gradually worse as the years go by, the pain coming on sooner. If the disorder is mistaken for a fixed disc protrusion and the patient put to bed for some weeks, he remains comfortable while recumbent, but as soon as he gets up, his symptoms return.

The diagnosis is made on the history and the patient's age. Pain felt after standing some while and *at no other time*, coupled with immediate relief on lying or sitting is characteristic. Confirmation is obtained by asking him to stand until his symptom has appeared. He then bends forwards, whereupon his pain ceases. He may have found this fact out for himself, walking with the spine flexed. Further examination reveals nothing; straight-leg raising is not limited and there is no neurological deficit. Only after some years is a toe likely to become lastingly analgesic or an ankle jerk absent.

Anterior protrusion proceeds silently for years. Since there is no sensitive structure lying at the front of the joint, the displacement increases in size without compressing any sentient tissue. As the disc is slowly ground to pieces, the gravel passes forward and bulges out the anterior longitudinal ligament during weight-bearing. Periosteum is raised up by the ligament and two huge osteophytes form. On the radiograph, these two beaks can be seen enclosing a round ball of anteriorly displaced disc substance (Plate XXI);

the disc becomes so narrowed that the vertebral bodies lie in apposition.

The mechanism of eventual pain is as follows: When the patient stands, the rubble of disc fragments exerts centrifugal force in all directions. Since attrition of the disc is complete, the ligaments, once spanning a joint 1 cm wide and now 1 mm wide, are much too long. They are therefore free to bulge abnormally far.

In front and at the sides, this does not matter since there is nothing sensitive to compress; but the posterior component impinges against the dura mater via the ligament and finally also the nerve roots. Bending forward opens the back of the joint and tautens the ligament, whereupon contact between ligament and dura mater or nerve root ceases at once. This disorder has been named the 'mushroom phenomenon' (Cyriax 1950) since it depends on bulging backwards of a lax posterior ligament and is a late result of complete erosion of the disc. However, many patients with such erosion do not (yet) have symptoms; hence radiography can only indicate the level of the compression, once the mushroom phenomenon has been found present on clinical grounds. Radiography is most useful, for the only effective conservative treatment in unilateral root pain is provided by injection of a steroid suspension at the nerve root itself. Central backache calls for arthrodesis. Usually the X-ray appearance provides a good guide to the level.

The mushroom phenomenon must not be mistaken for younger patients' nuclear self-reducing herniation. However bad the pain in the former, lying abolishes it in less than a minute, whereas a self-reducing protrusion may take an hour or longer to return to its bed. Moreover, each morning, whatever a patient does for the first hour or two, he remains pain-free, whereas a night's rest does not alter the timing of a compression pain.

If a young patient gives a history of backache followed by bilateral sciatica brought on by standing spondylolisthesis is the probable cause.

## Anterior Protrusion in Adolescents

*Osteochondrosis.* Between the ages of 14 and 18, the nucleus pulposus may burrow forwards between the cartilaginous end-plate and the bone of the vertebral body, which suffers pressure erosion. If the protrusion reaches the anterior longitudinal ligament, a small triangle of bone may be separated at the anterior corner of the vertebral body, which enlarges anteroposteriorly. After osteochondrosis at a lower cervical level, the body may occasionally be seen on the lateral radiograph to be almost double the normal length. The phenomenon is common at lower cervical, mid and lower thoracic, and upper lumbar levels (Plate XVIII). Since excessive weight-bearing might well be supposed to help drive the nucleus pulposus into the bone. Wassman (1951) investigated the incidence of this type of anterior protrusion in the thoracic spine of young recruits. He found it eight times more common in those from the country than from a town.

The disorder causes no symptoms and requires no treatment unless, as a result of the kyphotic posture of the joint consequence upon the vertebral wedging, posterior protrusion of disc substance has begun. Manipulative reduction, which has to be repeated often at first, is then required.

## Vertical Protrusion

This beneficent protrusion occurs, unfortunately, at the very lumbar levels where it is least wanted. It is not uncommon at the upper lumbar and lower thoracic levels; it is rare at the lower two lumbar joints at which it would be welcome.

There are two varieties:

*Schmorl's Node.* The vertebra provides the only situation where articular cartilage rests on trabeculae of cancellous bone rather than thick subchondral bone. During weight-bearing, the nucleus impinges against the articular cartilage of the vertebral body; this finally gives way and nuclear material invades the cancellous bone. This fixes the nucleus and diminishes the intra-articular centrifugal force, thus rendering posterior herniation less probable. No pain whatever is felt during this slow erosion of bone, but the radiograph shows clearly the irregularity of the joint-line. The node is first seen at the age of 17. The X-ray appearances do not alter appreciably later. There is no increased frequency as age advances; vertical herniation is a purely adolescent phenomenon. Post-mortem studies by Hilton et al. (1976) showed nodes in 76% of ordinary individuals, predominantly at the tenth thoracic level and progressively less frequent down to the fifth level. Nachemson (1960) states that, after experimental fractures of the vertebrae, part of the nucleus pulposus may be forced through the end-plate. This diminishes the compressive stress within the disc, i.e. increased vertical and diminished tangential strain on the annulus. This eases the centrifugal force, as is shown by the fact that Schmorl's nodes are commonest at the upper levels where disc protrusions are the least likely.

*Biconvex Disc.* This phenomenon indicates softening of bone, and indicates past rickets, osteomalacia or senile osteoporosis. Normal pressure by the disc on soft bone results in a smooth curve at many adjacent bodies. These biconvexities are well shown on Beadle's (1931) microscopic sections, and the radiograph reveals that the causative force has been exerted diffusely so as to produce regular concavity at each surface of the affected vertebral bodies.

## Circular Protrusion

During compression, a damaged disc may widen and bulge all the way round the joint. Outward pressure on the ligaments pulls on the periosteum and lifts it off the bone. Bone grows till it meets its limiting membrane once more; hence osteophytes form. These bony outcrops are often large anteriorly and laterally, but slight or absent posteriorly; they cup the front and sides of the damaged disc and diminish the likelihood of displacement, but would clearly do so more efficiently if the posterior component were more marked. Moreover, they limit spinal mobility, and thus hinder the very movements that would otherwise have led the fragment of disc to move out of position again.

Osteophyte formation is a beneficent phenomenon, and is the chief reason why elderly patients seldom suffer lumbar pain.

# Disc Lesions at Each Level

Clear indication of which nerve root is pinched is afforded by electromyography (Wynn-Parry 1980). When fibrillation is detected at a particular part of the sacrospinalis muscle the level becomes clear.

Troisier (1962) analysed 182 cases of lumbar root palsy due to disc lesions. The muscles affected were: psoas 6; quadriceps 7; tibialis anterior 19; extensor hallucis 45; extensor digitorum 40; peronei 37; calf 18; hamstring 16; gluteus medius 12.

## First and Second Lumbar Roots

*Frequency.* Though radiological evidence of a narrowed joint space and/or osteophytosis is common in elderly patients at the first and second lumbar levels, disc lesions here causing symptoms are very rare. Semmes (1964) found only one first lumbar protrusion and only two at the second lumbar level in 1500 consecutive laminectomies. Collis's discography (1963), Armstrong's (1950), O'Connell's (1951), Aronson and Dunsmore's (1963) and Gurdjian and Thomas's (1970) findings on upwards of a thousand cases each are set out below:

| Collis | | Armstrong | O'Connell | Aronson and Dunsmore | Gurdjian and Thomas |
|---|---|---|---|---|---|
| L1 | 0 | 2.1% (L1–L3) | 1.6% (L1–L3) | 0.29% | 0.09% |
| L2 | 1 | | | 1.46% | 0.30% |
| L3 | 44 | | | 3.72% | 2.80% |

The reason why root pressure is so seldom encountered at these two joints is anatomical. The roots emerge high up in the intervertebral foramen, and have passed too far laterally for a disc protrusion low in the foramen to reach them. Disc lesions at the upper two joints behave quite differently from those at the other three levels. They are nearly always of the nuclear type, the symptoms gradually appearing when a certain posture has been maintained, and ceasing when the patient alters his position. Except when they are secondary to a lower lumbar arthrodesis, they seldom respond to manipulation, but often do well on traction.

*First Lumbar Root.* The patient complains of pain in the back radiating to the region above the trochanter and to the groin. Since this is a commonplace in low lumbar disc lesions, not only as a result of extrasegmental dural reference but also in pressure on the third sacral root, at first no suspicion of the unusual level is aroused. However, the patient may complain that if he maintains the posture that causes the pain in the groin, he develops numbness there, but I have yet to meet paraesthesia in the outer buttock, where the greater part of the first lumbar dermatome lies.

Examination shows that the patient points to the upper lumbar 'forbidden area' as the site of pain. The lumbar movements set up lumbar pain in the ordinary way, but it is felt in the upper lumbar region. Examination of the nervous system reveals no muscle weakness or alteration in reflexes, but cutaneous analgesia may be detectable at and just below the inner half of the inguinal ligament.

I have made this diagnosis only a few times (Plate XIX shows the radiological appearances in one such case). Since the diagnosis was made before the X-ray picture was available, and the two correspond well, it seems to have been correct.

*Second Lumbar Root.* The symptoms come and go according to compression. Standing for some time causes pain in the back radiating to the front of the thigh as far as the knee; sitting down abolishes it, or vice versa. In disc lesions this may go on for years without change.

The lumbar pain is at an upper level; the lumbar movements hurt locally in the expected way. The root signs are weakness of the psoas and cutaneous analgesia from groin to patella. Whereas weakness of the psoas muscle as part of a third lumbar root palsy is not a sign of serious disease, an isolated second root palsy is seldom the result of a disc protrusion. Especially if it is bilateral, spinal metastases should be considered. However, I have seen one case of a patient fixed in flexion by severe pain felt only at the front of one thigh. Any effort to straighten up or to walk was impossible, and she had been confined to her room for six months; during this time her condition had not altered. Manipulative reduction failed; sustained traction succeeded, and this elderly lady has now remained well for several years. Surprisingly, traction was also most successful in a case in which the psoas muscle was weak.

Only one of my cases of second lumbar disc lesion came to laminectomy. The patient was 46 years old and complained of anterior pain in the right thigh on lifting for four years. After two years he had noticed pins and needles in the right knee at night. His symptoms had been regarded as psychogenic. Examination showed a gross deviation of the lumbar spine to the left and trunk extension hurt in the thigh. Provisional diagnosis was a neuroma at the second lumbar level and myelography suggested the same. At operation, however, a second lumbar disc protrusion was disclosed. In a very similar case, a neuroma was present.

The common cause of upper lumbar disc lesions is arthrodesis at a low lumbar level. Some years after the operation, the joints above the fusion, which have been over-used owing to the immobility below, develop disc trouble. Less common causes for upper lumbar disc lesions are fracture of a vertebral body or osteochondrosis, each with coincident damage to the discs, either occurring at the time of the accident or resulting from the kyphotic posture of the joint secondary to the wedged body. Secondary malignant deposits favour the upper rather than the lower lumbar spine; here, they cause a gross limitation of lumbar spinal movements, together with such weakness of the psoas muscle (often both) that the patient may be seen to lift his thigh with his hands when he wants to shift his leg in bed. Lymphadenomatous invasion is a rarity. Meralgia paraesthetica must be considered, but the analgesic area occupies the outer aspect of the thigh, and posture, coughing and the lumbar movements do not affect the pain when the lateral cutaneous nerve of the thigh is at fault.

## Third Lumbar Root

Some 4–8% of all lumbar disc lesions affect this joint; the figures vary considerably. In 1500 laminectomies, Semmes (1964) found a protrusion at the third lumbar level in only 2%, but this merely implies that third lumbar disc protrusions very seldom require laminectomy (which is, in fact, my experience). In 88 cases of root pain in the lower limb, 7 had a third lumbar root palsy (Cyriax 1965) and Troisier (1960) found 7 of 182 cases of root weakness to be third lumbar. Collis (1963) found that 44 of 1014 patients submitted to discography had a lesion at the third level. Gurdjian and Thomas's (1970) operative figures are lower, since third lumbar lesions seldom require laminectomy—2.8%. In 2% of their cases a protrusion was found at both the third and the fourth levels. In 44 cases studied by myelography by Masif (1975) four out of 144 defects were seen at the third level.

The early symptoms are usually felt in the mid-lumbar region. The root pain occupies the upper buttock, the whole front thigh and knee, spreading down the front of the inner side of the knee to just above the ankle and, for the first few nights, the patient may have to try to sleep sitting in a chair (so as to relax the root). Numbness may be mentioned at the inner knee or anterior leg. The lumbar movements hurt the back in the expected way, but since the third root is stretched on trunk extension and relaxed on flexion, the usual effect of these movements is reversed. Trunk extension usually hurts in the anterior thigh. Flexion is of full range; though sometimes painful, it may be stated to relieve the pain; such patients sleep with their knees bent up towards the thorax. The full root syndrome is: weakness of the psoas, weakness of the quadriceps; sluggishness or absence of the knee jerk; pain at the front of the thigh on full straight-leg raising;

limitation of prone-lying knee flexion; cutaneous analgesia extending from the patella along the front or inner aspect of the leg to just above the ankle.

## Fourth Lumbar Root

About four-sevenths of all disc lesions occur at the fourth lumbar joint. Collis (1963) states that they comprised 42% and fifth lumbar 37% of his patients undergoing discography. At operation, Gurdjian and Thomas (1970) found 42.4% of protruded discs at the fourth level, 32.3% at the fifth, and 15.6% at both, but O'Connell (1951) found the opposite—fifth lumbar 49.6%, fourth 39.6% and double 9.2%.

The patient points to the mid-lumbar area or the iliac crest as the level of his lumbar pain. When root pain supervenes, it occupies the inner quadrant of the buttock, the outer aspect of the thigh and leg, and, crossing over the dorsum of the foot, it reaches the big toe, which often tingles.

Marked lateral deviation, consistent or alternating, characterizes fourth lumbar disc lesions, and, in such cases, gross limitation of one side flexion movement is to be expected. In less severe cases, a painful arc on side flexion is often experienced. The full root syndrome is: limitation of straight-leg raising, often bilateral, the pain in the limb being further increased by neck flexion; weakness of the tibialis anterior and extensor hallucis muscles; cutaneous analgesia at the outer part of the lower leg and the big toe. Neither the knee nor the ankle jerk is affected. In 88 cases seen by me with root paresis, the tibialis anterior was weak in 12.

## Fifth Lumbar Root

About three-sevenths of all lumbar disc lesions occur at the fifth joint, but disc protrusions at either the fourth or the fifth level may equally compress the fifth root. A protrusion just off centre at the fourth level catches the fifth root, whereas one lying more laterally impinges on the fourth. Hence the discovery of a fourth root palsy indicates a fourth lumbar protrusion, and of a first sacral palsy a fifth lumbar protrusion. However, the discovery of a fifth lumbar palsy has an equivocal significance and it is by noting the presence or absence of lumbar deviation and pain on crossed-leg raising that the probable level is selected. As the patient stands, the lumbar spine may be seen to deviate towards or away from the painful side. An attempt at trunk flexion may increase the deviation, leave it unaltered or abolish it. Alternatively, the patient may stand with his lumbar spine vertical, but deviate when he bends forwards.

The lumbar movements hurt in the expected way. The full root-syndrome is: unilateral limitation of straight-leg raising, with increase in root pain on neck flexion, weakness of the extensor hallucis, peroneal and gluteus medius muscles, cutaneous analgesia at the outer leg and inner three toes; sluggish or absent ankle jerk. Occasionally, a protrusion may compress the inferior aspect of the fifth lumbar root and the superior aspect of the first sacral root. In this event, weakness of the extensor hallucis and peroneal muscles is accompanied by paraesthesia at the outer border of the foot and fourth and fifth toes.

## First, Second and Third Sacral Roots

The first and second sacral roots can be compressed by a fifth lumbar disc protrusion. Straight-leg raising is limited. The calf and hamstring muscles are weak; when the first sacral root is compressed the peronei are also weak. Though weakness of hip extension cannot be demonstrated, the gluteal mass is markedly wasted, and the patient cannot contract it. The outer two toes, the outer foot and the outer leg as far as the lateral aspect of the knee are analgesic.

In second sacral root palsy, the signs are the same except that the peroneal muscles escape and the cutaneous analgesia ends at the heel.

In third sacral root pain, no palsy is detectable. The patient has pain in the groin running down the inner aspect of the thigh to the knee. Straight-leg raising is not limited and no muscular weakness occurs. Although the bladder is innervated also from the second and third sacral roots—the main supply is from the fourth—it is not my experience that the bladder or rectum is affected in second or third sacral root syndromes.

## Fourth Sacral Root

The twinges that are felt in the back in lumbago may be experienced deeply in the lower sacral area, and the patient may attribute his pain to rectal spasm. When this happens, the pain of proctalgia fugax is simulated. I regard this event as an example of extrasegmental dural reference. The same misleading reference may well lead to pain felt at the lower sacrum or coccyx, but again this is not evidence of pressure of the fourth sacral root. This sets up pain felt to reach the penis, vagina, perineum or testicles (one or both), often with paraesthesia. Hence pain in the perineum or genitals, weakness of the bladder or rectum, pins and needles felt in the saddle area, scrotum or vagina, analgesia of the anus, or impotence—all indicate that the fourth sacral root is compressed. This is serious. It is important in this connection to establish whether a patient's frequency of micturition is caused by such weakness of the bladder that he cannot hold his water, or by a strong urge. If the latter, the fourth sacral root is not at fault. In all cases of lumbago, the state of vesical function or presence of perineal paraesthesia must be ascertained, since the impact of a disc on the fourth sacral root occurs at the preganglionic extent and may therefore set up an irrecoverable palsy.

Since it is central protrusion that endangers the fourth sacral root, the pain is felt all over the sacrum and in an isolated palsy does not radiate to the lower limbs. Nothing, therefore, arouses suspicion until the patient mentions that during his attacks of lumbago he has difficulty in passing, or retaining, urine, or he gets pins and needles in his scrotum, or his saddle area feels numb or his rectum lacks expulsive power. These symptoms suggest a considerable bulging of the posterior longitudinal ligament; indeed, it may be on the point of rupture. By contrast, the signs may be very slight and the discrepancy between the severe pain and the minor signs may suggest that the patient is exaggerating. Examination reveals rather minor articular signs indistinguishable from those of ordinary cases of unimportant lumbago. In lumbago straight-leg raising may be limited as a coincident dural phenomenon, but the fourth sacral root is not stretched by this test; hence it is often of full range and painless. It is therefore a full history rather than the examination which inspires caution.

Bilateral sciatica suggests that the fourth sacral root is menaced, particularly if the second or third sacral roots are affected on each side. This event shows that the posterior ligament is being subjected to pressure from both sides, and may well have become overstretched, then torn at each side; finally, the central strands rupture. When this occurs, massive sequestration of disc substance—sometimes the entire disc—forces the cauda equina backwards against the laminae. Severe backache forcing the patient into flexion and bilateral sciatica then appear at the same time as the fourth sacral palsy becomes manifest. Now straight-leg raising becomes bilaterally limited, neurological signs appear in both limbs and the situation becomes obvious. In Jennett's 25 cases (1956) of discogenic paralysis of the bladder, 14 began with bilateral sciatica.

Pressure on the fourth sacral root is exerted at a level proximal to the posterior ganglion and permanent paralysis of the bladder function can ensue. So far, I have encountered 12 cases, in all of which a laminectomy was performed within 24 hours; all recovered bladder function. Jennett (1956), reviewing 1000 cases of laminectomy, of which 25 were for paralysis of the bladder, noted that operation some months later cured only four. Matheson (1960) mentions four cases, two coming on immediately after manipulation under anaesthesia; and one of my patients developed severe bilateral sciatica and vesical paralysis with retention some hours after manipulation by an osteopath. She had been seen the day before when she requested manipulation, but was refused because the fourth sacral root was in danger. Richard (1967) and Hooper (1973) each describe one instance, both brought on by chiropractors. In Richard's case, laminectomy after a week restored power to the anus and both legs and, by eighteen months later, the only residue was a numb thigh and slight diminution of vesical sensation. O'Laoire et al. (1981) analysed 29 cases of sphincter disturbance secondary to central disc protrusion (L3:3, L4:14; L5:12). Laminectomy cured 18 patients though this was delayed for two months in two of the cases. Fair results were obtained in 6 cases. Five operations proved failures, though in 2 cases the interval between starting the sphincter weakness and the operation was only two and four days.

*Any suggestion that the fourth sacral root is menaced by a disc protrusion provides an absolute bar to manipulation* by any method, and even traction is not wholly safe. Bilateral sciatica especially with third sacral root pain, should make one cautious about manipulation except in patients over 60. Once a fourth sacral paresis has begun, however slightly, laminectomy is indicated. Even if bladder function is returning as the sacral numbness is wearing off, this remains the correct treatment, for there is no guarantee that lasting incontinence may not follow the next attack of lumbago.

Those anxious to deprecate spinal manipulation emphasize the danger of permanent urinary incontinence, as the result of pressure on the fourth sacral root. Those who do not wish to investigate the effects of manipulation, excuse their neglect by sheltering behind this remote (and avoidable) contingency. When manipulation is carried out without anaesthesia and with the safeguards recommended here, such a catastrophe has never yet occurred in the practice of myself and of the thousand physiotherapy students whom I have taught. Even if it did, the situation can still be reversed by immediate laminectomy. Penny (1888) in his lecture 'On Bone-setting' puts it in a nutshell: 'We should not, for a very remote danger of bad consequences condemn a large number of patients to a lifelong suffering.'

Three interesting, perhaps unique cases, are recorded:

The patient began lumbago at the age of 32. Aged 40, while standing, she felt a sudden click in her perineum. Instantly her left labium went numb, together with a small area to the left of the anus. This analgesia had persisted unchanged when she was seen 13 years later. From the moment of the click she lost her libido, which never returned. There was neither dyspareunia nor bladder weakness.

A medical man, aged 23, fell heavily on to his buttocks and hurt his back severely. It ached for a week and intermittently after that. A year later, numbness appeared on the left at the medial aspect of the lower buttock and the uppermost 3 inches of the inner thigh. The left side of his penis and scrotum became analgesic; when erect, his penis deviated to the left. Libido was little affected and the bladder did not become weak. His anus became anaesthetic on the left and defaecation was felt as a unilateral phenomenon only. These symptoms largely disappeared after two years, but when he was seen for his recurrent lumbago at the age of 33, slight cutaneous analgesia at these areas was still detectable.

The third case was similar. Another medical man developed analgesia of the left side of the penis and anus at the age of 26. He too noted leftward deviation during erection. The condition lasted two months. He began frequent attacks of severe lumbago, and at the age of 42 he was suffering from right-sided sciatica with a severe fourth and fifth motor root palsy. Laminectomy was performed.

## ADHERENT ROOT

Ordinarily, sciatica without appreciable neurological deficit gets well spontaneously in about a year. The herniation, projecting beyond the edge of the vertebra, and thus deprived of its nutrient synovial fluid, shrivels and laminectomy years after an attack of sciatica reveals a normal appearance at the posterior aspect of the joint originally affected. When, with the passage of time the projection recedes, straight-leg raising reaches its full height again. However, the disorder occasionally continues past the allotted period for no clear reason; cases of sciatic pain and very limited straight-leg raising may continue indefinitely. However long-standing, epidural local anaesthesia often restores the full range of straight-leg raising within a few minutes, thus indicating that the root is not adherent. By contrast, rare cases occur of adherence of the nerve root to the posterior margin of the joint. The patient's sciatica gets slowly less and after about two years his pain may be gone, but he complains that he cannot bend forwards and examination shows about 45° range of straight-leg raising on the affected side. Attempted trunk flexion causes no pain; he just cannot bend, and heavy work produces no symptoms in the back or limb. The condition can last a lifetime.

Root adherence is suggested when a sciatica, particularly in a young man, goes on and on, the symptoms abating but signs continuing; hence nothing special suggests this event during the first year or so of a root pain. Continuation after that arouses suspicion; if so epidural anaesthesia is diagnostic. Although the patient feels the root pain down the limb during the injection, the anaesthetic solution cannot force its way between two adherent surfaces, but only between two surfaces in free contact. Hence, the injection does not alter such root pain as is present nor restore for the duration of local anaesthesia the range of straight-leg raising. There is no other method of diagnosis—apart from inspection during laminectomy.

## SPONDYLOLISTHESIS

This was first described as a cause of obstructed labour by Kilian in 1854. In 1888 Neugebauer of Warsaw maintained that spondylolisthesis could be either congenital or acquired. Nevertheless, all this century it was regarded as caused by congenital lack of fusion at the neural arch, leading to elongation at the defect and a consequent forward shift of the vertebral body during adolescence. This concept was challenged by Batt (1939) who examined 200 fetal spines and found none with two centres of ossification. He concluded that it was not a congenital defect. Hutton et al. regard spondylolisthesis as an ununited fatigue fracture (1977). Newman and Stone (1963) described five types of this disorder. Analysis of 319 cases led to the following conclusions:

*Congenital.* 66 patients, 20 male, 46 female. The cause was poor development of the articular facets at the upper surface of the sacrum, often associated with spina bifida. This defective engagement led to forward displacement during childhood or adolescence, without elongation of the neural arch.

*Attrition of the Facet Joints.* 80 patients, 22 male, 58 female. None of the patients was under 40 years old, and the cause was advanced degeneration of the facet joints, the erosion allowing the vertebra to slip forwards until the displacement was arrested by engagement of the superior facets against bone, nearly always at the fourth lumbar level. In consequence the shift was never severe. No defect was present at the pars intermedia.

*Defective Neural Arch.* 164 patients, 93 male, 71 female. This is the common variety, and the defect in the pars intermedia enables the vertebra slowly to elongate during childhood and adolescence. In consequence, the vertebral body gradually moves anteriorly, while the facets still engage in the normal manner.

*Trauma.* Three cases.

*Generalized Bone Disease.* Six cases.

This abnormality sets up pain in two separate ways: (*a*) commonly, by causing a disc lesion at the unstable joint; (*b*) rarely, by stretching the ligaments and the nerve roots. It should not be forgotten that spondylolisthesis may cause no symptoms during the whole of a patient's lifetime. Crow and Brogden showed that 4.5% of normal young adults who have never had backache have radiological evidence of spondylolisthesis, and a further 7.6% have spondylolysis. My own figure for the incidence of spondylolisthesis in patients with symptoms attributable to the lumbar spine is 3.9%.

Blackburne and Velikas (1977) found that if the forward slip was less than one-third it did not increase as age advanced. This fraction was calculated on the distance that the posterior edge of the fifth lumbar vertebrae had shifted on the posterior edge of the sacrum in relation to the maximum width of the upper sacrum. In fact the degree of spondylolisthesis increased in only 12 of the 126 cases.

## Prophylaxis

Since it has become clear that spondylolisthesis is an acquired deformity in more than half of all cases the question of prevention arises. Repeated strains fall on the lowest two lumbar vertebrae when a baby is about a year old. Stress fractures form between the two halves of the vertebral arch, but cause no appreciable discomfort. No one realizes their presence and union by bone seldom takes place. Fibrous tissue fills the gap—a stretchable structure. After years of tension, some time during adolescence, the defect enlarges. The vertebra becomes longer and grows to project in front of the one below it. An unstable joints forms between these two vertebrae. In consequence a precocious disc lesion results, often during the patient's teens. The fatigue fracture is the result of the baby, not yet able to walk, learning to propel himself seated. At each push, the buttocks are bumped against the floor while the lumbar spine is held flexed. Alternatively, when a baby first learns to walk, after a few steps upright, his legs give way and he lands on his buttocks with the lumbar spine convex. Babies should be discouraged from pushing along seated and the mother should see to it that they go on crawling till they can walk. The baby who keeps falling seated should be provided with a thick napkin to cushion the fall and give him less far to go. There is a great deal to be said for the various walking machines now on the market, which enable the child to stay upright as he pushes himself along with his feet. The earliest example that I have encountered is on show at the Tezcuco Villa (Burnside, Louisiana), dates from 1860 and is made of mahogany. It comprises a triangular saddle suspended by three long springs from a large horizontal wooden ring. This is supported on convex legs, fitted with castors.

## Spondylolisthesis with Secondary Disc Lesion

The symptoms in spondylolisthesis are far more often caused by a disc lesion appearing precociously in the unstable joint, than by the spondylolisthesis as such (Key 1945). If so, nothing in the history arouses suspicion unless the patient states that he has had trouble since childhood. He suffers backache or attacks of lumbago, unilateral or bilateral, indistinguishable from those occurring without spondylolisthesis, merely beginning at an early age. If he later develops sciatica, this is unilateral. Epidural local anaesthesia abolishes the backache for the time being. Laminectomy occasionally shows that the disc lesion lies at the non-spondylolisthesic joint, just above or below.

It is only when inspection and/or palpation discloses the irregularity of the spinous processes that the presence of spondylolisthesis is suspected and confirmed by X-ray photography. The lumbar movements hurt in the manner characterizing a disc lesion; indeed, the signs and treatment are those of the disc lesion causing the symptoms. The only difference is the much enhanced liability to recurrence for slight reasons.

## Spondylolisthesis of Itself Causing Symptoms

The production of backache by spondylolisthesis shows that the ligaments about the lumbar intervertebral joints are not wholly insensitive. After years of stretching, they begin to set up discomfort. The ache is always central and largely unconnected with exertion; some days the back aches, other days it does not, for no clear reason. Prolonged standing is apt to cause either backache or discomfort at the outer aspect of both thighs; sitting or lying abates the pain. The patient may suffer vague crural numbness at night, but awakes comfortable. Thus the history may suggest a pulpy self-reducing disc lesion, but the aggravation by standing rather than by stooping or lifting should provide the warning.

Inspection may reveal the irregularity. When the patient's lumbar movements are tested, unlike the effect when a displaced fragment of disc impairs articular mobility, usually none hurts, even though the back is aching at the time of examination. This finding should lead to renewed scrutiny and palpation of the lumbar spinous processes as the patient stands. When he lies prone, this palpation is repeated, in order to discover if the irregularity continues or disappears when weight-bearing ceases; the latter is a rarity. Epidural local anaesthesia cannot reach the ligaments about the intervertebral joint and does not affect the pain.

Spondylolisthesis also causes bilateral sciatica, with or without premonitory backache. After standing for, say, half an hour the patient develops increasing sciatic pain and paraesthetic feet, sufficient to compel him to sit or lie down. This may continue unchanged for years; the symptoms are the same as in the mushroom phenomenon, but the patient is much younger. The forward movement of the listhetic vertebra drags on the nerve roots, which engage painfully against the shelf formed by the stable vertebra below. Alternatively, Gill et al. (1955) showed that a fibrocartilaginous mass is apt to form at the defect in the pars interarticularis, leading to adhesions about and compression of the nerve root. Good results followed removal.

## Concealed Spondylolisthesis

The patient describes the typical history of backache, perhaps followed by bilateral sciatica, brought on by standing for some time, abolished by sitting or lying. Inspection of the back shows the irregularity; its presence is confirmed by palpation. When the spinous processes are palpated later with the patient prone, no irregularity is detectable. Relief from weight-bearing has allowed the bone to slide back into place again. Since most lumbar radiography is carried out in recumbency, the patient brings with him radiographs that disclose no abnormality (Plate XXXVI). Unless he is X-rayed standing up, the displacement is not revealed.

## Posterior Spondylolisthesis

This is usually symptomless and is more often seen at the upper lumbar and lower thoracic levels than at the fourth or fifth lumbar joints. It results from congenital laxity or gradual stretching of the ligaments at the lateral articulations.

During spinal extension the lateral facets of the upper vertebra tend to move backwards, partly owing to the force of gravity and partly because the surface of the lamina slopes downwards and backwards and thus, when the end of the articular surface is reached by the point of the facet, this is carried backwards until the stetched ligament becomes taut. By bending his trunk forwards, the patient approximates the surfaces of the facet joints once more. This instability is well shown in Morgan and King's paper (1957). Such instability at these lateral joints, although itself symptomless, leads to attrition of the disc. At the upper lumbar levels, this is usually a benign phenomenon but, particularly at the fourth level, may give rise to disc symptoms—backache, lumbago and sciatica.

In the case illustrated in Plate XXIII, which followed interference with the lateral articulations at laminectomy, considerable bilateral root pain had been present for years, disappearing only when the patient lay down.

### Spondylolysis

This is not an uncommon condition, Willi (1931) dissected 1520 cadavers and found defects in one or both laminae in 79, i.e. 5.2%. It causes no symptoms unless a secondary disc lesion with protrusion results. It is detectable only radiologically, when the defect in the pars intermedia on one or both sides is shown in the oblique views. In the case illustrated (Plate XXIII) there had been considerable intractable backache for some years; arthrodesis was advised but refused.

## WEDGING OF A VERTEBRAL BODY

This results from fracture, osteoporosis, adolescent osteochondrosis, neoplasm, osteitis deformans and tuberculous caries.

### Fracture Causing Wedging

A vertebral body withstands one second's acceleration of 1000 kg vertical load before fracturing (Ruff 1950). Wedging occurs at the upper rather than the lower lumbar vertebrae. Until the fracture has united, there is bone pain; it is severe for only a week or two and has certainly ceased in three months. Any pain after that is due to a coincident disc lesion. Naturally, force sufficient to break bone often also damages the discs above and below the fracture. Hence recurrent attacks of pain follow the injury. Moreover, there is now a permanent kyphosis at the joints above and below the wedged bone. This explains why some patients with a fractured body later have severe trouble, while others are symptom-free. It is not what happens to the vertebral body but the state of the discs, not visible radiologically, that determines whether symptoms persist after the fracture has united.

Inspection reveals a small angular kyphos; slight limitation of movement may be detected. The kyphos is palpable and, as the supraspinous and interspinous ligaments have sometimes ruptured, a depression can be felt between two spinous processes. Radiography identifies the wedged vertebra.

Many patients who know a vertebral body has been fractured allege pain; in some it is organic, but in many it is assumed or psychogenic. Examination to detect neurasthenia is then required. Such cases provide thorny medicolegal problems on which no light is thrown by mere inspection of the radiograph, which only shows the vertebral body united with minor angulation. The radiograph cannot show whether a disc is damaged or not; only detailed, possibly repeated, clinical examination enables an objective opinion to be formulated.

### Senile Osteoporosis

Elderly patients, usually women, with marked generalized rarefaction of the spine may sustain a pathological fracture of one or more vertebral bodies. This is more frequent in the thoracic than the lumbar region. The wedging may come on slowly; it is then often symptomless unless a secondary disc lesion develops on account of the upper lumbar kyphosis at the joints to either side of the collapse. If wedging comes on suddenly, bone pain results; it may be severe for a week or two and ceases in two or three months. The kyphosis is visible and palpable; radiography discloses the reason. Osteoporosis itself does not appear to me to cause aching unless fracture supervenes, but frequent bouts of lesser pain may well be caused by repeated microfractures.

### Adolescent Osteochondrosis
(Scheuermann 1936)

In Crow and Brogden's (1959) series of 935 normal men who had never had backache, evidence of past Scheuermann's disease in the lumbar region was present radiographically in 20.7%. It comes on between the ages of 14 (Plate XVII/1) and 18, as the result of anterior disc protrusion. The end-plate is perforated, often at more than one upper lumbar level. Bone is eroded by the nuclear protrusion and wedging results. Since osteochondrosis at other sites causes discomfort and at the spine involves bone, I used to suppose that this was a painful condition. However, 30 years ago, when examining a girl of 15 with osteochondrosis of six months' duration, a painful arc was found present. This was inconsistent with the concept of bone pain, and it seemed possible that the cause of symptoms was disc pressure at one of the affected and, therefore, kyphotic joints. This proved so; for manipulative reduction was heralded by a click with instant disappearance of pain. This concept has since been confirmed on further cases.

The harmless nature of vertebral osteochondrosis was emphasized by Ross (1962) who X-rayed the spine of 5000 police candidates aged 20. He found evidence of osteochondrosis in two-thirds, but only 4.2% of this group had had backache. Schultze's figure (1971) for 1000 normal men aged 19 to 22 was 77%. Stoddard (1973) carried out yet another such survey and found radiological changes in 63.2% of his patients with backache, twice as frequent as in his control series without backache. Clearly, the resultant wedging of vertebral bodies might well be regarded as leading to enhanced likelihood of the development of a disc lesion at the now kyphotic joint, as Stoddard's figures and my experience suggest, but these two earlier surveys show that this result is infrequent. What the statistics do prove is that, of itself, osteochondrosis is symptomless. Much harm is done to parents' peace of mind, however, when, without further explanation, they are told that a youngster is suffering from so ominous-sounding a condition as Scheuermann's disease, merely on account of a radiographic finding often at entirely the wrong level.

### Calvé's Disease

This is an obscure condition in which one vertebral body flattens out and remains flat, without affecting the vertebra plana. The joint surfaces remain parallel and once the pain due to collapse of bone has ceased no further symptoms are to be expected. In the case described by Weston and Goodson (1959), a girl of 3 became unable to walk because of increasing backache in the course of two weeks. Recovery ensued after six weeks recumbency in a plaster bed and she had remained comfortable by five years later. In the course of fifteen days her fifth lumbar vertebra had collapsed to a wafer less than 6 mm thick. Five years later this remained unchanged but the flattened body projected forwards 12 mm further than originally.

### Neoplasm

Rapidly increasing backache, usually in an elderly patient or one who is known to have had an operation for cancer, arouses suspicion. Limited movement due to muscle spasm and neurological signs in the lower limbs without root pain or limitation of straight-leg raising make the suspicion a virtual certainty. A palpable kyphos confirmed by radiography completes the picture.

### Osteitis Deformans

One vertebra may collapse leading to a palpable kyphos. Radiography to determine the cause reveals Paget's disease in the isolated vertebra and in the pelvis.

### Tuberculous Caries

The symptoms are often slight at first, but inspection shows the beginnings of an angular kyphos or, if one side of the body is eroded alone, acute lateral deviation of the same type as occurs with hemivertebra. The lumbar spine is kept extended when the patient is asked to bend forward and the range of both side flexions is markedly limited. These findings naturally call for immediate radiography, which usually reveals the lesion clearly. Four times in my experience, however, the disc was affected alone at first and the original radiograph revealed nothing. Harrison in 1821 had pointed out that vertebral tuberculosis could begin in bone or in cartilage.

## LESIONS UNCONNECTED WITH DISCS

A large number of non-disc lesions give rise to pain in the back, groin and lower limb; they are much less common than a disc lesion, and are considered below.

## Backache with Fever

Staphylococcal osteomyelitis may come on suddenly with severe pain and fever. In such cases, infection is immediately suspected.

### Brucellosis

Chronic backache accompanied by minor fever suggests brucellosis. Most British cases appear to stem from Wales or the Midlands, farmers and veterinary surgeons being the most frequent victims. In January 1980 Scotland was declared free from brucellosis in cattle.

The outstanding symptoms are fatigue, breathlessness and sweating after minor exertion, headache and pain in the back. In such chronic cases the sedimentation rate is not raised and the radiograph uniformative. The diagnosis of infection is confirmed by complement-fixation and by the antihuman globulin tests. Unfortunately high titres are common in farming communities in symptomless patients (Henderson & Hill 1972), and such an individual might easily develop disc trouble. Zammitt's (1958) paper on the vertebral lesions illustrates the radiological appearances well. These become visible one to six months after the infection began in 1.8% of all cases. The first change is rounding of the anterior corner of a vertebral body, most often the fourth lumbar, in a manner closely resembling adolescent osteochondrosis. In the course of the next few months the lateral ligaments ossify, joining the two bones with a bridge. Localized destruction of a vertebral body may come on before healing with sclerosis ensues.

The best way to arrive at a diagnosis in an uncertain case is therapeutic. The patient is given tetracycline 0.5 g 6-hourly for six weeks and a daily injection of 1 g streptomycin for a month. If sensitivity tests are favourable, septrin (a mixture of trimethroprim 80 mg and sulphamethoxazole 400 mg) in a dose of six tablets a day for two or three months is indicated. Should antibiotics fail, levamisole was used with success in chronic intractable cases by Thornes (1976). Seven out of ten patients got well on 150 mg daily for a month, then two consecutive days a week for a further six months.

# Lumbar Pain

## Fractured Transverse Process

This occurs only after direct injury to the back. The pain is unilateral, localized, and in the mid or upper lumbar region, since the fifth process is scarcely ever broken. The history and the discovery of pain elicited by resisted movements when the patient lies prone give the clue, and the radiograph is diagnostic. If pain persists for more than a fortnight, it must be remembered that force sufficient to break a transverse process may also have injured a disc; alternatively, the idea of a 'fractured spine' may also be so attractive to a patient that psychogenic symptoms supervene. A rare cause of fracture is manipulation of the back. The snap is felt quite clearly, and a week's discomfort is to be expected.

## Ankylosing Spondylitis

If, as occurs in seven-eighths of all cases, the preceding sacroiliac arthritis has caused no symptoms, the first complaint may be backache. It comes and goes according to its own vagaries, and is often worst on waking; exertion, however severe, does not bring on an attack although it may aggravate pain already present. As a rule, all the lumbar spinal joints become involved at much the same time. Hence the patient, instead of indicating one spot, points to the whole lumbar region centrally. Examination shows a flat lumbar spine with, perhaps, the beginning of an upper thoracic kyphosis, combined with limitation of side flexion at the lumbar joints. By now active inflammation in the sacroiliac joints has ceased and clinically they are painless, but X-rays of these joints—*not* of the lumbar spine—reveal the tell-tale sclerosis.

## Osteitis Deformans

In advanced cases the pain is all over the elderly patient's back. On inspection, the trunk has a shortened appearance as if the thorax had come too far down towards the pelvis. Genu varum may be visible. Movement of the lumbothoracic spine is grossly restricted. Palpation of femur or tibia may show expansion. The radiograph of the pelvis is diagnostic.

Sometimes one vertebra is affected alone. If so, the body softens, broadens and collapses just as occurs on invasion by neoplasm, but does not proceed beyond cortex touching cortex. Localized backache results and inspection shows the angular kyphos. Plate XVIII shows the typical appearances. The differential diagnosis is made largely by seeking evidence of osteitis deformans elsewhere.

## Neoplasm

Neoplasms are nearly always secondary, although myeloma is encountered. In myeloma the sedimentation rate is seldom less than 100 mm in the first hour. There may be a history of previous operation for malignant disease, but undue weight must not be given to this fact, for such patients, like other individuals, often suffer from ordinary disc lesions. Much distress is caused, and effective treatment not given, when a disc lesion is mistaken for secondary malignant deposits; hence it is an error hardly less grave than the converse.

In disc lesions, the neurological signs are minor and the root pain severe; in neoplasm the reverse obtains.

The first suggestion of malignant disease lies in the history, which is not of pain varying with exertion but of steady aggravation irrespective of activity. A short period of increasing central backache in an elderly patient is always suspect. Then the pain spreads down both lower limbs in a distribution not corresponding to any one root. Moreover, the backache becomes worse when the sciatica, soon bilateral, appears. In a disc lesion, the backache eases when unilateral root pain comes on. If examination does not yet reveal a kyphos, muscular spasm markedly limiting movement is seen at the lumbar spine, most obvious on attempted side flexion. Neurological examination reveals signs that more than one nerve root is involved, e.g. the knee jerk is affected as well as the ankle jerk; the psoas muscle is weak together with muscles of lower lumbar derivation; the muscle weakness and the site of cutaneous analgesia belong to separate segments; the signs are bilateral and asymmetrical.

In a disc lesion causing muscle weakness, the patient must have had considerable root pain in the lower limb. Severe weakness without root pain is very suggestive of spinal metastases. So is gross weakness with a full range of straight-leg raising, without a history of recent acute sciatica. At the upper two lumbar levels, neoplasm may interfere with the sympathetic nerves; if so, the foot on the affected side is warmer than its fellow. These signs often appear before the radiograph shows erosion or collapse of one or more vertebral bodies. Indeed, there may be no X-ray changes only a few weeks before vertebral bodies can be crushed by the fingers post-mortem. Hence, *in the short run*, X-ray photography is not reliable. In a doubtful case, epidural local anaesthesia abolishes temporarily the pain due to a disc lesion, but not that due to metastatic invasion. The patient must be observed and X-rayed at monthly intervals until the diagnosis becomes clear, while a search for the primary growth is initiated.

## Sacral Neoplasm

This is more difficult to detect than lower lumbar metastasis, because the spinal joints retain a full and painless range of movement. The patient complains of sacral pain, sometimes of coccygodynia only. However, invasion of the nerve roots at the front of the sacrum, although (as the dural sleeve is not affected) it does not provoke root pain or limitation of straight-leg raising, gives rise to gross weakness of the muscles of one or both feet. Such paresis in the absence of root pain suggests a tumour, and the radiograph usually discloses a sacral defect. The symptoms are slight at first and the patient is apt to present himself late in the evolution of the disease.

## Lumbar Neuroma

These are rare, considerably rarer than cervical neuromas, and need be considered only if the case has unusual features.

When a spinal space-occupying lesion gives rise to first or second lumbar root pain, metastasis or neuroma is suggested merely because first and second lumbar disc lesions are so uncommon.

At first, neuromas at the lower three lumbar levels are very difficult to detect. However, certain features in the history should arouse suspicion. Most root pain in the limb becomes fairly rapidly worse, reaching a peak within one to four weeks. Severe symptoms may then persist for a month or two. Then improvement sets in slowly and, at the end of a year, nearly all patients have recovered. Though the onset in young people's primary posterolateral sciatica is more gradual, even so full evolution does not take more than three or four months at the most. Any root pain that is still getting worse at the end of, say, eight months is suspect. In disc lesions backache often precedes root pain, ceasing when this comes on. Neuromas may cause root pain only, but if they do cause backache, this continues. The fact that a cough hurts is no guide, of course, but if a cough does *not* hurt, neuroma is unlikely.

Some help is derived from a study of the lumbar movements; in a disc lesion one or two movements may well prove limited, but not all four. Root pain with gross limitation of every lumbar movement suggests metastasis but, if no evidence of malignancy is found on further examination, the question of a benign neuroma arises.

The range of straight-leg raising is not much help, since a neuroma near the foramen may cause marked restriction. If it lies more centrally, straight-leg raising may not be appreciably limited, but this is often the case also in long-standing disc protrusions with considerable neurological deficit.

When a disc protrusion causes root pain with neurological signs, these usually evolve within one to four weeks. They then continue unchanged for, say, six months, whereupon the beginning of recovery may be expected. Gradual increase in signs of impaired conduction month by month is most improbable and suggests a neuroma. Unlike the strictly uniradicular palsies that arise from cervical disc lesions, one lumbar protrusion often compresses two adjacent nerve roots, nearly always the fourth and fifth lumbar, or the fifth lumbar and first sacral, or the first and second sacral. Triple palsies or asymmetrical bilateral palsies more often result from metastases or neuralgic amyotrophy, whereas a palsy affecting two non-adjacent roots suggests a long neuroma.

The first step in all cases of suspected neuroma is to induce epidural local anaesthesia. Since the fluid cannot insinuate itself between the neuroma and the nerve root, the injection, though it sets up the root pain, has no effect on the symptoms or on the range of straight-leg raising when tested some minutes later. If this proves so, a myelogram is indicated (see Plate xxx/1). Intrathecal tumours have a smooth edge; extrathecal, a fringed edge.

There are four conditions that resemble a neuroma. Metastasis is not included, since progress is then much more rapid and in no way resembles the long drawn out aggravation of a neuroma.

*Adherent Root.* There is a superficial resemblance, for epidural local anaesthesia provokes the root pain as the injection proceeds, and has not altered the pain or the range of straight-leg raising by some minutes later. However, the sciatic pain is slight and has not increased over a year or two, nor has appreciable neurological deficit resulted, certainly not an increasing one. The range of straight-leg raising is limited, without any change from year to year. A full and painless range of spinal movements, except towards flexion, remain.

*Old Root Atrophy: Increased Protrusion.* Patients are encountered who had severe short-lived sciatica some years previously, losing their symptoms by root atrophy. Irreversible necrosis of many fibres in one or two nerve roots resulted and considerable weakness and numbness (usually of the foot and the muscles controlling it) persist. One day, without pain, the patient notices increased weakness and more extensive numbness. This is the result of further protrusion of disc substance at the original level, but it impinges against an insensitive nerve root; hence, there is further loss of conduction but no pain. This development is often regarded as connoting serious disease. True, the increased palsy is permanent, but, that apart, the disorder is unimportant.

*A Second Disc Protrusion.* A patient suffers sciatica with, say, a fourth lumbar root palsy. This is taking its expected course and after some months the pain is easing. Some time later, the pain gets worse, the range of straight-leg raising decreases, and a fifth lumbar root palsy is now found to have supervened. Weakness extending to an adjacent root after some months' sciatica does suggest a neuroma, but the myelogram shows either nothing or a disc lesion. Laminectomy now reveals large fourth and fifth disc protrusions, the latter obviously the cause of the more recent palsy.

*Neuralgic Amyotrophy.* This is rare in the lower limb. Straight-leg raising cannot become limited since this is a parenchymatous lesion not affecting the dural sleeve. The pain comes on suddenly and the palsy is maximal within the first few days, and the distribution of the weak muscles may include members of three or four roots. The pain eases in the course of four to six months and the muscles gradually strengthen.

## Afebrile Osteomyelitis

*Acute.* Afebrile osteomyelitis may come on quickly—in the course of, say, a week. The history is then identical with nuclear lumbago: rapidly increasing lumbar pain. After some days, when asked to stand for a moment to have his back examined, he cannot do so owing to severe pain. This is perfectly consistent with severe lumbago. But in central protrusion as marked as this, the dural signs are as conspicuous as the articular. Examination, however, reveals a full range of straight-leg raising; moreover, no pain is felt on coughing. This combination is typical of a severe spinal lesion, not affecting the mobility of the dura mater. Infection is suspected, and epidural local anaesthesia is induced at once diagnostically. This has no effect on pain caused by osteomyelitis, thus confirming the diagnosis. The only objective sign is usually a raised sedimentation rate (40–60 mm). The last such patient I saw lay in bed for two months before the abscess in the body of his fourth lumbar vertebra was revealed radiologically and was drained (Urquhart).

*Chronic.* The patient, always in my experience male, complains that a slight, constant, central backache came on some months previously and gradually became more severe. Examination at this stage reveals no diagnostic signs, but a disc lesion is excluded when epidural local anaesthesia fails temporarily to abolish the pain. Fever is absent. Radiography reveals no abnormality, but the ESR is raised. Under observation, the pain gradually worsens while restriction of side flexion at the lumbar spine appears. The pain on movement and the increasing limitation of range may suggest ankylosing spondylitis but the onset is too swift, and the X-ray shows the sacroiliac joints to be clear. The history is too long for a radio-invisible neoplasm. Once these points are established, the patient should be regarded as suffering from chronic osteomyelitis.

Plate XXVI/2 shows the appearance at the end of a year in a patient first seen six months after the onset of symptoms. Although the clinical signs were clear, the radiograph was still normal. In due course X-ray evidence of septic infection of the joint appeared.

Typhoid fever and brucellosis can give rise to spinal osteitis.

## Posterior Osteophytosis

The early history is that of a disc lesion, since it is damage here that is responsible for the bulging of the posterior longitudinal ligament that in due course draws out the osteophyte. When this becomes large enough, a constant backache sets in (as often happens also in disc lesions without osteophyte formation). Clinical examination is not distinctive, the pattern of articular and dural signs suggesting a minor disc protrusion. The diagnosis remains obscure until inspection of the lateral radiograph shows a large osteophyte jutting out backwards from the margin of the vertebral body and forming a bony projection (Plate XXVI/1).

During the early stage of its formation the osteophyte causes no symptoms, but when it is large enough to irritate the dura mater, the constant backache can be relieved only by removing it at laminectomy.

## Ligamentous Overstretching

This is most uncommon except in spondylolisthesis. In myopathy or anterior poliomyelitis affecting the muscles of the lower trunk, the patient has to balance himself bent slightly backwards. This puts a severe strain on the anterior longitudinal ligament; after some time a backache results that is immediately abolished by sitting down or bending forwards. Occasionally after laminectomy a flexion injury may painfully overstretch the fibrous tissue replacing the interspinous ligaments.

Rupture of a supraspinous or interspinous ligament increases the range of flexion at an intervertebral joint, thus predisposing to, or aggravating, damage to a disc. These ligaments are grossly overstretched on either side of a vertebral fracture with wedging. This tension may set up a central ache abolished for the time being by local anaesthesia.

## Gastric Ulcer Adherent to Lumbar Spine

The symptoms are often remarkable, being connected both with eating and with posture. The pain may be lumbar or felt in one or other iliac fossa; it is not in my experience epigastric. One patient had to eat standing by the mantelpiece; another could not stand up straight after a meal. One patient with only upper lumbago pain obtained ease by frequently drinking hot water. He had twice had his stomach investigated by a barium meal, and it was only when this was repeated in the Trendelenberg position that the ulcer on the lesser curvature was revealed.

Trunk extension stretches the scar tissue at the front of the spine and may cause central discomfort—a most misleading finding. However, the lumbar symptoms are felt in the forbidden area; they are not brought on by exertion although they are influenced by posture, and they are clearly connected with abdominal visceral function. This combination brings the diagnosis to mind.

## Aortic Occlusion

Filitzer and Bhanson (1959) pointed out that occlusion of the lower aorta or of the common iliac arteries may cause backache. Usually the claudication in one or both limbs overshadows the minor backache, which is felt in the upper lumbar region—the 'forbidden area'. The patient is regarded as suffering from sciatica, but the history is characteristic—limb pain occurs *only* on walking. The femoral pulse is absent and the diagnosis obvious. One patient with aortic thrombosis merely complained of numbness without pain at the front of both thighs after walking 50 yards. This symptom was pointed out by Sturge (1882) who described a heavy feeling and numbness in the left arm during an attack of angina.

Difficult cases are those with central upper lumbar or lower thoracic backache, unaltered by any movement of the spine. I examined such a patient once a week for a month before the femoral pulses ceased, clarifying the diagnosis. Another disorder difficult to identify is pressure, usually on the left third lumbar root, exerted by a slowly dissecting aneurysm. Severe left-sided pain in the back and limb without articular or root signs in an elderly patient should lead to suspicion. No relief is afforded by epidural local anaesthesia and myelography is, of course, also negative.

## Spinal Claudication

In 1958 Blau and Rushworth showed that exercising the hind leg of a mouse gave rise to dilatation of the blood vessels of the spinal cord on that side. Hence pressure hindering such increased bloodflow can set up cord symptoms, as was recognized by Déjerine in 1906. In such cases, the patient's lower limbs feel heavy during exertion and during this period the plantar response becomes extensor. If the neural canal happens to be smaller than usual (spinal stenosis) the likelihood of claudication is increased.

Rest makes the symptoms and signs disappear. Clearly, this phenomenon can affect also the cauda equina, e.g. by pressure from a disc protrusion. As a result the nerve roots claudicate, resulting in root pain and distal paraesthesia. Hence, in spinal claudication, walking causes backache and discomfort usually in both lower limbs, which ceases as soon as walking stops, but the pain is associated with pins and needles in both feet. Attention is thus drawn away from the vascular system and towards the nervous system, and this is reinforced when all the pulses are present on examination of the lower limbs. However, the symptoms, including the paraesthesia, come on only after walking a distance, and can be induced by exercising the limbs in bed. In 1961, Blau and Logue described six such cases of anoxia of the cauda equina. In five, removal of a central disc protrusion at laminectomy was followed by relief lasting up to five years. The sixth patient recovered spontaneously. Four protrusions lay at the fourth lumbar level, one at the third. Two of the patients had spinal stenosis.

## Vertebral Hyperostosis

This rare disorder was first described by Forestier and Rotes-Querol in 1950. Elderly patients developed an ache in the entire trunk, with marked limitation of movement at every spinal joint. The radiological appearances are different from discogenic osteophytosis since the disc spaces are well-preserved and different again from ankylosing spondylitis in that ossification is confined to the anterior longitudinal ligament. Ott (1953, 1967) found that 21.8% of such patients have concomitant diabetes.

My youngest patient was 48 years old at his first visit, and had diffuse backache for 14 years. Ossification of the anterior longitudinal ligament was confined to the first and second lumbar levels.

## Nutritional Osteomalacia

Female immigrants from Asia may live on a largely vegetarian diet, grossly deficient in lime salts, They lose a considerable amount of calcium if they bear a child, and more still by breast-feeding. Backache and bilateral sciatica then begin accompanied by complaints of lassitude. Since no physical signs are detectable on clinical examination, it is easy to dismiss the case as neurosis.

The early clinical sign—indeed often the only sign—is the characteristic waddle with which the patient walks. Even in the Punjab and West Pakistan where the disease is common, Vaishnava and Rizvi (1967) report that the condition is often missed. They see three or four cases a week, previously labelled psychogenic rheumatism, etc. One patient in five is pregnant and one in ten develops tetany as the first symptom.

The gait is diagnostic; the patient walks in with the feet turned outwards, dipping in the Trendelenberg way. Yet no abnormality of the lumbar spine, of the hip joints or of the muscles controlling them is found to account for this phenomenon. Radiography may not reveal rarefaction of bone at first, but the levels of calcium and phosphorus in the blood are low. In one such case of mine kindly investigated by Professor Prunty, the calcium level varied between 7.5 and 8.9 mg while the plasma phosphorus varied between 2 and 3.1 mg.

Osteomalacia occurs in Europeans after gastrectomy.

## 'Gonorrhoeal Fasciitis'

This is alleged to cause 'poker back' but is an entity copied from one textbook to another. I have never encountered such a case and, short of the fascia turning into bone, I do not believe that any such disorder could produce appreciable limitation of movement, in particular towards extension, which relaxes the fascia. Clearly, the idea of gonorrhoeal fasciitis depends on the coexistence in a single patient of gonorrhoea and ankylosing spondylitis—both diseases to which young men are prone. Moreover, spinal ankylosis is a well-known complication of Reiter's disease. Up to half of all cases of this disorder have radiological signs of sacroiliac involvement, and in them there is an increased incidence of advancing spondylitis compared with the general population.

### Pain Referred to the Back

When pain is referred to the back from an intra-abdominal or pelvic viscus, the outstanding finding is a full and painless range of movement at the lumbar spine. This finding focuses attention on the non-moving parts of the body, the kidney, colon, ovary, uterus and rectum. In cases of doubt, epidural local anaesthesia should be induced since it provides a clear, immediate answer.

## Root Pain

A common cause of pain referred to the groin is misleading dural reference from a low lumbar disc lesion. Alternatively, third sacral root pressure may be responsible. Far less often, it results from a lowest thoracic disc lesion. Pain in the groin was for a few months the only and, throughout, a prominent symptom in the case of fourth lumbar neuroma illustrated in Plate xxvi/1.

Osteoarthrosis of the hip, psoas bursitis and muscle strain may set up pain felt at first only in the groin. Intestinal and renal disorders, an ovarian cyst or a hernia may also cause pain felt chiefly in the groin. A gastric ulcer adherent to the lumbar spine sometimes causes puzzling symptoms there.

### Second Lumbar Pain

Pain at the front of the thigh reaching as far as the knee occurs in lesions of structures developed from the second and third lumbar myotomes. These include the second and third lumbar nerve roots, the hip joint, the psoas, adductor and quadriceps muscles, the psoas bursa, the femur and the bones about the acetabulum.

It must not be forgotten that obscure symptoms of numbness or weakness, not necessarily pain, felt in the anterior crural region after walking a short distance, may result from thrombosis of the lower aorta or external iliac artery. In the former case, both femoral pulses are lost; in the latter, only one. Although pain in the thigh brought on by walking naturally suggests a lesion in the moving parts, examination of the back and joints, muscles, etc., of the lower limb reveals no abnormality. This combination brings to mind the likelihood of claudication.

Pain at the front of the thigh which examination suggests has a local origin, but not in muscles, joints, etc., calls for radiography of the femur, which may disclose an osteoid osteoma.

*Weakness of the Psoas Muscle.* If the weakness is unilateral and is accompanied by lumbar pain on lumbar movements, a second lumbar disc lesion may be responsible. This is so rare, however, that the diagnosis should be unwillingly reached. If the weakness is considerable and pain felt in one iliac fossa is brought on when the muscle contracts, neoplasm invading the posterior abdominal wall should be suspected. If it is accompanied by increased pain in the thigh, metastatic invasion of the upper femur is likely, except in adolescents when avulsion of the epiphysis of the lesser femoral trochanter occurs. Unilateral weakness is rarely the first sign of interference with the pyramidal tracts; if so, the resisted movement does not increase the pain. Bilateral weakness characterizes neoplasm at the second lumbar level; if so, the feet are apt to be hot because of sympathetic paralysis.

*Meralgia Paraesthetica.* This is an interesting condition (Figs 86, 87). The patient complains of pain and paraesthesia in the area of skin supplied by the lateral cutaneous nerve of the thigh. This nerve emerges from the outer border of the psoas to cross the iliacus muscle. It passes under the lateral aspect of the inguinal ligament, and 5 cm below the anterior superior spine of the ilium pierces the fascia femoris. It emerges superficially 5 cm lower down, and it would seem that it can be irritated in any part of its course. The nerve may be nipped if, owing to congenital abnormality, it passes through the inguinal ligament instead of deeply. The difficult distinction between meralgia and a second lumbar root lesion rests on the following. (*a*) A history of pain in the back or upper buttock preceding the appearance of the numbness. (*b*) Finding that one or more of the lumbar movements hurt in the trunk or provoke the pins and needles. (*c*) Careful delineation of the paraesthetic area. Comparison of Figs 87 and 19 shows that the two areas correspond well laterally, but only the second root supplies the front and inner aspect of the thigh. (*d*) The degree of analgesia. Since the second and third root territories overlap, the numbness is very slight in root lesions, but may amount almost to anaesthesia with a clearcut edge in pressure on

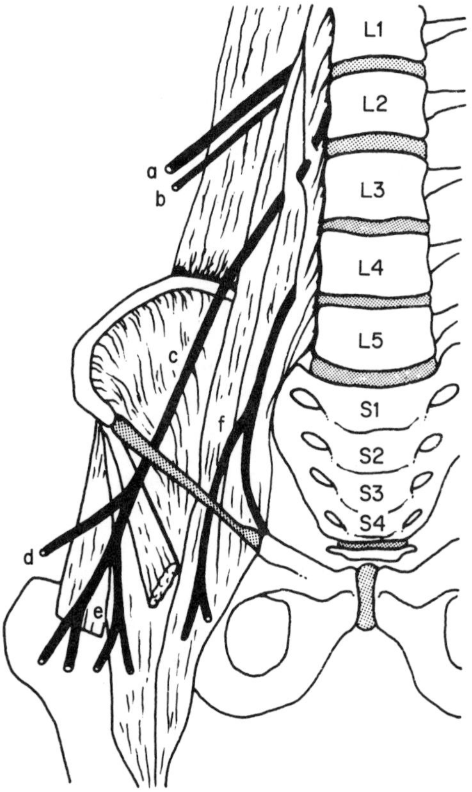


**Fig. 86.** Minor branches of the lumbar plexus, *a*, Iliohypogastric nerve. *b*, Ilioinguinal nerve. *c*, Lateral cutaneous nerve of the thigh with gluteal (*d*) and femoral (*e*) branches. *f*, Genitofemoral nerve. Note that the middle part of the lateral cutaneous nerve crosses the iliac crest and can suffer compression there during pregnancy.

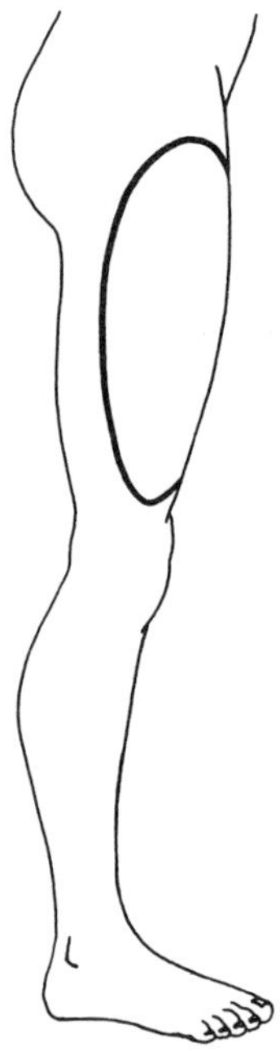

**Fig. 87.** The area of skin supplied by the lateral cutaneous nerve of the thigh. The anterior edge does not reach to the midline of the thigh in front. Contrast the distribution of the second lumbar nerve root which is shown in Fig. 19.

the cutaneous nerve. (*e*) The induction of epidural local anaesthesia. Naturally this injection abolishes symptoms only in a root lesion.

In cases of friction at the fascia tunnel, injection of 10 ml of 0.5% procaine suffices. The difficulty is to find the right spot, since the position of the nerve varies considerably. A thin needle 5 cm long is inserted superficially in line with the nerve and the point moved about until the prick induces the familiar paraesthesia. The whole injection is given here. If the nerve perforates the inguinal ligament, the deep fasciculus should be divided. If necessary, the nerve can be avulsed (Hager 1885).

*Meralgia during Pregnancy.* The upper extent of the analgesia in compression of the lateral cutaneous nerve of the thigh ends accurately at the level of the greater trochanter. If the analgesia reaches above that line, reaching to the iliac crest, pressure on the femoral cutaneous nerve where it crosses the iliac crest is probable and the uterus palpated. Such numbness is a rare complication of pregnancy. At the fourth month, the mother begins to feel discomfort at the front of one thigh and a few days later the anterolateral aspect of the thigh goes numb down to the patella. The symptoms disappear spontaneously in about three months. Since the symptoms are always unilateral, the cause would appear to be pressure from a small fibromyoma of the uterus, projecting posterolaterally. As the uterus enlarges, this impinges against the upper extent of the lateral cutaneous nerve close to its emergence at the lateral border of the psoas muscle. An overtight bandage round the pelvis after an operation can compress the nerve just medial to the anterior spine of each ilium.

*Haemophilic Meralgia.* Haemorrhage into the iliopsoas muscle may compress the lateral cutaneous nerve close to the inguinal ligament. In consequence, the outer thigh becomes analgesic. Stewart-Wynne (1976) describes such a case in a patient on warfarin subjected to manipulation by an osteopath for sciatica.

*Anterior Cutaneous Nerve.* This emerges through the fascia of the thigh some 7 cm below the inguinal ligament. Here, it may be compressed by the edge of a corset pushed downwards when the patient sits, or by the clasp of a suspender when the patient leans, say, against the edge of a table.

The cutaneous analgesia occupies the whole of the front of the thigh as far as the knee, and has the characteristics of local pressure. There is a defined edge to the numb area which becomes almost anaesthetic at its centre. Examination reveals an absence of all other signs and inquiry elicits the cause. The patient has to await spontaneous recovery.

*Obturator Nerve.* An obturator hernia may compress this nerve and give rise to an area of cutaneous analgesia at the inner side of the thigh just above the knee.

## Third Lumbar Pain

Apart from the nerve root itself, the common cause of a third lumbar pain is osteoarthrosis of the hip joint, whose capsule is usually developed wholly within the third lumbar myotome. Indeed, it is a commonplace that, especially in children, pain at the knee may originate from the hip. Strain of the psoas muscle, psoas bursitis and a loose body in the hip joint also give rise to pain of third lumbar extent. Pain felt at the front of the thigh can, of course, originate from the quadriceps muscle or the femur itself. If a third lumbar pain is described and there are no signs of any lesion of muscles, joints, nerves, etc., the femur should be X-rayed. Osteoid osteoma, early sarcoma or osteitis deformans may be disclosed.

*Long Saphenous Nerve.* This may suffer irritation analogous to the lateral cutaneous nerve. It is exposed to friction at the foramen by which it pierces the fascia just below the inner side of the knee; alternatively, its sheath may be damaged by a direct blow or by kneeling. The pain may start at the knee, later spreading down the inner side of the leg to the medial aspect of the foot. In other cases it may begin at the inner side of the heel and then extend up to the knee. This is a most deceptive story, drawing attention away from the knee and suggesting that the pain originates at the foot. The symptoms seldom include paraesthesia and walking may increase the pain since the nerve is shifted in its foramen at each knee flexion movement. Signs of loss of conduction are absent. The only physical sign is a small tender area situated at the inner side of the tibia an inch or so below the knee joint. This is present on the affected side only, at the foramen where the nerve emerges. Local anaesthesia here destroys the pain, which seldom returns appreciably.

*Dissecting Aneurysm.* Third lumbar pain, accompanied by severe backache, both left-sided, may result from a dissecting aneurysm of the aorta. Increasing pain accompanied by severe backache in an elderly patient should arouse suspicion. Epidural local anaesthesia affords no relief; myelography and laminectomy disclose no abnormality. Aortography reveals the lesion and should not be delayed.

*Painless Weakness of the Quadriceps Muscles.* When weakness is confined to the third lumbar myotome, without sensory changes, metastasis at the third vertebra is unlikely. Two other disorders have to be considered—localized myopathy and myositis. In either case, the weakness is bilateral and affects the quadriceps muscles only. By the time the patient has begun to notice that his legs are weak, very considerable loss of power is detectable clinically. Wasting is obvious, but the knee jerks are preserved and paraesthesia absent.

Distinction is important, since myositis can be halted by steroid therapy whereas myopathy cannot. Biopsy should be undertaken at once, so that the cases capable of arrest can be singled out.

## Fourth and Fifth Lumbar Pain

Sometimes the capsule of the hip joint is derived largely or wholly from the fourth lumbar segment; if so, arthritis gives rise to 'sciatic' pain. Acute lumbago, arthritis of both hips, spondylolisthesis, the mushroom phenomenon and malignant disease of the spine all set up bilateral pain in the limbs. Thrombosis of the external iliac artery may give rise to a cold foot and sciatic pain only after walking. This holds for outpatients only, for a day or two in bed restores equal warmth to the two extremities. A tight fascial compartment for the extensor group of muscles in the leg may mimic a root lesion, especially if pins and needles are felt. A loose body at the back of the knee may compress the tibial nerve, causing pain at the back of the knee and pins and needles in the adjacent surfaces of the first and second toes. Spinal claudication causes bilateral root pain with pins and needles in the feet, as do spondylolisthesis and the mushroom phenomenon.

Pressure on the peroneal nerve is usually postural; rarely is it caused by an osteoma at the head of the fibula. The patient habitually sits with his legs crossed, or with the outer aspect of his knee pressed against a hard edge. In due course, discomfort may be felt from the knee down the outer side of the leg to the foot. Distally, paraesthesia may be a prominent feature; as a rule weakness of the dorsiflexor muscles and diminution in cutaneous sensibility are not marked. Spontaneous recovery begins as soon as the cause of the disorder is explained to the patient.

*Root Atrophy.* The patient describes slight sciatica for some days or weeks; then he develops agonizing pain down the limb for anything between some hours and some days. Morphine is well justified. Then, quite suddenly the foot goes numb and the pain ceases. Rarely the protrusion becomes maximal instantaneously, the blinding pain down the leg lasting only a few seconds before the numbness comes on and the pain goes.

The patient has become symptomatically better by getting anatomically worse. The posterolateral protrusion has reached its maximum size and compresses the nerve root hard enough to render it ischaemic and thus insentient to the sustained impact. Hence pain ceases and full straight-leg raising provokes no discomfort, at the same time as the root palsy becomes complete in the course of a few minutes.

It is important to examine any patient who loses his pain in this way, since such an account suggests not reduction but further protrusion. If the fourth root is out of action the question of laminectomy arises since lastingly weak dorsiflexion of the foot is a disability and early decompression much enhances the likelihood of full restoration of muscle power. It is not, however, certain (Hakelius 1970). If a fifth lumbar or first or second sacral palsy has resulted laminectomy is less often called for, since some weakness of the peroneal or calf muscles, even if permanent, causes the ordinary person little annoyance. Unless the muscles are fully paralysed, adequate recovery within a year is to be expected, especially if the palsy is monoradicular. Complete paralysis may prove lasting.

If the patient decides to put up with the weakness and take his chance on spontaneous recovery, he need not wear a belt nor be particularly careful what he does, for the protrusion is already maximal.

*'Sciatic or Peroneal Neuritis'.* This is the name given to sudden foot-drop, occurring unilaterally in elderly patients. The true nature of the condition is unknown; paralysis is the marked feature; the disorder is entirely painless. Careful examination usually reveals some weakness in the hamstring muscles and slight gluteal wasting as well. The likely cause of this condition is a low lumbar disc protrusion that has passed more laterally than backwards, thus impinging against the nerve root just beyond the distal extremity of the dural sheath. Discomfort is therefore absent and a painless root palsy, usually permanent, results. Peroneal atrophy is painless and leads to bilateral weakness of tibialis anterior and peroneal muscles.

*Obstetric Palsy.* This results from pressure exerted on the lumbosacral cord at the brim of the pelvis. Since the pressure is exerted on a nerve trunk beyond its dural investment, local pain is absent and straight-leg raising neither painful nor limited. If full foot-drop occurs, the patient naturally reports the fact soon after confinement; but if only vague numbness and some weakness of the calf muscles are present, the paresis may pass unnoticed until she is up and about again. These cases are uncommon and recover spontaneously in a few months.

## First Sacral and Second Sacral Pain

The sacroiliac joints are derived from the first and second sacral segments, hence in early spondylitis ankylopoetica the ligamentous pain often radiates to the posterior thigh and calf. Intermittent claudication gives rise to pain in the calf and posterior thigh only on walking. Bilateral pain results from spondylolisthesis, the mushroom phenomenon, spinal claudication and secondary neoplasm. Gluteal bursitis, being a deep-seated lesion occurring at the upper extent of a low lumbar segment, can give rise to pain radiating from buttock to ankle.

Neuromas are usually benign and sometimes multiple. Some are found lying superficial to the sciatic nerve trunk in the thigh or lower buttock. Others are incorporated in the nerve, expanding it from within. Benign neuromas set up pressure effects when they form within the spinal canal. Hence the existence of multiple intraspinal neuromas can be inferred when they are found in the trunk or at a limb in conjunction with signs of impaired conduction at a higher level.

Deep phlebitis, osteitis deformans, neoplasm of the ilium or femur and various traumatic lesions of the muscles locally complete the list.

### Fourth Sacral Pain

Rectal, penile, scrotal, testicular, vaginal and bladder disorders are by far the commonest causes, but a low lumbar disc lesion compressing the fourth sacral root is a possibility. These cases may be ascribed to 'testicular' or 'vaginal' neuralgia. If the diagnosis is in doubt, the induction of epidural local anaesthesia provides an immediate answer.

## Multiple Root Palsy

### Neuralgic Amyotrophy

This affects the lower limb quite rarely. I have encountered only a few cases, all in men aged 50 to 70. There is no premonitory backache (in contradistinction the neckache when the upper limb is affected). The pain is considerable for about three months, and then slowly eases in the course of another three months. Pins and needles or numbness are rare, and then only in the cutaneous area corresponding to the muscles most severely affected. The pain is usually unilateral, and third, fourth and fifth lumbar weakness is encountered. Alternatively the fourth and fifth lumbar and first and second sacral roots are all affected.

Examination discloses a complete absence of lumbar articular signs and a full and painless range of straight-leg raising. When muscle power is tested a triple or even quadruple motor root palsy comes to light. Spinal metastases are of course suspected but though in pain the patient feels well, his lumbar spine moves well and the straight radiograph reveals nothing relevant. Moreover, the palsy is maximal from the first, does not increase nor spread to the other limb and there is little or no sensory loss. After six months muscle power begins to return and after a year recovery is complete.

Diagnosis is really retrospective. However, in any patient with a marked unilateral palsy of the third, fourth and fifth lumbar roots, or the fourth and fifth lumbar and first and second sacral roots, neuralgic amyotrophy should be suspected as soon as neoplasm has been excluded.

## UNDIAGNOSED BACKACHE

There is at least one—there may be many—cause of backache yet to be discovered. In a review of a thousand cases seen in 1956 (Cyriax 1965) with symptoms attributed to the lower back, 80.2% were certainly disc lesions, but in 4.8% no diagnosis was ever made. In nearly all, epidural anaesthesia had been induced diagnostically because of uncertainty and had shown that a disc lesion was not responsible.

Three possibilities arose: (*a*) That a variant of spondylitis ankylopoetica might exist starting at the lumbar joints without previous sacroiliitis. Follow-up for ten years showed no extension of the symptoms or signs. (*b*) That a primary rheumatoid arthritis existed at the lower lumbar joints. Again, follow-up showed no tendency to the development of arthritis elsewhere as the years went by and cortisone had no beneficial effect. (*c*) That the chiropractors had stumbled upon a correct ascription in shifting from their displaced vertebra to internal derangement at a lateral facet joint. In the former two instances, the pain would be central; in the third, unilateral.

These 48 patients were, therefore, carefully studied, but with very disappointing results. No common factor, no consistent pattern of pain or of physical signs emerged. The pain was as often in the lower limb as the back, and the backaches were neither all central nor all unilateral. One patient with unusual signs was seen only once, being asked to return next day for further examination. This he did not do, and he died a short time later of an unstated cause; he doubtless had spinal metastases.

Of the remaining 47 patients, 15 complained of central backache, one with numbness down the fronts of both thighs as well. Three patients had purely unilateral backache and four had pain in one buttock. In 16, the backache spread to one lower limb; in six, to both limbs. Six patients had pain in one limb without backache, with no local cause discernible in the limb itself. Neurological signs were present in three cases. In three, marked limitation of movement at the lumbar joints suggested spondylitis, but the sacroiliac joints were radiographically clear and cortisone brought no relief. Little change in symptoms or signs occurred as time went by, and they appeared not to suffer from undetected neurosis, nor could they have been missed neuromas, etc., or the lesions would have declared themselves by now. In none was the X-ray appearance then or later of any significance.

## NEUROSIS

Since most people suffer slight backache on and off, it is to be expected that the neurotic patient, when searching—doubtless subconsciously—for an acceptable peg to hang symptoms on, should choose the back; for this is where his only suitable symptoms are felt. Depression causes patients to attribute their mood and their disinclination to activity to a somatic symptom in preference to an outright admission of misery. It seems to them more respectable, and it certainly engenders a more satisfactory attitude in family and friends. Admitted depression is apt to elicit exhortation—'pull yourself together'—whereas severe backache evokes a suitable degree of commiseration. In this way the patient, to his or her own disadvantage, misleads the doctor, and treatment directed to the actual disorder present is avoided.

Thus, it is common for neurotic patients with little or no backache to receive physiotherapy or osteopathy rather than the psychological assistance that they really need.

When a patient with backache is examined on the lines described—articular signs, dural signs, nerve root signs, combined with tests for other joints and muscles—the patient who has no organic lesion answers at random and produces multiple inconsistencies and the self-contradictory pattern typical of neurosis emerges. It is not the absence of signs that enables a diagnosis of neurosis to be made; it is the presence of incongruity between what hurts and what does not hurt, and where; what is limited and what is not limited from one moment to another. In order that this pattern can emerge, a large number of movements, some relevant, some irrelevant, must be tested, consistency or inconsistency being noted throughout. This is important, for many depressed or nervous people have perfectly genuine backaches. The actual emotional state of the patient is not relevant in reaching a diagnosis, although it weighs considerably in reaching a decision on treatment. Clearly, active measures are unsuited to patients too nervous to bear any discomfort, even in the presence of a slight organic lesion. Considerable care should be taken not to confuse genuine backache in a neurotic patient with neurasthenic pain; hence inquiries concerning the patient's domestic circumstances and attitude to life are made only *after* the physical examination. For the same reason, whether a compensation claim is pending is not asked until after the examination is completed, so as to avoid prejudice.

In the survey of a thousand consecutive patients, 5% were of slight organic lesion in a neurotic patient and only in a further 2.7% were the symptoms wholly psychogenic. The clinical impression was that they were much commoner than that—a notion that clearly reflects the much greater time that such patients need to relate their history, and the concentration of the doctor's effort when they are examined, often several times, before a firm conclusion can be reached.

My psychological colleagues at St Thomas's report that the type of case which reaches the orthopaedic physician because of somatic symptoms due to depression is particularly difficult to help. Although they confirm the diagnosis regularly enough, they find the prognosis poor.

## COCCYGODYNIA

This may be referred or may arise locally.

### Referred Coccygodynia

Coccygodynia can arise from a lumbar disc lesion as a result of both segmental and extrasegmental reference (Cyriax 1954). This view was confirmed by Bohn et al. in 1956, who found that stimulating the fourth sacral root gave rise to coccygeal pain. In 0.5% of Fernström's cases, coccygeal pain was provoked at lumbar discography (1960) and adhesions about the dura mater at the fifth lumbar level were found by Gill et al. (1955) to be associated with coccygodynia. One patient of mine, a woman of 48, had had five years' increasing coccygodynia, without any root pain or signs, the result of a third lumbar neuroma.

Referred coccygodynia is distinguished from a local disorder firstly by the fact that it is present not only when the patient is seated, but also at other times. Moreover, it does not necessarily follow a fall seated, although this is a possible cause both of damage to the coccyx and to a low lumbar disc. Secondly, in referred coccygodynia coughing, some of the lumbar movements and, often, straight-leg raising, increase the pain. Trial of the relevant movements, coupled with those that detect psychogenic pain, provides the diagnostic criteria. A search for local tenderness affords no assistance; for this is to be expected whichever variety of coccygodynia is present (referred dural tenderness). This ascription must always be confirmed by epidural local anaesthesia, since this happens also to be the most reliable conservative treatment. Rarely, invasion of the sacrum by neoplasm of the prostate or rectum gives rise to coccygeal pain only, but the relentless increase in pain and early loss of ankle jerk affords the clue.

## Local Coccygodynia

This mysterious complaint is in reality perfectly simple. The common cause is a flexion injury or direct contusion of the coccyx, usually as the result of a fall in the half-sitting position. When an individual sits upright on a hard surface, the weight of the body is borne by the two ischia. The coccyx lies 2 cm above this plane. It is only when the body is tilted backwards to an angle of 45° that the coccyx can become contused. Alternatively, the coccyx can receive the impact if he falls on an uneven surface or on a projection less in width than the distance between the ischia (12 cm). Less often childbirth causes an extension strain. In spondylitis ankylopoetica, fixation of the coccyx affords a minor additional discomfort.

Since the coccygeal segments occupy a restricted local area, the pain cannot spread in any direction and is felt at the coccyx only. Sitting, and the act of becoming seated, bring on the pain. Standing and lying do not hurt; walking causes pain only when the coccygeal fibres of the gluteus maximus muscle are involved. Defaecation sometimes hurts. In repeated subluxation, the patient experiences a painful click on getting up after sitting.

As the diagnosis rests on the subjective basis of the elicitation of tenderness, the elimination of psychogenic cases is a matter of importance. These are, however, much less common than is supposed. The history may help; the usual cause is aversion to coitus. Coccygeal pain of local provenance cannot spread; patients with neurotic symptoms are usually eager to describe radiation in various directions. Except in referred coccygodynia, the lumbar movements are painless. In all cases the tests for the sacroiliac joints and lower limbs are negative; hence, psychogenic symptoms are not difficult to detect if the patient is given enough rope. When tenderness is sought, it is well to start at mid-sacrum.

Four varieties of coccygodynia occur:

1. Sprain of the posterior fibres of the sacrococcygeal joint capsule.
2. Contusion of the tip of the coccyx and the tissue immediately about it.
3. Contusion of the posterior intercoccygeal ligaments.
4. Strain of the coccygeal fibres of the gluteus maximus muscle. The patient states that the pain is perceptibly unilateral, and walking may set up discomfort.

*Treatment.* Massage is almost always quickly effective (see Volume II). The alternative is the injection of triamcinolone.

A few people are born with a rigid pointed coccyx devoid of anteflexion. They sit on a spike which eventually comes to hurt. The curious fact is that these individuals start getting pain only during their thirties. The bone should be excised.

CHAPTER 18

# THE LUMBAR REGION: MANIPULATION AND TRACTION

No more controversial subject exists in medicine than the treatment of backache. Certainly, there is none in which a body of scientific men allow their judgement to be so strongly swayed by emotion. Some doctors would never allow a patient of theirs to be manipulated at all; others would themselves manipulate every case of lumbar pain. Obviously there must lie a rational way between these two extremes, which this book in the last 30 years has tried to express.

It is perfectly possible for a patient with backache to visit six different consultants on six consecutive days and be advised: rest in bed, exercises, corsetry, traction, injections into tender areas and manipulation under anaesthesia respectively. There is no other disorder in the world on which such extreme contradictions exist among equally competent medical men. There is no other disorder in which the temperament of the consultant rather than the nature of the condition determines selection of treatment. This chaos stems from failure to realize that the lumbar joints are insensitive to internal derangement (see Chapter 15). Since the lumbar joint is insensitive to displacement within it, it follows that the joint itself requires no treatment. This is indeed fortunate; for, were the state of the joint the important factor, doctors who regarded backache as incurable would be right. Moreover, spontaneous cure with advancing years would not be possible. No criterion on choice of treatment is afforded by inspection of the radiograph to discern whether the disc is thick or thin, degenerate or not, with or without osteophytes about it. What matters in disc trouble is any projection beyond the vertebral margin; since the disc itself contains no nerves, symptoms arise only when the displacement is large enough to compress adjacent sensitive tissues, i.e. the dura mater and the nerve root. Hence, the treatment of disc trouble may be directed to the disc, to the dura mater or to the nerve root, never to the joint itself. Once the concept of dural pain is accepted, hitherto inexplicable phenomena become intelligible, and treatments thought unreasonable become logically feasible. It is for these reasons that the radiograph of the bones and joints is irrelevant.

## 'Therapeutic Automatism'

An extraordinary unquestioned association exists in all—at least British—doctors' minds linking backache with physiotherapy. Asher calls it 'therapeutic automatism'. This notion is so ingrained that most medical men order physiotherapy (by which they mean heat and exercises) for any lumbar pain, without further thought or ado. When asked on what logical grounds this connection rests, they are more pained that such an awkward question should be asked than prepared to offer any justification. All back troubles pose difficult problems—there is no such thing as a simple case of backache—but the answer to none of them is conventional physiotherapy. I feel sure the association rests on the obsolete idea that physiotherapy is the treatment of intractable pain when it does not endanger life. If only doctors would abandon this notion and realize that most backache is not intractable, rational treatment would come within their purview.

Public despondency is enhanced when television programmes and newspaper articles (of which there were several in 1973) appear emphasizing what is *not* known about backache, how difficult to overcome it is, and advocating obsolete measures such as heat, rest in bed and exercises. The result is that ordinary people realize more and more that it is no good going to doctors about backache; they just are not interested and end by telling the sufferer to 'live with it'. Public media should go out of their way to lay emphasis on the great deal that exists on the positive side. Otherwise we merely give laymen a free advertisement, patients not unreasonably inferring that they can do something whereas medical men either cannot or will not do anything.

## Therapeutic Nihilism

Indications on choice of treatment in disorders stemming from the lower back are contained in the history and are also derived from clinical findings. Often these two sets of criteria carry the same suggestion, but if they conflict it is hard to decide on the best approach.

The main confusion that exists is on the conservative treatment of disc lesions. This diagnosis has left a therapeutic hiatus, largely filled today, alas, by lay manipulators. On the one hand, the realization that backache, fibrositis, lumbago, and sciatica result largely from disc lesions has deprived of the last vestige of theoretical justification the traditional measures: drugs (apart from analgesics), vitamins (particularly B1), hormones, radiant heat, diathermy, massage, exercises, injection of myalgic spots and nodules, and 'taking the waters'. On the other hand, little has replaced these obsolete types of 'treatment'; and the distress of doctors and patients at the apparent absence of effective conservative measures is heightened when told that the only radical treatment is an operation, by no means always successful, and warranted only in extreme cases. Indeed Professor Cochrane's report on back problems (1979) declares that currently available services for their treatment are insufficient and that the cost to the nation is £220 million in lost output, £40 million in sickness benefit and £60 million in drugs. He proposes no remedy apart from clinical trials!

This therapeutic nihilism is quite unjustified, for there are a number of simple treatments, none a panacea, each with its due proportion of successes. Few patients remain wholly unrelieved if conservative means are intelligently employed, and it is only for some of these few that surgery need be contemplated at all. In order to show that the phrase 'therapeutic nihilism' is justified, the following quotation from the report of the October 1954 meeting of the Orthopaedic Association is appended. A panel of seven experts sat under the chairmanship of Professor McFarland.

*Q.* 'One-third of all orthopaedic out-patients complain of low backache. Has the panel any suggestion for coping with this vast number?'

*A.* 'The panel has none.'

# TRADITIONAL TREATMENT

Myrin (1967) contrasted a series of cases of lumbar trouble treated by conventional methods (i.e. rest in bed, physiotherapy, corsetry) and by manipulation. His results were:

| | Well | Slight symptoms | Moderate symptoms | Unable to work |
|---|---|---|---|---|
| Conventional treatment | 4% | 21% | 49% | 26% |
| Manipulation | 23.5% | 23.5% | 53% | — |

Conservative treatment of the conventional type will soon become obsolete. It comprises: (*a*) analgesics, (*b*) rest in bed, (*c*) heat and exercises, (*d*) less often, heat and massage, (*e*) muscle relaxants, (*f*) support and (*g*) embrocations. These measures depend on the hope that the patient will improve with the passage of time, and the endeavour is merely to keep him as comfortable as possible meanwhile. If playing for time fails, laminectomy is often advised.

## Analgesics

These are necessary when immediate treatment directed to the lesion fails to relieve the pain adequately.

## Rest in Bed

In lumbago and minor sciatica the compression strain on the joint exerted in the erect position ceases during recumbency. Except in the elderly, the vertebral bodies tend to move apart during rest in bed, applying suction; also, the bulging posterior ligament is tautened, again with centripetal effect. Since Nachemson has shown the pressure on the disc to be one-third as great when the patient lies on his back as on his side, the supine position is to be preferred. It is often an adequate but slow, treatment. Again, in many cases of sciatica, lying down diminishes symptoms; hence, to stay in bed while awaiting spontaneous recovery passes the time more pleasantly for the patient. It is probable that much of the time lost by treating lumbago by mere recumbency could be obviated by the application of a weight-relieving corset.

## Heat, Massage and Exercises

These treatments are anachronisms, left over from the time when back troubles were thought to be muscular (Gowers 1904). But now that sciatica (Dandy 1929) and lumbago (Cyriax 1945) are widely accepted as articular lesions, it is to the disc and not to the muscles that treatment should be directed.

Originally, patients were given flexion exercises because it was thought that, if a patient could not bend forwards, mobility in this direction would be enhanced by constant endeavour. Had the lumbar joint been stiff from extra-articular causes, e.g. adhesions, this would have been reasonable, and in those days it was not realized that the limitation was caused by an intra-articular block. When disc lesions were accepted, extension exercises were substituted on the mistaken view that increasing muscle strength encourages reduction and diminishes the liability to internal derangement. One has only to consider who ruptures the meniscus in his knee—the footballer with superb muscles—to realize that vigorous use, such as fractures fibrocartilage, is more, not less, likely to be performed by the individual with really strong muscles. Moreover, during active prone extension the intra-articular pressure is almost doubled (Nachemson 1976).

Heat is a treatment for sepsis and also affords temporary comfort in incurable disorders. In disc lesions, heat and massage though futile are quite harmless, but this does not apply to exercises which are contraindicated. If the displacement is in being, exercises grind the projection against sensitive tissues and increase pain. If it is no longer present, the main object of treatment must be to keep the joint motionless in a good position, so as to avoid recurrence. Exercises maintain mobility and are therefore harmful. By contrast, teaching the patient to keep his lumbar joints still by muscular effort is most helpful. This is how exercises should be used in cases of recurrent spinal internal derangement—the inculcation of a constant postural tone that keeps the joint still. This important difference must be explained to physiotherapists, who have all learned to administer the very exercises that, for the above reasons, are so deplorable.

## Support

A fracture, once reduced, is then often immobilized in plaster. The same should apply to all suitable disc lesions. Reduction, followed by maintenance of the affected lumbar joint motionless in a good position, is logical treatment. After reduction, to keep the lumbar spine in lordosis by an effort of memory, a corset, a jacket of plastic or plaster is most reasonable.

Supports have a poor name with many patients, since they are often applied with the displacement still in being. This violates the orthopaedic principle of reduction, followed by the maintenance of reduction.

## Muscle Relaxants

The idea still persists that the pain of lumbago is the result of muscle spasm; Capener held this view as lately as 1961. It follows from this notion that the treatment should be directed to relaxing muscle spasm. Unfortunately, one glance at a patient's back during lumbago will show that he is fixed bent forwards, not in extension as he would be if the sacrospinalis muscles were really in spasm. The muscles about a spinal joint with internal derangement contract to protect it, but it is the articular lesion, not the secondary muscle guarding, that hurts. No one considers that the treatment of displaced meniscus at the knee with a springy block on extension is a drug that relaxes the hamstring muscles. To give an ambulant patient a muscle relaxant diminishes his power to keep the joint voluntarily as still as possible and thus to avoid pain. Such drugs are, therefore, contraindicated. By contrast, there is no harm in giving a relaxant to a patient in bed, when the compression strain is off the joint. It can then be hoped that the drug will enable him to move the deranged joint more during the recumbency and thus initiate reduction the sooner. A far more direct way of securing this mobility is to abolish the pain, and the secondary muscle guarding with it, by means of epidural local anaesthesia.

## Weight Loss

Patients are often advised to lose weight in order to diminish the compression stress on the lumbar joints. But fat usually accumulates in the abdomen, buttocks and thighs, thus causing little added strain on the lumbar spine. Indeed, Kelsey (1975) found that the incidence of sciatica was not influenced by weight or body bulk.

### Embrocations

Lumbago is not a skin disease; hence rubbing something into the skin is as valueless as heating the skin. Nevertheless, various ointments are regularly prescribed. I have written to the vendors of various unguents, who maintain that their product relaxes muscle spasm, to explain that the flexed posture (immortalized in the picture for 'Doan's Backache and Kidney Pills') cannot be caused by spasm of the sacrospinalis muscles—the very muscles over which the embrocation is to be rubbed. In several cases the medical adviser to the company has had the illustration changed, but not the recommendation that the liniment should be applied.

## ORTHOPAEDIC MEDICAL TREATMENT OF DISC LESIONS

The scope for conservative treatment was set out by Benn and Wood (1975). They stated that National Health Service statistics showed 13.2 million days' work to be lost each year owing to back troubles. Each year 2.7% of the entire population consults a doctor about backache. The number of disc operations each year is 5100, whereas the number of family doctors' consultations is 1 126 000. This gives plenty of opportunity for conservative treatment. The Minister of Health (Owen 1976) estimated the economic loss from back troubles at £100 million a year. It is not, therefore, an unimportant disease.

The aim of conservative treatment is threefold: to get the patient well while (*a*) out of hospital, (*b*) out of bed and (*c*) at work. Hence conservative treatment consists of: (*a*) postural prophylaxis; (*b*) manipulative reduction; (*c*) reduction by traction; (*d*) the maintenance of reduction; and (*e*) epidural local anaesthesia. These measures are set out in Volume II.

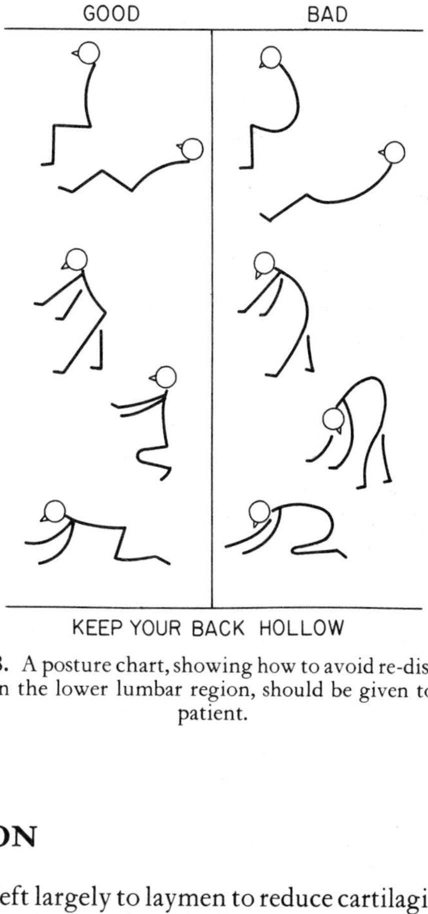


**Fig. 88.** A posture chart, showing how to avoid re-displacement in the lower lumbar region, should be given to each patient.

## MANIPULATION

Naturally, if something is out of place the obvious treatment is to restore it to its proper position; it must then be maintained there. This is clinical orthodoxy throughout the body and applies also to the lumbar joints. Therefore, unless some good reason exists, manipulative reduction should be attempted as soon as the diagnosis of a disc lesion is made. This measure is universally adopted when a torn meniscus in the knee joint has moved, but it has, till recently, been left largely to laymen to reduce cartilaginous subluxations at the spinal joints.

Schiötz's research has revealed that the first mention of this possibility was by a French doctor. Lieutand (1703–89). It was said of him, that when he had reached a diagnosis of '*entorse lombaire*', he '*savait la réduire*...' This is the first account embodying the concept of reducing a displacement as distinct from merely advocating manipulation in a non-specific way. Harrison

(1821) regarded spinal displacement as resulting from lax ligaments and also advised reduction. Nicaise (1890) states 'la bosse soit traité et reduit avec les mains'.

## Indication for manipulation

This is simply the diagnosis of a displacement and the absence of contraindications. *The positive indication is a cartilaginous displacement*, not too large and not placed too far laterally. Particularly suitable cases are subacute lumbago and patients in whom trunk flexion, and/or extension, and/or side flexion away from the painful side are found to hurt in the back. A painful arc is an encouraging sign. Two further desiderata are that the patient is not too neurotic to accept active treatment, and that he is anxious to get well. Thus, not only the type of displacement but the type of patient has to be assessed and each finding given due weight. It is unfortunate that, in this sort of work, the patient's uncorroborated (and controvertible only with difficulty) statement is paramount. If a patient who has been fully relieved of all his organic symptoms, for example by manipulation, alleges that he has been made worse, whether on account of neurosis or a compensation claim, it is difficult to refute the statement. Hence, all active treatment is contraindicated unless there is a genuine intention on the patient's part to admit improvement.

Not all small disc displacements respond to manipulation. The reason is anatomical; the protrusion may be hard or soft, i.e. composed of fibrocartilage or nuclear tissue. Naturally, the former respond to manipulation, and the latter to traction. My teaching is: 'You can hit a nail with a hammer, but treacle must be sucked.' Young, in an analysis of cases coming to laminectomy, showed that in 56% of his cases the protrusion was cartilaginous, and in 44% nuclear. My impression is that in patients not requiring operation, the proportion is more like two cartilaginous protrusions to one nuclear. Manipulation can nearly always reduce a small cartilaginous displacement, but seldom affects a pulpy protrusion. Small and very recent nuclear herniations sometimes respond, provided that the technique of manipulation is changed from the jerk to sustained pressure.

The most amusing theory to date on the effect of manipulation comes from Pace (1978; personal communication). He states: 'It is reasonably certain that manipulation is beneficial, because of what it does to the joint, separating the two cartilage surfaces and creating a vacuum which fills with nitrogen. This pain-free period of 20–30 minutes while the joint rides on a nitrogen cushion permits movement . . .'

### Is Reduction a Possibility?

No one doubts, when a click is felt at the knee and the pain and limited movement caused by a displaced meniscus cease, that reduction has taken place. But many surgeons take the view that manipulative reduction is impossible in disc displacement. The opinion is in a way well founded; for it is based on operating on patients because this particular displacement *is* irreducible. Those in whom reduction can be achieved by manipulation do not require laminectomy and are not included in these surgeons' operative experience.

No one disputes that a click in the back, felt and heard by the patient and the manipulator, may afford instant relief. Something has moved in a therapeutically desirable way. It clicked and was, therefore, hard structure. The radiograph shows that the bone itself has not moved. The only alternative is a fragment of cartilage which obviously can move inside an intervertebral joint. This fragment must, therefore, go back into place or move to a position right outside the joint. If it goes back into place it can, as at the knee, come out again and, in fact, lumbago is recognized as a very recurrent phenomenon. If it shifted farther outside the joint, lying at a point where it no longer compressed a sentient tissue, there would be no tendency to recurrence. Moreover, when a patient who had had 20 attacks of lumbago in 20 years finally came to laminectomy, 20 small extruded fragments of fibrocartilage would have to be found lying at the edge of the joint or free in the neural canal. They are not. There can be no doubt that the click, which all sides admit heralds relief from symptoms and signs, results from reduction of the loose fragment of cartilage. This was shown radiographically by Chatterton in 1949, when he demonstrated by myelogram that the defect was visible when the patient stood, but receded when he lay down. Young, at laminectomy, has reduced protrusions under direct vision, and Jirout (1969) by applying compression to a lumbar joint during laminectomy has watched a reduced displacement emerge again.

Mathew's epidurograms have demonstrated (see Plate XXXII) the flattening out after manipulation of the shadow indicating a protrusion.

Just as Jirout shows increased displacement during compression, so does Mathew's show diminished displacement after traction or manipulation.

## Historical Note

There is nothing new about manipulation, nor indeed about traction, nor even manipulation during traction. Hippocrates in the fifth century BC and Galen (AD 131 to 202) both practised it and wrote about it. About the year 1000, Avicenna in Bagdad used and taught Hippocrates's methods. Paré (1510–90) in France pointed out that severe backache could be brought on by heavy work with the spine held flexed, and included pictures on manipulative technique which have a very up-to-date flavour. Charaf Ed Din (1465) in Turkey (see Plate III/1) and Vidio (1500–69) advised and illustrated manipulation during traction. In Spain, similar illustrations are found in Mercado's book (1599) on bonesetting. The authoritative history of manipulation was written by Schiötz (1958), and the interested reader cannot do better than read his erudite and entertaining book (Schiötz & Cyriax 1975).

A book called *The Compleat Bone-Setter*, written by Friar Moulton, appeared in 1656, but it does not deal with bonesetting as it is understood today (i.e. the manipulation of joints). Wiseman in *Severall Chirurgical Treatises* (1676) states: '... I have had occasion to take notice of the inconvenience many people have fallen into through the wickedness of those who pretend to the reducing luxated joints by the peculiar name of bonesetter who that they may not want employment do usually represent every bone dislocated that they are called to look upon.' This was the very opinion that Paget deplored in his lecture 'Cases that Bonesetters Cure' (1866).

This first attempt to describe bonesetters' manipulations systematically was by Hood, a medical man who published a book *On Bonesetting* (1871) describing the methods of a bonesetter called Hutton. He makes a remark in the preface of his book that holds today as it did over a hundred years ago. 'When I first knew Hutton, I often tried to argue the point with him, and to explain what it really was that he had done. I soon found, however, that, if I wished to learn from him, I must content myself with simply listening and observing. He had grown old in a faith, which it was impossible to overturn.' As recently as 1935, osteopaths showed the same obstinacy at the inquiry in the House of Lords, though it led them into a series of untenable positions. Even today, although osteopaths have changed the lesion that they are manipulating four times since Still (1874) first enunciated the hypothesis that a displaced vertebra compressing an artery was the cause of all disease—displaced vertebra pinching a nerve, displaced sacroiliac joint, displaced disc, displaced facet—they hold fast to the hypothesis stated in the current edition of the 'Osteopathic Blue Book': Osteopaths maintain that the presence of spinal lesions exerts an influence upon the systems of the body through nerves and blood circulation, and it is held that removal of these lesions alleviates much physical disability and ill-health. Hood goes on to say: 'If surgeons will only give proof of the knowledge of the good that bonesetters accomplish, the public would then be ready to listen to any reasonable warning about the harm.' So little notice was taken of this sensible advice that I wrote in 1947, 'Clearly nothing is easier than to dismiss osteopathic theory as pure fancy. Indeed, this negative attitude has governed doctors' views in the past. But this is not enough; for there remains on the positive side the discovery of the real way in which manipulators achieve their undoubted results.' I might well have added that, if we want to obviate manipulation by laymen, this will be achieved not by denigrating the method, but by improving on these laymen. Doctors' informed selection of suitable cases and use of techniques more successful than osteopaths' will alone return manipulation to medical hands. Indeed, at the Copenhagen Congress of Manual Medicine in 1977, Brodin (Sweden) and Rasmussen (Denmark) described trials in which lumbar manipulation gave a four-fold advantage over the control group.

In 1978, Szechenyi et al. treated 50 patients with unilateral sciatica by the standard means in Hungary for six weeks (rest in bed, anti-inflammatory and muscle relaxant drugs, vitamins and physiotherapy) without improvement or alteration on the epidurogram. Protrusion was seen in 46 of these patients, at L4 and 5, 21 cases; L4, 11; L5, 11; L3–4 and 4–5, 3 cases; 2–3, 3–4, 4–5, 2 cases. Then they were all subjected to 'Cyriax's Torsical Extension'.

The results were:

1. Immediate complete relief: 18 cases, of whom the second epidurogram showed recession of the protrusion in 12.
2. Immediate improvement; full relief in three weeks: 12 cases, of whom 4 showed recession of the protrusion.

3. Improved; symptom-free in 6 weeks.
4. No better. Laminectomy.

They maintain, and I agree, that these facts indicate that one third of all patients with sciatica recover in one manipulative session.

## Reducible or Irreducible?

### History

This is often indicative. For example, a patient bends forwards and feels some aching in his back, which gets worse later in the day; next morning he finds himself unable to get out of bed because of severe lumbago. This history indicates a protrusion that has gradually increased in size—that is, one consisting of nuclear material. By contrast, the patient who is subject to attacks, initiated by a click in the back followed by sudden agonizing lumbar pain fixing him in flexion, has clearly suffered an abrupt cartilaginous displacement, suited to manipulations. Since the nucleus pulposus has ceased to exist by the age of 60, nuclear protrusions do not occur in the elderly. Hence, the older the patient with a small displacement, the more certain that it is cartilaginous and will respond to manipulation, whether causing lumbar, gluteal or sciatic symptoms.

*Primary posterolateral protrusions* causing sciatica are nearly always irreducible by manipulation. This is indicated when a patient with a low lumbar disc lesion states that his pain began in the calf or thigh without previous backache. Naturally, a central displacement impinges first against the dura mater, thus causing backache before it sets up sciatica; primary posterolateral protrusions never touch the dura at all, hence premonitory backache is absent. By contrast, secondary posterolateral protrusion (i.e. pain in the back followed by root pain is often suited to manipulation unless gross lumbar deviation or neurological weakness has supervened.

The *self-reducing disc lesion* is characterized by a different history. The patient wakes comfortable but, as the day goes on, backache develops. This becomes worse, especially after exertion or stooping. A night's rest once more abolishes the pain. Naturally, if the posterior bulge at the joint recedes spontaneously as soon as the compression strain on the joint is released, only to recur when the joint bears weight again, the reduction brought about by manipulation is equally unstable and ephemeral. Alternatively, the patient may describe backache coming on after sitting some time, relieved by standing up. Many state that they have to get out of a car every half hour for a few minutes—an indictment of the shape of car seats. Clearly, if restoration of the lordosis results in the nuclear protrusion receding again, the problem is not reduction but its maintenance, and ligamentous sclerosis is called for.

The *mushroom phenomenon* results from compression; it, too, is not amenable to manipulation, since no manoeuvre can relieve the affected joint of the compression due to body weight during standing. *Spondylolisthesis* with a secondary disc lesion is treated in the same way as an uncomplicated disc lesion, but the tendency to recurrence is much enhanced. When ligamentous stretch secondary to spondylolisthesis is the cause of backache, manipulation is of course useless. *Recurrence after laminectomy* is not a contraindication to an attempt at manipulative reduction, but it seldom succeeds if the lesion at the joint operated on, but often works well if another joint contains the displacement.

### Physical Signs

Manipulative reduction is so regularly successful in recent lumbago that it should always be attempted unless the pain is so severe that the endeavour proves impossible to bear; if so, epidural local anaesthesia is substituted. The appearance of the patient's back is most informative. If no deviation is seen while he stands or during as much flexion as he is capable of, one session of manipulation often suffices. If he stands symmetrically but deviates on trunk flexion, reduction will probably take two sessions. If he deviates considerably as he stands, the displacement is large and two to four attempts may be required; some relapse between sessions is to be expected. Displacements at the fourth level do best on rotation strains, the ilium on the painful side being drawn forwards, whereas at the fifth level the prone extension manoeuvres are usually the most effective. Just about half of all cases of lumbago get well in one treatment. Barbor (1955), dealing only with recent cases, fully relieved 57% in one treatment. This was confirmed by Fisk (1971) who found that 170 out of 369 patients were put right by one session of manipulation (46%). MacKenzie has written an entire book on the treatment of backache by lumbar extension (1981).

Nuclear protrusion causing acute lumbago presents a difficult problem. The patient wakes unable to get out of bed because of severe lumbar pain the day after doing much stooping and lifting. However, effective mechanical traction makes acute lumbago considerably worse, and no one with twinging lumbago should ever be given strong traction. While he lies stretched on the couch the pain ceases, but when the pull is abated he suffers a series of agonizing pains. In consequence, the traction may have to be released very slowly and it may take three or four hours to get the patient off the couch, none the better for this ordeal. Hence the best must be done with manipulation by sustained pressure followed by making the patient lie deviating in the way that reverses his lateral deformity. Alternatively the effect of epidural local anaesthesia must be tried followed by getting him to stand and practise side flexion repeatedly in the hitherto impracticable direction. MacKenzie's and my manoeuvres are strongly indicated (See Volume II). If all else fails, constant pelvic traction in bed is called for, kept up for some days until the symptoms have abated considerably. Only then can daily traction on the couch be cautiously begun.

In lumbago, the choice between manipulation and traction does not arise. In backache however, this is the constant problem. A sudden onset, a click, or the existence of a painful arc, with or without momentary deviation, suggests a small mobile fragment and augurs well for manipulation. If one of the lumbar movements other than flexion hurts in the thigh or calf rather than in the back or upper buttock, manipulation seldom succeeds. Reduction by manipulation may prove difficult or impossible in patients under 60 years old who have their greatest pain on pinching the lesion, i.e. on side flexion towards the painful side. → nuclear lesion.

Impaired conduction along the relevant root shows the protrusion to be larger than the aperture whence it emerged. Hence this finding should be regarded as an indication of irreducibility, whether the lesion was originally of cartilage or nucleus. The only exception to this rule is in recurrent sciatica, when the weakness, etc., may have continued since a previous attack and be irrelevant to the present bout, which may well be caused by a small and recent protrusion, quite easy to reduce. In backache the sign that suggests that manipulation will succeed easily is the partial articular pattern, i.e., some lumbar movements hurting at their extreme, some not, the pain being felt in the centre or at one side of the lower lumbar region or upper buttock. A typical pattern would be trunk flexion hurting (it does not matter whether flexion is limited or of full range); extension merely uncomfortable; side flexion towards the painful side not painful, whereas away from that side does hurt. A painful arc is favourable. In sciatica, reduction seldom proves difficult if: (*a*) the backache continued when the root pain came on; (*b*) the lumbar movements other than flexion hurt in the back rather than the limb; (*c*) there is no gross deviation or neurological weakness; (*d*) the root pain is recent and straight-leg raising only moderately limited.

When, as may happen, the symptoms and signs point in opposite directions, the one suggesting traction the other manipulation, it is always worth while making one attempt. During the first session of manipulation, it usually becomes quickly clear whether reduction by this means will prove feasible or not. By contrast, traction often has to be continued daily for a good week before its effectiveness can be ascertained.

If then neither the patient's age, nor physical signs afford a pointer to the consistency of the displacement, manipulative reduction should be attempted forthwith. If it fails, traction is substituted the next day. The reverse policy wastes a great deal of time.

## Contraindications to Manipulation

Manipulation is contraindicated in all lumbar disorders not caused by a disc lesion. Other contraindications are as follows.

### Danger to the Fourth Sacral Root

A complaint of bladder weakness causing frequency of micturition without a strong urge affords an absolute bar to manipulation. Pain in the perineum, rectum, scrotum; impotence; paraesthesia in the genital area, saddle area or anus, all suggests that the third and fourth sacral roots are menaced by the protrusion and that the posterior ligament is bulging considerably and possibly partly ruptured. If so, manipulation may rupture it completely and allow massive extrusion of the entire disc. This has happened, but not (so far, I am happy to say) at our hands.

### Hyperacute Lumbago

Ordinary patients with reasonably severe lumbago stand manipulation well, and most receive immediate relief. If the twinges of severe pain are such that no movement at the lumbar spine is possible, the patient holding himself quite rigid, manipulation is intolerable and the attempt unkind and unreasonable. In such cases: (*a*) when asked to turn to lie prone, it takes the patient some minutes to roll over; (*b*) when gentle pressure is applied to the patient's back, unbearable pain is set up. These patients should all be treated by the immediate induction of epidural anaesthesia.

*Oscillatory techniques.* Percussion was practised by Balfour in 1819 and Recamier in 1838. Manual vibrations (about ten a second) were given to patients immobilized by severe lumbago from the turn of the century by Edgar Cyriax, but they were altogether too gentle to have much effect. Osteopaths use a coarser oscillation which they describe (with cheerful disregard for English usage) as 'articulating'. Maitland (1964) also moves the affected joint by a series of small pressures, about two a second. In my experience, in these severe cases, this type of manoeuvre has to be carried on for a long time, e.g. on and off for half an hour, but persistence affords relief. Maitland, however, assures me that it is seldom necessary to go on for longer than five minutes.

## Pregnancy

During the first four months, the pregnancy can be disregarded. During the next four months, the supine and side-lying rotation manoeuvres can still be employed. During the last month, manipulation is impracticable, and rest in bed or epidural local anaesthesia should be substituted.

## Spinal Claudication

In this disorder, the cauda equina is compressed sufficiently to impair circulation within the nerve roots themselves. The existence of this syndrome must therefore imply considerable bulging of the posterior longitudinal ligament, possibly spinal stenosis as well. Hence manipulation, though it has not been tried by us, must be regarded as contraindicated.

## Anticoagulant Treatment

Intraspinal haematoma formation has been described after chiropractic manipulation for sciatica in a patient taking warfarin (Dabbet et al. 1970). The haemorrhage extended from the sixth to the twelfth thoracic vertebra and required surgical removal.

## Aortic Graft

No case of rupture of the junction of an aortic graft has been reported, but this can reasonably be regarded as a contraindication.

## Neurosis

It is very tempting to manipulate the back of a psychoneurotic patient when examination discloses a genuine minor disc displacement. The patient assures the physician that his or her nervous state is not as serious as all that and the treatment is given, the patient leaving the department happy and pain-free. That evening, he or she has doubts about the consequences of the symptoms ceasing, and by midnight severe pain is alleged and the family doctor is called during the night to cope with an hysterical attack. Naturally, this does not endear him to manipulation.

The patient should be warned, in the presence of a relative, not to succumb to a 'post-manipulative crisis' and the doctor warned that, if he is sent for on this account at night, he should not go. These precautions will usually prevent the family doctor being put to trouble for what is really the manipulator's fault; for he should have noticed the neurosis as well as the disc lesion and taken corresponding care.

Neurotic patients whose backache has no organic basis should not be treated by manipulation. It is useless; and if the patient's emotional state happens to get worse about this time, the treatment will be blamed. The family doctor should be apprised of the state of affairs and the hospital social worker asked for a report on what can be done to help. Psychological referral may prove necessary. Quite apart from the fact that manipulation is treating a non-existent disorder, there are three further disadvantages: (*a*) Proper treatment to relieve the patient's depression is being withheld. Though he prefers treatment to the lesion not present than to the lesion present, it is the physician's duty not to offer a placebo when effective treatment may well exist. (*b*) It harms the reputation of manipulation when patients without an organic lesion report, as they so often do, years of futile manipulation by laymen. (*c*) At training schools for physiotherapists, manipulation, or, indeed, any other form of physical treatment given for psychological reasons has the unfortunate effect of bewildering the student and of fostering the pernicious notion that physiotherapy is a second-rate form of psychotherapy.

Compensation neurosis should not be treated by manipulation or physiotherapy. The patient has no desire to get better—indeed, he would be the poorer if he did; he attends hospital because his solicitor considers his case weakened if the client alleges severe symptoms and is not receiving 'hospital treatment'. Alternatively he wishes to be able to say that even treatment advised by an expert has failed or had aggravated the disorder. Such cases should be left until the suit is concluded; but few plaintiffs bother to visit the doctor again afterwards.

## Manipulation is Useless

Manipulation is useless but not harmful and thus not exactly contraindicated in the following types of disc lesion:

### Too Large a Protrusion

This declares itself in three ways:

*Neurological Signs.* Signs of impaired conduction along the nerve root, i.e. muscle weakness, sluggish or absent reflex, cutaneous analgesia, indicate that the protrusion is larger than the aperture whence it emerged and manipulation will fail. So will traction.

*Lumbar Deformity with Sciatica.* Protrusion in patients with sciatica (i.e. root pain with little or no backache, *not* backache with slight sciatic radiation) coupled with a considerable lateral deviation at the lumbar spine nearly always prove irreducible whether they cause neurological deficit or not. Side flexion in one direction barely reaches the vertical and shoots a pain down the lower limb.

*Sciatica in Flexion.* The pain is in the lower limb and the patient is reasonably comfortable sitting or standing slightly flexed. An attempt to stand erect shoots a severe pain down his leg and lumbar extension is markedly limited. Whether neurological signs coexist or not, manipulation is painful and useless.

When the lumbar spine is fixed in flexion or in side flexion deformity owing to root pain, all conservative treatment is likely to fail, and the only successful measure is laminectomy.

### Too Soft a Protrusion

Nuclear protrusions do not respond to manipulation but do well on traction, except in acute lumbago. They identify themselves by a gradual onset, the pain slowly increasing after—not during—stooping or sitting, sometimes not till the next day. In these cases, side flexion of the lumbar spine towards the painful side often hurts, and is a sign that manipulation is likely to fail. Pulpy protrusions do not occur in the elderly, in whom the nucleus has degenerated and is no longer soft.

Primary posterolateral protrusions (i.e. sciatica without immediately preceding backache) all appear to be nuclear; for manipulation always fails whereas, during the first few months, traction is regularly successful. However, recurrence soon after full reduction is a commonplace.

### Too Long Duration

There is no time limit in backache. However long the displacement has persisted, there is always some chance of successful reduction; my maximum to date is a constant displacement of 36 years' standing and my previous record was 22 years. In root pain, without backache, six months is the limit, counting from when the pain in the limb became established, not from the onset of the preceding lumbar pain. After the age of 60, there is no time limit, especially in those who retain some backache after the root pain has appeared.

### Compression Phenomena

The elderly patient who gets pain in the back or leg after standing for, say, ten minutes is suffering from the mushroom phenomenon, i.e. posterior bulging when the joint is compressed. This cannot be altered by manipulation. The patient with a pulpy self-reducing disc lesion awakes comfortable and is without pain for the first few hours. Then the ache comes on and continues for the rest of the day, but is once more abolished by the decompression of a night's rest. Since reduction takes place every night, manipulation, even if it secures reduction, proves equally transient.

### Post-laminectomy

Manipulation seldom succeeds in recurrence after laminectomy, but there is no harm in trying, particularly if the signs suggest that this is a fresh protrusion at another joint. Traction is often successful in recurrence after operation. By contrast, mid or upper lumbar disc displacements secondary to a low lumbar arthrodesis often reduce quite easily.

### Unfavourable Trunk Movements

In patients under the age of 60, when trunk flexion hurts on the side towards which the patient leans, manipulation usually fails in backache, but not in lumbago. If any trunk movement other than flexion hurts in the lower limb instead of the back, manipulation is almost certain to fail. Over the age of 60, these rules no longer apply. If pressure on the lumbar spine gives rise to root pain in the lower limb while the patient lies prone, the manipulation is clearly pressing the protrusion harder against the nerve root, and the attempt should be abandoned at once.

## Dangers of Manipulation

### Aggravation

As long as anaesthesia is avoided, this is a rare event since, if unfavourable signs show themselves, the examination which follows each manoeuvre discloses them. Manipulation is discontinued.

### Fracture of a Transverse Process

When pressure to left or right of the lumbar spine is applied, a transverse process may snap. The click is felt much more sharply than that of a fragment of annulus shifting. This accident is of very little moment, since the pain is never severe and lasts only a week or two. The incidence is about 1 in 10 000 cases.

## Technique of Manipulation

Manipulation should be carried out unless some contraindication exists. In practice, it is found that about two-thirds of all cases of backache, and one-third of all cases of sciatica, prove amenable to manipulative reduction. The patient lies prone on a low firm couch and the extension and rotation strains described in Volume II are applied. The more the lumbar spine deviates, the more reliance should be placed on the rotatory manoeuvres. After each attempt, the effect is estimated by, if coughing hurt originally, asking the patient to cough; if straight-leg raising was limited, ascertaining its range again; if one or more trunk-movements hurt, asking the patient to stand and try them again. Manipulation is successful quickly or not at all; hence one, two or three, or at the most four sessions are required. Each lasts about 20 minutes; for no patient, however willing, can relax adequately after this time and it is useless to go on.

Since patients with backache and lumbago are so often sent to a physiotherapist for treatment, and most of them require manipulation, it is clear that during her undergraduate time, she must learn how to manipulate. At St Thomas's Hospital during my 35 years there, I taught these methods to all my students, and the patients were treated by them. This is a policy that I recommend to all schools. After all, most doctors in general practice clearly have not the time, inclination, assistants, or a proper couch for carrying out such manoeuvres themselves. It must, therefore, be made possible for them to send suitable cases to every graduate physiotherapist for this purpose.

## Anaesthesia for Manipulation

For a *set* manipulation, anaesthesia is often an advantage, By 'set' is meant a manipulation during which the operator knows what he is proposing to do and requires no assistance from the patient. The reduction of a fracture, of a dislocation and of the cartilage at the knee, affords examples of a set manipulation.

General anaesthesia must not be employed for disc lesions. The disc lesion that has previously been reduced under anaesthesia is, in my experience, at least as easily reduced on another occasion without. When manipulation under anaesthesia is attempted because it has failed without, renewed failure is to be expected, for it is not the manipulation that is at fault, but the protrusion which is irreducible.

When reduction is attempted at any spinal joint, the manipulation is *not set*. The reason is that examination can show that a displacement is present, but cannot indicate whence it emerged, i.e. whether reduction involves pushing it to the left or right or centre. Therefore, one manoeuvre is tried and its result on the physical signs assessed. If it has done good, it should be repeated. If it has not, another technique should be used, and the result assessed again, and so on. This is repeated until in successful cases the patient can move the affected joint in each direction painlessly. This can be determined only in the conscious patient, who cooperates throughout. Under anaesthesia, none of this knowledge is available to the operator, who has no means of knowing even whether he is making the patient better or worse. This deprivation is much more important than additional relaxation. Most orthopaedic surgeons warn about the dangers of spinal manipulation, and in so far as this relates to the practice of manipulating under anaesthesia. I fully agree with them. But these warnings do not apply when manipulation is performed with due safeguards on selected conscious patients.

Lay manipulators seldom employ anaesthesia, and to that extent are reasonably safe, but their lack of medical knowledge prevents their exercising proper selection of cases. Hence they are forced to manipulate all comers, whatever the lesion present, and just await events.

## SUSTAINED TRACTION

Just as the first approach to a displaced fragment of cartilage is manipulative reduction, so does a nuclear protrusion call for immediate reduction by traction, unless some contraindication exists. Traction for the reduction of pulpy disc protrusion was first suggested many years ago (Cyriax 1950), but was used long before discs had ever been heard of. MacKinney's book (1965) contains a reproduction of lumbar manipulation during mechanical traction taken from a fourteenth-century translation of Albucasis's *Surgery*. In Charaf Ed-Din's manuscript (1465) is shown a traction-couch for spinal trouble (Plate III/1). Schiötz (1958) reproduces in his paper the method of traction employed by an Arabian physician, Abü Qàsim (AD 1013–1106). Plate IV/1 shows the Hippocratic method of applying a sharp jerk to all the spinal joints, as described by Appolonius of Kitium 2000 years ago. The patient hangs head downwards with his feet tied to the top rung of a ladder. By ropes over a pulley, two men hoist the ladder vertically, well clear of the ground, and suddenly let go. The bottom of the ladder hits the ground, and the patient's momentum imparts a strong distraction to all his spinal joints. This is the same jerk as is used today by osteopaths lifting the patient back to back. Guidi illustrates a traction table in his *Chirurgia* (1544) and Plate III/2 shows one of his machines, now in the Wellcome Historical Museum, London. Riadore (1843) states that Chesher's method of stretching a patient by pulleys attached to a cervical collar and a pelvic belt cause 2–7 cm lengthening owing to ligamentous elasticity. Similar results were obtained by Worden and Humphrey in 1964. They found that traction of 60 kg for an hour resulted in an increase in the length of the body of 1 to 30 mm. The individual then lost height at the rate of 4 mm an hour. The ages of the patients were not stated but the photographs all show young men. This was confirmed by Levernieux (1960) who found that, in an excised lumbar spine, traction of 10–30 kg increased each joint space by 1.5 mm.

Distraction at the affected joint has three effects: (*a*) Increasing the interval between the vertebral bodies, thus enlarging the space into which the protrusion must recede. (*b*) Tautening

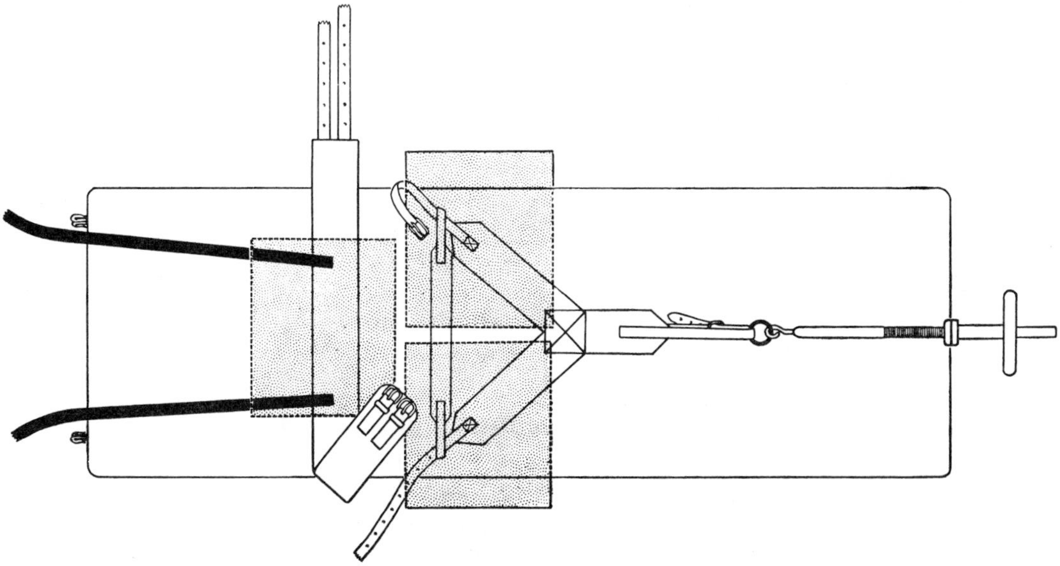

**Fig. 89.** The position of the straps before the patient lies down.

the posterior longitudinal ligament. Naturally, when the slack is taken up, the ligament joining the vertebral bodies tightens and exerts centripetal force at the back of the joint. (*c*) Suction. This draws the protrusion towards the centre of the joint.

Traction is likely to achieve positively what recumbency achieves in a neutral manner. In the erect position, the joint is compressed, and lying down avoids this squeeze. Traction affords positive decompression. It represents a way of achieving quickly, while the patient remains up and about, what would otherwise take perhaps weeks in bed. Since the intention is to bring about more reduction in half an hour than the ambulant patient can reverse by making his joint bear weight all the rest of the day, the distracting force must be (*a*) as strong as possible, (*b*) given daily and (*c*) continuous (see Levernieux's discograms before, during and after traction in Plate XXXIX). Continuous traction fatigues the muscles; they relax and the strain now falls on the joint. For this reason, the rhythmic traction that so many osteopaths use is impressive rather than effective. It takes three minutes for electromyographic silence to be attained after traction begins; hence, pulls of shorter duration merely elicit the stretch reflex and exercise the sacrospinalis muscles without distracting the joint surfaces. Electromyography (Wyke 1980) shows that as the distracting force is increased, so does motor activity increase. This continues until the traction stimulates the mechanoreceptors in the tendons. As soon as this inhibitory effect starts, motor activity falls and the joint takes the strain. Hood et al. (1981) found that electromyography showed the activity in the sacrospinalis muscles to be the same after continuous or intermittent traction continued for longer than 3 minutes. Technique of traction is described in Volume II.

## Indications for Traction

At the lumbar joints, manipulation and traction are to some extent interchangeable. While it is true that some protrusions prove irreducible by traction yet reducible by manipulation and vice versa, others respond to both measures. However, since manipulation is so much the more quickly effective, if the choice is in real doubt, manipulation should be tried once. If it fails, no time is lost, and the patient feels assured that he is attending for the slower method of securing reduction with good reason. Sometimes, considerable improvement may be achieved by manipulation, the residual displacement not proving amenable to further attempts. Even so, such partial reduction saves the patient several sessions of traction.

### Nuclear Protrusion

The patient is under 60 years old and describes the gradual onset of pain in the back or lower limb, appearing or increased after stooping or sitting. The lumbar spine has to be maintained in kyphosis before the symptoms increase; the aggravation may start next day. The signs of irreducibility (e.g. neurological deficit) are absent.

The signs suggesting that traction will succeed but manipulation fail are: trunk side flexion towards the painful side increases pain; trunk movements, other than flexion, hurt down the lower limb; primary posterolateral protrusion.

### Indeterminate Protrusion

The consistency of the protrusion is uncertain; manipulation has been tried and has failed or proved only partly successful.

It may happen that, although the protrusion consists of annular material, the adjacent vertebral surfaces have closed in behind it and the path for its return no longer exists. In such cases, the separation of the articular surfaces by traction restores the original width of the joint space and suction then induces reduction.

### Fourth Sacral Reference

If reduction is to be attempted in cases with pain referred to the genital area or coccyx, traction must be attempted with caution at first. Even this measure is not entirely safe, for marked weakness of the bladder developed immediately after traction for sciatica in one patient (unhappily not seen by myself, so I do not know if any contraindications to traction were present or not). Laminectomy was performed the next day, and full control was restored.

### First and Second Lumbar Disc Lesion

At these levels, in primary disc lesions, manipulation has always failed at my hands, whereas traction is regularly successful. In disc lesions secondary to lower lumbar arthrodesis, however, manipulation often succeeds.

### Recurrence after Laminectomy

Manipulation is seldom successful, but can safely be attempted. Traction is more often effective, but the prognosis is, of course, less favourable in those who have, than in those who have not, had the operation.

## Contraindications to Traction

### Acute Lumbago

This is *the* contraindication to traction, and unwisely giving this treatment in such cases is responsible for most of the reports of severe unfavourable reactions. Lumbago with twinges is made much worse for several days by one session of traction. As soon as the force is applied pain ceases, straight-leg raising reaches full range and all seems to be going well, but as soon as the tension is diminished even slightly, the patient gets such agonizing twinges that the force cannot be reduced. It may take a patient three or four hours to get off the couch, and at the end of this ordeal he is as bad as before starting. Surprisingly enough, the twinges are abated but not abolished by the induction of epidural local anaesthesia, and are best treated by a rotation manipulation as the patient lies there. But he should never have been given traction in the first place.

### Cartilaginous Displacements

Sustained traction is not suited to small annular displacements which should be reduced on the spot by manipulation.

### Certain Cases of Sciatica

In patients with neurological deficit or gross lumbar deformity maintained by root pain, the attempt at reduction will fail whether manipulation or traction is tried, and for the same reason: the protrusion is larger than the path by which it emerged. The uselessness of traction in sciatica with neurological deficit was confirmed in a controlled trial by Weber (1973).

Sciatica in a patient aged under 60 years old which has persisted for six months has passed the time limit. It is too late for traction or manipulation.

### Fixation in Flexion

Most patients fixed in flexion are suffering from acute lumbago and are therefore unsuited to traction. If fixation in flexion is present with more chronic pains in the back or lower limb, it is usually impossible to give traction, since no position can be found in which the pain is not increased as soon as the stretch is applied.

### Protrusion in Old Age

In patients over 60, the disc has undergone degeneration and the nucleus has ceased to exist. Hence, manipulation, not traction, is the treatment of choice. Elderly patients, the emphysematous or those with impaired cardiac or respiratory function may find the thoracic harness an embarrassment.

### Embarrassed Ventilation

Patients with cardiac failure, emphysema or asthma may not be able to lie down at all, let alone tolerate the thoracic harness. By contrast, a healed laparotomy scar provides no bar, for the tension on the abdominal muscles during traction is less than on merely bending backwards.

### Long-standing Primary Posterolateral Protrusions

Primary posterolateral protrusions all consist of nuclear material and respond very well to traction, whereas manipulation has no effect. Hence such a protrusion of a month or two's standing should be reduced by daily traction. However, in this type of lesion, the tendency to relapse after reduction is considerable. If then this is a second attack or the protrusion has continued for three or four months, it is sounder to leave it where it is, especially in a young patient with slight pain only—the common situation. Spontaneous recovery usually takes nine months from the onset of root pain, and the strong tendency to recurrence is largely obviated by allowing the patient to get well of himself. He should be kept under observation until the protrusion is stable at its maximum size, i.e. the range of straight-leg raising has stopped decreasing and is found unaltered at two examinations a fortnight apart. This is the moment for one or two inductions of epidural local anaesthesia which usually abolish the root pain in a few weeks.

### Manipulation has Failed

Traction should not be given immediately afterwards, or it may make the pain worse. The patient should attend the next day, unless he has been treated early in the morning, when he can return in the late afternoon.

### Traction in Bed

Patients with acute lumbago, the result of a nuclear protrusion, set a very real problem. They cannot, as in nuclear backache or sciatica, be treated in the logical way, i.e. by daily traction, since this measure makes acute lumbago worse. An attempt at manipulative reduction may not achieve much and epidural local anaesthesia also fails, affording some hours' relief only. Apart from leaving the patient in bed for as long as fortune dictates in the old-fashioned way, only one alternative exists—sustained traction during recumbency.

The foot of the bed is fitted with a pulley and raised 30 cm on blocks. A pelvic belt is applied, to which a cord with a 20 kg weight is attached. Traction is sustained continuously for up to a week—until a cough no longer hurts, straight-leg raising has become full and the constant ache has ceased. The patient is left free in bed for a day and then tries getting up for increasing periods daily. During the first few days up, he may stand or lie but not sit.

This method of traction works well in nuclear acute lumbago, getting the patient on his feet again in, say, a week instead of a month. It has nothing in common with adhesive plaster on one or both legs and, usually, 3 kg weights. So small a distracting force does not overcome the frictional resistance of the leg on the bedclothes and is indentical with lying in bed without traction—a view endorsed by Jennett (1974). Moreover, this way of applying even a useless degree of traction carries with it an appreciable risk of venous thrombosis; hence, it should be abandoned.

## THE VERTETRAC MACHINE

The vertetrac traction belt was invented by Stabholz in Israel. He kindly lent it to Miss Hickling at St Thomas's Hospital and to me. It consists of two U-shaped steel bars, strapped to the patient so that the lower bar rests on the iliac crests and the upper bar engages against the lower ribs. These bars are strapped on by anterior bands to make a tight fit. They are held apart by two vertical rods posteriorly. These are lengthened by a ratchet device whereby the thoracic harness is moved upwards on the stationary iliac harness as the patient stands. Posteriorly, there is also a screw attached to a lumbar pad for increasing the lumbar lordosis if necessary.

This machine was lent to us to try to test if it was in any way superior to our traditional method of giving traction lying flat (Cyriax 1949). We had little success with it and we abandoned it after a two-months' trial.

## COMMENT

There is a stage in the development of almost every disc lesion when it is reducible. The early cartilaginous displacement responds to manipulation, the nuclear to traction. If these two simple and logical measures were employed at once as a routine, the immense amount of invalidism caused by back troubles would be reduced to a tiny fraction of today's figures. (This has already been proved in Germany and Norway.) Patients would benefit; so would industry; sickness insurance would be saved large sums of money.

CHAPTER 19

# THE LUMBAR REGION: EPIDURAL LOCAL ANAESTHESIA

The most effective treatments for low lumbar disc lesions are manipulation, traction and epidural injection. Manipulation or traction is called for in a reducible displacement. The epidural injection is suitable to those cases in which the protrusion cannot be shifted, and the endeavour is then to deal with the dura mater and the nerve root instead. It provides a most valuable method of dealing with lumbar disc lesions, with both diagnostic and therapeutic intentions. I have used this method since 1937 over 50 000 times on unprepared out-patients without disaster.

In France, Sicard and Cathelin devised the technique of the injection separately in 1901; and by 1909, Caussade and Chauffard claimed cures of sciatica after one injection. The next favourable report came from Viner in Canada (1925). There is thus nothing new about the method, except in its application. I first began to use epidural local anaesthesia in 1937, purely diagnostically, with the idea of finding out if the cause of backache and sciatica lay outside or inside the vertebral column. It was only when a proportion of patients came back after the diagnostic injection declaring themselves permanently improved that I realized I had stumbled on a method also with therapeutic applications.

## DIAGNOSTIC INDICATIONS

It is chiefly in early cases with slight symptoms, and physical signs difficult to interpret, that epidural local anaesthesia is so helpful diagnostically. This often has medicolegal importance, too, since it may be alleged that the backache is muscular or ligamentous in origin and, therefore, likely to get well without sequelae, whereas injury to cartilage is permanent and the risks of recurrence must be taken into account when damages are assessed.

### Uncharacteristic Backache

Cases are quite frequent in which neither the history nor the physical signs clearly define any one lesion. There have been no frank attacks of internal derangement; the symptoms do not vary according to posture or exertion in the discish manner; the lumbar movements cause aching in a way not much like disc trouble; there is no painful arc. To make matters worse, other tests prove contradictorily positive, e.g. of the sacroiliac joints, when the lumbar movements have already indicated that the lesion, though indeterminate, is lumbar.

### Referred Pain

There may be no backache at all, the question being whether a pain, say, in the groin has a low lumbar origin or results from perhaps chronic appendicitis or an ovarian cyst. Since extrasegmental reference from the dura mater is not widely appreciated, when a pain felt in the twelfth thoracic or first lumbar dermatome is attributed to a low lumbar disc lesion, the orthopaedic physician may well be met with incredulity, which it may need an epidural injection to dispel. Or a pain in the buttock, thigh or calf may have an undetectable origin, no lumbar movement hurting, but no abnormality being detectable in the limb itself either. This is particularly apt to happen in slight but persistent bilateral sciatica, the question in each case being whether the symptoms have a local source or are referred from the back.

### Contradictory Opinions

Various medical men, perhaps in a medicolegal case, have stated that a disc lesion is present, and others have disagreed. There is no point in taking sides in this argument since judge, patient and family doctor alike are not going to be impressed by words, of which they have already had a surfeit. The matter is resolved and confidence restored when the patient himself is made the arbiter of the diagnosis. He is kept in the dark on the same lines as for psychoneurosis (see below).

### Psychoneurosis

Then there is the patient with psychoneurosis in whom it is uncertain whether a small underlying organic lesion is present or not. In such cases, when the injection is given diagnostically, no mention is made of the nature of the fluid to be injected. After the induction, it is well to wait for at least ten minutes (since 0.5% procaine works rather slowly to achieve its full effect) and the patient must in any case be given time to recover from any giddiness caused. The question is then put misleadingly: 'I am afraid this injection may have made you a bit sore; how is your back (or limb) now?' If the patient, after so broad a hint of what to expect, nevertheless maintains that his pain has gone, and when he later stands and the lumbar movements are tested these are now painless, he clearly has a minor disc lesion.

## Diagnostic Response

The fluid runs up the neural canal and along the external aspect of the lower lumbar nerve roots (Plates XXXI, XXXIV). It does not enter any joint. This is theoretically impossible; for Nachemson (1962) has shown that even in excised specimens of the lumbar spine the ligaments exert a pressure of 0.7 kg/cm—a far greater force than that at which the solution drips into the sacrum. Moreover, the radiographs show that it does not. Nor can the solution bathe the anterior aspect of the posterior longitudinal ligament, where pressure from a protruded disc would be exerted. Procaine 1:200 is a surface local anaesthetic only; it does not penetrate the dural membrane nor the sheath of the nerve root; no lower motor neurone lesion results. The lumbar muscles and those of the lower limbs are unaffected, and the skin (except rarely over the sacrum) retains its sensitivity. The only structures rendered anaesthetic are the exterior surface of the dura mater and nerve roots. Presumably the posterior surface of the posterior longitudinal ligament and the anterior surface of the ligamentum flavum are numbed too, but the effect of 0.5% procaine does not penetrate to the substance of such tissues. If, then, a patient has a lesion of the moving parts of the back and epidural local anaesthesia affords one to two hours' relief, the cause must be pressure on the dura mater or dural root sleeve without adherence. The solution can pass between two adjacent surfaces if they are merely pressed together, but cannot percolate to the point of impact if adherence or invasion has occurred. Cessation of symptoms after the injection shows that the solution has been able to pass between two surfaces and there is only one tissue apt to protrude posteriorly without invasion: a disc lesion.

In conditions like sacroiliac strain or arthritis, ankylosing spondylitis, afebrile osteomyelitis, neuroma, secondary neoplasm, claudication of the cauda equina or in the buttock, gluteal bursitis, spondylolisthesis without a disc lesion, the injection makes no difference to the pain for the time being. The response is also negative in some 5% of patients with backache whose cause remains obscure to me (see p. 348).

## THERAPEUTIC INDICATIONS

It is fortunate that epidural local anaesthesia is often an effective treatment for just those cases unsuited to manipulation or traction. The way that permanent benefit results appears different in different disorders.

### Hyperacute Lumbago

If the patient has such a large protrusion impinging via the ligament against the dura mater that he experiences severe twinges on the slightest movement, an attempt at manipulative reduction is unthinkable and even rhythmic oscillations cannot be borne. A long period in bed is then often thought to provide the only hope of eventual relief. But there is one—only one—rapidly effective treatment: epidural local anaesthesia. Failing the injection, agonizing twinges force the patient to lie motionless, his muscles guarding and compressing the joint. Hence the immobility and muscle tension are such that the gradual reduction in the degree of displacement, that relief from weight-bearing is intended to secure, begins very slowly. By contrast, the injection affords immediate, complete relief and not much pain returns when the anaesthesia has worn off. It would seem that, as the patient lies prone, during absence of compression, the free movement rendered practicable for 90 minutes by the anaesthesia allows spontaneous reduction to begin days or weeks before it would otherwise have become possible. By next morning, he is usually fairly sore but able to get up and to travel up for manipulative reduction of any residual displacement. The immobilizing twinges have been abolished.

It follows that a patient treated for severe lumbago by this injection should not be permitted to get up from the couch and walk home. He should return, as he came, by ambulance; alternatively, the injection should be given in bed at home. The patient stays recumbent till next day.

It is interesting to note that immediately after the induction of local anaesthesia, all pain ceases, but, if marked lateral deviation has been present before the injection, it often continues for a while, the patient averring that painless stiffness restricts the movement. This is theoretically correct, since the displacement is still in being, limiting joint movement, but impinging against a now insensitive structure. By contrast, as is also to be expected, all the dural manifestations cease completely; a cough and neck flexion no longer hurt and straight-leg raising on each side becomes of full range and painless.

## Intractable Backache

When backache, the result of a low lumbar disc lesion, proves refractory to both manipulation and traction, it must be regarded as caused by an irreducible displacement. The best approach is then to attempt desensitization of the dural tube, in the hope that symptoms will thus be mitigated. They often are; the constant ache may be lastingly abolished, leaving only the momentary pain on certain movements which the patient learns to avoid, or can wear a corset to prevent.

## Chronic Backache

There is a type of chronic ache in middle-aged or elderly patients in which articular signs are virtually absent. The ache is constant, little altered by posture or exertion. Examination reveals that perhaps only one lumbar movement increases it slightly; sometimes no movement makes any difference. Such a symptom can often be permanently abolished by one induction of epidural local anaesthesia. If this should fail, ligamentous sclerosis offers the only other chance of relief.

## Matutinal or Nocturnal Backache

The patient can do everything, even heavy work by day but is regularly woken in the small hours by backache severe enough to force him out of bed to walk round the room. After half an hour or so the ache subsides and he can then sleep on. Other patients wake in the same sort of pain at, say, 7 a.m., which ceases after they have been up for about an hour, and are pain-free for the rest of the 24 hours. Examination during the day reveals nothing, but the patient may make one revealing statement: that during the time his back is hurting, a cough causes pain—not otherwise. This suggests dural compression of some sort and gives the injection its theoretical justification. Often one epidural injection is curative. One patient who had to get out of bed nightly for 27 years, had two months' relief, but then relapsed after a day's digging. Failure is encountered, of course; if so, ligamentous sclerosis is indicated.

## Pregnancy

During the last month of pregnancy, backache or sciatica caused by a disc lesion is best treated by either rest in bed or epidural local anaesthesia.

## Root Pain with Neurological Signs

Signs of interference with conduction show that the protrusion has reached a size that makes reduction impossible; the bulge is larger than the aperture whence it emerged and cannot return. Desensitization of the nerve root at the point of impact is then strongly indicated by epidural local anaesthesia. It might well have been supposed that adding a steroid to the solution would enhance the desensitizing effect, but this was not so when tried out originally (Cyriax 1957) and in two recent cases, epidural local anaesthesia afforded immediate lasting relief some days after hydrocortisone by the lumbar route had no effect.

The relative value of recumbency and epidural local anaesthesia was estimated in a series of 50 patients (Coomes 1963). All the patients had sciatica with severe pain and signs of impaired conduction along the nerve root. Half the patients were admitted to hospital for bed rest; the other half received one or two epidural injections and rested at home. The conclusion was that the injected patients had largely recovered in ten days, whereas the recumbent took 30 days to reach the same degree of comfort. The injection thus saves the patient almost three weeks' pain, and the Health Service about £200 per patient. In Canada, Fraser (1976) contrasted the duration and the cost of acute lumbago treated by epidural local anaesthesia and by traditional measures, e.g. recumbency, traction in bed, heat, analgesic pills. His figures were:

| | | |
|---|---|---|
| Epidural | 3.8 days | $352 |
| Other | 15.6 days | $1448 |

The injection then is the main weapon for treating root pain with absent or sluggish reflex, one or more weak muscles, analgesic skin (not mere pins and needles). Indeed, there is no other treatment possible, unless, exceptionally, laminectomy is indicated. In hospitals where a surgeon exists who removes protruded discs but there is no physician skilled in inducing epidural local anaesthesia, numbers of avoidable laminectomies are inevitable. If laminectomy were always successful and left the patient with a strong back afterwards, this would not matter much; it would merely represent a waste of money and hospital beds. However, after operation, the patient must be permanently careful of his back, whereas those who get well with the epidural injection can go back to reasonably heavy work. Moreover, if laminectomy fails, subsequent epidural local anaesthesia is seldom effective, whereas if the injection fails, laminectomy is in no way embarrassed.

Patients in whom lumbar extension is markedly limited by pain shooting down the limb, and patients with marked lumbar deviation in whom attempted side flexion in the limited direction is restricted by severe root pain, are often refractory to epidural local anaesthesia. Indeed, it is these two types of case that often end with operation. Prognosis is impaired when the patient stands in a symmetrical posture and deviates on trunk flexion. The greater the list, the less likely the injection is to afford lasting benefit. It is my practice, when the issue is uncertain, to give the injection and wait a week. If there has been no improvement, laminectomy is indicated.

Patients with severe neurological weakness usually lose their pain fairly quickly as the result of root atrophy. Occasionally, the pressure of the protrusion falls just short of producing the requisite degree of ischaemia, and in spite of marked signs they continue to have root pain. Most such patients are permanently relieved by the epidural injection. If this does not succeed, and the root pain has continued for some months, it is no good waiting further, laminectomy being indicated at once.

Patients with sciatica who are over 60 do not respond as favourably to epidural injections as do younger people, but this is not universal, and an occasional good result is seen in patients even over 80. In third lumbar disc lesions with root pain, the injection works less well than in lesions at the fourth or fifth lumbar levels. The immediate relief is often not quite complete; a greater number of injections is required, and the failure rate is higher.

There is no theoretical limit to the number of epidural injections that can be given. However, since they are usually very effective at once, many injections are seldom required. The likely number is two or three. If the first injection has afforded no lasting benefit, there is no point in repeating it. A sinuvertebral block should be substituted. In severe sciatica, a daily injection may be required for the first two or three days, but in most cases repetition is called for only four or five days later. After a second injection in chronic sciatica it is well to wait about three weeks, since further treatment is seldom necessary. Cases do present themselves in which each injection affords a little improvement only; if so, they are continued until adequate relief has been achieved, which very seldom amounts to more than six.

One type of sciatica often requires more than the usual number of epidural injections, up to, say, five. The patient has had unilateral root pain for, say, six months and on examination does not deviate, has slight or no neurological signs but straight-leg raising is limited to 20° on the painful side and 45° on the painless side, both bringing on the unilateral sciatic pain. Immediately after the first epidural injection, the good leg rises to 90° but the range of straight-leg raising on the painful side is little increased. At the second visit, the range of straight-leg raising on the good side is found to have remained full. After the second injection, the leg on the bad side rises a little farther and progress is gradual thenceforward.

## Root Pain without Neurological Signs

There are four conditions that strongly indicate the injection.

*Root Pain that has Continued for too Long.* Root pain caused by a disc lesion at the third, fourth or fifth level should recover spontaneously in a year at the most if there is no neurological deficit and more quickly if impaired conduction is present. Cases occur in which spontaneous recovery is delayed, the pain and often limitation of straight-leg raising continuing. In these cases, the pain is not very severe but has persisted for so long that laminectomy is contemplated. These cases respond excellently to the injection, with only few exceptions. (These are the patients already mentioned with limited trunk extension causing pain in the lower limb, and those with sciatica and gross lumbar deviation while standing.) The patient has, say, 45° limitation of straight-leg raising; after the injection, full range is restored (if not, an adherent root is present). At his next visit ten days later, he states that his pain has been much less and straight-leg raising is now found only 20° limited. The injection is repeated and when seen a fortnight later, the patient has lost his symptoms and full straight-leg raising is at most slightly uncomfortable. No more need be done. The result appears to be achieved by mobilization of the nerve root during local anaesthesia, which may afford lasting desensitization there as well. The injection is very often entirely effective, and restores the patient's capacity for quite heavy work; hence, in these cases, laminectomy is strongly contraindicated until the injection has had an adequate trial.

*Full Evolution of the Root Syndrome.* This applies chiefly to young people with primary posterolateral disc protrusions at the fourth or fifth level. The patient may attend complaining of increasing pain in the calf and/or thigh after sitting which, in a month or two, becomes a constant ache. The range of straight-leg raising is diminishing and the discomfort in the limb—there is none in the back—is becoming more persistent. Epidural local anaesthesia affords no benefit in a case that is still evolving, and the choice lies between reduction by traction, or awaiting stabilization of the protrusion in the position of maximum displacement and then giving the injection. In the very early case, reduction by traction may well be preferred, but the recurrence rate is high and reduction seldom lasts a year. Since the patient is never in severe pain, it is better practice to wait and to examine him each few weeks until his range of straight-leg raising becomes stable (usually 30°–45° range); and once this point has been reached to give the epidural injection. If this is done, he is likely to recover in six months instead of spontaneously in twelve, and, having come out of his sciatica on the far side, as it were, he is much less likely to suffer recurrence. This is all explained to the patient and the choice left to him. Sometimes, there is a compromise; reduction by traction is carried out with agreement that, if the root pain recurs soon, it will then be left to evolve on the second occasion.

*Recurrent Sciatica after a Root Palsy.* Recurrence at the same level from sciatica with neurological signs is uncommon following recovery, whether spontaneous or after an epidural injection. However, it can happen that a patient who lost all his pain after a couple of epidural injections gets another attack of sciatica within a year. It might well be argued that this is a small recent protrusion and should, therefore, be treated by manipulation or traction. This is logical, but both these measures are apt to fail, whereas epidural local anaesthesia usually succeeds. This does not apply if a patient gets sciatica again many years later or at a new level.

*Root Pain without Physical Signs.* Sometimes a patient has a root pain, with or without backache, and the history suggests a disc lesion. Examination reveals a full range of painless lumbar movements, full painless straight-leg raising; no alternative cause for the pain is detected in the lower limbs either. Such root pain may be unilateral or bilateral (if bilateral, spondylolisthesis should be considered). Epidural local anaesthesia is necessary diagnostically. If the injection is successful in abolishing the pain for the time being, it is not uncommon for the relief to continue.

In these cases, one can only suppose that persistent bruising of dura mater or nerve root(s) has resulted from a past disc lesion, which has undergone sufficient reduction or shrinkage no longer to interfere with joint or root mobility. The local anaesthesia appears permanently to desensitize the tender tissue at the point of past impact. The same applies to the bruising of a nerve root giving rise to persistent sciatica after the offending disc has been removed.

## Recovering Sciatica

If there is sciatic pain without backache, even though neurological signs are absent and the case seems otherwise suitable, manipulation and traction are best avoided if reasonably intense root symptoms are subsiding. The patient has spent some days or weeks in bed and is over the worst, but still has a considerable ache in the limb and limited straight-leg raising. The treatment of choice is epidural local anaesthesia.

### Nocturnal Cramp

Severe cramp coming on each night may continue to wake a patient long after a sciatica has ceased. It occurs in the calf of the affected leg only.

Epidural local anaesthesia serves to desensitize the nerve root whence the stimulus to the cramp presumably originates, and gives the patient comfortable nights. The injection may need repetition about six months later. This approach often succeeds when muscle relaxants have failed.

### Coccygodynia

It is often difficult to know whether pain in the coccyx is local or referred, since the bone may be tender on sitting and on palpation (as a referred dural phenomenon) in either case.

Epidural local anaesthesia followed by asking the patient to sit again determines the issue at once; moreover, in referred cases it may prove curative.

## EPIDURAL INJECTION

This is a simple procedure, suitable for outpatient use. It is best to say that an injection will be given which passes between the disc and the compressed tissue (dura mater in backache, nerve root in sciatica), and will merely cause some aching. Patients who have heard alarming tales about lumbar puncture are informed that this is a different manoeuvre; that it is intrasacral, that the needle does not penetrate to the spinal fluid, and that no one has to rest in bed for 24 hours afterwards. Inquiry should be made about sensitivity to local anaesthesia. Since almost everyone has at one time or another had a local anaesthetic injection into the gum for dentistry, it suffices to ask if untoward symptoms were caused thereby. If apparent sensitivity is reported, it is more often due to adrenaline than to the anaesthetic agent itself, especially if the patient is taking an antidepressant drug. The patient is then given a test dose of 10 ml of 0.5% procaine without adrenaline into, say, the buttock. If nothing happens, the epidural injection is given next day. Technique is fully discussed in Volume II.

## CONTRAINDICATIONS

These are few, since local anaesthesia cannot itself do lasting harm.

### General Anaesthesia

It is dangerous to give the injection while the patient is unconscious; for he cannot then report that it is making him feel faint, etc. Moreover, the diagnostic action is lost, since he has only 90 minutes in which to report the effect on the pain and, even after a short-acting barbiturate, not all patients are composed enough to be sure. Moreover, it unduly complicates and makes inconvenient what is a simple measure.

### Local Sepsis

Since the introduction of bacteria into the neural canal is a disaster, the risk must not be taken. Injection must be postponed if the neighbouring skin is not clear from sepsis. If a needle has to be reinserted, a fresh one should be used.

### Previous Sepsis

Old septic adhesions at the lower end of the theca may be disturbed by the infiltration, which in one case temporarily reactivated an undiagnosed febrile neurological infection from which recovery had been complete six years before.

### Previous Laminectomy

Sterile gloves used to be packed with talcum powder, which consists of 90% anhydrous magnesium silicate, with small amounts of magnesium carbonate and zinc oxide to make up the remaining tenth. During laminectomy, enough of this powder came off the surgeon's gloves to set up a diffuse fibrosis, akin to chronic pulmonary talc silicosis. In consequence, the whole neural canal soon became filled with dense white fibrous tissue adherent to the dura mater and nerve roots and indistinguishable from them. A second laminectomy thus became extremely difficult and time-consuming and epidural injections could not reach the right area. The cause of this fibrosis was elucidated in 1946 by Lichtman et al. and their recommendation that talc should be abandoned was universally adopted within a few years. Hence, in patients whose laminectomy took place after 1950, the epidural local anaesthesia solution stands a good chance of getting to the right spot. However, postoperatively, the likelihood of lasting relief is diminished. By contrast, arthrodesis has no deleterious effect.

### Recent Myelogram

It is probably best to wait a few days before epidural local anaesthesia is induced. Whether the displacement lies above or not is immaterial.

### Sensitivity

Patients may state that they are sensitive to procaine. This is a very rare event; they are sensitive instead to adrenaline. However, in order to be certain, 10 ml of 0.5% procaine are injected into, say, the buttock. If nothing untoward happens, the epidural injection is given the next day.

### Excessive Volume of Fluid

Clark and Whitwell (1961) injected two patients suffering from sciatica with 120 ml of isotonic saline epidurally under general anaesthesia. Blurred vision caused by intraocular haemorrhage resulted. Hoffman (1950) had already reported two cases. These events provide no contraindication to the slow injection of a reasonable volume of fluid without anaesthesia, using the correct technique.

### Anticoagulant Therapy

In contrast to the importance of bleeding at the cervical and thoracic spinal levels, this does not appear to matter within the sacrum. The insertion of the needle may puncture a vein but the consequent haematoma causes no trouble then or later. I doubt if anticoagulant treatment provides a valid contraindication to epidural local anaesthesia.

## DANGERS OF EPIDURAL INJECTION

These have been grossly exaggerated. Provided the precautions outlined here are conscientiously observed, little trouble is to be expected. My experience includes four misfortunes, but no disaster, i.e. less than 1 per 10 000 injections. No sepsis has resulted.

### Hypersensitivity

One patient was highly sensitive to procaine and had, in fact, fainted several times after dental injection, a fact which he neglected to mention and when interrogated before the induction. He took 20 minutes to become unconscious, which excludes an intrathecal injection, which would have taken less than a minute. He had to be given artifical respiration for two hours before he recovered completely.

### Semipermeable Dura Mater

Two patients developed a paraplegia to the mid-thorax, which took a quarter of an hour to appear. Diaphragmatic breathing was retained, and in two hours each recovered, but in one case the injection was a therapeutic failure.

### Chemical Meningitis

Two other patients possessed a semipermeable dura mater and developed a paraplegia from the lower thorax downwards; they had to lie for two hours until muscle power returned. Some hours later, each patient complained of headache, nausea and neck rigidity. Meningism was present, next day there was fever. Lumbar puncture showed 400 mg of protein and 4000 white cells/$mm^3$. Culture was sterile. As a precaution, both patients were treated with penicillin and recovered in a week, without sequelae.

Both these cases occurred 30 years ago before central sterilization, when syringes were boiled before use. The dural inflammation was probably caused by some chemical, possibly an antiseptic, polluting the water in which the instruments lay. There had been no case in recent years.

## EXTRADURAL STEROIDS

Hydrocortisone added to the local anaesthetic solution and introduced by the sacral route was not found to help (Cyriax 1956). Using the same approach, injection of 10 ml of the suspension undiluted did not help either. However, hydrocortisone introduced extrathecally at a lumbar level has since been advocated by Barry and Kendall (1962). Harley (1966) has made an interesting film of the technique and its results. Unfortunately he used a mixture of hydrocortisone and local anaesthetic, thus leaving the issue in doubt which agent was responsible. In 1972 Harley informed me that he has now adopted the technique described in this chapter as his first choice, reserving the lumbar route for those that do not respond. Using 6 ml of 1:200 xylocaine solution mixed with 4 ml of hydrocortisone acetate (i.e. 10 ml in all) he secures relief in 70% of cases. Swerdelow and Sayle-Creer (1970) employed epidural injections in 325 unselected cases of lumbosciatic pain, using a local anaesthetic agent or methyl prednisolone. In acute cases the results were equally good with either drug but in chronic cases the steroid proved the better—the opposite of my experience. A further series of 500 unselected cases was reported by Warr et al. in 1972. They obtained 63% good results from epidural local anaesthesia followed by manipulation under general anaesthesia. This double treatment leaves the issue in doubt, but I feel sure the injection should be given the major credit. Nevertheless the combination lacks logic, since manipulation is for reducible, and epidural local anaesthesia is for irreducible, disc protrusions.

## INTRADURAL STEROIDS

The effects of steroid suspension introduced outside and inside the theca was compared by Winnie et al. (1972) in 20 cases of sciatica. They found that in each series of 10 patients, 8 were relieved by the injection of 2 ml of methyl prednisolone, whichever route was chosen. They recommend the intradural approach after repeated laminectomy or in arachnoiditis caused by contrast medium, usually pantopaque.

The theory underlying intrathecal steroid injection in sciatica is obscure, but Mathews (1972) stated that post-mortem studies of patients who had had repeated laminectomies showed evidence of root sleeve fibrosis spreading right up to the spinal cord. In such cases, and in sciatica aggravated by myelography, he too recommends intradural methyl prednisolone.

## SINUVERTEBRAL NERVE BLOCK

It sometimes happens that a patient with root pain to all appearances well suited to the therapeutic induction of epidural local anaesthesia fails to benefit. Though his pain eases and his range of straight-leg raising is increased immediately after the injection, he returns a week or two later with his symptoms and signs unchanged. Repetition of the injection, this time with added triamcinolone, yields the same long-term negative result.

In such cases the next approach is a sinuvertebral block, which has to be induced at the correct level. The main difficulty is to distinguish between the fourth and fifth lumbar levels. Since only 2 ml of 2% procaine are used, the injection is given at the likelier level; if straight-leg raising has not risen to full range a few minutes later, the injection is repeated at the other level. It may well happen that this method has lasting success after epidural injection has proved temporary only. If lasting benefit is achieved, one or two more such local injections should afford full recovery. It is surprising that this difference should exist, for the solution reaches the same spot in each case, but is in one instance in a 2%, the other 0.5%, solution of procaine.

The reverse also holds. Patients in whom a sinuvertebral block has had an ephemeral result only may be lastingly benefited by the epidural approach. On the whole, patients under 60 are likely to do best with epidural injections, but as old age advances local anaesthesia at the sinuvertebral nerve becomes increasingly effective. Again, cases of second lumbar root pain which do not respond to traction do better with a sinuvertebral block than an epidural injection.

CHAPTER 20

# THE LUMBAR REGION: OTHER TREATMENTS

The three mainstays in treatment are manipulation, traction and epidural local anaesthesia. In this chapter other methods are discussed.

## REST IN BED

In 1947 Asher wrote on 'The dangers of going to bed'. Browse (1965) agrees, stating that 'the bed is often a sign of our therapeutic inadequacy, rather than a therapeutic measure deserving of praise. The bed is the non-specific treatment of our time, the great placebo'. This is certainly so in low lumbar disc lesions. Yet rest in bed, the traditional management for lumbago and sciatica, is still universally practised. In lumbago, though tedious and time-consuming, it nearly always succeeds in the end, but this is not always so in sciatica. Resorting to rest admits failure and should be the doctor's last thought, not his first. In fact, it is seldom called for, to be contemplated only when adequate conservative methods do not succeed. Yet it is still advocated (e.g. Mathews 1977).

It has been alleged that gradual reduction by rest in bed, by causing less trauma to the joint and to the disc, results in a 'better' reduction than that secured by manipulation. This is merely an excuse for inactivity, for once the loose fragment is back in place, the agency is immaterial, except that the more quickly this is achieved, the shorter the time during which the posterior longitudinal ligament remains stretched. The idea that rest in bed allows the disc to heal is a chimera; cartilage is avascular and cannot unite.

Rest in bed in lumbago serves a double purpose; reduction and relief from pain, but in sciatica, there are two different situations; one, reduction and consequent relief; the other, relief without reduction.

### Lumbago

There is only one way of achieving recovery in lumbago: reduction. As soon as the body weight is off the joint, the centrifugal force on the disc eases greatly; hence, in lumbago the protrusion recedes to some extent and the pain is correspondingly lessened as soon as the patient lies down. The marked difference between the range of trunk flexion and of straight-leg raising illustrates this point well. The patient with lumbago may scarcely be able to bend forwards at all whereas, if the attack is not too severe, when compression on the joint stops and allows the protrusion to recede somewhat, he may regain a full range of straight-leg raising. The same applies to cough, which may hurt standing and sitting, not lying. Often, a deviation seen while the patient stands ceases when he lies down. Staying supine in bed, therefore, has three immediate effects: (*a*) the cessation of centrifugal force acting on the protrusion; (*b*) tautening of the posterior ligament as the vertebrae move apart, and (*c*) relief from pain as the bulge caused by weight-bearing recedes slightly. Hence the stress bulging the disc out backwards diminishes at the same time as relief from pain enables the patient to move more easily, and thus assist reduction.

The patient stays in bed as long as is necessary, usually one to four weeks, and is fit to get up when the attempt ceases to be unduly painful and remaining up does not cause the symptoms to return. So long as coughing hurts and straight-leg raising remains limited, recumbency continues. During the first few days he should not sit up at all. The supine position is the best since Nachemson has shown that, if the weight on a lumbar intervertebral joint of the individual standing is taken as 100, it is 25 when he lies on his back, 75 when he lies on his side.

That recumbency will effect reduction is by no means certain after the age of 60, for by then osteophyte formation and ligamentous contracture often combine to prevent the vertebral bodies moving apart when the compression of weight-bearing ceases. Hence, the older the patient is, the more his lumbar movements are limited, and the more osteophytes the radiograph shows, the more he needs manipulation rather than rest in bed for his lumbago—the reverse of what would be expected and indeed of what is commonly believed. The warm regard for lay manipulators expressed by some elderly members of the House of Lords in 1935 at the inquiry into osteopathy clearly stems partly from this fact.

*Recurrence after Recumbency.* It has been argued that rest in bed allows the disc to heal—an impossibility in an avascular structure—and that patients treated by recumbency achieve a more stable reduction than those treated by manipulation. The opposite is to be expected since immediate reduction spares the posterior longitudinal ligament prolonged stretching and thus should obviate instability due to ligamentous laxity. In fact, the figures for recurrence after either treatment are very similar and it would seem that recovery allowed to proceed gradually carries an identical prognosis with swift reduction.

My series (1957), followed up for three years showed a recurrence rate of 44% for lumbar pain and 40% for sciatica. Pearce and Moll (1967) describe 43% recurrences and Dillane et al. (1966), who treated all their lumbagos by rest in bed, also reported a 44.6% recurrence rate in four years.

*Comment.* Before lightly putting a patient with lumbago to bed, the doctor should pause to ponder the harm that results to the patient, to the community and to the doctor. The patient has a displacement that can be reduced, by one manipulation in 50% of cases. Alternatively, if the pain is too severe for that, epidural local anaesthesia can be relied on largely to abort the attack. Mere recumbency thus often condemns the patient to days or weeks of avoidable pain. Moreover, during the time that, mentally active, he lies there deploring his plight and the absence of effective treatment, ideas of industrial compensation begin to take root, as would never have happened if brisk treatment had returned him to his work in a few days. There is also the financial loss to the community, the cost of avoidable time off work being borne by either the patient or sickness insurance. Finally, there is the loss to the doctor himself in esteem and time. If the patient consults a lay manipulator who makes him more comfortable, the medical profession is regarded the less. If the doctor pays two visits the first week and one a week after that for a month (five minutes' journey there, five minutes back and ten at the bedside), this adds up to 100 minutes. Adequate examination, followed by a manipulative session, cannot take more than half this period. Hence recumbency wastes the doctor's time too.

## Sciatica

In sciatica, there are four ways in which recovery can ensue. One is reduction.

### Relief from Pain by Reduction

In minor sciatica, the patient is put to bed in the hope that relieving the compression stress on the joint will result in gradual recovery, the signs and symptoms ceasing together. The mechanism is the same as in lumbago, i.e. reduction. But if reduction is going to take place gradually during relief from weight-bearing, why not actively decompress the joint by traction? It was this argument that originally made me contemplate traction as an ambulant treatment (Cyriax 1950).

### Relief from Pain without Reduction

In major sciatica, the question of reduction does not arise. The patient gets well eventually by shrinkage of the disc, by vertebral erosion or by root atrophy; hence, the object is relief from pain during the process. The general rule is, therefore, to avoid anything that sets up the root pain; apart from that, the patient can do what he likes.

Most patients suffer less pain while in bed, and should thus be kept there until the root pain has largely abated and getting up does not return the pain appreciably. Some patients cannot lie in bed, being obliged to walk the room at night; they need morphine. Since the protrusion is fixed and maximal, getting out of bed will not increase its size, but merely cause additional pain. When the worst symptoms are over, it is for the patient to decide which he dislikes more—not doing what he wants or getting increased pain if he does. He should realize that any activity that causes ephemeral exacerbation will do him no harm, merely make the period of awaiting recovery more disagreeable. This can be succinctly explained to the patient by the injunction 'Don't do anything that hurts the leg much'. There is no point in keeping a patient of this sort in bed any longer than he wishes, or making him wear a corset.

The treatment of choice in most major sciatica is epidural local anaesthesia. This was confirmed by Coomes (1963) who found that the injection reduced the period of recumbency by two-thirds and often obviated the need for complete bed rest.

Rest in bed should not be continued for too long. If six weeks recumbency and epidural local anaesthesia both fail, laminectomy is nearly always indicated, unless there is a large neurotic element in the symptoms.

## AWAITING SPONTANEOUS RECOVERY

### Shrunken Protrusion or Vertebral Erosion

Backache shows little tendency to spontaneous cure. A possible reason is that a central protrusion remains intra-articular, covered as it is by the posterior longitudinal ligament. Posterolateral protrusion, since no ligament confines it, becomes extra-articular. In consequence the fibrocartilage loses its nutrient synovial fluid and slowly shrinks.

Backache eases only in the very long run. Between the ages of 50 and 60, the spinal joints tend to lose their range of movement owing to ligamentous contracture; moreover, at this age, osteophytes, both cupping the disc and further limiting articular movement, make their welcome appearance. Hence intermittent backache or attacks of lumbago often cease at this time of life. By analogy with lumbago, which does regularly recover spontaneously, patients are often told that their backache will soon go. Any backache may recover, it is true; but it often does not, and intermittent or constant aching over several decades is a commonplace. To await spontaneous recovery in lumbago is, therefore, a waste of time but, up to a point, reasonable. However, in backache, or in backache with a minor degree of root pain, the main symptoms remaining lumbar, it is fraught with disappointment.

In root pain the position is quite different, and spontaneous recovery is to be expected, *provided that the backache ceases when the pain shifts to the limb.* Time is counted from the appearance of the root pain, not from the onset of lumbar symptoms, which may have continued for months or years.

Shrinkage of the protrusion or its accommodation in a neutral position by vertebral erosion takes from 8 to 12 months. As at the cervical spine, the larger the displacement, the sooner the patient recovers. This is understandable in erosion, when it can be argued that, the larger the protrusion, the more pressure it exerts and the sooner it nests itself in; but it applies also to recovery by shrinkage. Sciatica of three months' standing with, say, 45° of straight-leg raising and no neurological signs, is unlikely to become well in less than another nine months, unless epidural local anaesthesia is induced. The same situation, but with some neurological deficit, may well indicate recovery in another three or four months, assuming that an epidural injection is not given. Spontaneous recovery is rather quicker at the third level than at the fourth and fifth.

These rules do not apply once the patient has reached 60 years of age. In sciatica in the elderly, the backache is seldom lost and no limit can be placed on the natural history of the pain. Even if the backache does cease when the root pain comes on, the older the patient is, the less certain it is that it will not continue indefinitely.

By contrast, root atrophy may come on in the course of seconds or weeks. A patient may awake with an excruciating pain in one lower limb that lasts for a few seconds; then his foot goes numb, his pain ceases and he falls asleep again. Next morning his foot feels weak and examination shows a disc lesion without limitation of straight-leg raising but a complete root palsy. Another patient may lie in bed with increasing root pain for days or weeks and then suffer several days' agony before the numbness and the relief appear.

Patients who have recovered with the passage of time, by shrinkage, erosion or root atrophy, do not need to be particularly careful afterwards. The displacement has not been reduced with the restoration of the status quo; hence the likelihood that what has moved once may move again does not arise. They are, of course, neither more nor less likely to develop a disc lesion at a fresh level than any other individual, and disc lesions are so common that everyone should always maintain his lordosis during lifting whether he has had trouble in the past or not. But they need not wear a belt or avoid reasonably strenuous work.

### Recovery from Palsy

Recovery is the rule, especially in those patients

who get well slowly by shrinkage or erosion. If it has not begun after a year, time is unlikely to bring recovery; after two years, no further change is to be expected. Usually, after some months, often before the root pain has wholly ceased, the muscles begin to strengthen and the skin to regain its sensitivity. The ankle jerk is permanently lost in about half of all cases; the knee jerk returns more often. Root atrophy may lead to a little permanent weakness, especially when two roots are compressed, when the muscle common to both roots may never recover, e.g. the extensor hallucis in a combined fourth and fifth lumbar root paresis. In general, weakness confined to one root recovers; affecting two roots, largely so. However, if disc protrusion gives rise to complete paralysis of a muscle—this is most uncommon—the loss of power is apt to be permanent. If a root palsy is developing or has just occurred, laminectomy would doubtless lead to swift restoration of conduction, but patients are well advised to risk the minor disability of a weak muscle rather than operation. A professional footballer may insist that his foot must not be allowed to weaken, but, after laminectomy, he is permanently unfit for football. There is no guarantee that laminectomy will restore muscle power if carried out late, since actual pressure necrosis of some nerve fibres may lead to permanent paresis.

Recovery does not necessarily occur at the nerve root itself; for Woolf and Till's muscle biopsies (1955), based on van Bogaert's findings, show that reinnervating fibres wander out from the intact nerves within the muscle; hence, such recovery occurs as the result of this distal mechanism. Excellent microphotographs are contained in Coomes's (1959) paper showing the branching out of new terminal neurones to supply several adjacent non-innervated muscle fibres. He regards this as brought about by terminal branching within 1 mm of the motor end-plate of healthy nerve fibres derived from another root supplying the same muscle. They grow down the empty endoneural tubes of the fibres that have lost their central connection and new end-plates are formed. Yates (1964) studied 48 patients with radicular weakness due to disc protrusion. In only one of eight multiradicular cases did full recovery ensue, but he found that in all 40 patients in whom one root was only involved, full recovery was completed in an average of seven months.

The speed of recovery is very variable. Sometimes a root palsy recovers inexplicably in a month or two, even before the pain has ceased, and cutaneous analgesia may begin to diminish after only a few weeks. Since regrowth of nerve is at the rate of 1.5 mm a day, this cannot be the mechanism. Normally a root palsy recovers slowly in 6–12 months, i.e. at the expected rate of nerve regeneration, and improvement goes on for two years in all. When patients with a palsy involving even two roots are seen again for some other disorder years later, it is remarkable how few have any muscle weakness or appreciable cutaneous analgesia. If an ankle jerk was lost, it often remains absent, but the knee jerk nearly always returns within a year. Estimates based on short follow-up periods tend to excessive pessimism.

It is well to realize that muscle weakness is a sign that is detected by the doctor rather than a phenomenon apparent to the patient. In fourth lumbar paresis, he may notice the foot flopping after he has walked some distance; in fifth lumbar paresis he is apt to turn his ankle over easily; in first or second sacral paresis he cannot rise on tiptoe on the affected leg. But he notes rather than minds, and certainly—and rightly—prefers this slight and temporary inconvenience to laminectomy. In fact, most patients with weakness are quite unaware of it.

### Aggravation of the Palsy

This is rare. Past compression has induced root atrophy which time has not improved. Laminectomy has sometimes been performed in vain. There is no change for years; then the patient suddenly notices increased painless weakness in the foot. Examination confirms that further loss of power has taken place, sometimes to the point of complete paralysis. This finding clearly implies that the protrusion has become even larger but, pressing as it does against the dural sleeve rendered insensitive by ischaemia, the phenomenon evokes no pain.

The condition is best left untreated except, perhaps, by an orthopaedic boot.

## LAMINECTOMY

This should not be lightly undertaken, but should not, on the other hand, be unreasonably withheld. It is apt to be recommended far too readily, without adequate weight being given to the effectiveness of conservative treatment and also to the passage of time. There is also a smaller group of patients who do require laminectomy but for the same reasons are denied it. In the view of Shealy of Minnesota only one in ten of the laminectomies performed in the USA today is justified.

Even in the best hands, the results of laminectomy in sciatica are not perfect; immediate relief is secured in about 90% of patients but recurrences bring this figure down to 80% within five years. This tendency to recurrence—which may, of course, result from displacement at another level—should prohibit patients from ever resuming heavy work.

Laminectomy in the presence of lumbar symptoms alone carries only half the cure rate obtained when root pain is present. Hence, in such a case, if there is nothing for it but operation, the patient is asked to exert himself, e.g. dig, in an endeavour to induce root pain and to have the operation at a time when this is present. If he cannot bring on any sciatica, the chances of a successful result are diminished. Nelson (1975) reviewed the surgical literature in 2423 operative cases and confirmed these figures. The follow-up period was 1–25 years and he found sciatica lastingly relieved in 8 out of 10 cases, backache in 5 out of 10. In 1975, H. J. Goald began microlumbar discectomy, following the method of R. W. Williams of Las Vegas, who claims 91% cures in 530 patients. They use a 1 inch skin incision and a surgical microscope. A small amount of ligamentum flavum is removed, the nerve root is held to one side, and the nucleus removed. The patient goes home 2½ days later. The operation takes less than 40 minutes. Schwartz of California has adopted a technique invented in Japan for removing a disc protrusion under local anaesthesia. Through a needle pushed into the disc, a pair of small forceps is introduced as far as the protrusion. The disc protrusion is nibbled away until the patient reports that the sciatic pain has ceased. He is securing 60% cures at present (personal communication 1981).

Laminectomy is seldom required in young adults. My youngest patient was 17 and was found at operation to have a large protrusion at both fourth and fifth levels. Laminectomy is also seldom required at the third lumbar level. The pain when this root is affected may be fairly severe for some weeks, but scarcely ever reaches the agonizing pitch that raises the question of operation. Out of 913 patients operated on by Young (1952), only seven had the third disc removed; 20% of his patients had a double protrusion.

Patients without severe root pain who, after, say, six months, are getting weary of their symptoms, should be told that spontaneous recovery will take another three months at the third level and another six months at the fourth or fifth level. A patient who believes that he will be in discomfort for life—this is not an unreasonable idea after six months—will accept laminectomy unless the non-operative prognosis is explained to him. Laminectomy—even more, laminectomy without even trying the effect of epidural local anaesthesia first—is not an easy way out and does the patient real disservice. He stands a 90% chance of immediate relief it is true, but the cure rate of epidural anaesthesia or merely waiting another six months is higher. When he gets well without operation, he can return to heavy work; after the operation he must be permanently careful of his back. It is worth recalling that the patients who had sciatica in pre-laminectomy days were not operated on and nearly all recovered notwithstanding. Time healed all but a few. If, then, a patient suffering from tolerable root pain does not respond to conservative treatment, especially local anaesthesia at the nerve root, he should be advised to wait till a year has elapsed since the root pain began. Only the very few who are not well by then need surgery.

Laminectomy has one important disadvantage: it abolishes the tendency to spontaneous recovery in sciatica and third lumbar root pain. Hence, if the operation proves unsuccessful, the normal recovery from root pain with the passage of time can no longer be counted upon.

After laminectomy, no patient should be allowed to do heavy work again. Recurrence takes place (not necessarily at the same level) in at least 10% even of those who are careful of their lumbar joints. Renewed root pain after laminectomy is difficult to treat and shows little tendency to spontaneous cure with the passage of time. It may prove intractable, and a second laminectomy is a formidable operation. Hence, a patient who proposes putting his back in jeopardy again must be given a stern homily. All patients should be warned not to do exercises while in bed after the operation, nor afterwards at home.

In California, laminectomy is not popular with the Workman's Compensation Board. Leavitt et al. (1971) discovered that the cost of compensation and treatment when laminectomy was contemplated and *not* performed was $5414, whereas when contemplated *and* performed it was $10 017, i.e. double.

Laminectomy followed by immediate fusion has proved to have the same result by some years later as laminectomy alone. The combination is not recommended. The same applies to myelography; whether the herniation shows or not is immaterial. Indeed in 5 of 17 patients requiring laminectomy (Bihaug 1980) the myelogram was normal in spite of large disc protrusions.

## Indications

### Severe Intractable Root Pain

*It is not the severity of the lesion but the severity of the pain that matters.* Identical disc protrusions and identical signs may be present in patients with severe root pain or merely slight aching in the limb. Hence, the problem must be approached subjectively. The simple idea that sciatica with neurological signs warrants operation, and without such signs does not, must be entirely abandoned; nothing could be more fallacious. Burton (1978) has calculated that the neurosurgeons of the USA of whom there are 2614, between them performed 117 630 laminectomies in 1974. Since some 20% have recurred within five years, this implies the creation of over 23 000 cripples a year. Third and fourth laminectomies are successful in only 10%. First, the size and level of the protrusion must be estimated, then the amount of pain alleged must be set against the patient's sincerity and sensitivity to pain; then the likelihood of time bringing relief (and, if so, in how long a time) and the possibilities of conservative treatment must be assessed. This is not the work of a few minutes, and requires experience if errors are to be avoided. Care is taken to ensure that the physical signs are consistent with each other and compatible with allegations of severe pain.

Intractable pain may mean that part of the annulus has protruded posterolaterally upwards or downwards and has come to lie on the posterior surface of the vertebral body; in such a case, conservative treatment, however prolonged, is bound to fail. It is also possible for more and more of the nucleus to escape past an intact annulus and form a large bulge with a thin neck; then, as the joint space in consequence narrows, the herniation is trapped by contact between annulus and vertebral body—the collar-stud phenomenon. Unless erosion of the vertebral body allows the protrusion to nest itself away, lasting root pain results.

The worse the symptoms and signs, the better the results of the operation. A history of previous attacks also augurs well, for it implies that the lesion is as mature as possible. In particular, by operating late, ample opportunity is given for protrusion at both levels to develop. If so, both discs are dealt with and the likelihood of recurrence is correspondingly diminished.

The cases in which laminectomy most often proves necessary are those of sciatica, with or without neurological signs, in which either trunk extension is markedly restricted by pain felt in the lower limb, or there is a considerable lateral tilt of the lumbar spine, with side flexion in the limited direction inhibited by severe root pain. Bihaug (1980) found that 33 out of 123 patients with sciatica felt pain in the calf when digital pressure was applied to the lower lumbar area. In these the laminectomy rate proved to be 51% whereas in the other 90 it was 24%.

### Gross Lumbar Deformity

A gross side flexion or flexion deformity, or both, kept in being by sciatic pain so severe that the patient cannot stand up straight, very seldom responds to any conservative treatment. Nor does it often lead to spontaneous relief by root atrophy or even by the passage of many months. Trunk flexion often relieves the pain and straight-leg raising is often full and painless. Extension is completely blocked. Side flexion of the lumbar spine one way is of full range and painless; attempted the other way the spine does not even reach the vertical. Often there is no neurological deficit. These patients require laminectomy. In a border-line case one epidural injection is worth trying but if no improvement is manifest a week later the operation should not be delayed.

### Incipient Drop-foot

A patient who develops weakness of all the muscles controlled by two adjacent roots must be warned of the possibility of permanent weakness of the muscle common to both roots. Moreover any completely paralysed muscles (e.g. the peronei) usually remain permanently so. But, the athlete or ballet-dancer who insists on the importance of a strong foot cannot return to heavy sport or dancing after laminectomy, whereas this is possible in recovery without operation. Hence, it is better to wait, relying on the considerable probability that the muscles will recover. Though seldom indicated on the grounds of muscle weakness alone, immediate laminectomy does afford the best hope of rapid restoration of muscle power. It is not however a certainty, for necrosis of the root fibres may have supervened; if so, nothing will restore strength, and even peripheral reinnervation is no longer probable. This persistence of neurological signs after laminectomy comes out clearly in Hakelius's (1970) statistics. He studied 583 patients with sciatica of whom 166 were operated on. Residual paresis continuing six months after removal of the disc occurred in 20%. This was confirmed by Weber in 1978. He followed up 64 patients for four years. All had had sciatic root palsies and half had had laminectomy and the others conservative treatment. No difference between the recovery from the palsy was found.

When pressure atrophy causes complete insensitivity of the nerve root, pain is abolished and straight-leg raising quickly reaches full range at the same time as the palsy becomes complete. The patient is apt mistakenly to believe himself to be improving; so he is, subjectively, but the true position must be explained to him. Extreme weakness or full paralysis of two or three muscles is apt to prove permanent, whereas considerably weakness usually disappears to the point where it is no longer perceived by the patient in 6 to 12 months.

## Third and Fourth Sacral Root Palsy

Weakness of the bladder with incontinence or retention of urine (usually the former) during an attack of lumbago or sciatica calls for immediate laminectomy. Since the impact of the protruded disc is applied in a pre-ganglionic position, severe maintained pressure on the third and fourth sacral roots may well lead to permanent incontinence. Moreover, late laminectomy usually fails (4 cures in 25 cases in Jowitt's series) to restore vesical control. Hence, operation is urgent, though Dandy's (1929) first two cases of removal of the central protrusion succeeded three and ten weeks after the supervention of the vesical palsy. One was a case of bilateral sciatica and recovery took six months. The other followed manipulation under anaesthesia by an orthopaedic surgeon and urinary control returned in ten days, rectal in one month. In 15 cases seen by me, all early, postoperative recovery was complete.

If a patient with lumbago is improving and power is returning to the bladder or rectum, or his sacrum is becoming less analgesic or the impotence is waning, there is no urgency. Nevertheless, prophylactic laminectomy is indicated; for there can be no guarantee that the next time he gets lumbago his protrusion will not transect the fourth sacral root, and this may happen in a country where urgent laminectomy is unobtainable; alternatively the importance of acting quickly in this type of lumbago may not be appreciated, since this is after all very seldom a dangerous disease. All my patients have accepted prophylactic laminectomy and, so far, all have remained free from further trouble.

## Adherent Root

If the symptoms warrant, the adhesions must be divided at laminectomy. In fact, after about two years the discomfort becomes slight or even ceases entirely, and the patient's only disability he cannot stand up and bend forwards. He is well advised to put up with this minor annoyance.

## Buckled End-plate

This is a rarity. The end-plate covering the vertebral body may become detached and finally double over on itself, forming a block at the back of the joint. When the patient attempts to bend backwards, he cannot, and when he tries he squeezes the cartilaginous displacement and is seen to recoil forward again in a characteristic manner suggesting the springy block of a meniscal displacement at the knee. Only laminectomy discloses the state of affairs, and there is no other cure.

## Arterial Obstruction to the Cauda Equina

Spinal claudication leading to bilateral root pain with paraesthetic feet has not in my experience responded to traction; manipulation is clearly contraindicated. Hence laminectomy provides the only answer.

## Arterial Obstruction to the Cord

A lumbar disc protrusion may interfere with the arterial flow at the lower segment of the spinal cord. If the branch running upwards from the low lumbar or the iliolumbar artery is compressed, sciatica accompanied by spasticity of the lower limb on the painful side results, together with an extensor plantar response. The mechanism is explained in Fig. 90.

Should this phenomenon supervene in a case of sciatica, laminectomy should be considered, in order to preserve the blood supply in the spinal cord.

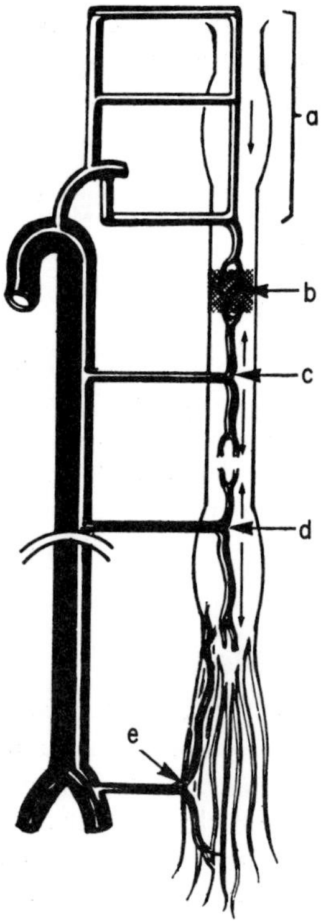


**Fig. 90.** The arterial supply of the spinal cord. *a*, Cervical and upper thoracic cord supplied by branches of the vertebral ascending cervical and superior intercostal arteries. *b*, 'Watershed' at the level of the fourth thoracic segment. *c*, Mid-thoracic cord supplied from a single intercostal artery. *d*, Thoracolumbar region supplied by a large vessel near the diaphragm (arteria magna). *e*, Cauda equina supplied from the lower lumbar, iliolumbar and lateral sacral arteries, which occasionally supply the distal part of the cord also. Note that pressure at a low lumbar level may interfere with the artery as it passes upwards to the lowest segment of the spinal cord. (*Reproduced by kind permission of R.A. Henson and the Editor from The Quarterly Journal of Medicine, 1967*).

## Repeated Crippling Attacks

These may occur so often and be so severe while they last, that the patient's life is a misery. Even if reduction is easily achieved, whether spontaneously or as a result of treatment, another attack follows in spite of adequate precautions for the maintenance of reduction.

In such cases, laminectomy may be indicated. If it is decided upon, the operation should be carried out at a time when maximum displacement is present, even if this has to be purposely induced just before the operation. However, arthrodesis is to be preferred.

# Contraindications

## Relievable by Conservative Means

If a patient can be got well by conservative means, or will clearly recover with the passage of a reasonable length of time, no operation is required.

## Neurosis

As has already been pointed out, it is not so much the severity of the lesion as the amount of pain experienced that provides the main indication for laminectomy. Moreover, the criterion of cure is largely the patient's own statement afterwards. It is thus essential to provide the surgeon with cooperative patients; for a patient anxious to make the worst of his disorder will not allow himself to be deprived of it by surgery, nor after an operation is it any longer feasible to convince the patient that the organic part of his trouble has ceased. Individual sensitivity to pain is gauged in two ways. First, by the assessment of personality afforded by listening carefully to the patient's account of his troubles, together with his digressions. Secondly, by noting the responses when irrelevant as well as relevant movements are performed. Since minor symptoms due to a low lumbar disc lesion are all but universal, it is not difficult for a patient credibly to describe and to exaggerate backache or sciatica, severe disablement being alleged to obtain sympathy or compensation or pension, or escape from some domestic situation. Such symptoms may appear confirmed when a narrow disc space (such as many middle-aged patients symptomlessly possess) is visible on the radiograph. These patients may welcome operation and, once it has been performed, it becomes very difficult to estimate how much of the patient's disablement has an organic origin, and impossible to get the patient to agree to the assessment.

It must be remembered that, when a complaint of backache is made, it is seldom wholly groundless. Some discomfort may well exist and careful examination may disclose signs of a past or present minor organic disorder. Purely psychogenic symptoms are easily detected; a slight organic disorder complicated by a large psychogenic overlay is more difficult to separate accurately into its two components. Prolonged disability after operation is to be expected in such patients, even if such organic trouble as was found was adequately dealt with. After all, any laminectomy, however successful, may be followed by some intermittent backache. Ordinary patients are so vastly improved that they ignore this slight symptom, but it is gladly grasped by the psychoneurotic. Unrecognized psychoneurosis is becoming, in my experience, increasingly treated by measures designed to affect a disc lesion, especially manipulation, immobilization in plaster and laminectomy. Hence, the operation should be avoided if the patient's character precludes the achievement of a good result.

## CHEMONUCLEOLYSIS

This is the term coined by Smith to describe attrition of the disc by means of an enzyme. At first it was hoped that this method would largely replace laminectomy. Chymopapain was isolated in 1941, but it was in 1963 that Smith of Chicago, after much experimentation with animals, treated the first human patient. By 1967, he and Brown had treated 75 patients and by 1969 these numbered 207 (Smith 1969).

### The Enzyme

Chymopapain is obtained from the fruit of *Carica papaya*. If the fruit is scarified while still green on the tree, a latex forms which contains crude papain. This is a mixture of protease enzymes from which chymopapain can be isolated.

Chymopapain is the main proteolytic component of papaya latex. Tsaltas had produced alteration in the cartilage of rabbits' ears by 1958, and in 1964 Murray had caused changes similar to human osteoarthritis in young rabbits' knees by means of injecting papain into the joint. But the first to suggest the injection of a chondrolytic enzyme was Hirsch (1959) when he proposed converting the disc into dense fibrous tissue by this means. In vitro experiments have shown that the nucleus pulposus is quickly dissolved by hydrolysis of the non-collagen protein (Stern 1969). Digestion brings about degeneration of chondromucoprotein and takes only some hours. The enzyme is well tolerated epidurally and intradiscally, but dangerous if it is introduced intrathecally. There it bathes thin-walled veins and capillaries, leading to haemorrhage and death from the consequent raised cerebrospinal fluid pressure, unless this is released promptly by draining the fluid off. There is no effect upon the dura mater, ligament, bone, nerve roots and large blood vessels (Smith et al. 1963). The minimal effective dose administered to the nucleus is 2–4 mg diluted as a 1:100 solution. For details the reader is referred to the Symposium on Chymopapain (1969). Troisier (personal communication 1977) found that four weeks after an intra-articular injection of chymopapain the width of the disc space had gone down by one-third to two-thirds: clear evidence of erosion. The same was found by McCulloch in Toronto (1977). He too showed that the disc space diminished within a week, and reached its maximum in a month. In 1975 he had two deaths but a case of anaphylaxis (1 in 480) was revived in 1977. There was only 10% failure in sciatica but a 73% poor result in backache.

In 1976, a double-blind trial showed that 49% of a placebo group, and 58% of those injected with chymopapain had good to excellent results. Since Travenol had withdrawn chymopapain at the suggestion of the FDA in 1975, they could not ban a product already off the market. Sussman says that chymopapain is the wrong enzyme; collegenase is safe, effective and should be substituted (Sampson 1978).

### Results of the Treatment by Chemonucleolysis of 150 Cases of Sciatica

In 1980 Troisier said: 'Chemonucleolysis was introduced in medical practice by Lyman Smith in 1963 with the Russian authors Osna, Kasmyn and Vetrile following soon after, during the years 1965–1968. North American, Canadian and more recently European authors followed suit; Bouillet was the first in Belgium, then Popovic in Yugoslavia, Anderson in England and various others, including myself, when I started in France in 1976.

The treatment consists in injecting an enzyme, mainly chymopapain, extracted from the fruit of carica papaya directly in the intervertebral disc.

Thus, polymucosaccharides included in the nucleus pulposus are depolymerised and both disc and prolapse shrink. Therefore this treatment diminishes the pressure exerted on the nerve-root and its sheath, providing two conditions are fulfilled:

1. There are enough polymucosaccharides in the prolapsed part.
2. The enzyme can actually reach it, which might not be the case when the fragment is extruded.

Patients are selected on three criteria:

1. The diagnosis of disc prolapse causing root pain must be ascertained by history, clinical examination and contrast X rays.
2. Conservative treatment has failed.
3. The intensity and/or duration of symptoms are sufficiently important to the patient that destructive treatment is called for.

The choice of chemonucleolysis rather than surgery is based on the absence of contra-indications.

The treatment is carried out in the X-ray department, in the same conditions as a surgical procedure.

Local anaesthesia is used but everything is in place for resuscitation as an anaphylactic shock is possible when the enzyme is injected.

Needles (a straight outer needle gauge 18, in which is secondarily thrust an inner straight or distally curved needle gauge 22, one inch longer) are thrust in extradurally, passing very near the *outer* aspect of the facet joints, and avoiding the nerve root. A very accurate stereotaxic method has been devised by the author so that penetration of the needle in L5–S1 is not complicated.

After a dural irritation (characterized by lumbar pain and increased straight-leg raise limitation, usually bilateral) has subsided, the patient gets up and starts his rehabilitation programme.

The results have been classified according to four items: two subjective; radicular pain and residual backaches and two objective; neurological deficit and lumbar mobility, measured with the Schober's test.

*Radicular Pain.* This is assessed 'well' if it has disappeared completely; 'much better' if it remains weakly on rare occasions and for a short time; 'slightly better' if it is constant but less than before the treatment; alternatively there is 'no change'.

*Lumbar Pain.* This is of non protrusive type I or II. It is 'well' if absent; 'much better' when easily controlled by the patient and does not interfere with either occupation or sport; 'slightly better' if it does not interfere with the patient's occupation but certain physical activities and sports are impossible or when pain-killers are necessary; there is 'no change' if it interferes with professional life and needs antalgic drugs.

*Neurological Deficit.* This is assessed 'well' if absent; 'much better' if a slight difference is noted with the other side; 'slightly better' if it is still there but somewhat improved; there is 'no change' if it is as before the treatment.

*Lumbar Mobility.* This is assessed 'well' if it equals or exceeds 6 cm; 'much better' if between 5 and 6 cm; 'slightly better' if it is found to be between 3 and 4.5 cm; 'no change' if below 3 cm.

## Results

Four periods have been studied: 2 to 4 months after the treatment (150 patients); 1 year (109 patients); 2 years (61 patients); 3 to 5 years (23 patients).

The table below shows the results on radicular pain. It is of interest to notice that with time the percentage of those 'well' increases whereas those 'much better' tends to disappear.

**Follow Up of Root Pain**

| Period of study and no. of patients | Well | Much better | Slightly better | No change |
|---|---|---|---|---|
| 4 Months 150 | 47.3% | 26.6% | 10.6% | 15.3% |
| 1 Year 109 | 56% | 21.1% | 5.5% | 17.4% |
| 2 Years 61 | 67.2% | 4.2% | 8.2% | 19.6% |
| > 3 Years 23 | 73.9% | — | — | 26.1% |

The same phenomenon occurs with the 'slightly better' results and the 'no change' results, so that cases after 3 years follow up are either 'well' or there is 'no change'.

The analysis of the 'no change' cases show that:

1. 3.3% have changed their addresses and could not be contacted.
2. 2.6% had definite signs of disc prolapse before treatment but were nevertheless considered as having psychogenic troubles.
3. 13.3% were operated on. Among these 7.33% had a remaining disc prolapse usually extruded, and adherent to the nerve-root; 4.66% were found to suffer from bony stenosis and in 1.33% the treatment was carried out at the wrong level.

This table shows the results on neurological deficit which is present in 62% of our 150 cases.

The addition of the 'well' group to the 'much better' group gives a rather constant figure (over 80%).

**Follow Up of Neurological Deficit**

| Period of study and no. of patients | Well | Much better | Slightly better | No change |
|---|---|---|---|---|
| 4 Months 93 | 53.7% | 34.4% | 5.3% | 6.4% |
| 1 Year 67 | 64.1% | 22.4% | 4.4% | 8.9% |
| 2 Years 41 | 68.3% | 19.5% | 2.4% | 9.7% |
| 3 Years 18 | 61.1% | 16.6% | 11.1% | 11.1% |

The table below gives the results on residual backache: this symptom remains constant with time as compared to radicular pain. It is totally absent in only a third of the patients, and is easy to control in another third; conversely it is a real problem in the last third.

**Follow Up of Backache**

| Period of study and no. of patients | Well | Much better | Slightly better | No change |
|---|---|---|---|---|
| 4 Months 150 | 30.6% | 32% | 21.3% | 16% |
| 1 Year 108 | 26.8% | 30.8% | 16.6% | 17.6% |
| 2 Years 61 | 31.1% | 37.7% | 14.7% | 16.3% |
| 3 Years 23 | 30.4% | 21.7% | 21.7% | 26.1% |

The table below shows the follow up of lumbar mobility: one can see that the mobility increases with time but does not reach 5 cm in nearly half of the cases.

**Follow Up of Mobility**

| Period of study and no. of patients | Well | Much better | Slightly better | No change |
|---|---|---|---|---|
| 4 Months 150 | 6.6% | 20% | 52.6% | 20.6% |
| 1 Year 108 | 12% | 31.4% | 37% | 19.4% |
| 2 Years 60 | 18.3% | 31.6% | 31.6% | 18.3% |
| 3 Years 22 | 22.7% | 31.8% | 18.2% | 27.3% |

### Comparisons Between the Four Items

This is of particular interest in the group of *radicular pain 'well'*. In this group we found that:

1. The neurological deficit is 'well' in 71% and 'much better' in 25.7%, and 'no change' in 2.8%.
2. In other words radicular pain and neurological signs respond to the treatment in the same way.
3. The lumbar pain is assessed 1 year after treatment. In almost 50% of the cases, it is 'much better' and 'slightly better' in about 30% which leaves a few cases with an excellent result on radicular pain and a somewhat important residual backache.
4. The mobility is found 1 year after treatment 'well' in 15%; 'much better' in 38.33%; 'slightly-better' in 35%; and 'no change' in 15%.

We also studied the group assessed *mobility 'well'* and noticed two interesting findings:

1. There was no 'no change' result on radicular pain.
2. There was no 'no change' result on residual backache. Furthermore only 8.5% were assessed 'slightly better' 1 year after treatment. The rest of them are either 'well' (44.7%) or 'much better' (46.8%).

Therefore one can say that the establishment of the mobility is a good objective element in order to appreciate residual backache.

In conclusion, chemonucleolysis, if not contra-indicated, should be considered *after* the failure of conservative measures, but *before* surgery in cases of sciatica due to prolapsed intervertebral discs. In our series of 150 patients, less than 15% were submitted to surgical treatment.

## ARTHRODESIS

By comparison with laminectomy, spinal grafting is a minor operation; for it is performed outside the spine without removing bone or exposing dura mater or nerve roots. An incision is made; the muscles on each side are separated from bone down to the bases of the spinous processes where periosteum is stripped up locally. Two grafts are laid in place and secured here. Originally this was regarded as a formidable operation, owing to the long period of convalescence. The patient had to stay in bed for three months until the grafts united, and spend another three months in a plastic or plaster jacket pending consolidation. The modern technique is to screw the vertebrae together before applying the grafts. A fortnight in bed now suffices since the screws maintain immobility until the fusion is solid. An alternative, practicable at the lumbrosacral level, is to copy nature and create a sacralized fifth lumbar vertebra. The periosteum on the sacrum and the tip of the fifth lumbar transverse process is stripped up and a column of bone chips inserted between these two surfaces. Only a week in bed suffices.

Transabdominal anterior arthrodesis has its advocates, but the reported results are on the whole less satisfactory and the rate of complications higher. Freebody keeps his patients in bed only three weeks, since the erect posture and any movement towards flexion squeeze the uniting surfaces more strongly together.

There is one great disadvantage to arthrodesis. The joint immediately above the fusion now takes double strain when the patient moves. After the operation many patients can still bend to reach their ankles, which must involve considerable stress at the lumbar joints. Hence, some years later a fresh disc lesion is apt to appear at the joint just above the graft. Indeed, the few disc lesions that are encountered at the first or second lumbar levels are mostly the result of lower lumbar arthrodesis.

The indications are as follows:

1. *Spondylolisthesis* causing ligamentous lumbar pain or bilateral sciatica. If enough callus has formed about the pseudarthrosis at the pars intermedia to compress the nerve root, excess bone should be removed and the raw surfaces screwed together.
2. *Anterior protrusion* (the mushroom phenomenon), the backache comes on after standing and ceases within a minute of sitting down or lying. Before arthrodesis is considered in these cases, ligamentous sclerosis (for backache) and a sinuvertebral block (for root pain) are worth trying.
3. *Nuclear self-reducing protrusions.* The patient wakes comfortable and can do everything soon after getting up. By noon, backache begins which gets slowly worse as the day goes on but is abolished again by a night's rest. The pain is not severe, but persists for years, until finally the patient, understandably enough, insists on the only effective treatment, i.e. arthrodesis.
4. *Unsuccessful laminectomy.* In the first place, it is important to steer away from further surgery patients who, even if made better, will not admit it. Secondly, if laminectomy has been performed on a patient in fact suited to conservative treatment, this should be tried before the second operation is contemplated. Traction and epidural local anaesthesia may well prove successful after laminectomy, as may ligamentous sclerosis and posterior ramus or sinuvertebral blocks. If a laminectomy has proved unsuccessful from the first, it may well be that the lesion was never reached and that the result of conservative measures will not be impaired.
5. *Intractable severe backache,* absent on lying. If this is so, the operation stops the compression strain on the joint otherwise present when the body weight falls on the joint.
6. *Frequent severe attacks.* One important point must be observed before spinal fusion is undertaken—namely, that no displacement exists at the time when the operation is performed. This precaution is sometimes neglected, especially in spondylolisthesis with a secondary disc lesion, with the result that the symptoms continue and later the graft has to be removed and laminectomy carried out.

   The abiding difficulty is to know at which level, or both, to perform the fusion. It should be borne in mind that at laminectomy Young found two protrusions in 20% of cases. Discography carried out at the fourth and fifth lumbar levels is very informative, and so are radiographs taken in full flexion and full extension. If these show a shift of one vertebra, it is highly probable that this is the unstable joint in which the damaged disc lies. If root pain is present, it may prove possible to abolish it temporarily by a sinuvertebral block. The level is determined by noting if success follows induction at the fourth or fifth lumbar foramen.
7. *Laminectomy followed by fusion.* This is not recommended. A ten-year survey (Frimoyer et al. 1978) showed that the late result of laminectomy was almost the same, whether arthrodesis was carried out at the same time or not.

## Inducing Posterior Contracture

Permanent shortening of the supraspinous, the adjacent part of the interspinous ligament and the ligaments that allow sliding at the facet joints would clearly prove beneficial in disc lesions by limiting the range of flexion at the affected joint.

## Ligamentous Sclerosis

This treatment was instituted by Hackett (1956). As a young surgeon, when operating on patients for hernia who had been treated years previously by sclerosing injections into the inguinal canal, he noticed hard lumps of fibrous tissue difficult to cut with a scalpel. Years later he applied this finding to the idea of ligamentous sclerosis. His original solution consisted of zinc sulphate and carbolic acid. R. Ongley, of New Zealand, decided to try these injections out on a large scale. He varied his method and his solution until he found the most effective; Barbor and I profited by his extensive experience. Barbor (1964) described Ongley's method in detail, giving indications, methods and results. Wyke has established that the solution does not cause tissue sclerosis, but protein coagulation. Hence it is more accurate to speak of tissue contracture.

Though I do not, it is only fair to add that Ongley and Barbor, the leading exponents of sclerosant therapy, do include the sacroiliac ligaments in their injection sites. It seems to me that the strain on an imperfect low lumbar joint can only be increased if such slight mobility as exists at the sacroiliac joint is diminished. Hence sacroiliac ligamentous sclerosis appears to me illogical. On the other hand, if these injections instead exert their effect by the mechanism described by Wyke (see Chapter 21), i.e. by abating the stream of subliminal impulses flowing to the spinal cord, the more tissues that are infiltrated the better, as long as they belong to the same segment as the lesion.

Scott-Charlton and Roebuck (1972) have put forward a similar theory. In cases of persistent backache, they found that local anaesthesia induced at the upper aspect of the posterior sacrum might abolish pain for the time being. When this proved so, they injected phenol under radiographic control at the point of exit of the posterior ramus from the sacral foramen. Permanent relief was secured, in their view, by the provocation of a localized peripheral neuritis.

## Pathological Investigations in Sclerosant Therapy

There can be no doubt that the fibrous tissue Hackett found in the inguinal canal was formed in response to sclerosant injections. Anderson and Dukes (1925) described the histological picture produced by injecting haemorrhoids with phenol in 10% solution of glycerine and water:

> Carbolic acid, being a powerful irritant to the tissues, initiates an aseptic inflammation, characterized by dilation of the vessels, emigration of leucocytes and transudation of lymph.
>
> By these means the alien liquid is diluted and removed; thereafter, the inflammation quickly subsides.

Troisier (1962) reported to me that visible ligamentous fibrosis could be provoked. A patient of his, who was to have his lateral meniscus removed, received three injections at weekly intervals of sclerosant solution into the coronary ligament at the knee two months before the operation. At meniscectomy, it was authoritatively agreed that the ligament had developed marked localized thickening, up to four times the normal, at the extent infiltrated.

In order to ascertain the sclerosing effect of the injection, a series of experiments were kindly carried out for me by Sarias, under Professor Trueta's direction. Unfortunately, the results were entirely negative. Twenty-two adult rabbits were used, aged about four months.

He reports as follows:

> Before injection the animal was given a general anaesthetic. The site of injection of the anaesthetic proliferent solution (1 ml) in each animal was the interspinous ligament between L 5 and L 4. In half the animals 1 ml of saline was injected in the interspinous ligament between L 3 and L 2, and in the other half 1 ml of alcohol was injected. Nothing was injected between L 4 and L 3 in any of the rabbits, so a normal interspinous ligament could be compared with the injected one above and below.

| | |
|---|---|
| 4 rabbits killed | 1 week(s) after injections |
| 3 | 2 |
| 4 | 5 |
| 1 | 8 |
| 5 | 12 |
| 5 | 13 |

> After being killed, each animal was injected through the upper abdominal aorta with a solution of 50 per cent micropaque and 50 per cent solution of 2 per cent Blue Berlin, so as to visualize radiologically and histologically the blood vessels. The whole of the lumbar spine was removed, fixed in formaline, decalcified, fine grain X-rayed, and sectioned and stained with haematoxylin eosin for histological examination.

*Results*

*Fine grain radiography.* No change was seen. *Histology.* The slides were examined under the light microscope at a low powered view. Attention was focused on the insertion of the ligament into bone, in the anaesthetic proliferent solution injected area, in the control area, and in the alcohol or saline injected area.

In the transitional zone into fibro-cartilage, no gross changes were seen in any of the three examined areas.

The proportion of collagenic fibres and amorphus intercellular substance in the 2 injected areas was like that of the non-injected area, as was the proportion of encapsulated fibroblasts and Sharpey's fibres. This picture remained constant irrespective of the time after injection in which the animals were killed. The dark areas seen in the fine grain X-rays proved, when examined under the microscope, to be a free extravasation of the micropaque Blue Berlin injection with no tissue reaction around them, and they have the same characteristics in the anaesthetic proliferent zone, as they have in the alcohol or saline zone.

## Others' Results

Borden's film of sclerosant technique shows histological changes in rabbit tissue removed for microscopy after such injections.

At St Thomas's Hospital, Sanford carried out a blind trial on sclerosant therapy for several years ending in 1972. He used three solutions: (*a*) 2 ml of sclerosant mixed with 8 ml of saline; (*b*) 10 ml of 0.5% procaine; (*c*) 10 ml of normal saline. He chose 100 cases, of whom only three were lost. (The only difficulty here is that, by diluting the sclerosant fluid to a quarter of its original strength, the osmotic pressure on which the sclerosant action depends must have been considerably impaired.) His results (1972) are set out below.

| Solution | Well | Much better | Slightly better | No change | Total |
|---|---|---|---|---|---|
| *a* | 6 | 10 | 4 | 11 | 31 |
| *b* | 10 | 6 | 2 | 16 | 34 |
| *c* | 7 | 3 | 5 | 17 | 33 |

These results show that the diluted sclerosant and the procaine solution were equally effective, largely relieving half the cases. By contrast, saline alone was helped less than a third.

It has been argued that the mere insertion of needles can of itself prove effective. There is nothing new in this suggestion. In Paris Berlioz wrote a book on acupuncture in 1816 and Churchill's *Treatise on Acupuncturation* appeared five years later. In 1826 Wansborough described cure in six cases of lumbago and sciatica. The following year Elliotson, physician to St Thomas's Hospital relieved 30 out of 42 patients by this means. Again, in 1830 Renten in Edinburgh had cured three more patients with sciatica by acupuncture but Sir William Osler failed to help a patient thus in 1879 (Cushing 1926). However, nowadays so many patients receive injections into their backs without benefit that this mechanism can clearly be discounted.

# DISC LESIONS IN THE ELDERLY

After the age of 60, most disc lesions are small and cartilaginous; therefore, they are nearly always reducible by manipulation. Moreover, they lie within joints at which movement, and therefore distraction, is very limited by osteophyte formation and ligamentous contracture. Hence, several months in bed, with or without traction, usually prove equally ineffective; for neither method achieves enough separation of the joint surfaces to let the displaced fragment slip back. Owing partly to the small size of the fragment of annulus and partly to sclerosis of bone at the joint margins, the young person's mechanism for spontaneous cure of root pain does not operate; hence, not only backache but also sciatica can go on indefinitely.

The history is distinctive in sciatica, for the backache seldom ceases when the root pain comes on. Examination shows some of the lumbar movements to elicit the backache in the expected way; trunk flexion and straight-leg raising are seldom restricted and may not even set up pain in the limb. Muscular weakness is uncommon, and the ankle jerk is apt to become sluggish only after many months; if so, it is even then worth while trying manipulation once.

In cases of this type, the orthopaedic physician's hand is forced. However unwilling he may be, however old and frail the patient, however fearful both may be, the choice lies between leaving the patient in pain, perhaps for life, and manipulation. If he agrees, manipulation must be attempted with adequate care but also with enough firmness to give the patient a chance of being helped.

Manipulative technique should be restricted to the prone-lying extension pressures and the rotation movements that are carried out with one hand on the buttock and the other on the thorax, since applying a rotation strain using the thigh as a lever might easily fracture the femoral neck.

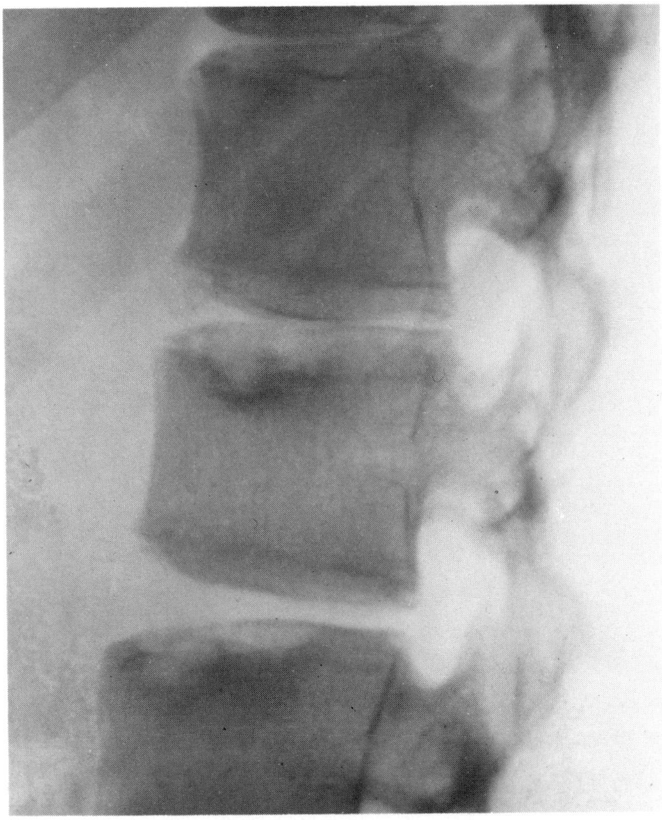

Fig. 1. Adolescent osteochondritis. The patient was a girl aged 14 with a history of 6 months' mid-lumbar backache. Note the anterior defect at the bodies of the third and fourth lumbar vertebrae, causing wedging at the affected levels. The symptoms were caused by a reducible disc lesion, secondary to the articular deformity.

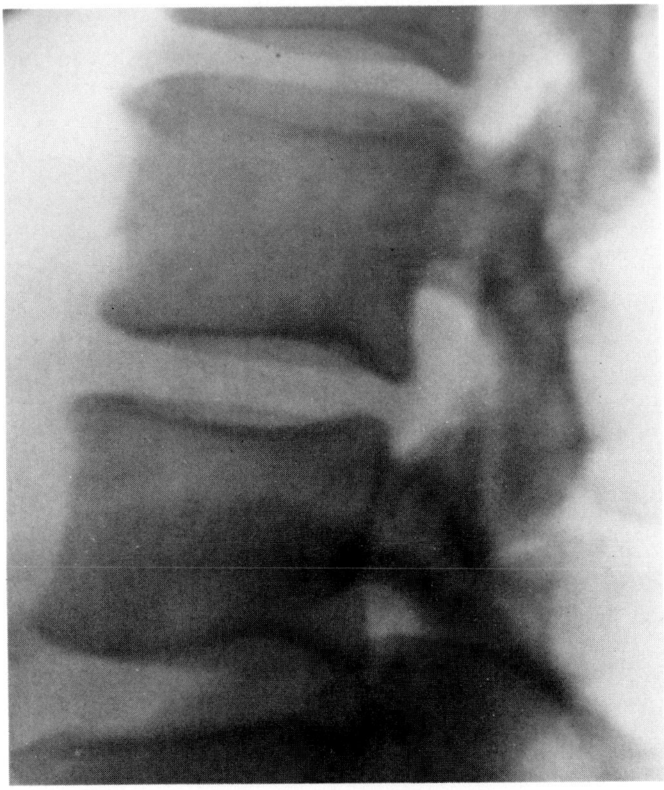

Fig. 2. Complete erosion of the disc at the fifth lumbar level.

PLATE XVIII

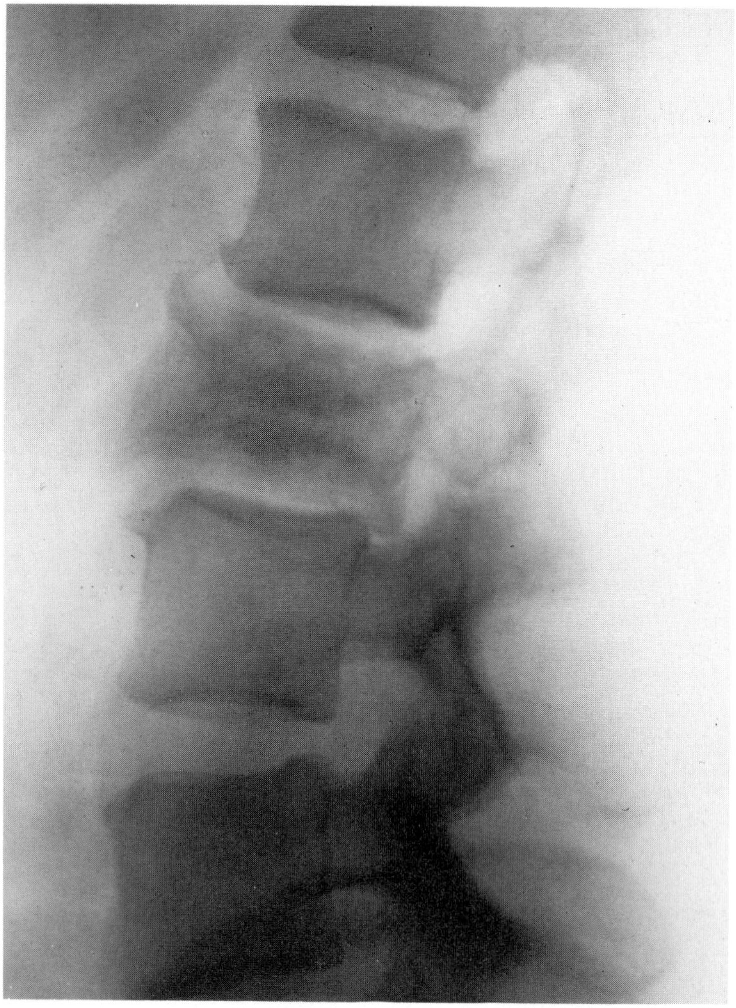

Localised osteitis deformans at the second lumbar level. This man, aged 46, had had 6 months' backache. An upper lumbar angular kyphosis was visible and palpable. Note that collapse continues until cortex touches at the vertebral body. The pelvis showed the typical appearances of osteitis deformans.

PLATE XIX

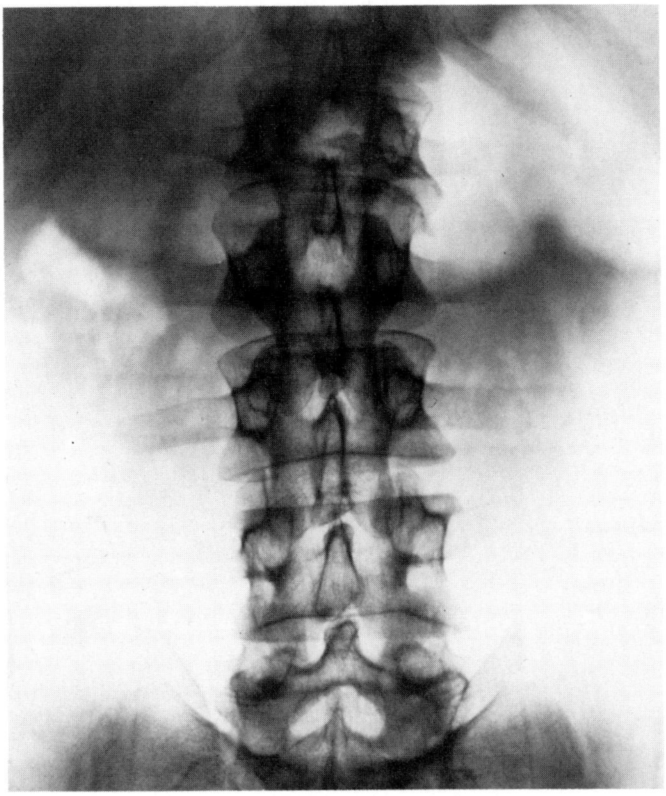

Fig. 1. First lumbar disc lesion. Radiograph of a man aged 31, whose upper lumbar pain and cutaneous analgesia in the groin were ascribed on clinical examination to this rare lesion.

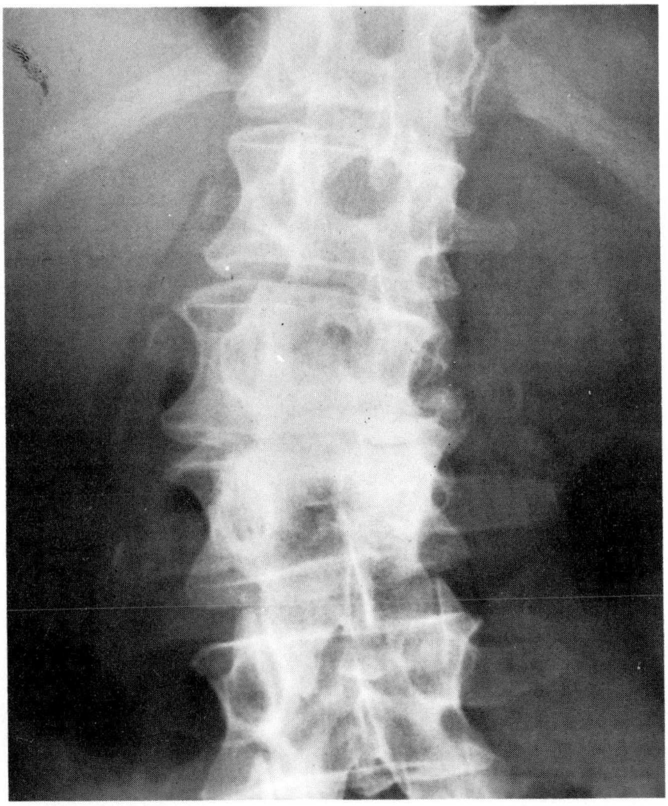

Fig. 2. Osteophytic compression of the second lumbar nerve root. A woman of 57 had for 2 years suffered pain and pins and needles at the front of the right thigh down to the knee, after standing for some time. Symptoms ceased as soon as she sat or lay down.

PLATE XX

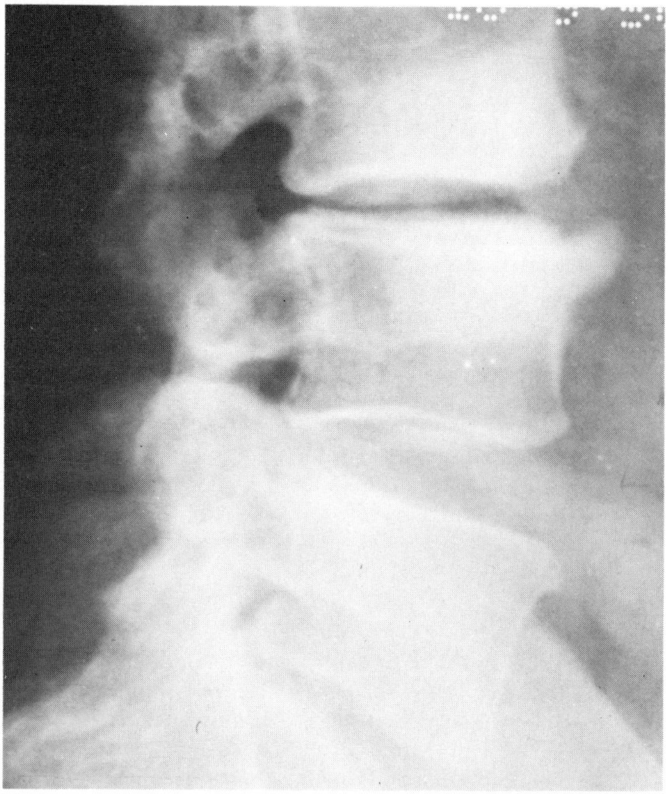

Fig. 1. Third lumbar root compression. A man aged 48 had for 6 months noticed pins and needles in the inner aspect of the lower thigh on standing, relieved at once by sitting or lying.

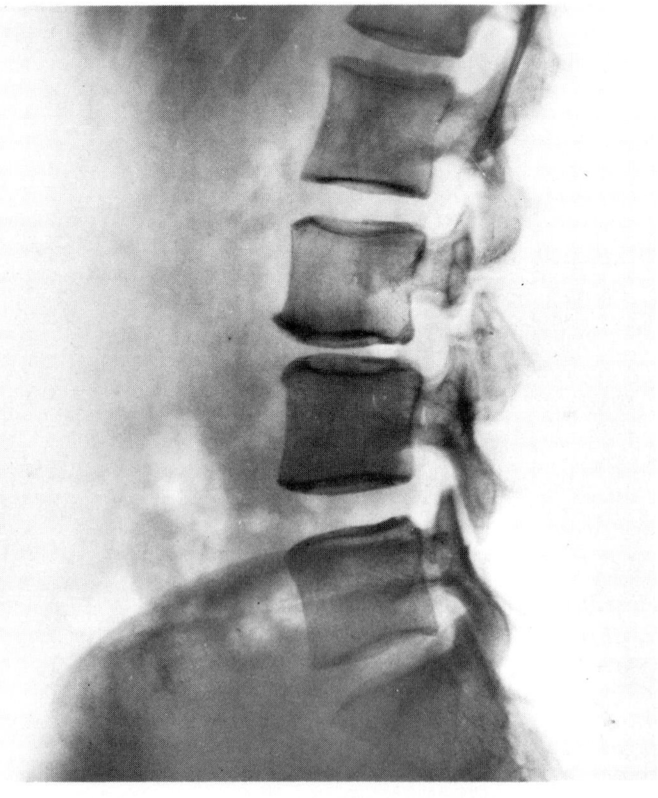

Fig. 2. Spondylolysis. Fibrous defect at the isthmus of the third lumbar vertebra without the deformity of spondylolysis. The patient was a woman aged 40 who had suffered from backache for 3 years. Though the radiograph suggests that the symptoms are due to a secondary disc lesion, examination showed capsular stretch to be responsible.

PLATE XXIII

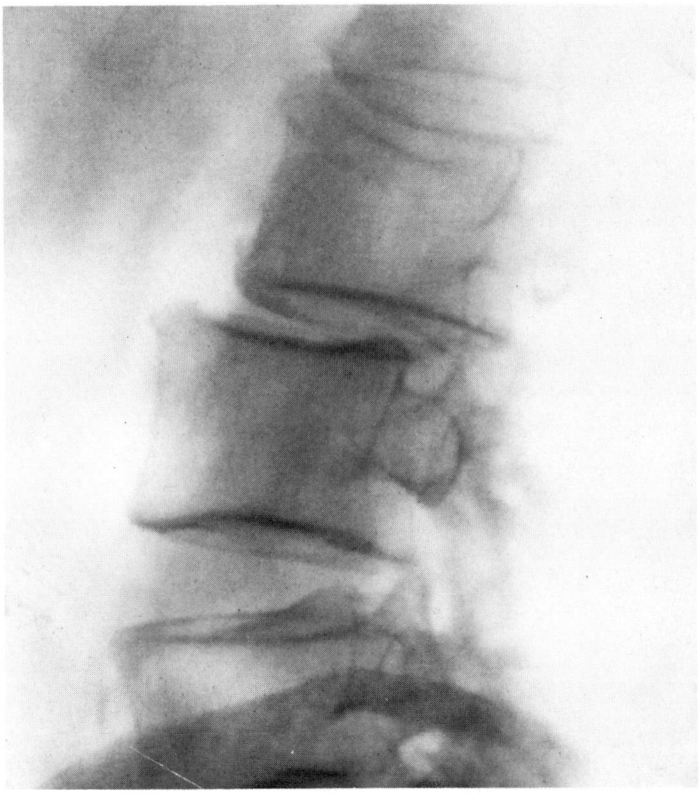

Fig. 1. Posterior spondylolisthesis at the third lumbar level. This followed a laminectomy at which the lateral articulation had been encroached upon. This patient had suffered several years' bilateral root pain at the front of the thighs.

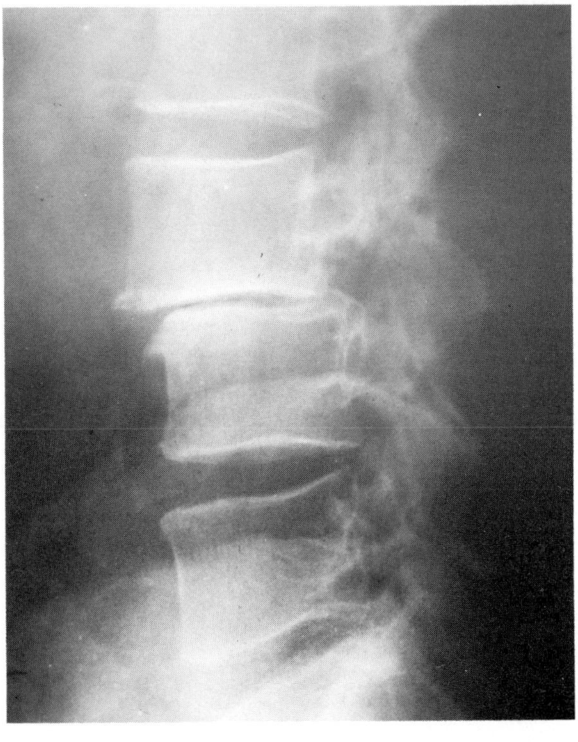

Fig. 2. Third lumbar spondylolisthesis. The patient, aged 54, had suffered for 11 years from pain at the front of one thigh only while standing, for which no cause had ever been detected. The condition was cured by arthrodesis.

PLATE XXIV

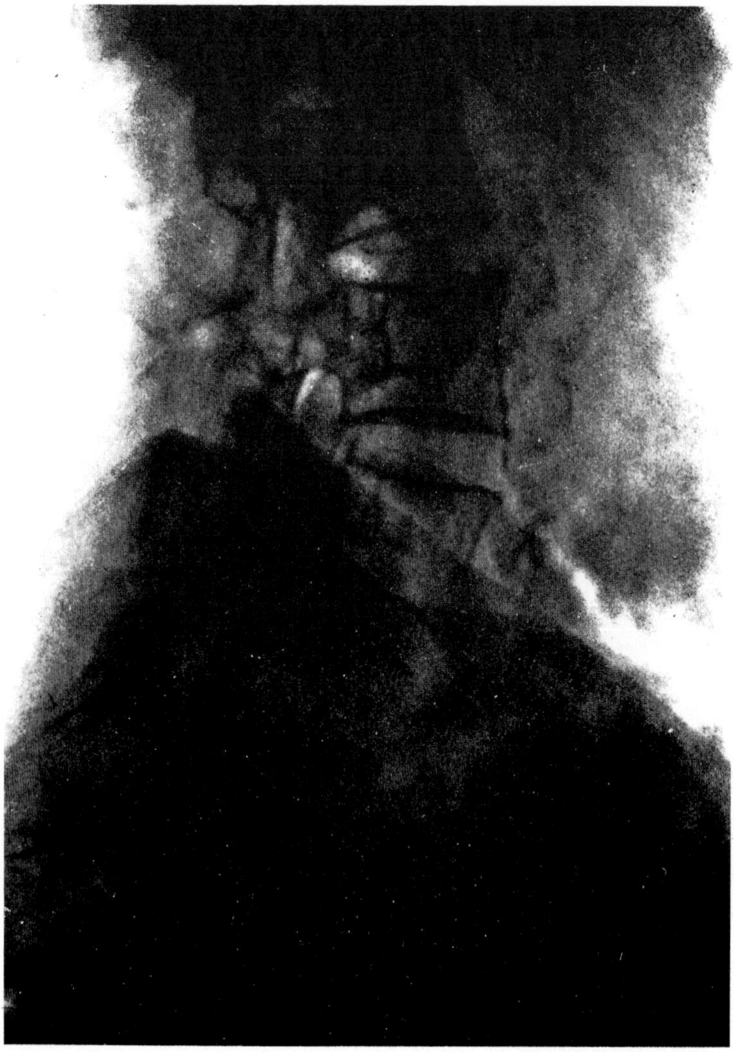

Senile osteoporosis. Note the extreme rarefaction of the lumbar vertebrae, contrasting with the calcified areas in the aorta. There were no symptoms.

PLATE XXV

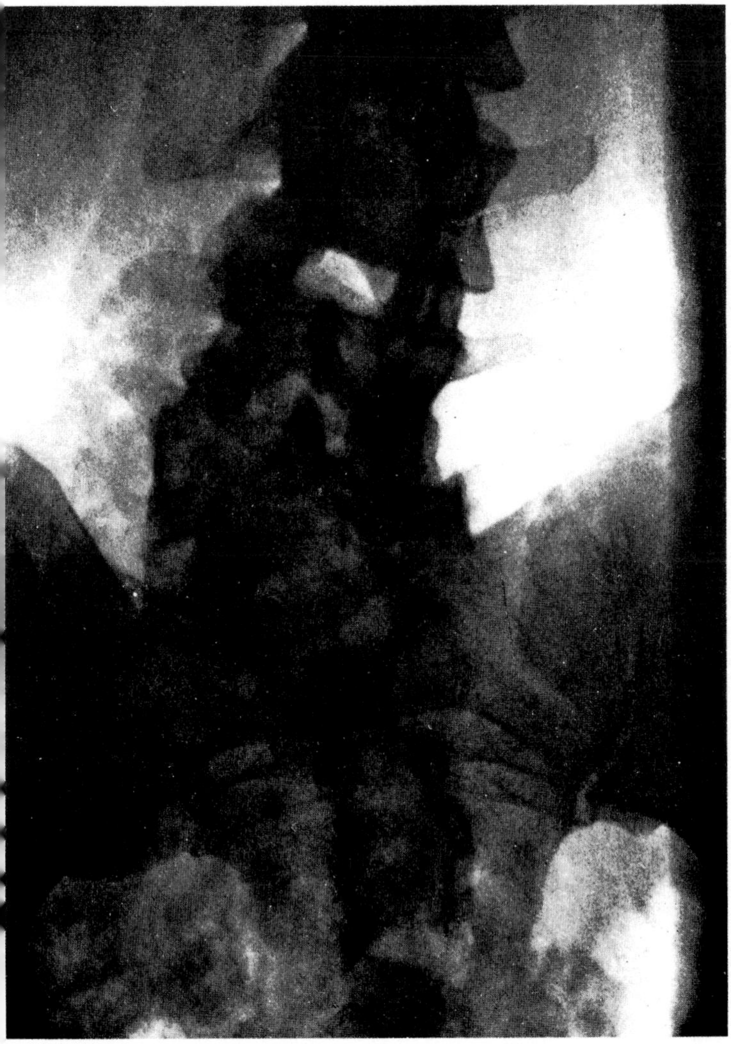

Lumbar hemivertebra. This patient had suffered from aching at the back of the thighs for 6 months.

PLATE XXVI

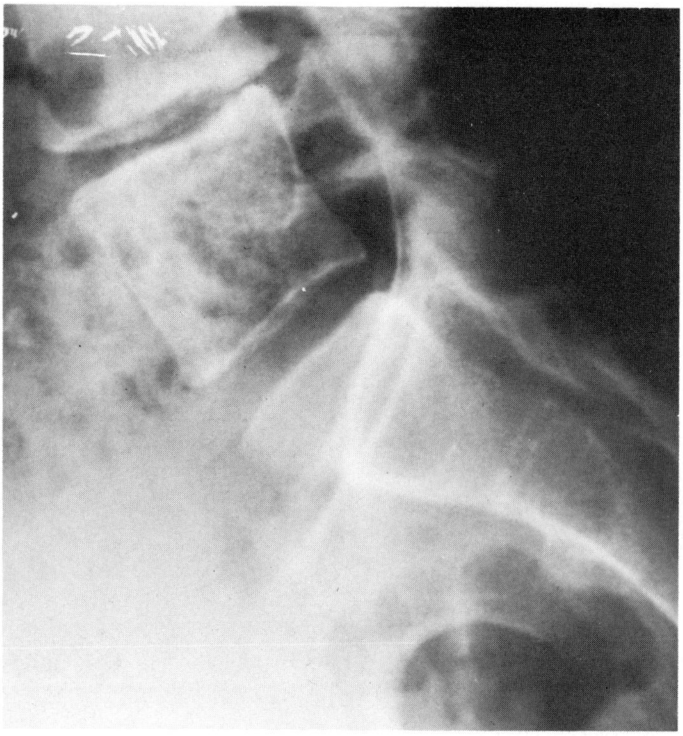

Fig. 1. Posterior osteophytosis. The osteophyte is clearly visible at the postero-inferior angle of the fourth lumbar body. The patient, a man aged 36, had recurrent lumbago for 15 years and constant backache for 2 years.

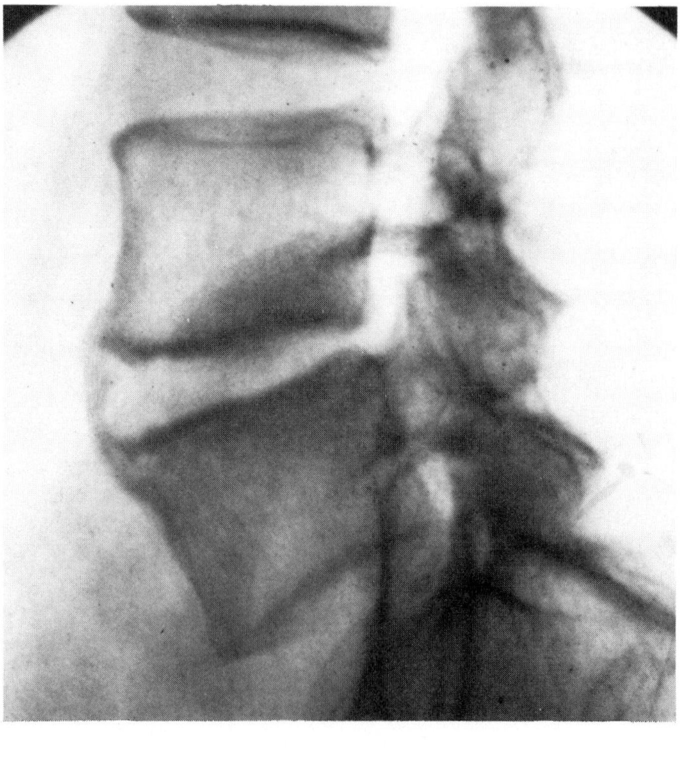

Fig. 2. Septic arthritis at the fourth lumbar joint. This man, aged 42, was first seen by me after 6 months of increasingly severe backache. The radiograph then revealed no abnormality, but the lumbar movements were markedly limited. At the end of a year the ankylosis by bone became clearly visible (see text).

PLATE XXVII

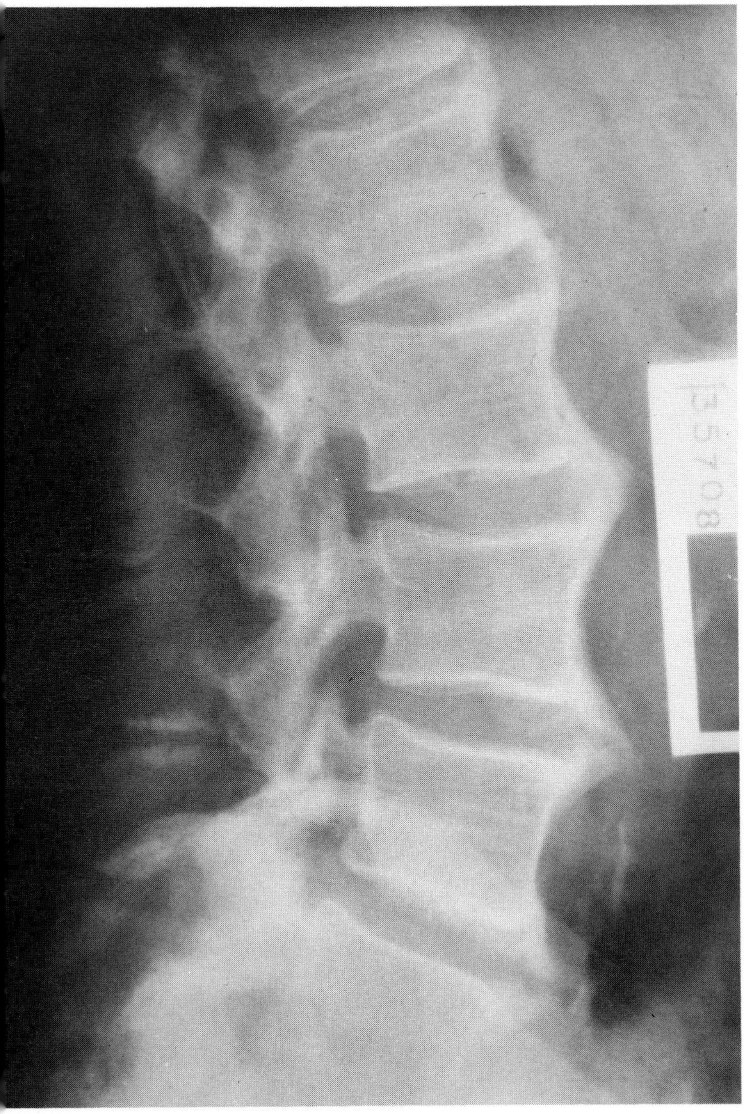


Vertebral hyperostosis. The patient, a man aged 58, had had lumbothoracic backache for 5 years. The anterior longitudinal ligament has ossified and the disorder had involved the adjacent margins of the spinous process.

PLATE XXVIII

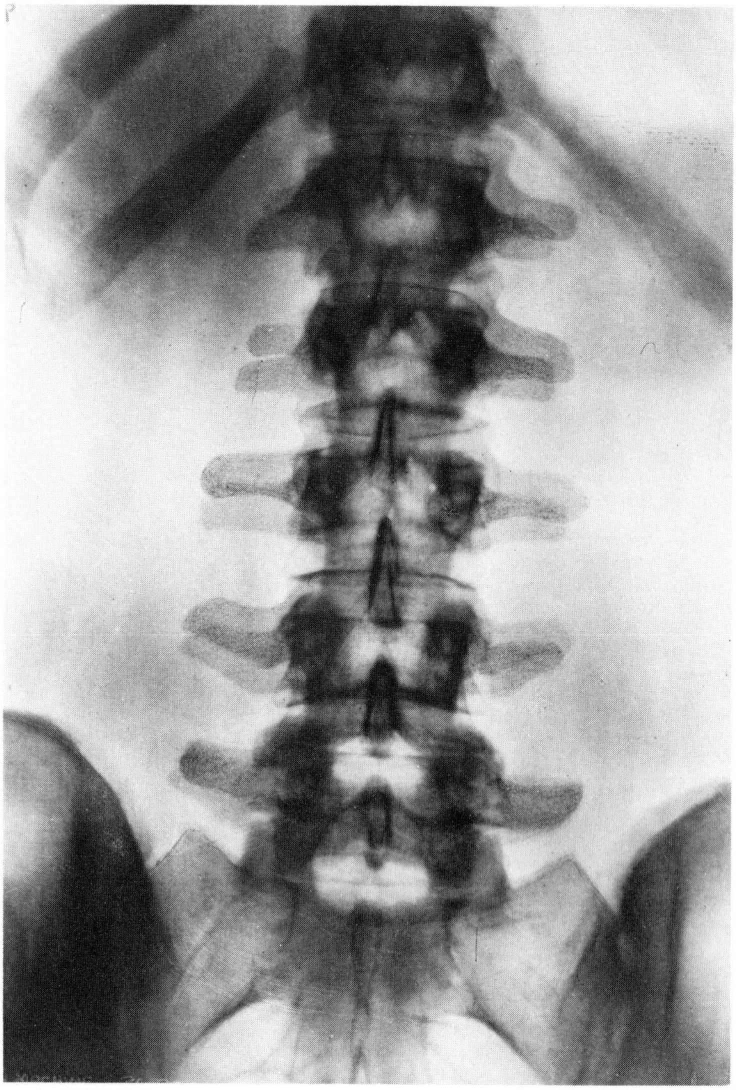

Traction on the lumbar spine. Two photographs have been superimposed, corresponding at the sacrum and iliac crests. The first was taken as the patient lay prone and the second after 10 minutes traction by 50 kg (100 lb). The amount of traction obtained is visible and can be seen to be less than that secured so easily by hand at the cervical joints (see Plate VI).

PLATE XXIX

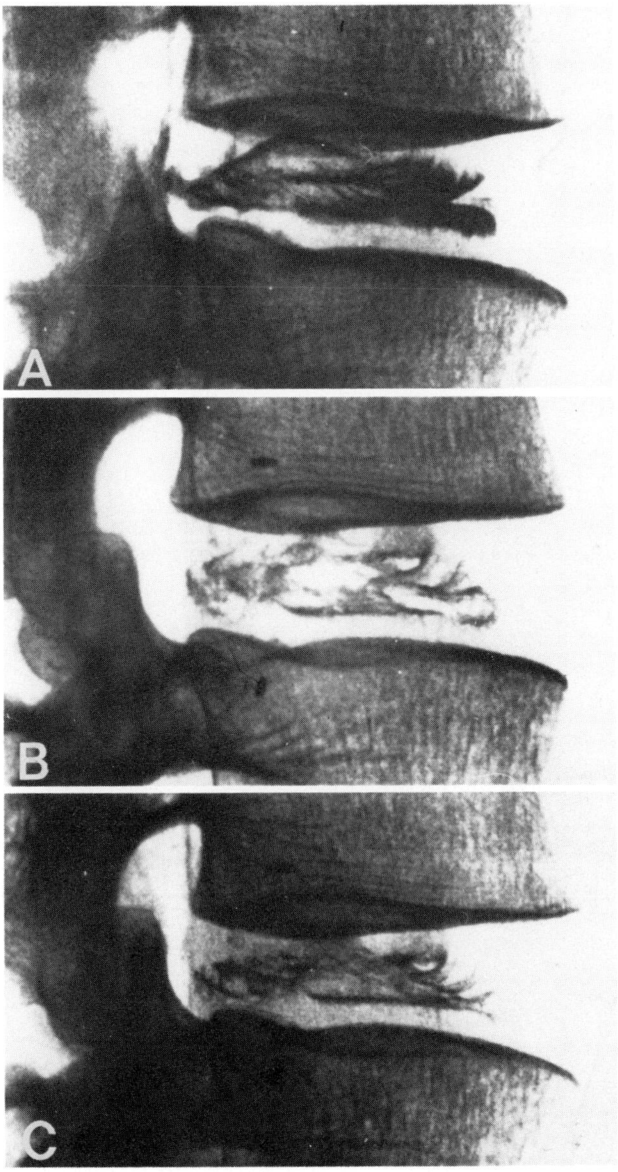


Traction discography. A, Before traction the constant medium outlines the posterior protrusion. B, During traction the joint space widens by 1.5 mm. The oil is sucked back level with the bone edges. C, After traction reduction is maintained.

PLATE XXX

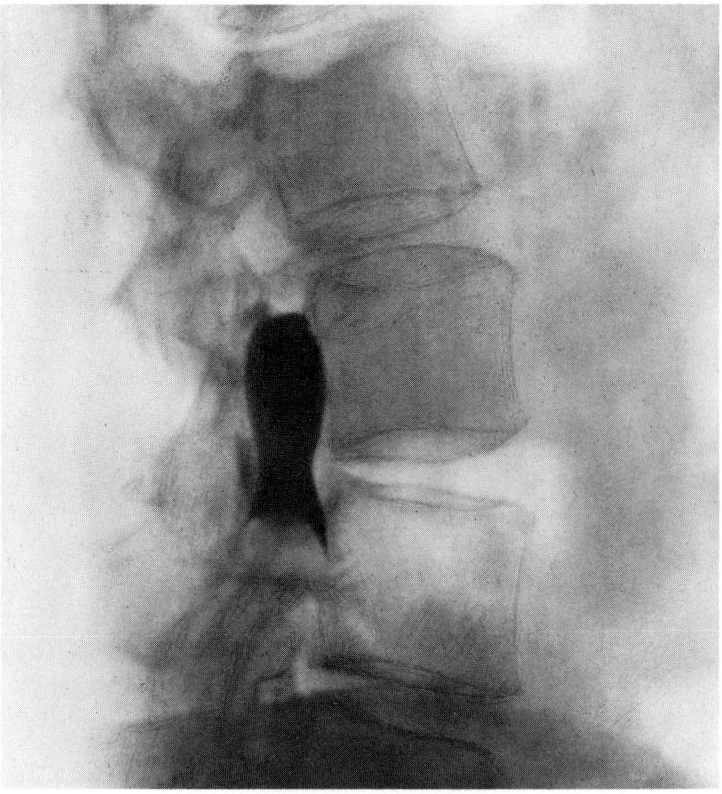

Fig. 1. Lumbar myelogram, showing a spinal tumour at the fourth lumbar level. The patient had had pain in the right groin for nine months and sciatica for six months. Straight-leg raising was limited on the right. No alteration of muscle power or reflex was detectable, but the patient's flexed posture aroused immediate suspicion.

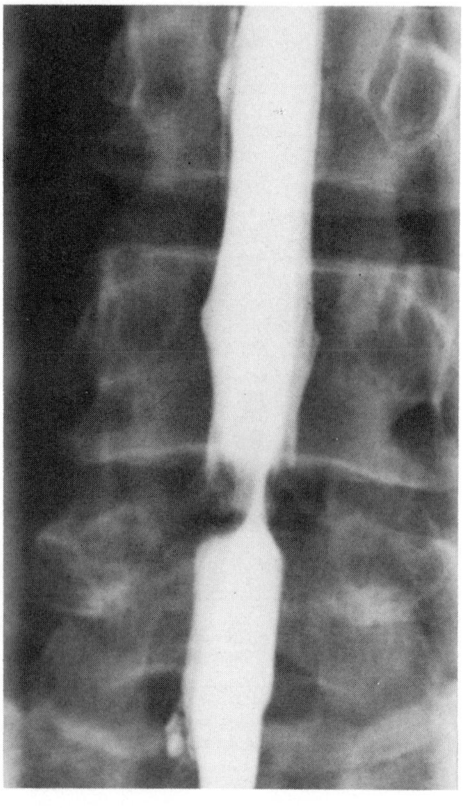

Fig. 2. A myelogram showing a fourth lumbar protrusion. The patient was fixed in flexion by right-sided sciatica. Note the fringed edge denoting extrathecal compression (cf. Fig. 1.).

PLATE XXXI

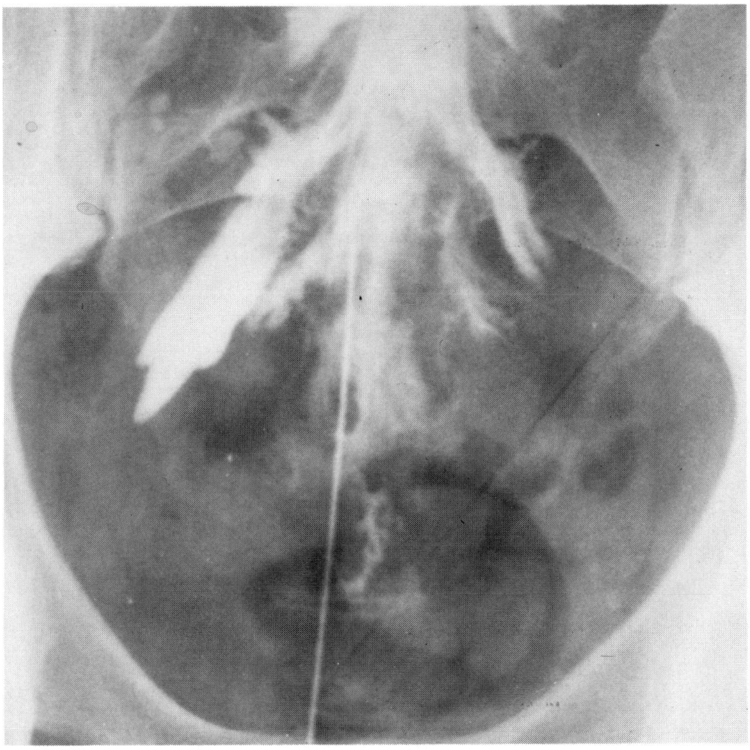

Fig. 1. Epidurogram. The needle is in situ and 10 ml of equal quantities of 1:200 procaine and urographin have been injected. The contrast medium is spreading down the sciatic nerve roots.

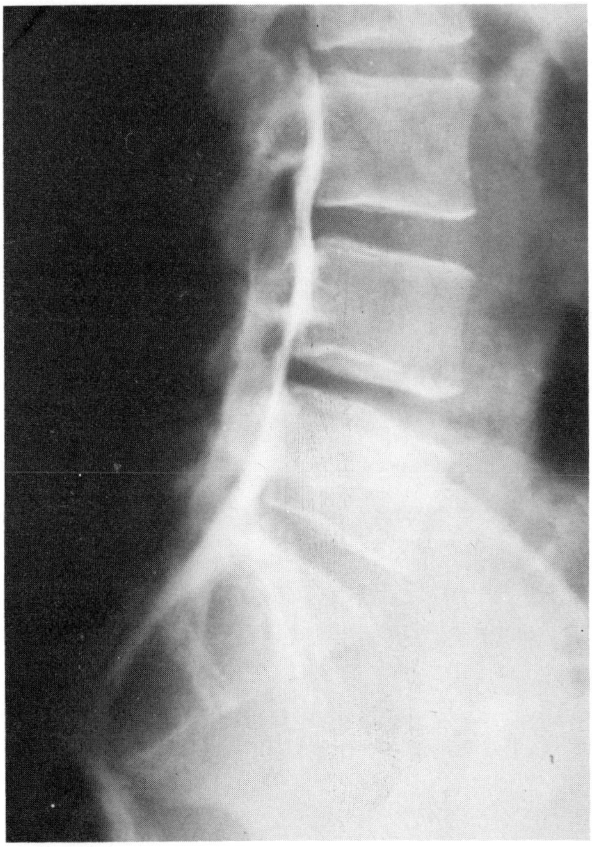

Fig. 2. Epidurogram. 20 ml have now been injected. The opaque solution has travelled extradurally as far as the third lumbar level.

PLATE XXXII

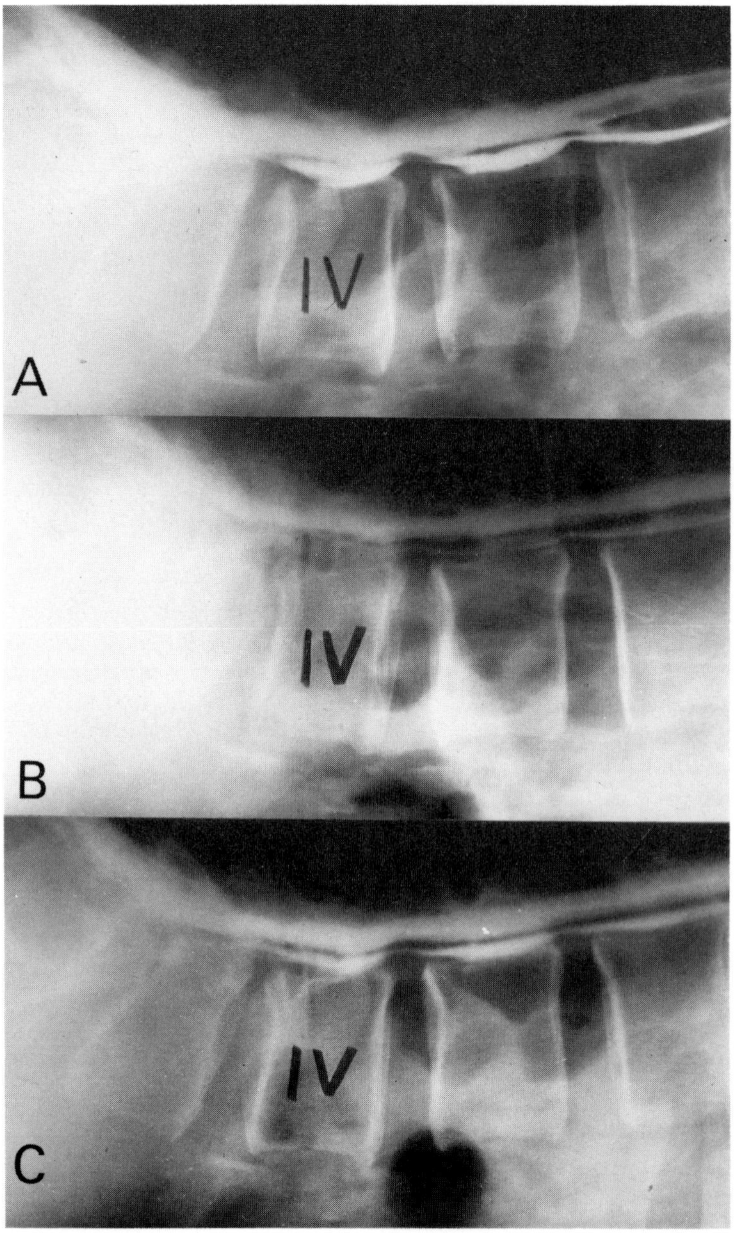


Epidurogram. Contrast radiography by J.A. Matthews (St Thomas's Hospital) before, during and after traction in a man aged 67 with root pain due to prolapse of disc material at the third lumbar level. A, Before traction. B, After traction of 65 kg for 20 minutes. C, Ten minutes after ceasing traction. The prolapse between the third and fourth vertebrae is seen to recede during traction, but to return partly after its release.

PLATE XXXIII

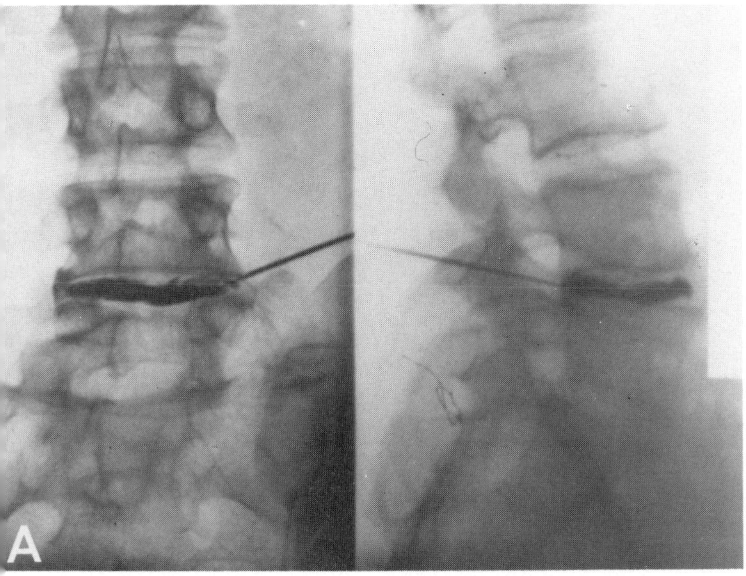


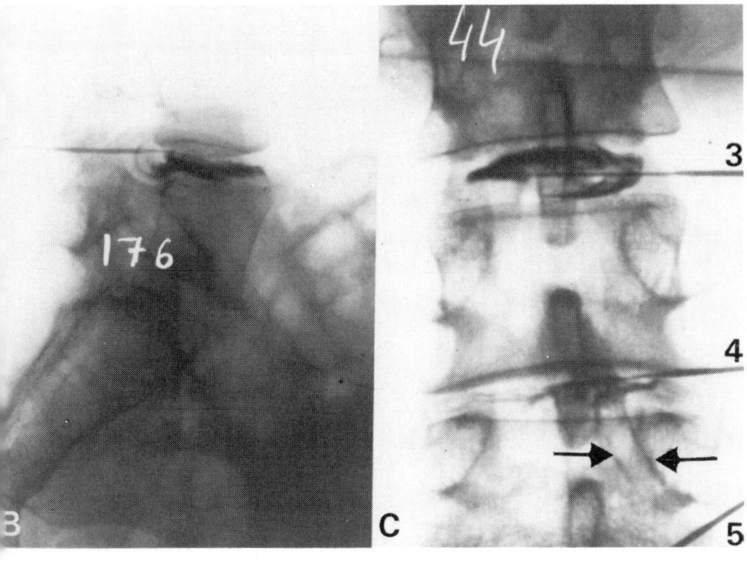


Discograms. A, Advanced degeneration of the entire fourth lumbar disc. B, Large posterolateral protrusion. The oil also outlines the bulging posterior ligaments. C, Extravasation of oil along the fifth nerve root. The dye has been injected into the nucleus and has emerged from the joint, outlining the fifth nerve root (arrowed). Note how this root can be compressed at the edge of the posterior ligament by a fourth lumbar protrusion. *(By courtesy of O. Troisier)*

PLATE XXXIV

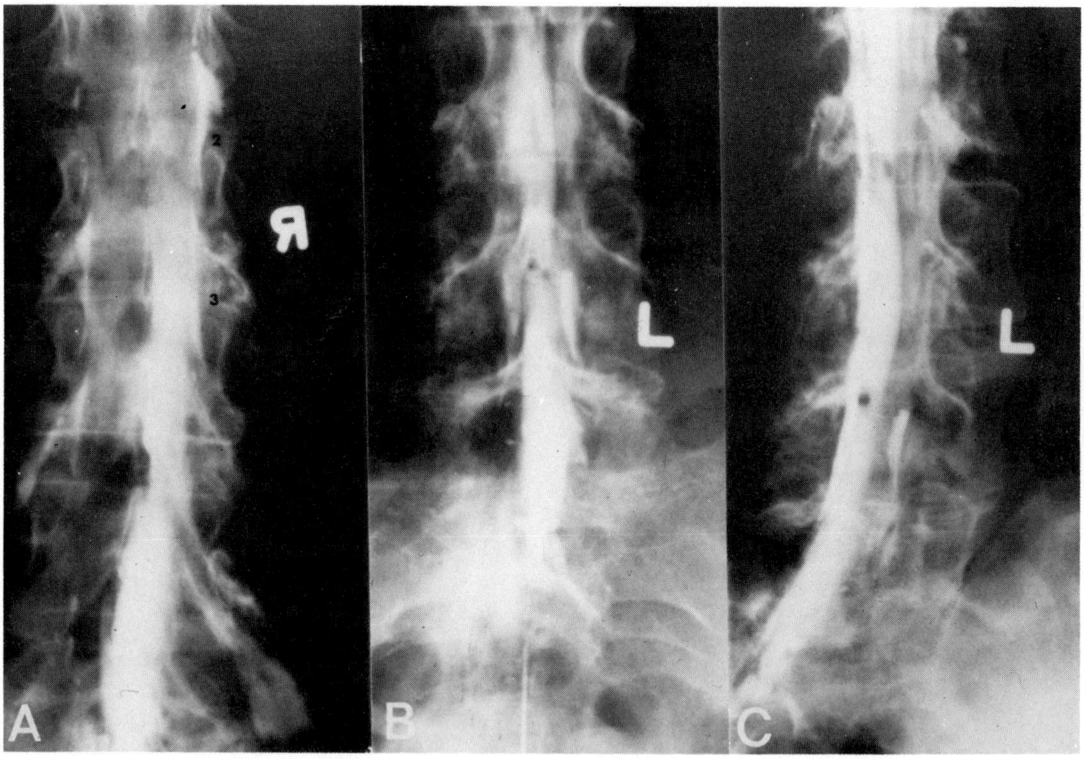


Caudal epidurograms. A, Disc protrusion in a man aged 29 at the fourth and probably fifth levels. The second root is outlined as far as the edge of the vertebra and the third slightly beyond. On the left side no oil is seen at the fourth and fifth roots, although they are well displayed on the right. B, The contrast material outlines the whole width of the intervertebral space and can be seen flowing along the first, second, third and fourth nerve roots, but there is none at the fifth level on either side, the site of previous laminectomy. C, Lateral view of the same patient as in B. Once again the second, third and fourth nerve roots are outlined by the oil. *(By courtesy of Richard Ellis)*

PLATE XXXV

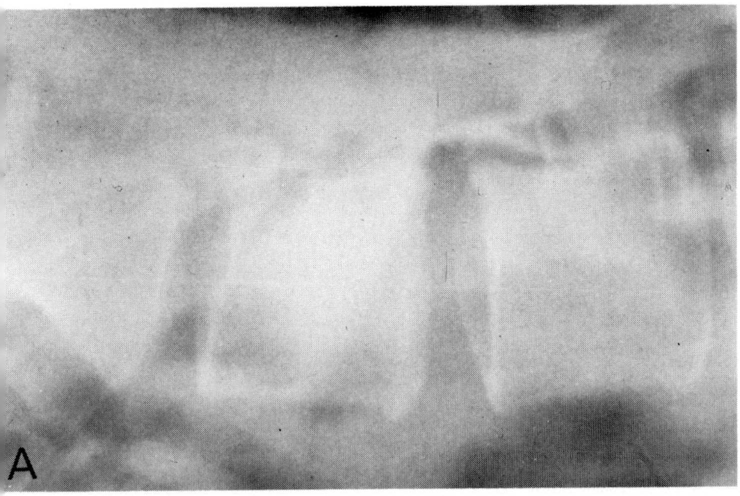


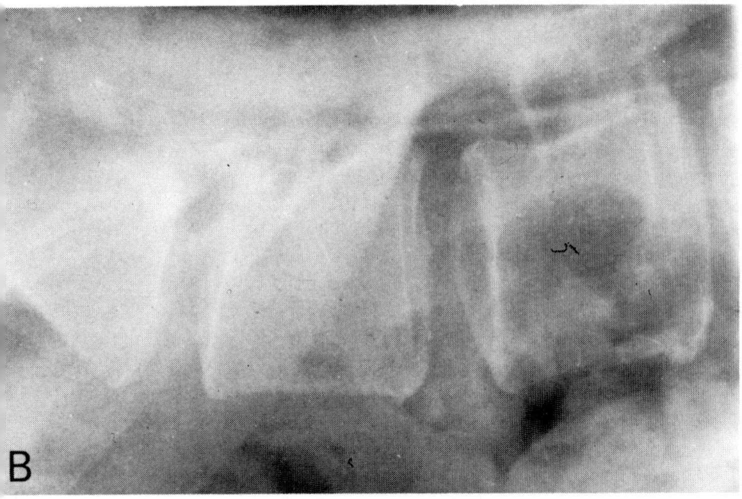


An epidurogram from a patient with acute lumbago. A, Contrast radiograph, showing the posterior longitudinal ligament at the fourth level bulging posteriorly on account of the central protrusion. B, A second radiograph, taken 30 minutes later, after manipulation reduction had succeeded. Note that the posterior ligament now follows a straight line. *(By courtesy of J.A. Matthews)*

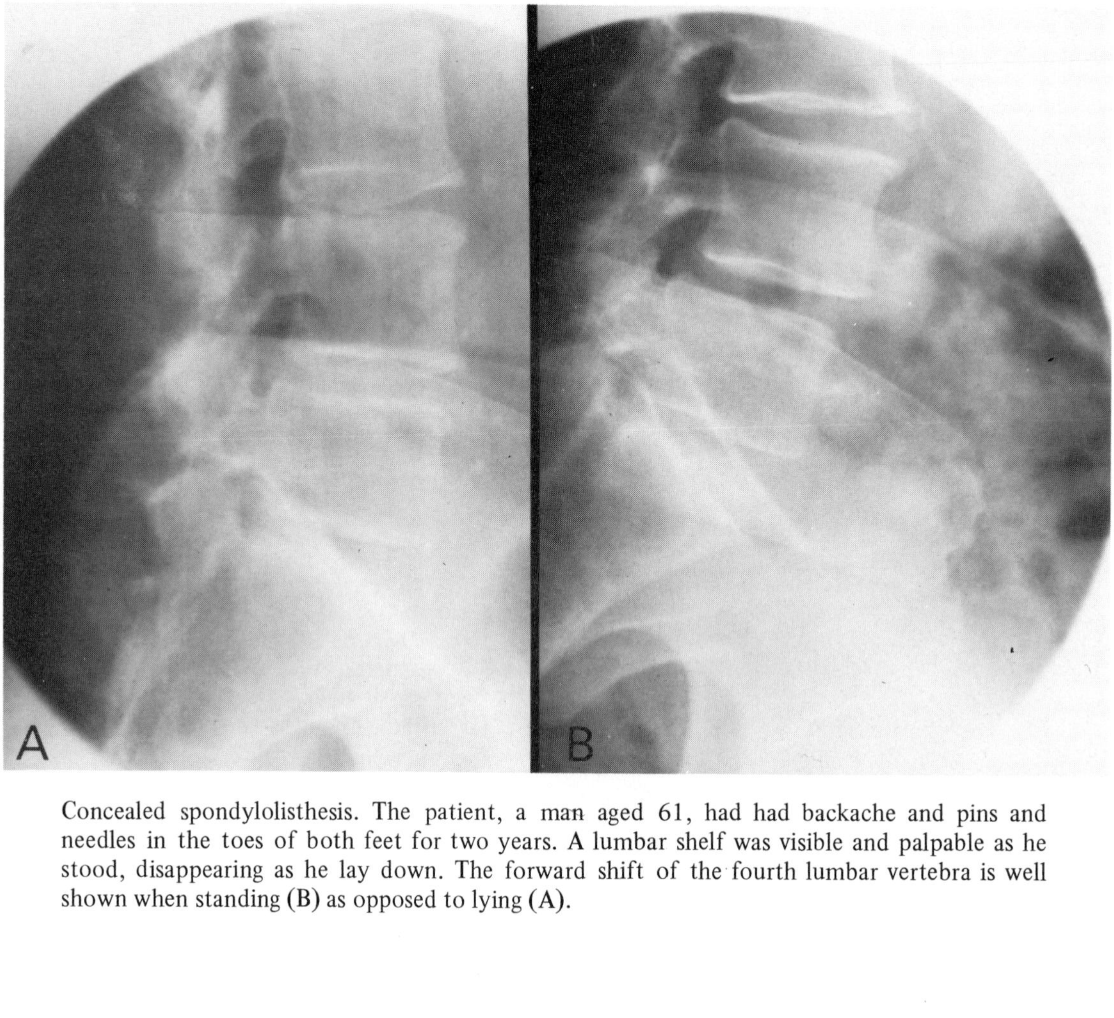


Concealed spondylolisthesis. The patient, a man aged 61, had had backache and pins and needles in the toes of both feet for two years. A lumbar shelf was visible and palpable as he stood, disappearing as he lay down. The forward shift of the fourth lumbar vertebra is well shown when standing (B) as opposed to lying (A).

PLATE XXXVII

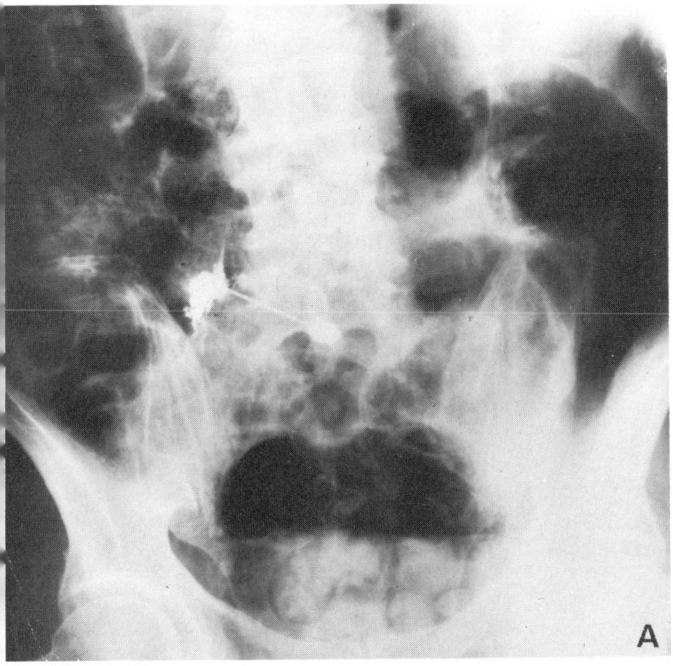


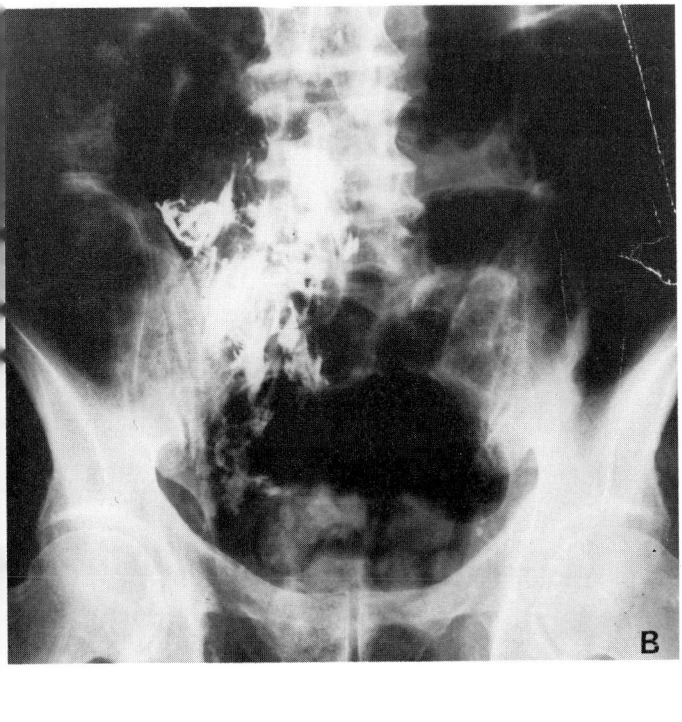


Sclerosant injection. A, The contrast medium is shown lying at the fifth lumbar transverse process, at the origin of the iliolumbar ligament. A needle 7-8 cm long is needed. B, The injection completed (for clarity on one side only). *(By courtesy of Dr P. Slatter, who carried out the infiltration)*

PLATE XXXVIII

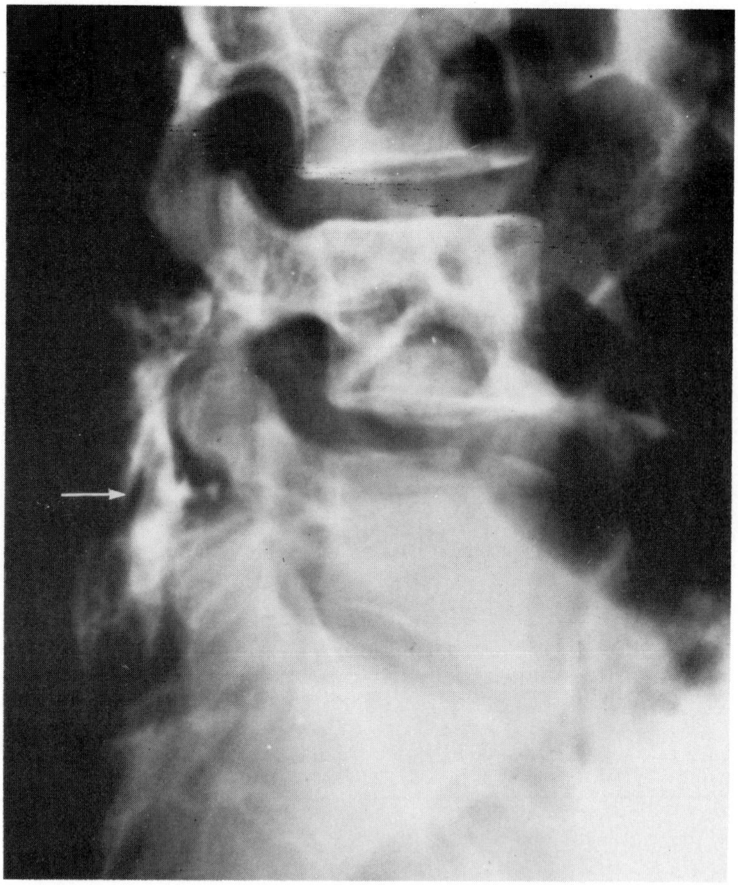

The spread of fluid injected at the edge of the lamina. 1 ml of urographin has been injected at the fourth lumbar level, and a further 1 ml at the fifth. The oils have joined, reaching the area where the lateral branch of the posterior ramus follows the deep lumbar fascia. None has passed forwards to the sinuvertebral nerve.

PLATE XXXIX

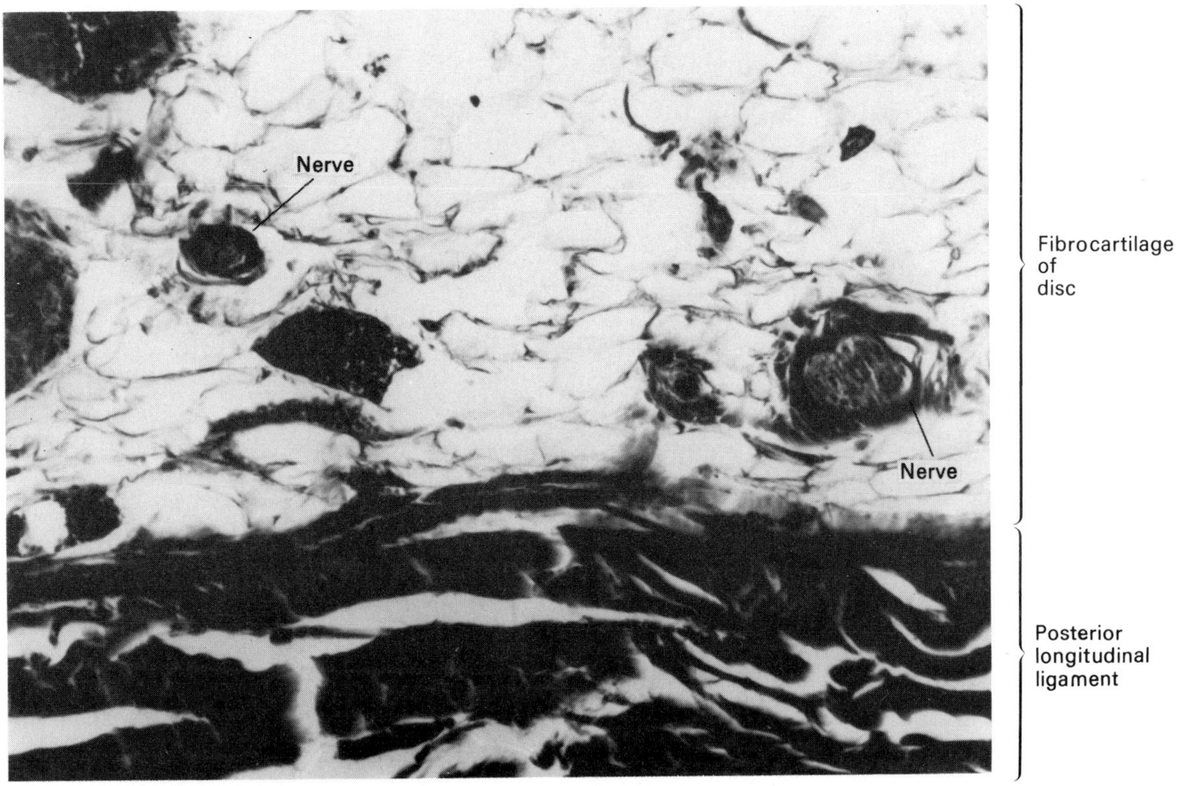


The innervation of the disc. Two twigs derived from the sinuvertebral nerve lie in the epidural tissue 3 mm beyond the posterior surface of the posterior longitudinal ligament. No nerves were discovered penetrating the annulus more deeply x 680 *(By courtesy of Professor K. Bradley)*

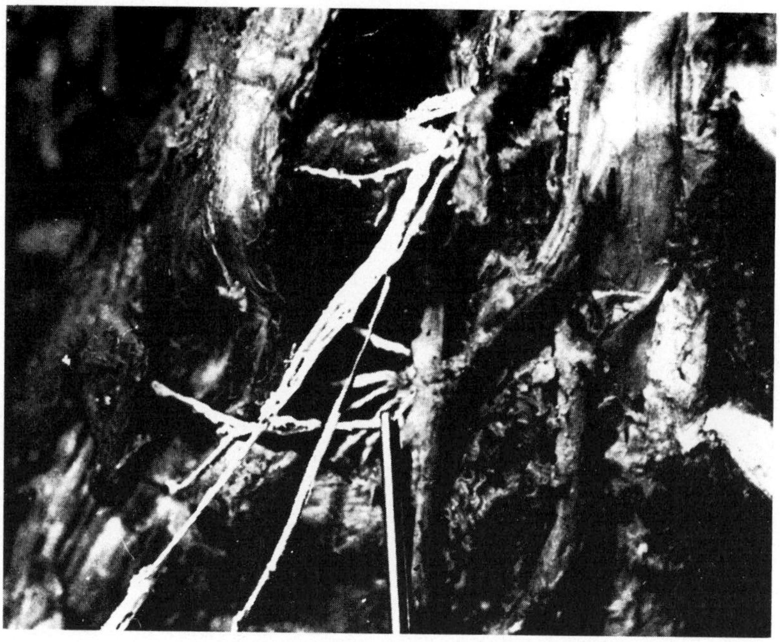

PLATE XL

Dissection of the lumbar nerve. Th nerve to the quadratus lumborun muscle (held in forceps) is derive from the second lumbar root an crosses the tip of the third lumba transverse process. *(By courtesy o Professor P. Sturniolo, Institutos Med icos Antartida, Buenos Aires)*

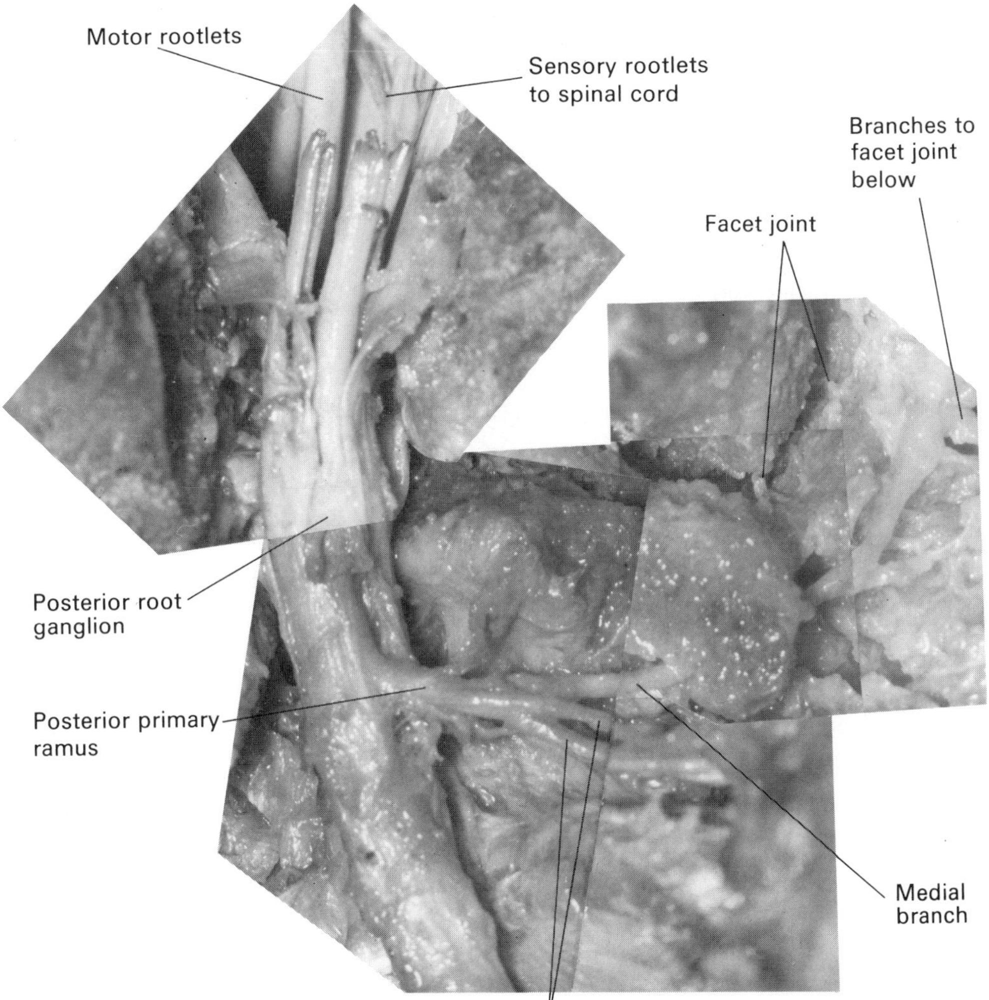


Dissection of the posterior ramus. The facet joint is innervated by the medial branch of the posterior ramus. This divides into two the longer filament running to the facet joint below and the lateral branches to the adjacent periosteum and muscle. The sinuvertebral nerve emerges from the ramus proximally and loops back into the foramen. *(By courtesy of Professor K. Bradley, University of Melbourne)*

PLATE XLII

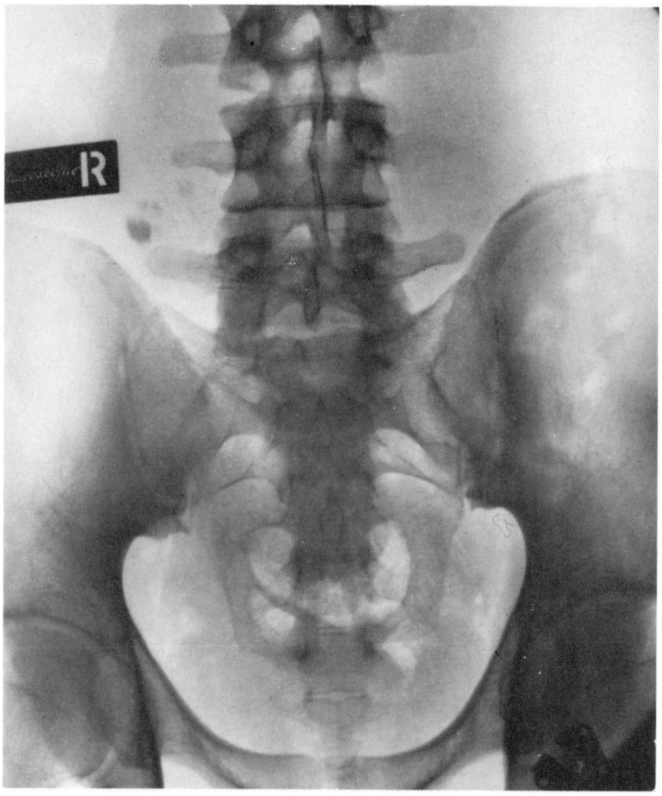


Fig. 1. Early ankylosing spondylitis. Sclerosis at the iliac side of the left sacroiliac joint is beginning. The patient was aged 19 and had had bouts of pain in one or other buttock for 18 months. Previous radiographs had revealed nothing.

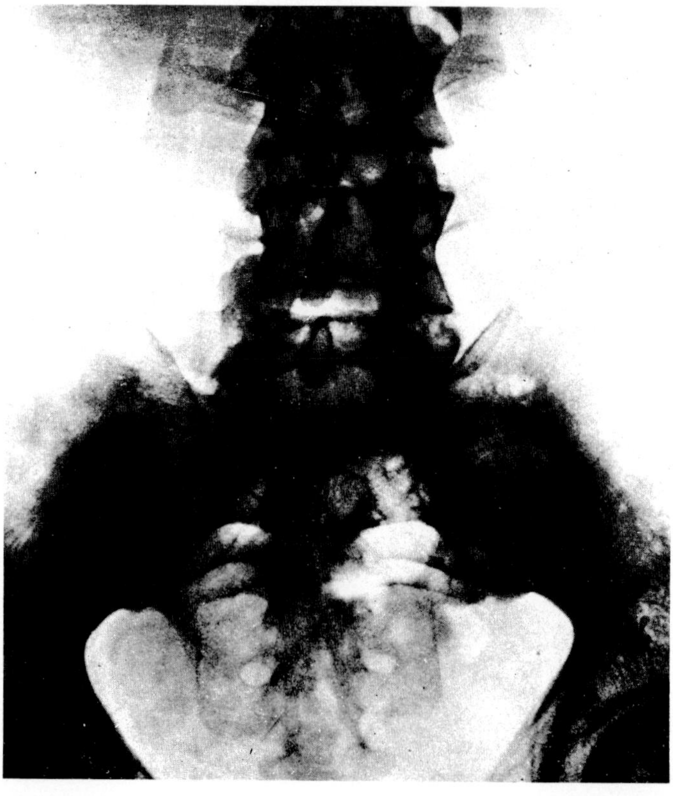

Fig. 2. Sacroiliac fusion. The sacroiliac joints have disappeared as a result of spondylitis deformans of 30 years' standing. Note the ossification of the left side of the second lumbar vertebra.

PLATE XLIII

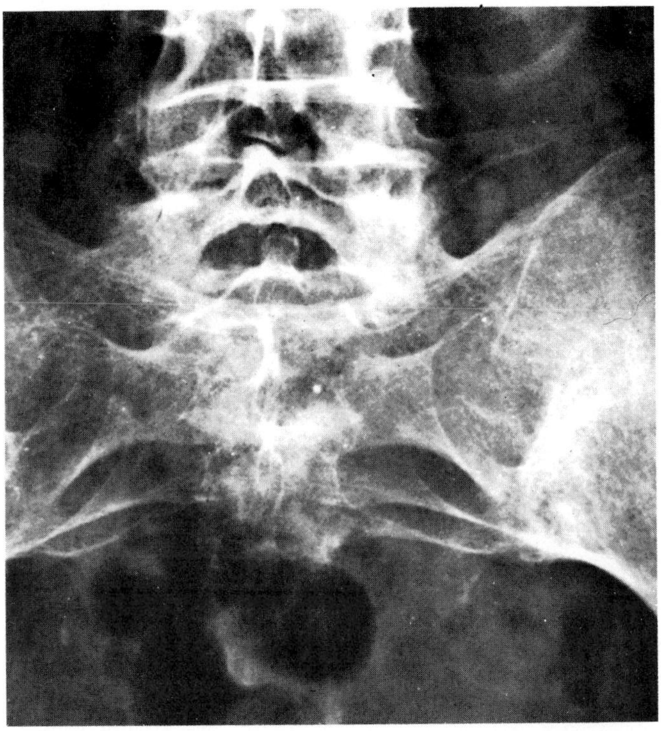

Fig. 1. Osteitis condensans ilii. The sclerosis occupies the central part of the joint whose margins are not blurred.

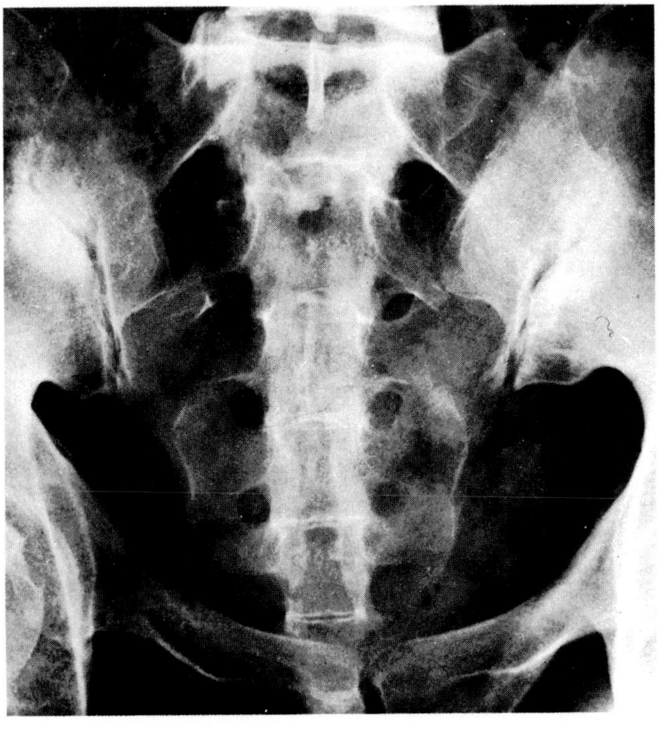

Fig. 2. Aborted spondylitis. A woman aged 65 reported intermittent sciatica from the ages of 17 to 27. She had had no subsequent symptoms and a good range of painless movement was present at her lumbar and thoracic joints.

PLATE XLIV

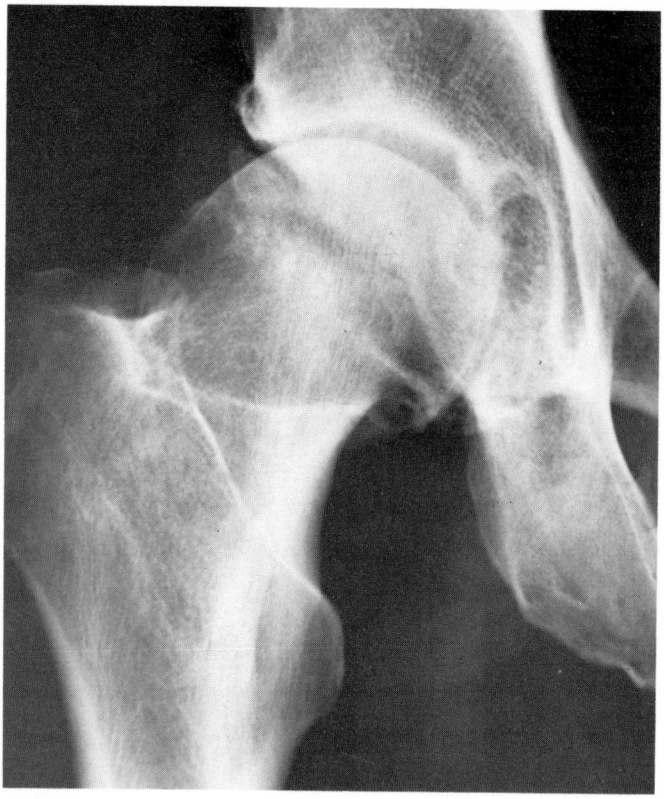

Fig. 1. Osteoarthritis of the hip. This type carries a good prognosis.

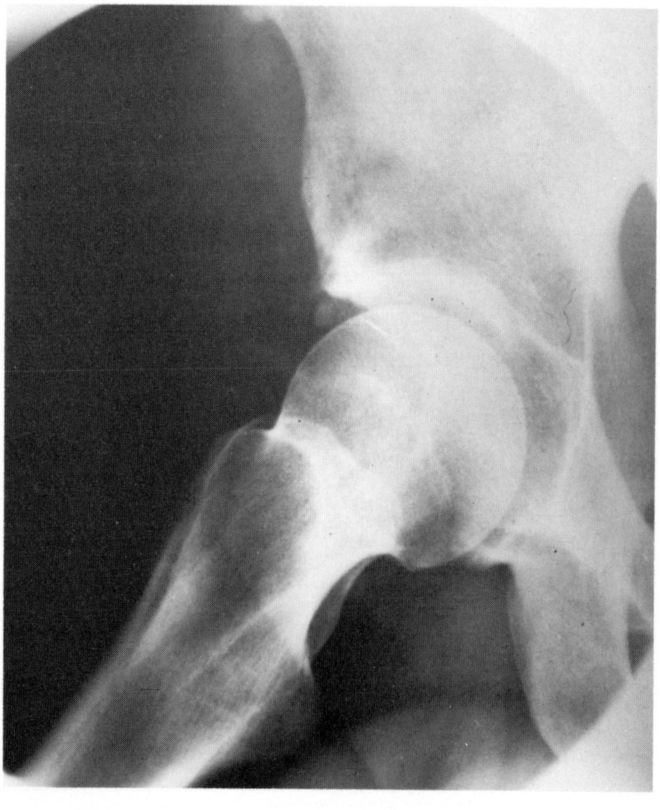

Fig. 2. A loose body in a normal hip joint. The patient, aged 38, had suffered twinges for 3 weeks.

PLATE XLV

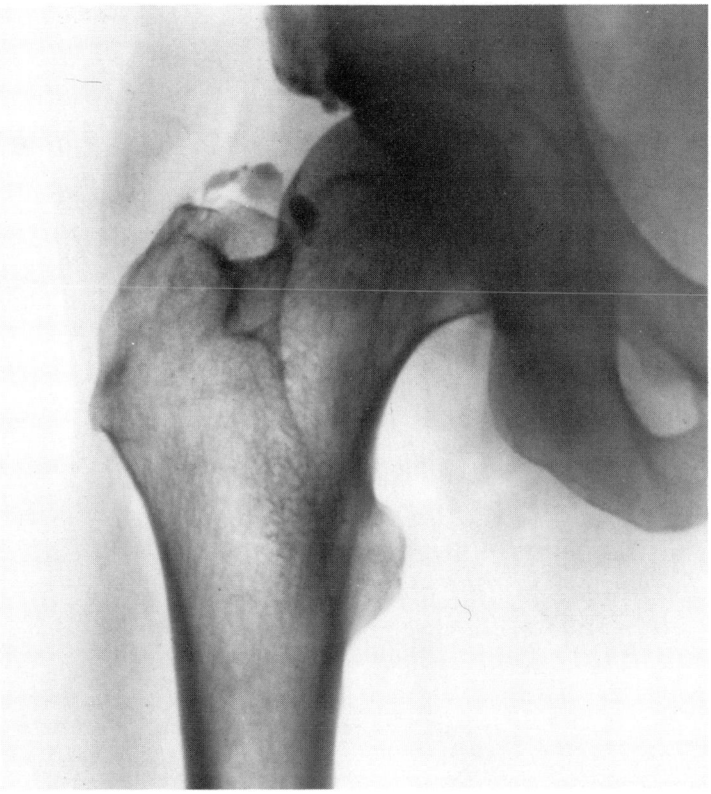

Fig. 1. Calcification in the gluteal bursa.

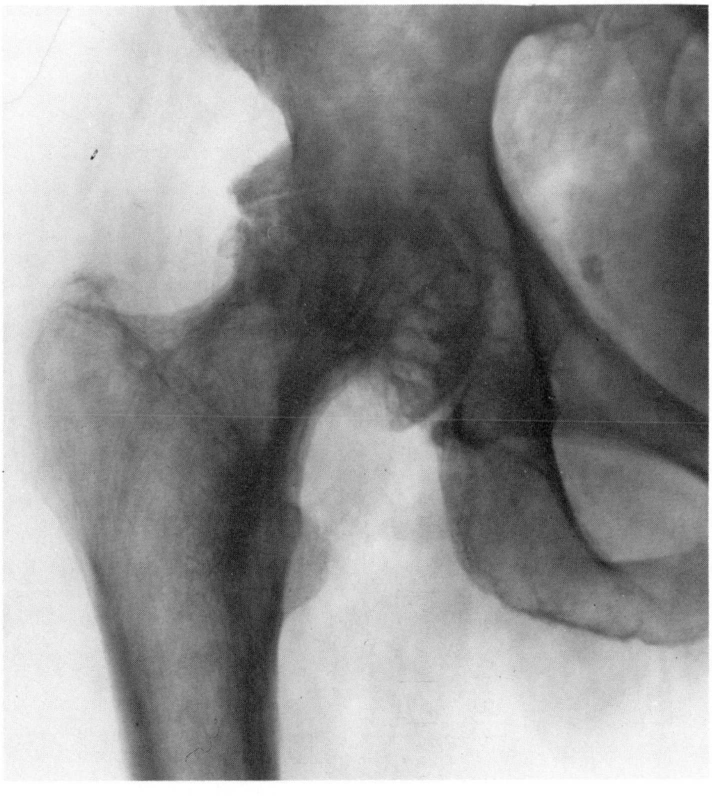

Fig. 2. Gonococcal arthritis of the hip. 20 years previously the patient, aged 66 at the time of the radiograph, had spent 6 months in bed with gonococcal arthritis at the hip. There is a striking contrast between the X-ray appearances and the full range of painless movement which was present at the joint. The muscles were considerably wasted.

PLATE XLVI

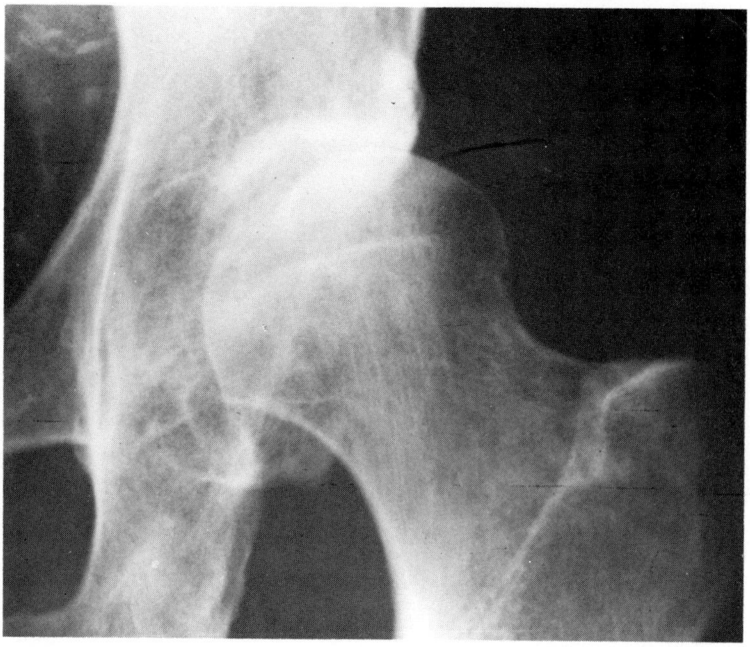

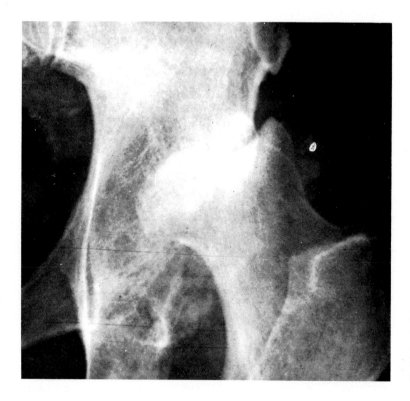

Radiographs from a man aged 68, suffering from pain in the thigh. A, After 1 month of symptoms. B, 3 months later. No steroids had been given orally or by injection.

PLATE XLVII

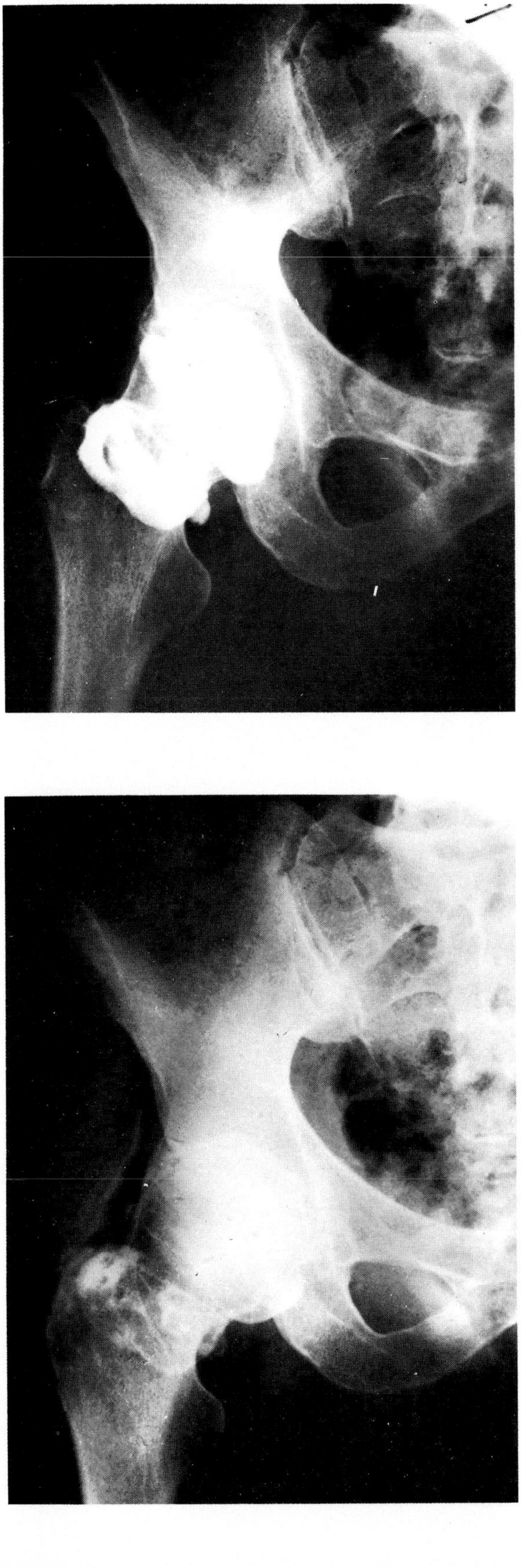

Intra-articular at the hip. A, Injection of 25 ml: the contrast medium remains within the joint. B, Injection of 40 ml: extravasation.

PLATE XLVIII

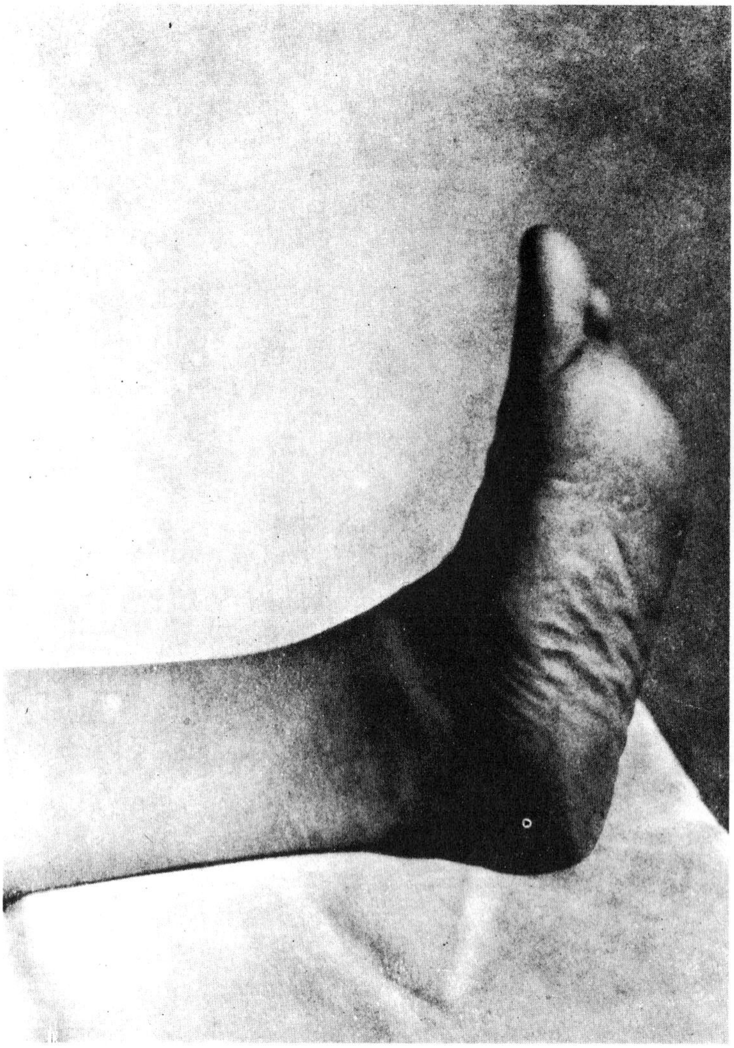

Metatarsus inversus. Note the medial rotation deformity of the forefoot on the hind-foot.

PLATE XXI

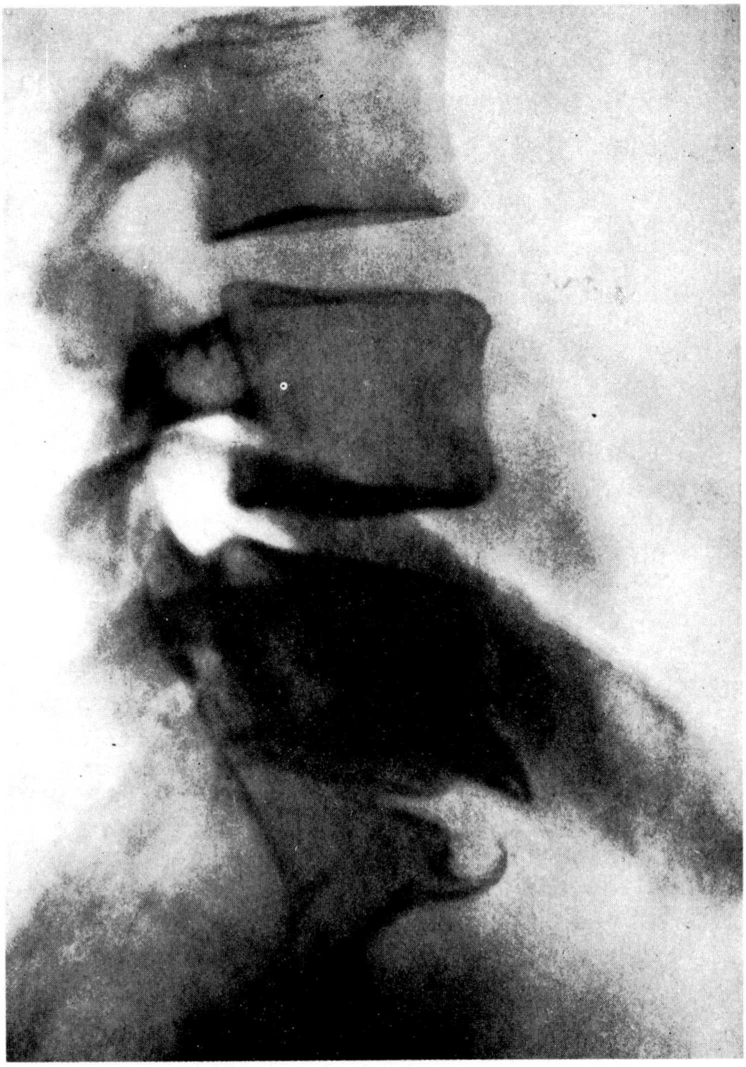

Anterior disc protrusion. The fifth lumbar disc had been reduced to rubble and the intervertebral bodies lie in contact. The remaining disc substance has become displaced forwards, where it lies enclosed by the two huge osteophytes that have formed in consequence of the traction exerted by the anterior longitudinal ligament. Since the protrusion does not impinge on a sensitive structure, no pain is felt for many years; finally compression causes the 'mushroom phenomenon' (see text).

PLATE XXII

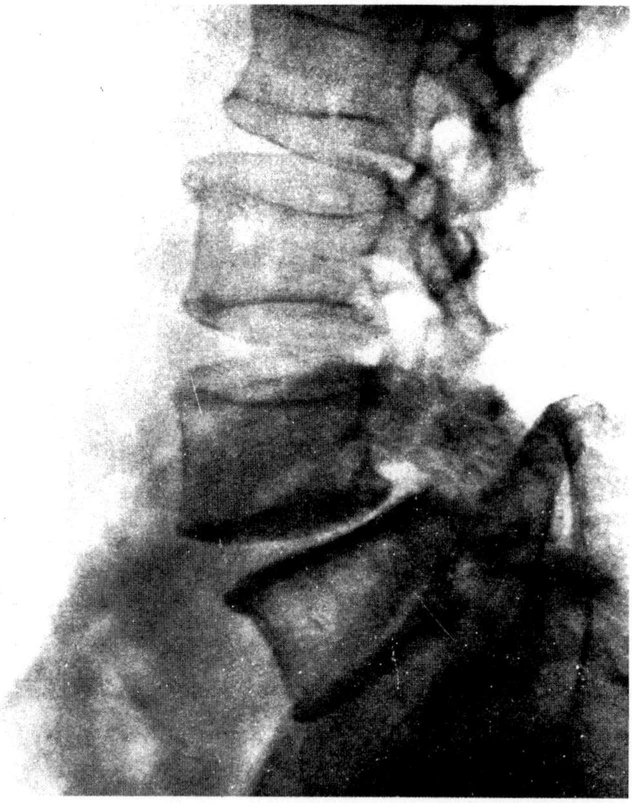

Fig. 1. Spondylolisthesis at the fourth lumbar level. This patient was a waiter whose deformity remained symptomless until it gave rise to bilateral sciatica at the age of 64 years.

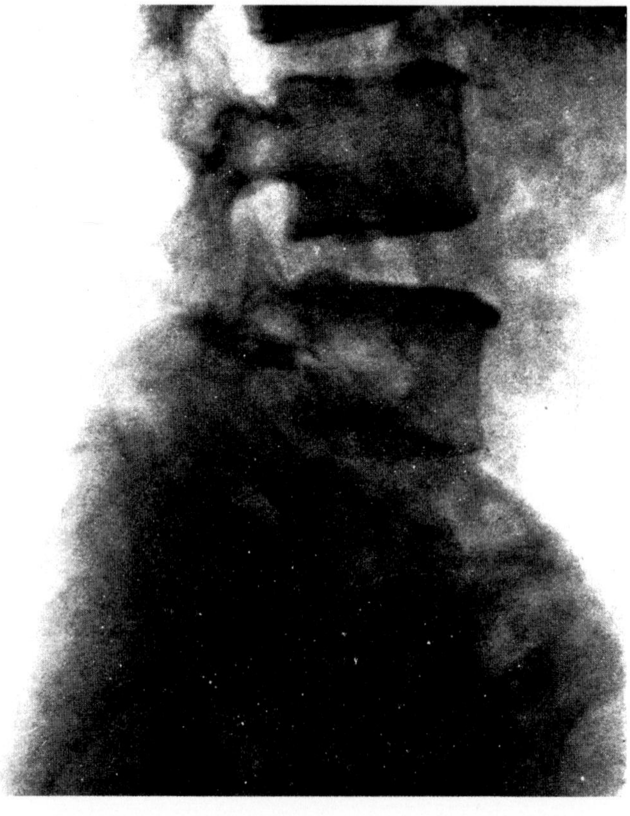

Fig. 2. Spondylolisthesis at the lumbosacral joint. The patient had suffered for 25 years from pain and paraesthesia in his right lower limb after standing for some time. As soon as he sat down the symptoms disappeared. Note the forward displacement of the fifth lumbar vertebral body on the sacrum and the long pedicle. There was no complaint of backache. The sciatica was ascribed to the stretching of the fifth lumbar nerve root against the shelf formed by the upper edge of the sacrum.

## DISC LESIONS IN PREGNANCY

Some women make room for the enlarging uterus by bending forwards over it, losing their lumbar lordosis. Others counterbalance the forward shift of their centre of gravity by bending backwards, increasing lordosis. The former alteration in posture may result in backache. In contrast, these women with low lumbar disc lesions who adopt extension, find to their surprise that they are more comfortable when pregnant than at any other time.

A young woman with a lumbar disc lesion can be assured that pregnancy will not harm her back, and that labour itself will not be affected. It is the stooping involved in looking after the baby after the puerperium that is apt to make the backache worse. An expanding lumbar corset may be prescribed. She should, however, be warned that her posture in bed during the puerperium is important. Proper support for her lordosis must be forthcoming throughout the period of rest in bed (see Volume II). She should turn to lie prone for several periods each day as soon as her condition permits.

During the first four months of pregnancy a disc lesion can be treated by manipulation or traction in the same way as if the woman were not pregnant. During the next four months, traction and the prone-lying manipulations cannot be employed, but side-lying and supine rotations are still practicable. During the last month, epidural local anaesthesia remains quite safe and is often effective. The injection must be given with the patient lying on her side (Fig. 91). Since the fluid injected tends to gravitate downwards, she must lie on the affected side during the induction.

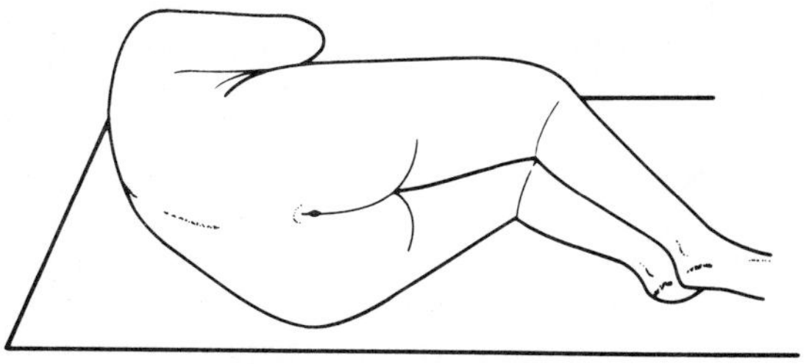

**Fig. 91.** The position of the patient for the induction of epidural local anaesthesia during advanced pregnancy. The patient lies on the affected side.

If the epidural injection fails, rest in bed is indicated.

## DISC LESIONS IN ADOLESCENCE

If patients in their twenties with lumbar disc lesions are asked when their trouble began, they often recall an attack of lumbago while at school, or describe recurrent minor backache beginning at 10 or 12 years old. During the early teens, though disc lesions are uncommon and usually dismissed as 'growing pains' or 'muscle strain', they certainly occur. Sciatica with limited straight-leg raising begins at 11 and, at this age, is much commoner in girls. The ankle jerk may be lost alone. My youngest patients with a root palsy so far are a boy of 12 with considerable fifth root weakness, and a girl of 16 with a first sacral sensory and motor root paresis. In the latter, the muscles recovered full strength in three months. An X-ray photograph must be taken, to make sure that no bony disorder is present, since a precocious disc lesion is often the result of spondylolisthesis, or of sacralization of the fifth lumbar vertebra with consequent double strain on the fourth joint.

Diagnosis is always difficult; for young people are just as likely as adults to use an ache to avoid a disagreeable situation, such as an overbearing parent who wishes all sorts of things done. But it is hard to be sure that the inconsistencies such children show on examination are not just the product of a child's willingness to say what he thinks is expected of him, merely from a wish to please. Nevertheless, when the examination discloses the same pattern of inconsistencies as for psychoneurosis in adults, attention should be directed to the parent. If over-solicitude or domination is a factor, reference to a Child Guidance Clinic often has a good result.

When one of the normal patterns for a disc lesion is found on examination, the diagnosis should not be shunned merely because of the patient's youth. At the Mayo Clinic five cases of disc lesion out of 6500 requiring laminectomy were in children under 16, and in 840 such operations in Oslo seven were in children aged 11 to 17 (Rugtveit 1966). The first recorded juvenile operation was in 1946 on a child of 12 (Wahren 1946). O'Connell's (1951) youngest was 11.

Hirschfeld (1974) collected fifteen patients, the youngest age 8. One was 10, two 11, two 12, one 14 and eight 15, of whom three had sciatica, two with neurological deficit. A 12-year-old and a 14-year-old required laminectomy. My youngest (1975) was a girl of 11, fixed in flexion with severe sciatica, bilateral limitation of straight-leg raising and a fourth and fifth motor root palsy. A fourth lumbar protrusion was removed.

In backache, manipulative reduction is the therapeutic standby, repeated as often as necessary, followed by the prevention of recurrence by postural training. When wedging of the vertebral body from osteochondrosis is present, manipulative reduction will require frequent repetition at first. It is useless merely to tell a youngster that he must not bend forwards; he forgets; his life must be so arranged for him that he does not have to do so, i.e. no gym or games; but swimming and running are encouraged. Unless it is absolutely necessary, a corset should not be advised particularly for boys during their time at boarding school; it is a great embarrassment.

Traction is seldom required, but is quite successful. One boy of 12 proved to have a protrusion irreducible by manipulation but recovered with traction and, by the age of 27, had had no further trouble. Rarely, a week in bed is indicated; this succeeded in a boy of 10 with backache referred to the back of one thigh, in whom manipulation failed. By the age of 23 he had had no recurrence. Nevertheless, most disc lesions in children do recur, although the fact that growth continues enables articular changes to occur that may prevent further trouble.

Treatment in disc lesions causing root pain is expectant. They are nearly always of the primary posterolateral type and it suffices to explain that the disorder will pass off in about nine months from the onset, leaving the child well and able to do everything. Since the pain is never severe, however marked the physical signs, this period of waiting is not particularly disagreeable. Once the disc protrusion has reached its maximum size and is stable, epidural local anaesthesia is indicated, and I have given it from the age of 15 upwards with consistent benefit. The last measure that should be considered in these young people is laminectomy; indeed, I have so far only twice found it necessary under the age of 17. One boy had had two months' unilateral sciatica and had 10° range of straight-leg raising on each side. He was found to have huge protrusions at both the fourth and fifth lumbar levels.

There is one very curious type of backache without sciatica that begins only between the ages of 15 and 25. The pain is persistent and central and continues unchanged for years. The only sign is limitation of trunk flexion and a corresponding *bilateral* limitation of straight-leg raising. It can be shown by epidural local anaesthesia to be caused by a low lumbar disc protrusion but, although a full range of straight-leg raising is restored for the time being, no lasting improvement follows. Only one such case of mine has come to laminectomy (Urquhart); a central disc protrusion at the fourth lumbar level was removed with excellent result.

Since the protrusion is central, its duration cannot be forecast; although straight-leg raising is limited, there is no root pain and thus no tendency to spontaneous cure, at any rate within five years. My most chronic case was 33 when I first saw him and had been in pain for ten years. Manipulation is quite useless; the only effective conservative treatment is traction, which has to be continued daily for at least two or three months. Neither doctor nor patient must lose heart if there is no improvement after the first month; persistence is essential and seldom fails to bring eventual reward.

## BACKACHE IN CHILDREN

Under the age of 10, the likelihood of backache being due to a disc lesion is remote. However, Young's earliest case of root pain was a girl of 7 who had two years' sciatica with limited straight-leg raising, and he has described a case of lumbago in a boy of 18 months. Fernström found post-mortem a partly ruptured fifth lumbar disc in a boy of 6. My youngest patient with lumbago was the daughter, aged 6¾ years, of one of my physiotherapy graduates; she recognized the disorder at once. The pain had lasted for five days after a fall; coughing hurt. Lumbar flexion and extension and full straight-leg raising hurt at the centre of the lower back and all my tests for psychogenic trouble proved negative. Manipulative reduction succeeded.

Backache in children is rare, and must be investigated thoroughly. If limitation of lumbar movement is present, the fact that the patient is afebrile does not rule out osteomyelitis or an extradural abscess, and the first X-ray photograph does not always disclose tuberculosis. Previous lumbar puncture should give rise to suspicion of an epidermoid implant.

Backache in children is very seldom due to neurosis; at that age such symptoms affect a limb.

## DISC LESIONS AND SPORT

The emphasis throughout is on the fact that the patient can do much of what he did before, but must do it differently. He must flex his knees rather than his lumbar spine.

Swimming is the only actively beneficial sport. While in the water, the swimmer keeps his trunk extended in order to raise his head to breathe; moreover, he is suspended in a fluid medium and all compression on the lumbar spinal joints ceases. Diving is dangerous, since patients liable to lumbago have been known to become fixed in flexion in mid-air and to experience great difficulty in reaching land again.

Tennis can be permitted to patients with pulpy herniations, for the quick movements of down and up do not allow enough time for the nucleus to ooze. Patients with an annular fragment, on the other hand, play at their own risk.

Riding is harmless as long as the patient does not tire. While he is fresh, he maintains his lordosis—the correct posture for riding. If he continues to the point of fatigue, he may slump into kyphosis. Hence he must work up to a day's hunting by degrees. He may well wear a corset, as did cavalry officers at the turn of the century.

A schoolboy can usually safely play rugby football as long as he is kept out of the scrum.

## OBSOLESCENT TREATMENTS

Four measures have been universally employed in the treatment of back troubles in spite of their manifest lack of success and contravention of first principles. They are: physiotherapy, mobilization under anaesthesia, rehabilitation and postural exercises.

### Physiotherapy

Physiotherapy, i.e. heat and exercises, is not indicated in any sort of organic backache. It is a mystery to me how the notion ever arose, except as an extension of the routine whereby incurable locomotor lesions ended up in the physiotherapy department. Acceptance was hastened, but not initiated, by Griffiths's work and is now so ingrained in doctors', patients' and physiotherapists' minds that the one prescribes, the second accepts and the third administers without question an entirely illogical measure. Physiotherapy is an expensive treatment. Glanville (1971) calculated that six applications of radiant heat cost the Health Service £5. Hence it is clear that huge sums are squandered daily because of this tradition. Physiotherapists are now well-paid experts in short supply. It is thus a sad waste of scarce time to ask them to give heat and exercises for lesions that do not respond, yet often do well on genuine treatment.

### Mobilization under Anaesthesia

The justification for this method of treatment rests on a misapprehension of the lesion present. Mobilization under anaesthesia, i.e. putting the joint through its full range of movement during complete muscular relaxation, is suited to rupturing adhesions. But in backache and sciatica no adhesions are present; a displacement exists requiring reduction. Admittedly, it can be reduced under anaesthesia, but only by good fortune and with difficulties and dangers that are avoided if the patient remains conscious. Reduction is not a set manipulation; each manoeuvre depends on what effect previous steps have had. Deprived by anaesthesia of the patient's active cooperation, the manipulator has no idea whether to go on or stop, whether to repeat a manipulation or avoid it. Moreover, incontinence has been described after such a blunderbuss manipulation as the result of pressure on the fourth sacral root. Another hazard under anaesthesia is death from rupture of an arteriosclerotic aorta during forced hyperextension.

Even worse is forcing a full range of straight-leg raising under anaesthesia. However haphazard, a lumbar manipulation *can* secure reduction; to treat the limb for a lesion in the back is unjustifiable. The only way benefit appears to follow 'stretching the sciatic nerve' is when the root is so tautened over the projection that an immediate pressure palsy results. Patients are encountered who lost their pain but acquired the weak numb foot of root atrophy; they form a moderately pleased minority.

### Rehabilitation after Back Injury

Griffiths's admirable work at the Albert Dock Hospital led to great advances in the rehabilitation of injured dock workers. In so far as this related to fracture, deformity after burns, head injury, amputation, stiff joints, weak muscles, nothing could have been more effective. He took the logical view (1959) that rehabilitation was a full-time job and arranged that dockers should receive a supplementary wage during their period of all-daily attendance.

Unfortunately, this application of rehabilitation to so many suitable disorders led to the inclusion of back injuries without damage to bone. His general advocacy led to a mistaken extension of its scope. Thus the treatment of those common accidents in which the brunt is borne by the disc was placed influentially on the wrong footing. Since a quarter of all dockers' injuries affect the spine, the error was not without importance, and persists today. In consequence, many hospitals run a 'back class' at which spinal exercises are carried out under physiotherapists' supervision. Many hospitals order extension exercises only; others insist on flexion exercises; the chaos is complete. Yet no one would order a footballer rehabilitation on this scale *before* menisectomy, in the hope that his cartilage trouble would cease. The inherent futility of rehabilitation after lumbago, for example, still awaits recognition. Mattingly (1971) followed up 38 dockers who had passed through Garston Manor and found that 31 had not been able to resume heavy work.

In my view, rehabilitation after the ordinary sort of trouble in a workman's back should be dealt with by measures to promote the maintenance of reduction. Those patients in whom the reduction proves unstable should be retrained for lighter work.

Great care must be taken not to include cases of neurasthenic or assumed pain in any programme of rehabilitation. Such patients are apt to damage the other patients' morale and seldom allow themselves to 'recover', however encouraging the atmosphere. Their treatment is economic disposal, not medical.

### Postural Exercises

It is widely believed that postural exercises are an excellent remedy for backache. This belief is so ingrained that doctors tend to dismiss as fanciful or prompted by laziness, patients' complaints that the exercises make the backache worse. Nevertheless, the patients are right. Postural exercises are harmful in backache; they are suited only to children with postural deformity without backache. Even then they are of doubtful efficacy. There is all the difference in the world between teaching the patient to hold a certain posture and giving postural exercises. Strengthening the sacrospinalis muscles does not increase the stability of the lumbar joints, which is dependent on ligaments and the interlocking facet joints. The huge strength of a footballer's quadriceps does not hinder a rotation strain on the joint from breaking the meniscus. If a joint subject to internal derangement is exercised, it is moved to its extremes of range; as a result mobility is maintained and, with it, the liability to intra-articular displacements. If a joint is kept still in a position unfavourable to the development of internal derangement, obvious benefit follows. Postural instruction in the use of the sacrospinalis muscles to immobilize the lumbar joint, yes; postural exercises, no. This was confirmed by a controlled trial (Aberg 1980) at the Ryginstitut in Sweden. In 353 cases of long-standing backache, no difference was found in the result of those receiving rehabilitation exercises and those not.

## FUTURE TREATMENTS

Suggestions, not altogether fanciful, are as follows:

### A New Disc

The restoration of the disc and its space is not a theoretical impossibility. A plastic substance in solution could be injected into the affected joint while traction kept the vertebral bodies apart. This would then set, enclosing the fragments of disc, during the time that the tautened capsule of the joint exerted centripetal force. The disc would then become one solid mass again, the hitherto loose pieces lying embedded in the plastic material.

This idea was put forward in the 1954 edition of this book and a year later Cleveland was filling the emptied joint at laminectomy with methylacrylic. This paste becomes solid by polymerization in about 10 minutes, producing heat up to 82°C. Hamby and Glaser (1959) also introduced the paste at laminectomy and compared 14 patients with and without acrylic implant. They detected no difference between the two groups in postoperative course or in the width of the joint spaces determined radiographically a year later. Then Fernström began replacing the nucleus pulposus with stainless-steel ball-bearings in 1962. His published results of 191 such insertions by 1966 show the considerable advantages of the prothesis, and the retention of a good range of movement, visible radiographically. His figures were:

| Post-laminectomy | Ball bearing | No ball bearing |
|---|---|---|
| Backache continued | 40% | 88% |
| Sciatica continued (protrusion found) | 14% | 50% |
| Sciatica continued (negative exploration) | 47% | 80% |

## Chemical Arthrodesis

An alternative is chemically induced arthrodesis. If a substance were discovered that promotes the formation of new bone and was introduced into the intervertebral joint, permanent fixation would be achieved without operation. Since capsular ossification occurs after bacterial arthritis, in ankylosing spondylitis and in fluorine poisoning, stimuli with this effect clearly exist. Roholm (1937) described osteosclerosis and joint stiffness in cryolite workers in Denmark, associated with deposits in ligaments and tendons, as the result of chronic excessive intake of fluorides. Animal experiments on the effect on joints of injecting various concentration of fluorides in solution might well prove the starting-point for discovering a safe method suited to human joints. Giving fluoride by mouth is not advisable. It was given in dosage of 100 mg daily by Cohen (1966) for myelomatosis. Unfortunately, nausea, vomiting and optic atrophy were apt to result. Matin's research on implants of vesical mucosa in guinea-pigs offers another approach on these lines. At the site of implantation a cyst formed containing a glairy fluid which, on escape into adjoining tissues, stimulated bone formation there. Should a similar phenomenon be reproducible in humans, a means of fixing the joint without operation in backache and arthritis at the hip may at last be in sight. Another relevant finding was made by Bridges and McClure (1968) who found that injections of lead acetate into animals led to the formation of persistent calcified plaques. Hence it might be possible to make the posterior spinal ligaments less pliable in this way.

## Simplified Arthrodesis

In the meanwhile, simplified techniques of arthrodesis not requiring appreciable postoperative rest in bed ought to be investigated. The adjacent surfaces of two spinous processes might be stripped of periosteum and the interspinous ligament excised. A wedge of bone could then be introduced between the spinous processes. The two spinous processes would now be tightly wired together squeezing the graft. After a few days the patient should be allowed up in a plastic corset holding the lumbar spine extended so as further to pinch the wedge. An alternative to this suggestion has now become a standard orthopaedic practice. The two vertebrae requiring fusion are fixed together by screws before the graft is inserted; these maintain immobility pending union. In consequence only a fortnight in bed is required postoperatively.

## A Lasting Anaesthetic Agent

Epidural local anaesthesia abolishes backache and sciatica due to a disc protrusion for an hour or two; then the pain often returns. If a local anaesthetic agent could be devised that lasted for several months, it would be well worth while for those patients who have an intractable constant backache due to a minor disc lesion to attend at whatever intervals proved necessary for repeated epidural injections. It is very galling that, although a remedy for chronic backache and root pain exists in theory, the agent appears no closer to discovery now than at the turn of the century.

## Erosion of the Disc

Smith (1969) introduced an enzyme into the intervertebral joint. Chymopapain disrupts polysaccharide–protein complexes, and can thus destroy the disc, without attacking bone or ligament. Wiltse et al. (1975) stated that since the disc consisted of four-fifths water, its extraction caused such marked shrinkage that subsequent laminectomy showed the intervertebral joint to be empty. A year after the erosion of the disc with chymopapain he reported good result in 75.4% of cases.

# TREATMENT OF OTHER LUMBAR DISORDERS

These are treated on standard lines.

## Simple Wedge-fracture

Contrary to general belief, uncomplicated wedge-fracture of a vertebral body does not require immobilization in plaster. Indeed, many such fractures are discovered years later on a radiograph taken for some other reason.

A fortnight in bed, during which prone-lying trunk extension exercises are prescribed, suffices. The patient must not, of course, lie with pillows in flexion. For a further month, he is up and about, but is not allowed to bend forwards. At the end of three months the fracture is consolidated. After that, whatever the shape of the vertebral body on the radiograph, the presence or absence of symptoms depends on what has happened to the adjacent discs and to the patient's state of mind.

## Fracture Dislocation

This is an entirely different matter. The spinal cord and cauda equina are in grave danger and surgery is usually required.

## Fractured Transverse Process

A fractured transverse process is really a muscle injury; it gives rise to muscle signs and strictly unilateral pain. Hence the diagnosis becomes clear if the patient, after a blow on his back, is found to have pain on resisted movement when the joints and muscles are tested separately.

It is an unimportant injury, spontaneous recovery without treatment taking at most a fortnight. Whether eventual union by fibrous tissue or by bone takes place is insignificant. If the patient is anxious for exceptionally speedy recovery, he can be made well in less than a week by local anaesthesia induced between the bone ends; then deep massage is given to the lateral aspect of the sacrospinalis muscle in the vicinity of the transverse process, followed by gentle exercises. Rest in bed, plaster and so on are all contraindicated.

Force sufficient to break bone may damage the disc. Hence pain persisting longer than two weeks almost certainly arises from a lesion other than the fracture visible on the radiograph.

## Adolescent Osteochondrosis

If this causes symptoms, these appear due to a disc lesion secondary to the kyphosis at the affected joint that results from the wedging. Manipulative reduction should be carried out as required.

The wedging never becomes extreme and wearing a plaster jacket or rest in bed is not required.

## Tuberculous Caries

For years, treatment has consisted of immobilization followed by arthrodesis. But Konstam and Blesovsky (1962), working on unpromising patients in Nigeria, achieved results quite as satisfactory by giving ambulant patients para-aminosalicyclic acid and isoniazid for at least a year. Abscesses were drained and only those who could not walk were put to bed for an average period of three weeks while costectomy was carried out (28 of 56 paraplegics). The result in patients without paraplegia were: 199 healed, 5 not healed, 3 died. In the 56 with paraplegia, 51 made a complete recovery; 2 others became able to walk; there were 2 operative deaths and no improvement in 1 case.

## Senile Osteoporosis

This does not itself cause symptoms and care must be taken that elderly women with a disc lesion or a mushroom phenomenon complicating symptomless osteoporosis are not regarded as suffering from the condition shown on the radiograph. If pathological fracture results, this causes bone pain for up to three months.

Calcium gluconate (1 gm a day) by mouth and anabolic steroids are said to arrest the disorder. Calcitonin, one of the hormones elaborated by the thyroid gland, diminishes the plasma level of calcium and may prove a suitable treatment for osteoporosis.

Pak et al. (1969) tried to suppress parathyroid function with corresponding enhancement of thyrocalcitonin secretion by repeated infusions of calcium and four of six patients were much improved for many months. Jowsey et al. (1972) have reported benefit from 50 mg of sodium fluoride, 0.9 mg of calcium and 50 000 units of vitamin D daily. The latest possible agent for increasing calcium absorption from the gut is 24,25 dihydroxycholecalciferol, a renal metabolite of vitamin D (Kanis et al. 1978). Nordin, Professor of Mineral Metabolism at Leeds, has pointed out that the vitamin is of doubtful value and that ethinyloestradiol (25 μg daily for three weeks out of the four), combined with 3 Sandocal tablets a day, provide the best basis for treatment (1973, 1979).

## Spondylolisthesis

If this causes lumbar pain of ligamentous origin, sclerosing injections may help. If not, and in bilateral sciatica, arthrodesis is required unless a corset affords adequate relief. A secondary disc lesion is treated on standard lines, disregarding the spondylolisthesis, but of course the liability to recurrence is much enhanced. Toakley (1973) found that the response to neurofasciotomy was as good in patients with, as it was without, spondylolisthesis.

## Chronic Osteomyelitis

Immobilization on a plaster bed is instituted at once and maintained until ankylosis is well advanced. This usually takes three or four months from the time that it becomes possible to make the diagnosis with certainty. Antibiotics are administered, but as these patients often remain afebrile throughout, the best criterion of when to stop is return of the sedimentation rate to normal. If pain continues, surgical evacuation of the abscess in the vertebral body is indicated as soon as it becomes radiologically visible.

## Osteitis Deformans

The basic abnormality in osteitis deformans is enhanced proliferation of osteoclasts and osteoblasts. In consequence the formation and resorption of bone is unduly rapid. Since calcitonin inhibits osteoclastic bone resorption, the bone pain nearly always ceases after the injections are begun (Woodhouse 1974) and persists for as long as administration continues. His paper illustrates regression of bone changes.

Calcitonin is clearly the treatment of choice, but lasting good results have been reported (Ryan et al. 1969) with mithramycin, an antibiotic causing hypocalcaemia. Another way of increasing the levels of blood-borne calcitonin is the administration of intravenous glucagon.

All these drugs need to be injected. However, Russell et al. (1974) found that sodium etidronate taken orally inhibits the excessive bone turnover which characterizes Paget's disease. After two to six months of a daily dose of 20 mg/kg body weight the alkaline phosphatase level had dropped to normal in half of all patients. Bone biopsy revealed suppression of the disease and pain had ceased. No side effects were anticipated since the drug is excreted unaltered. Relief lasted for up to two years after stopping the treatment.

## Osteomalacia

Leavened bread should be substituted for chupatty, which has a high phytin content. The diet should be supplemented with calcium carbonate.

## Anterior Longitudinal Ligament

Since this suffers when the abdominal and sacrospinalis muscles are weakened as the result of myopathy or anterior poliomyelitis, a stiff corset or a brace is indicated according to circumstances. In spondylitis and vertebral hyperostosis, phenylbutazone is indicated.

## Facet Joint in Spondylitis

Unilateral upper lumbar pain may result from invasion by the spondylitic process of one lateral articulation. Curiously enough, movement of the lumbar spine does not evoke or increase the constant discomfort and only the fact that the patient has sacro-iliac or lumbar spondylitis ankylopoetica brings the disorder to mind. The level must be ascertained as accurately as possible by palpation for tenderness.

One injection of 1 ml of triamcinolone suspension affords many months' relief, but several endeavours may have to be made before all the affected joints have been reached.

CHAPTER 21

# THE TREATMENT OF INTRACTABLE BACKACHE

Much of what is regarded as intractable backache is not intractable at all. Its persistence is due merely to the general belief held by medical men that all backache is incurable, and that to offer treatment verges on quackery. Concepts of 'spinal arthritis' and 'disc degeneration' help to reinforce this negativism, though statistics from many countries all agree that backache rises to a peak at 40 to 50 years of age and that after 60 the incidence declines sharply. This could not be so if arthritis, osteophytosis or degeneration were really responsible.

These mistaken concepts stifle endeavour, and prevent the institution of rational treatment. Inexplicably, they lead to wholesale prescription of heat and exercises, based on the therapeutic automatism whereby doctors unthinkingly equate backache with physiotherapy, though it is difficult to grasp how these measures could be thought to affect osteophytes or erosion of a disc. At a loss, many doctors acquiesce in a visit to one of various brands of lay manipulators. Here again, were the lesion osteophytosis or attrition of the disc, manipulation could have no effect. Yet some patients are relieved—clear evidence that the cause of symptoms was neither spinal arthritis nor degeneration of the disc as such. These were what the radiograph showed, but it must be remembered that these appearances existed before the pain began, persisted during the attack and continued unchanged after the attack was over—further proof that the lesion was not spondylosis. Other patients, not relieved by manipulation, can be helped by traction. If so, the same argument applies.

By 'intractable backache' I mean pain, occurring in a patient without neurosis or tendency to exaggeration, which has defied logically defensible methods. These are: manipulation, traction, epidural local anaesthesia, ligamentous sclerosis, corsetry and rest in bed. (I do not regard heat, massage and exercises as logically defensible—they are merely an expensive way of playing for time.) When these justifiable treatments have failed, or examination shows that none is applicable, the tendency exists either to tell the patient he must 'live with it', or to jump to surgery: laminectomy or arthrodesis. However (quite apart from chemonucleolysis with chymopapain), there exist further simple and innocuous measures that merit consideration. These are: peripheral nerve block (posterior ramus and sinuvertebral); posterior ramus sclerosis; infiltration of a steroid suspension about the nerve root; and neurofasciotomy. All these measures can be carried out at four levels—third lumbar to first sacral. The possible alternatives, therefore, number 20.

## Historical Note

Ever since 1956, when Hackett's book on ligamentous sclerosis in the treatment of backache first appeared, these injections have become increasingly popular. In the early days of this century, patients with hernias were given sclerosing injections into the hernial sac with the intention of provoking widespread adhesions leading to obliteration of the neck. In his early days, Hackett, a surgeon in the USA, operated on such patients and found that in the course of years the sclerosing agent had provoked round fibrous masses, so tough that a scalpel could cut them only with difficulty. Several decades later, he was confronted with numerous patients with backache, many of whom he considered to be suffering from lax ligaments. This theory led him to treatment by chemically induced ligamentous sclerosis. I read his book and started a trial, but became discouraged at initial lack of success, and by the painful reaction provoked by the fatty acid proliferant solution that he advocated. Working with me at that time was Ongley, who shortly afterwards returned to New Zealand. There he experimented with alternative solutions and different approaches. His techniques and his standard solution are now widely used. His improved methods enabled Barbor (see Volume

II) to achieve 52% full relief in a consecutive series of 67 patients picked out by myself in 1966 as wholly intractable. Barbor's latest figures (1972), based on 2000 cases followed up for one to seven years, are 90% of men and 86% of women either wholly pain-free or able to live a satisfactory life with only minor symptoms easy to ignore. Even this achievement leaves a hard core of incurable patients, not bad enough for surgery, not likely to benefit from surgery, or in whom surgery had already proved a failure.

A curious event cropped up from time to time, when ligamentous sclerosis was being induced by me with the intention of provoking a contracture that would stabilize the affected intervertebral joint. It was surprising to hear a patient declare at his next visit that, as from the day after his first sclerosant injection, he had lastingly lost his pain. This naturally suggested neurosis, but examination did not bear out this ascription. Yet relief had been achieved long before any ligamentous contracture could possibly have started. This puzzled me considerably, but led me to consider if such an immediate success could be caused by unintentional blocking of peripheral nerves. Substance was lent to this idea by the fact that an analgesic area, lasting several months, was occasionally provoked at the inner upper quadrant of the buttock by a sclerosant injection, clearly as the result of interference with one of the cutaneous nerves of first to third lumbar derivation where they cross the iliac crest, by infiltrations about the ilio-lumbar ligament.

In 1972, a similar effect was described by Scott-Charlton and Roebuck. They decided that intractable lumbogluteal pain after spinal surgery might stem from the sacroiliac joint, at which they therefore performed arthrodesis. To their surprise, some of the patients reported full relief from the day of the operation. They concluded, just as I did, that such an immediate result could only be brought about by interference with nervous conduction, in my case from the chemical induction of peripheral neuritis, in their case from actual division of nerves. They therefore decided on inducing a peripheral neuritis at the lateral aspect of the sacral foramen, where the posterior ramus lies. Our solution has, since 1960, contained 2% phenol; they bettered this by dissolving the phenol in myodil to form a 5% solution, whose radiopacity allowed injection under X-ray control.

Though our weaker solution had an occasional immediate effect, this usually became manifest only after a few weeks, indicating the slow onset of a peripheral neuritis. Until then, I had accepted the idea of the gradual onset of ligamentous contracture stabilizing the joint. I partly subscribe to this view even now; for in my hands sclerosing injections and nerve blocks have not proved interchangeable. Sometimes the blocks have secured relief after sclerosis has failed, but in other cases a sclerosant injection given with Ongley's technique has succeeded, after a posterior ramus block had failed.

Therapeutic peripheral nerve blocks were originated in the Argentine by Sturniolo in 1961 and he explained his views to me a year later, but I did not at that time grasp the mechanism whereby he obtained his good results. He had found that local anaesthesia induced at the apex of the third lumbar transverse process could lastingly relieve both backache and sciatica. He named the condition the 'apico-transverse syndrome'. He considers the relief to be due to relaxation of the quadratus lumborum muscle, consequent upon the peripheral motor nerve block. In 1964, his results were confirmed by di Miglio et al. in Italy. In recalcitrant cases, he goes on to open division of the tendon that runs laterally from the tip of this transverse process, and through which the nerve passes. Sometimes he removes the apex of the bone itself. Of 131 cases of pain in the back and lower limb submitted to this open operation, all but four were a success (Sturniolo 1971).

Then I met Rees in 1970. For the previous ten years he had had excellent results from subcutaneous tenotomy of the deep lumbar fascia. He divided it at the fourth and fifth lumbar levels on each side, thus severing the lateral branch from the posterior ramus that lies along its surface. He combined this neurofasciotomy with the induction of epidural local anaesthesia and secured over 99% success in both backache and sciatica (Rees 1971). This combined approach is unfortunate from the scientific point of view, since it leaves the issue in doubt which of the two methods was the effective one. My experience of epidural local anaesthesia in the type of case he described would lead me to expect less than 50% successes. Since he claims 99%, the neurofasciotomy should be accorded the major credit. There is a certain irony here. The 1947 edition of this book contained a description of subcutaneous tenotomy of the deep lumbar fascia, which I had found occasionally successful. Those were the days when I still regarded lesions of the soft tissues as contributing to backache. But, logically enough, wishing to release a supposed contracture, I unfortunately divided the fascia transversely. The cut was thus made parallel to the nerve, which was clearly seldom severed. The results were indifferent, and I abandoned the method, the more readily once it had become clear that no fascial contracture existed, but that the limitation of movement was due to a disc protrusion blocking one side of the joint. Rees's work now made me wonder what part unsuspected denervation had played in securing relief.

## NERVE BLOCK

### Indications

However successful, peripheral nerve block should not be regarded as the treatment of choice for all backache. There is the theoretical objection that, if the injection succeeds by making the patient unaware of his minor disc protrusion, he may unwittingly go on exerting his back and give himself a major displacement, leading to root palsy, including possibly that of the third and fourth sacral roots innervating the bladder and anus. This is a valid argument, but Rees's results over a 12-year period show that this is not a real danger. Though it is difficult to maintain a complete follow-up of a thousand patients, severe subsequent trouble could not fail to have been brought to his notice.

Another objection might be that denervation of the facet joints might in due course lead to neuropathic arthropathy. This would not set up pain but would lead to the development of the adult type of spondylolisthesis. However, section at the deep lumbar fascia divides only the lateral branch of the posterior ramus, leaving intact the medial twig supplying the facet joint. Hence, Rees's neurofasciotomy would not have this danger since the divided nerve runs merely to adjacent periosteum and fibres of the sacrospinalis muscle. Clearly then the practical benefits of peripheral nerve blocks outweigh theoretical objections in *otherwise intractable chronic backache*, i.e. when the lesion present is fairly static.

Suitable lesions thus are:

1. *Unprogressive lesions.* When certain activities or postures always bring on the same ache, whether the result of a small unstable fragment of disc or to recurrent bulging of the nucleus, and there has been no change for some years, a good chance exists that the damage has reached a static level. Abolishing the pain, while the patient remains careful of his back, is an apparently safe and practical solution.
2. *Chronic constant backache.* Even more does this argument apply when the ache is constant and unaltered whatever the patient does. Sometimes it is worse at night and relieved by movement. This is particularly likely to happen in elderly people after years of recurrent trouble with the back.
3. *Compression phenomenon causing root pain.* When root pain is present only on standing—the mushroom phenomenon—steroid injection about the affected root is remarkably effective. Relief lasts six months to several years and repetition is equally effective.
4. *Postlaminectomy symptoms.* Search for the spot where local anaesthesia abolishes the pain for the time being may involve several infiltrations in unlikely places, but perseverance often brings its reward. The patient must be warned that patience is often required.
5. *After arthrodesis.* Relief is much more difficult to achieve, since the graft gets in the way of the needle and the first sacral foramen is often covered over.

As from March 1971, I have treated all intractable backache in the first place by posterior ramus blocks and all intractable root pain by sinuvertebral blocks. My original idea was to copy Rees, but without the epidural injection and in a more selective way, performing his neurofasciotomy not in four places as a routine, but at the spot identified as relevant by the responses to local anaesthesia of the posterior ramus. This obvious precaution was also adopted by Brenner (1973), who in this way, out of a total of 270 patients singled out 100 suitable cases. Of these 75 benefited from the neurofasciotomy.

If no such spot could be singled out, the idea of neurofasciotomy was abandoned. Occasionally, to my surprise, it turned out that the mere induction of local anaesthesia had a lasting effect. When it proved transient, a sclerosant injection about the peripheral nerve or a steroid infiltration about the nerve root, sometimes afforded lasting relief. Neurofasciotomy turned out seldom to be required. In any case, epidural local anaesthesia was never induced simultaneously. If there was any hope that this would help, it was carried out at least a week before the next step in treatment.

## Anatomy

The classic account of the spinal nerves is contained in Hovelacque's book (1927). Further studies were carried out by Stilwell on monkeys in 1956. The dura mater and the dural sleeve of the nerve root receive sensory fibres from the sinuvertebral nerve which passes back into the foramen again (Luschka 1850). Edgar and Nundy (1966) showed this nerve to supply the anterior aspect only of the dura mater. This nerve also reaches the posterior longitudinal ligament (Pedersen et al. 1956). The facet joints are supplied by the medial branch of the posterior ramus (Lazorthes & Gaubert 1957), which Bradley (1973) showed to divide into two, the longer supplying the facet joint at the level below (see Plate XXXIX). The lateral branch crosses the deep lumbar fascia superficially, and supplies sensory fibres to adjacent periosteum and motor fibres to the adjacent multifidus spinae muscle.

## Relevant Nerves

Four nerves and six nerve roots are relevant to backache and root pain. At four levels—third lumbar to first sacral—the peripheral nerves can be blocked. The intention is then to denervate the tissue proved by the response to local anaesthesia to be connected with the patient's pain.

The roots themselves range from the third lumbar to the third sacral. Since impingement against the dural sleeve causes the discomfort, the intention is now to desensitize the dural sheath of the relevant nerve root.

The method adopted has therefore been to apply local anaesthesia, then if necessary a sclerosant solution to a peripheral nerve. Alternatively, local anaesthesis has been followed by an injection of triamcinolone about the nerve root. No sclerosant solution is injected close to a nerve root for fear of a phenol radiculitis.

The relevant peripheral nerves are:

1. The branch of the posterior ramus where it crosses the apex of the third lumbar transverse process (Sturniolo).
2. The medial branch of the posterior ramus, lying at the junction of the transverse process with the superior articular facet.
3. The lateral branch at the medial edge of the deep lumbar fascia (Rees).
4. The loop of the sinuvertebral nerve.

## Technique

Throughout, 2 ml of a 2% solution of procaine was employed. No interference with conduction was discernible after any of these injections, including at the nerve roots. Clearly the root sleeve is too dense to allow the solution to soak through. In contrast to the root pain nearly always evoked by epidural local anaesthesia in cases of sciatica, only local discomfort was provoked, nothing being felt down the limb. This might well have been thought to indicate that the dural sleeve of the nerve root had not been reached, but this was shown not to be so when, in many cases of stubbornly limited straight-leg raising of many months' standing, this became of full range and painless within a few minutes. After a posterior ramus block, no cutaneous analgesia nor sacrospinalis muscle weakness was detectable.

To start with, the patient stands. He is asked if he has any constant discomfort. He performs the four lumbar movements and states whether any of them alters or brings on his pain. One block is then carried out. After a minute (2% procaine acts quickly), the patient stands and declares the effect on his abiding discomfort and

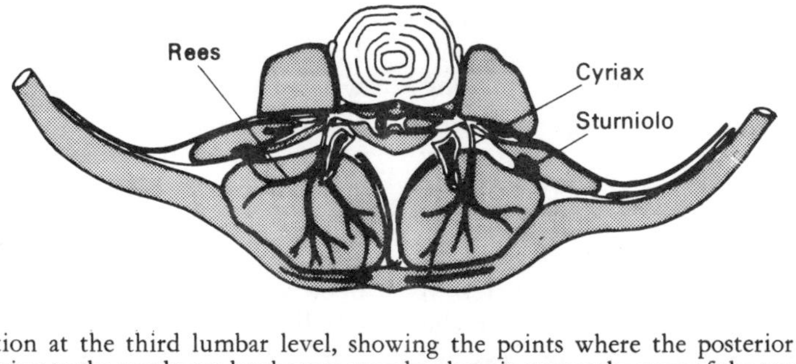


**Fig. 92.** Transverse section at the third lumbar level, showing the points where the posterior ramus can be attacked. Sturniolo: the nerve running to the quadratus lumborum muscle where it crosses the apex of the transverse process. Rees: the lateral branch of the posterior ramus where it lies along the deep lumbar fascia. Cyriax: the posterior ramus just before it divides, where it crosses the deep lumbar fascia at the edge of the lamina. (*After Sturniolo 1963*).

on the aggravation by lumbar movements. If there has been no change, the block is induced at the next level, and so on, until the right spot is found or it becomes clear that this approach has failed. In unilateral cases it suffices to carry out the blocks on that side only; if central, both sides must be infiltrated. The patient is seen again a week later. If relief was secured and persists, no more is done; if the pain has returned after a peripheral nerve block, 2 ml of sclerosant solution is injected at the same spot. This injection works slowly and may take a week or two to produce its full effect. Post-injection soreness is not great and has gone by next day.

A sclerosant injection must be given time to work; hence the patient is seen again after two weeks. If the anaesthetic solution secured full relief but the sclerosant solution has not been followed by lasting benefit, neurofasciotomy follows at once.

At a nerve root, if local anaesthesia affords full relief for the time being and straight-leg raising rises to full range, lasting improvement is to be expected. In such cases, one or two repetitions often prove curative. If the relief does not last, triamcinolone is substituted.

## Injection Technique

### Apex of the Third Transverse Process

The fourth vertebra lies level with a line drawn between the upper edges of the two iliac crests. The intervals between the second to fifth spinous processes are defined and the third process identified. As the patient lies prone, the upper edge of the spinous process lies level with the transverse process. Its length varies considerably; the distance from its tip to the centre of the spine is measured on the radiograph. A spot is chosen along this horizontal level the correct distance from the midline and a thin needle 5 cm long inserted vertically downwards. Its angle is altered until its tip reaches bone. The angle is now altered again so that it follows the bone along, finally passing just beyond the edge. The needle is moved back to its previous spot and an injection made at the exact edge of the vertebral process. Unexpectedly, a procaine block at the apex of the third lumbar transverse process has proved particularly suited to midlumbar pain associated with osteoporosis.

### Lateral Branch of the Posterior Ramus

This emerges at the medial edge of the deep lumbar fascia halfway between two adjacent transverse processes (Rees 1971). The level lies midway between two supraspinous ligaments, and a 5 cm needle is inserted vertically downwards 2 cm from the midline. It strikes the lamina, whereupon the tip is moved laterally by repeated insertions of increasing obliquity until contact ceases. Here is the edge of the deep lumbar fascia.

The needle is not passed any further in, for it then approaches the nerve root emerging at the foramen. When procaine is used, this does not matter, but a sclerosant solution containing phenol should not be allowed to bathe a nerve root for fear of persistent pain.

When procaine is used, the injections cause very little discomfort or after-pain. When a sclerosant is substituted, the solution, being a chemical irritant, causes smarting as it is injected and the patient feels sore for the rest of the day.

### Medial Branch of the Posterior Ramus

This crosses the vertebra at the angle between the base of the transverse process and the superior articular facet.

The supraspinous ligament is identified at the selected level. The distance of the facet from the midline is measured on the radiograph—usually 2.5 cm. A vertical insertion is made until the tip of the needle reaches bone. The injection is made here. In 1976 Lora and Long described satisfactory relief from electrocoagulation in 40% of cases that had had no operation performed, but only 26% after surgery.

### Sinuvertebral Nerve and Nerve Root

Local anaesthesia here can be practised both when the pain in lumbar and when it is felt in the limb, since the procaine blocks conduction along the sinuvertebral nerve and numbs the adjacent surface of the dural investment of the nerve root.

A spot is chosen at the requisite level halfway between two supraspinous ligaments. A thin needle 7 cm long is fitted to a syringe containing 2 ml of 2% procaine solution, and introduced obliquely downwards at a point 3 cm from the midline. At a depth of 3–4 cm it strikes the lamina, if so the needle is partly withdrawn and thrust in again in a less medial direction. At nearly full length, the needle can be felt to halt at the posterior aspect of the vertebral body. If it engages against the disc, the tough resistance of cartilage can be felt, but the needle will pass further in, as in discography. As soon as bone or cartilage is felt, the needle is drawn back 5 mm. After aspiration, to make sure the tip is neither inside the theca nor in a blood vessel, 2 ml of 2% procaine are injected.

All patients with root pain who appear relievable by epidural local anaesthesia but in whom the injection has unexpectedly failed, should receive a sinuvertebral block at their second attendance.

When root pain results from a compression phenomenon (Cyriax 1950) epidural local anaesthesia always proves a failure therapeutically. By contrast, 2 ml of triamcinolone suspension, introduced at the nerve root by the same technique as for a sinuvertebral block, is very often successful. This discovery has proved a great boon to those elderly patients who used to require arthrodesis.

## First Sacral Root

This may require infiltration via the first sacral foramen. This is a large aperture, not hard to find with the point of a needle. It lies about 1 cm above the apex of the first sacral spinous process and some 3 cm from the midline. First the edge of the ilium is identified, for the needle must be inserted as obliquely as possible. A vertical insertion can traverse the sacrum, emerging anteriorly, where it can puncture the bowel and bring infection back along its track when withdrawn.

The needle should be 6 cm long and inserted as far from the midline as the ilium allows. It meets the surface of the sacrum at about 4 cm. It is then manoeuvred about until no resistance is felt and it suddenly passes in freely another 2 cm. There it impinges intrasacrally against the body of the first sacral vertebra. It may pierce the dura mater just there, and aspiration before injection is particularly essential before the injection is given. Since pressure on the first, second or third sacral roots is exerted at the lumbosacral level, infiltration via the first sacral foramen is suited to all three roots.

# NEUROFASCIOTOMY

This was first performed by Rees 12 years ago but as long ago as 1842 Riadore was dividing the tendons of origin of the spinal muscles in the treatment of scoliosis. My adaptation of his procedure consists merely in determining the site requiring the division by previous local anaesthesia, and then establishing that neither the diagnostic block itself nor a sclerosing injection there has had any lasting result. If there exists any chance that epidural local anaesthesia will help, this is induced at least a week previously.

The patient lies prone on the couch and 5 ml of 2% procaine are introduced 2–3 cm from the midline at the level already known to be correct, into the skin and down to the deep lumbar fascia. If the pain is central, this procedure should be

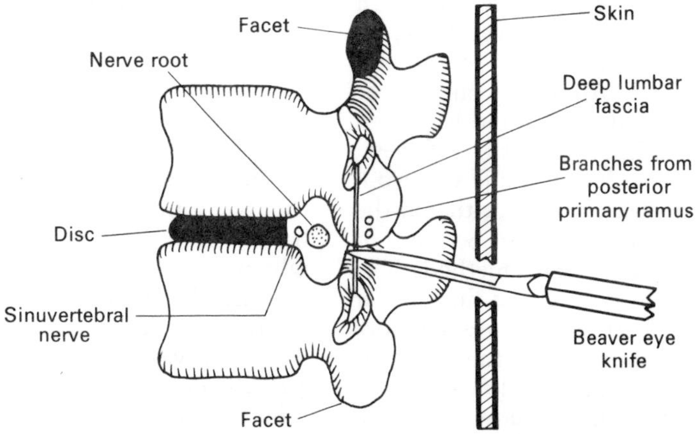


**Fig. 93.** Rees's neurofasciotomy, laterial view. (*By courtesy of W. S. Rees*).

carried out on each side. A cataract knife with a blade 3 cm long is now introduced obliquely downwards until it reaches the correct depth. This has already been ascertained by noting how far the needle had to pass before reaching the surface of the outer edge of the lamina and the depth at which it could be felt puncturing the fascia.

Rees has devised a thin scalpel particularly suited to this little operation by virtue of its slightly curved point, which catches the nerve (eye-knife 52L manufactured by R. Beaver). The knife, after insertion, is moved so that the point of the blade describes an arc about 2 cm in extent, cutting from the base of one transverse process to the other. It is then half withdrawn, turned through 180° and reinserted with the opposite obliquity. The division is now repeated from the opposite side with an equal sweep. Section of the nerve gives the sensation of a thread being stretched and cut. The scalpel is now withdrawn. The incision is only 2 mm long and bleeds little. Pressure is applied for a couple of minutes, then Elastoplast is applied, whereupon the patient walks home. He is seen again a week later. Bogduk et al. (1977) have shown by dissection that Rees's incision does not divide the nerve he intends to cut.

Patients feel next to nothing and are quite prepared to have the 'nerve snicked' once they are reassured that it has no appreciable useful function, yet has been demonstrated to be involved with their pain. The soreness afterwards amounts to no more than a day's nuisance.

## Results

In the course of the two years starting in May 1971, 2354 patients were seen by me with symptoms attributable to the lower back, in whom one or other type of disc lesion was regarded as responsible. All had seen one or several consultants already and some had been operated on. Most had had osteopathy. Of these, 226 (9.2%) were regarded as sufferers from intractable pain in the back or limb, either at the time of the first examination or because of unexpected failure of our standard methods. The length of history was in no case less than a year and in many dated back 10, 20 or 30 years. Before 1971, I would have abandoned treatment at this point. However, as the figures below indicate, the results, though not brilliant, show that these additional methods of dealing with chronic pain are worthwhile.

**Analysis of Cyriax's Cases**

| | *No. of cases* Male | Female | Total | Average age |
|---|---|---|---|---|
| Full relief | 12 | 17 | 29 (13%) | 46 (24–75) |
| Worthwhile relief | 58 | 57 | 115 (51%) | 48 (24–73) |
| Little or no relief | 44 | 38 | 82 (36%) | 48 (20–78) |

| | *Complaint* Back pain | Root pain | Both | *Previous treatment* Laminectomy | Arthrodesis |
|---|---|---|---|---|---|
| Full relief | 11 | 10 | 8 | 2 | — |
| Worthwhile relief | 49 | 20 | 46 | 5 | — |
| Little or no relief | 31 | 21 | 30 | 3 | 2 |

| | *Treatment employed* Post-ramus block | Post-ramus sclerosis | Sino-vertebral block | Steroid infiltration | Neuro-fasciotomy |
|---|---|---|---|---|---|
| Full relief | 6 | 3 | 6 | 10 | 3 |
| Worth-while relief | 33 | 20 | 43 | 7 | 9 |
| Little or no relief | 23 | 11 | 39 | 6 | 3 |

### Rees's Results

Rees claims a very high proportion of cures, indeed, over 99%, thus inviting immediate scepticism. However, two independent surgeons in Australia have both achieved over 80% improvement in previously intractable cases of chronic pain in the back. Hence, the operation is clearly an important addition to the approaches available. It should be made plain that Rees regards his incision as dividing the medial branch of the posterior ramus: the nerve that supplies the facet joint. This is not so; it severs the lateral branch running along the deep lumbar fascia which merely innervates adjacent periosteum and muscle. Hence, any relief that ensues is not the result of denervating the capsule of the facet. This fact was corroborated by Bogduk et al. in 1977. They established that the nerve to the facet joint lay against the bone of the lamina, emerging from the ramus at the angle formed by bases of the superior facet and of the transverse process.

This is not where Rees makes his cut, and they added further proof that his idea how his incision succeeds must be mistaken. Indeed, they dissected three cadavers on which Rees's neurofasciotomy had been performed, and found that none of the 18 incisions had the medial branch of the posterior ramus or its articular branches been severed.

Inexplicably, he calls his operation 'rhizolysis' i.e. freeing of the nerve root, whereas the most it can do is to afford peripheral denervation. In a later publication he alleged that the manoeuvre springs open the facet joints, increasing the size of the intervertebral foramen. This is not a tenable hypothesis either; for this effect is secured much more by lumbar side-flexion away from the painful side, a movement that very seldom abates the pain in sciatica.

### Results of Toakley, Francis, Hutton, Houston and Oudenhover

Toakley (1973) reported on 200 cases on which he had performed Rees's operation under local anaesthesia without the epidural injection. Of these, 116 were aged 40–60, and the average duration of pain was nine years, with extremes of one and 30. The main complaint was pain in the back, though in 152 cases there was also discomfort in the groin or thigh, radiating in only 60 instances down the leg to the ankle. The ache in the limb was the lesser complaint, and straight-leg raising was seldom limited. Many patients had had past attacks of severe sciatica, and in 90 residual neurological deficit was present; 48 had already been operated on; 175 had radiological evidence of attrition of the disc and 14 had spondylolisthesis.

Toakley found that clear discogenic sciatica did not benefit from neurofasciotomy, neither did ankylosing spondylitis. By contrast, the presence of spondylolisthesis made no difference. His results were: good 125; fair 37; unchanged 36; worse 2. Considering the intractable nature of these selected cases, such results indicate remarkable success. One cannot but agree with his assessment of 'very worth while'.

In 1973, Francis of Perth reported on a further 97 cases of lumbar pain subjected to Rees's neurofasciotomy. His figures were 82% fully relieved and a further 11% improved. He too found that the operation did not help in fully developed root pain. By contrast, Hutton (1973), reporting on 200 cases treated by Rees's operation, found 57% of backache well or much improved but also 49% of those with root pain.

Houston's figures (1975) are 45% excellent, 35% good and 17% failure. McCulloch and Organ (1977) obtained relief by radiocautery in 67% of their cases of backache without root pain and no previous surgical intervention. Oudenhoven (1977) obtained 80% successes due to denervation of tissues supplied by the posterior ramus.

## Coagulation

Rees's tenotomy was adapted by Shealy (1973) with excellent results. Instead of division with a tenotome, he coagulates by heat. He thrusts a needle down to the deep lumbar fascia and confirms its position by X-rays. The tip of the needle is heated electrically and is kept at 70°C for 90 seconds, thereby destroying the posterior ramus. In his series there were no complications, and in spite of the chronicity of his cases, the results below were obtained.

| | *Results* | | | |
|---|---|---|---|---|
| Category | Failure | Good | Excellent | Total |
| Previously unoperated* | 6 | 24 | 30 | 60 |
| Previous lumbar surgery† | 9 | 8 | 13 | 30 |
| Lumbar fusion‡ | 25 | 17 | 8 | 50 |
| Total | 40 | 49 | 51 | 140 |

* This is a very mixed group of patients including those with compression fractures, discogenic pain, etc. About half had had a myelogram. At least 10 of these had myelographic defects compatible with a 'bulging' disc.

† These patients had had one or more lumbar laminectomies for 'ruptured' discs.

‡ Many of these patients also had arachnoiditis.

## Cryotherapy

Intense cold also inhibits conduction along a nerve, but not lastingly. Cryotherapy is used by Lloyd at Abingdon Hospital, Oxford, in the same way as Shealy uses electrocoagulation. He inserts a needle at whose tip a bubble of compressed nitrous oxide is allowed suddenly to expand, causing a fall in temperature down to −70°C. Though the nerve recovers in some twelve days, conduction of pain impulses may cease for several months.

## Theoretical Aspect

The theoretical aspect of a posterior ramus block raises problems. In cases of backache of uncertain aetiology, I have for the last 40 years induced epidural local anaesthesia diagnostically. The surface of the dura mater and of the lower lumbar nerve roots is bathed by the procaine solution, and I did, and still do, regard cessation of pain for the time being as proof that a disc lesion is responsible for the pain. Procaine of a strength of 1:200 is used and is too weak to penetrate tissues, it merely numbs surfaces. In lesions of bone or ligament, no alleviation follows the local anaesthesia, e.g. spondylolisthesis, neuroma, metastasis, abscess, ankylosing spondylitis. Many of the patients treated by posterior ramus block had already had this diagnostic injection and the local anaesthesia had abolished the pain for the time being. No palsy results at the lower limb or of the sacrospinalis muscles. It remains obscure to me how any block carried out at the posterior ramus could have the same result as an epidural injection, since the solution does not reach the same nerve or the same tissues. It is even more obscure how Rees's division of a nerve that to all appearances has no connection with any tissue causing backache can serve a useful purpose. The possibility crossed my mind that, by accident, some of the solution might percolate anteriorly to reach the loop of the sinuvertebral nerve that projects just beyond the edge of the intervertebral foramen (see Fig. 75). A nerve block there would lead once more to local anaesthesia of the dura mater, since the sinuvertebral nerve is responsible for the sensitivity of its anterior surface.

In order to test this hypothesis, 2 ml of urographin were injected at the point where the deep lumbar fascia stretches between the transverse processes at the edge of the lamina. The radiograph (Plate XXXVIII) showed no oozing of oil anteriorly nor towards the intervertebral foramen. On the contrary, the solution travelled downwards following the contour of the bony surfaces. Certainly, unintentional block of the sinuvertebral had not taken place.

Undoubtedly, Rees divides the peripheral nerve distal to the branch supplying the facet joint, whence in his view the pain stems. The only observation that can be invoked to explain the relief resulting from neurotomy at that point is Kibler and Nathan's (1960). They established the surprising fact that blocking a nerve by local anaesthesia induced *distal* to the site of the lesion could abolish pain, sometimes lastingly. This result is known to be infrequent, as is testified by the well-known failure of interference with the supra- or infraorbital nerve in trigeminal neuralgia. None the less, this possibility offers one hypothesis to account for Rees's successes, and fits in with Ritchie-Russell's contention (1959) that 'many chronic pains are effectively relieved by attention to the periphery'.

Though the mechanism of relief following the measures described in this chapter may be obscure, this fact provides no reason for failing to give them a trial. The methods are simple and harmless, and are strongly indicated after operations have failed. They must also be contemplated in cases not really suited to surgery, when complaint of persistent pain is beginning to force the physician's reluctant acquiescence to an uncertain last resort.

## Wyke's Contribution

Much light has been thrown on pain-mechanisms, especially spinal, by Wyke's brilliant experimental work.

Pain can clearly be relieved in six ways. This result can follow:

1. A lesser input of stimuli from the peripheral source to the spinal cell.
2. A lesser input of stimuli reaching that same cell from normal tissues developed within the same segment.
3. A greater input of competing or inhibiting stimuli converging on the same spinal cell from the mechanoreceptor system.
4. Interfering with the spinal afferent pathway.
5. Stimulating the inferior part of the reticular nucleus with, e.g. valium or librium.
6. Ensuring cerebral disregard, e.g. leucotomy. Those who work themselves into a frenzy and can then slash themselves without feeling pain are apparently inducing the release of a polypeptide called 'endorphin' which acts like morphia. This substance was first discovered by Hughes and Kosterlitz in Aberdeen in 1975, but it is not yet clear how the brain manufactures or utilizes it.

Wyke has kindly contributed the following summary of his conclusions. His novel concepts go far towards explaining many hitherto incomprehensible phenomena. One obvious example is the patient, usually with sciatica, who has found a spot on his back or buttock which, when touched, brings on the pain down his limb. This previously puzzling statement is now seen to imply that, when the appropriate spinal cell receives this extra stimulus, it is further filled even by that small amount and the impulses from the nerve root now spill over and pass upwards to the sensory cortex. The concept of competing impulses may serve to explain the phenomenon of painless operations during acupuncture. If the impulses by the tissues pricked by the needle overshadow the impulses arising from the surgical manoeuvres, no pain there will be felt. I know of a healer who employs this fact; he puts the patient into a small room and so suffuses the patient's consciousness with enormously loud music that, while there, he can feel nothing.

### Rocking-chair

Since impulses from mechanoreceptors take precedence over sensory impulses, Wyke has utilized his observation that sitting in a rocking-chair keeps up a constant gentle stream of impulses from the moving parts. Since these have priority, for as long as the rocking continues, transmission of pain impulses to the brain is blocked. He advises all patients in chronic pain to adopt this simple method for relief.

He also reminds that barbiturates and caffeine are to be avoided, since they increase reticular sensitivity and thus enhance the appreciation of pain. Diazepam and carbamazepine have the opposite effect on this nucleus.

The inquiring reader should consult Wyke (1969, 1973).

## PAIN

*by B. D. Wyke**

Neuro-anatomical and neurophysiological studies (Melzack & Wall 1965; Brodal 1969; Wyke 1969; Melzack 1972) have shown that the activity of the cells in the spinal grey matter that relay nociceptive afferent impulses of peripheral origin into the central nervous system to evoke the experience of pain is also modulated by coincident inputs from tissue mechanoreceptors. In normal circumstances this latter influence is inhibitory, so that the minor tissue traumas of everyday life do not give rise to pain; and in like manner, moderate degrees of pain may gradually be abolished by massage, vibratory stimulation or passive manipulation of the painful tissues—which procedures stimulate tissue mechanoreceptors, and thereby block the centripetal flow of nociceptive activity at its synaptic entry into the central nervous system. Conversely, selective loss of the normal mechanoreceptor afferent input from tissues renders them exquisitely sensitive to what would otherwise be relatively innocuous stimuli (Noordenbos 1959; Melzack & Wall 1965)—as occurs in patients with causalgia and postherpetic neuralgia for instance—whereas selective local anaesthetic blockade of the small diameter afferents in the nerves supplying a tissue renders that tissue analgesic but not anaesthetic (Wyke 1969).

Individual relay cells in the spinal grey matter receive convergent inputs from receptors in all the tissues (both somatic and visceral) that are segmentally related to them, no matter where those tissues are located in the mature body (Brodal 1969). Continuous irritation of nociceptive receptor systems in a particular tissue eventually creates a state of persisting hyperexcitability in the related relay cells (Melzack & Wall 1965; Melzack 1972); and when this state is established, any afferent input from receptors in other segmentally related tissues (especially the skin) gives rise to pain that is felt to be in these latter tissues—which is the mechanism of so-called 'referred' pain (Brodal 1969). It is for this reason that local anaesthetic infiltration of tissues (or the nerves innervating them) that may be anatomically remote from the site of primary pathology may diminish or even abolish the patients' pain, for such a procedure reduces the global afferent input to the hyperexcitable relay cells and thereby reduces the frequency of their centripetal discharge into the central projection systems whose activity ascends into the brain to evoke the experience of pain.

*Senior Lecturer at the Royal College of Surgeons of England.

## Summary of Wyke's Work

At a lecture† delivered at the *VIth Reunion sobre la Columna Vertebral* in Spain (1977), Wyke summarized some of the neurological mechanisms involved in spinal pain.

He emphasized that the experience of pain is not a primary sensation but an unpleasant emotional state experienced in the limbic system of the brain; this is in response to activation of a specific nociceptive afferent system within the neuraxis. In the case of the spine, this central nociceptive afferent system is linked, through

†Published in *Patologia de la Columna Vertebral* (1977), ed. Hernández Conesa, S. and Seiquer, J., pp. 45–46. Ferrer Internacional: Murcia. Full details and references are given in Wyke's Chapter 10 in *The Lumbar Spine and Back Pain* (1976), ed. Jayson, M. I. V., pp. 184–256. London: Sector Publishing Company.

fine diameter nerve fibres traversing the spinal nerves, with a nociceptive receptor system distributed through some, but not all, of the spinal tissues. This receptor system consists of a tridimensional plexus of unmyelinated nerve fibres; these are in the facet joint capsules, the spinal aponeuroses, the vertebral periosteum, the epidural adipose tissue and the anterior (only) aspect of the dural tube, and in the walls of the spinal blood vessels (arteries and veins) and of free nerve endings (in the spinal and sacroiliac ligaments, and in tendons attached to the spine). There are no nerve endings of any description in articular cartilage, synovial tissue or mature intervertebral discs—the only place where a nociceptive receptor system is directly related to the discs is in the region where the posterior edge of the annulus fibrosus is attached to the expanded portions of the posterior longitudinal ligament by dense fibro-elastic tissue (in which a nociceptive plexus is embedded).

In normal circumstances, the spinal nociceptive system is quiescent; but it becomes active when the receptor endings in the above tissue are irritated mechanically or chemically, or when the related nociceptive afferent fibres in the spinal nerves or dorsal nerve roots are activated directly. Mechanical nociceptive stimulation occurs when the spinal tissues containing the nerve endings are sufficiently stressed by stretching, compression or tearing. Chemical stimulation occurs when the nerve endings are exposed to sufficiently high concentrations of irritant chemicals such as lactic acid, potassium ions, 5-hydroxytryptamine, polypeptide kinins, histamine and some of the prostaglandins, in the surrounding tissue fluid—as occurs in inflammation, for example.

The afferent fibres linking the various parts of the spinal nociceptive receptor system with the central nociceptive pathways, traverse the related branches of the spinal nerves into the dorsal roots. All the tissues lying posterior to the plane of the intervertebral foramina at each level (i.e. the facet and costotransverse joint capsules, the vertebral arch periosteum, the related tendinous and aponeurotic attachments, and the flaval and interspinous ligaments) are innervated from the posterior primary rami, whereas the more anterior tissues (i.e. the vertebral body periosteum and marrow, the costovertebral joint capsules, the two longitudinal ligaments, and the anterior spinal dura) are supplied through branches of the anterior primary rami and the sinuvertebral nerve. Wyke drew special attention to the fact, however, that in no region of the spine is this innervation segmental but instead, at every level, is intersegmental—the receptor systems in the tissues of each spinal segment being supplied not only from the numerically related dorsal root but also by descending and ascending branches of rostrally and caudally located dorsal roots—to a degree that varies with the particular region of the spine. Any attempt to determine the level of a spinal lesion causing pain that is based on an assumption that the spinal tissues are segmentally innervated is therefore fallacious.

The nociceptive afferent fibres in the above nerves traverse the dorsal spinal roots to the apex of the spinal grey matter. At this point they give off branches that run anteriorly to synapse with neurones in the basal spinal nucleus at the root of the dorsal horn. The axons from these latter neurones then ascend in the anterolateral tracts to the thalamic and brain stem reticular nuclei, whence activity is further relayed to the cerebral cortex. In order to reach the brain and evoke the experience of pain, then, nociceptive activity in the spinal nerves must traverse the synapses in the basal spinal nucleus—which therefore constitutes the nociceptive gateway into the central nervous system.

It was for a long time assumed that the intensity of any painful experience was determined solely by the intensity of irritation of the peripheral nociceptive system (receptors or their afferents). However, this is not so, for the centripetal transmission of nociceptive activity is modulated by many influences, facilitatory and inhibitory, that operate on the central synaptic transmission of such activity. One of the important sites at which such synaptic modulation operates from both peripheral and central sources is on the gateway synapses in the basal spinal nucleus. The peripheral source is of major concern to practitioners of orthopaedic medicine.

This peripheral modulatory mechanism is operated, among other things, from the low-threshold corpuscular mechanoreceptors embedded in the spinal tissues—particularly those in the capsules of the facet and rib joints. The large diameter afferents from these mechanoreceptors (as well as from those in the related spinal musculature and overlying skin) enter the spinal cord and give off branches that synapse with neurones in the apex of the dorsal grey horn (the apical spinal nucleus); these then project anteriorly into the basal spinal nucleus where they terminate in inhibitory synapses on the presynaptic terminals of the nociceptive afferents therein. Through this intraspinal inhibitory relay system, then, mechanoreceptor afferent activity exerts a suppressive effect on the centripetal transmission of activity through the basal spinal nucleus (i.e. at its portal of entry into the neuraxis) and thus on awareness of pain in the back. Deliberate stimulation of the highly-sensitive mechanoreceptors in the tissues of the back (as by massage, passive manipulation of the spine, the oscillating activity of a rocking chair or the application of vibrators) can therefore be employed in the palliative treatment of many types of back pain.

CHAPTER 22

# THE SACROILIAC JOINT

Lesions of the sacroiliac joint are as rare as pain at the medial aspect of the buttock and the side of the sacrum is common.

## NOMENCLATURE

The uncertainty that surrounds the vexed question of 'sacroiliac strain' results purely from loose nomenclature. This is often used to designate any pain felt at the side of the sacrum, whereas it should be reserved for pain arising from the sacroiliac ligaments in the absence of rheumatoid inflammation. When such inflammation exists, the condition is correctly named 'sacroiliac arthritis'.

The disagreement between those who hold sacroiliac troubles to provide a common cause of backache and sciatica and those who doubt their very existence is based on differences in clinical examination and interpretation of signs. Little agreement exists on the criteria that justify a diagnosis of sacroiliac strain. When pain felt at the upper inner quadrant of the buttock accompanied by local tenderness suffices, such 'strain' is not uncommon, but when the diagnosis is restricted to cases in which stretching the sacroiliac ligaments hurts, the incidence has proved in my hands to amount to only one in 230 patients with lumbogluteal symptoms.

The term 'sacroiliac strain' should be reserved for cases of pain arising from the sacroiliac ligaments in the absence of arthritis. This creates a difficulty, for in 14% of cases of early sacroiliitis the pain and clinical signs precede the appearance of radiographic sclerosis. Unless, therefore, the pain has lasted for some years, negative X-ray appearances do not preclude arthritis. Help is afforded by the fact that sacroiliac strain never alternates, whereas this is mentioned in one-third of all ankylosing cases.

## SACROILIAC MOBILITY

Whether or not movement occurs at the sacroiliac joint has long been a vexed question. If it can move, then the fixed subluxation so dear to lay manipulators is at least a possibility. In fact, a small range of rotation does exist between the sacrum and ilium, elicited at the extremes of flexion and extension of trunk on pelvis. The axis is horizontal and transverse, and lies about a third of the way down the auricular surface, where a small prominence on the ilium fits into a corresponding depression on the sacrum. This rotation enables the individual to bend a little farther forwards and backwards than would otherwise have been possible. When the patient stands and bends forwards, contraction of the psoas and rectus abdominis muscle draws the upper part of the sacrum forwards as far as the sacrotuberous and sacrospinous ligaments will allow. Mobility at the sacroiliac joint therefore relieves part of the flexion strain on the lumbar spine by providing rotation elsewhere; this is clearly beneficial and no endeavour should be made to diminish it, particularly if a lumbar lesion is already present.

Mobility doubtless decreases with age; for elderly patients often possess osteophytes at the lower margin of the sacroiliac joints. Clearly such ligamentous ossification must diminish the range of movement and may eventually fix the joint, as does the fusion in ankylosing spondylitis.

The possibility of a fixed sacroiliac subluxation causing symptoms is very dubious; no evidence for it exists. It is hard to grasp how the displacement could be maintained if it did occur; for no muscles span the joint that, by their contraction, could keep it displaced. The joint contains no intra-articular meniscus; hence, it cannot suffer the type of internal derangement

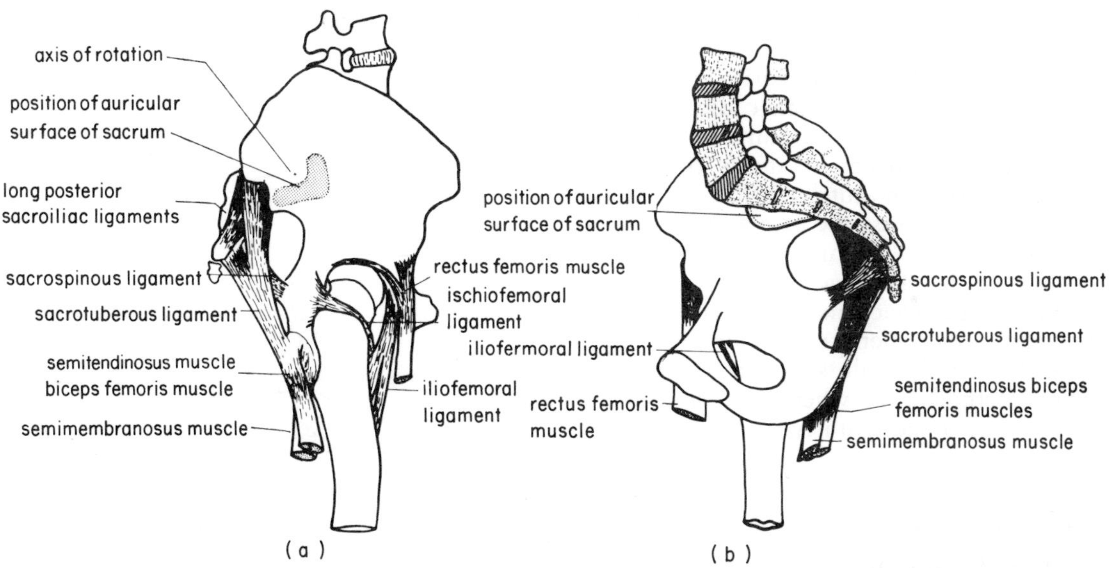


**Fig. 94.** Median section (*a*) and lateral view (*b*) of the bony pelvis showing the ligaments and muscles acting on the sacroiliac joint. The position of the axis of rotation is also defined. (*By kind permission of Professor Duckworth*).

that is so common at the spinal joints and the knee, where muscle guarding does militate against reduction. It is not to be denied that pain can arise in the sacroiliac ligaments from strain in cases of excessive ligamentous laxity or from spondylitic inflammation, but I find no evidence for the concept of pain arising from fixed subluxation.

Stimulated by a conversation with Barbor in 1965 on tests for sacroiliac mobility, Professor Duckworth of Toronto carried out a series of post-mortem studies on fresh specimens, and has kindly sent me a summary of his findings (1967).

*Movement at the Sacroiliac Joints.* The normal movements that occur at the sacroiliac joints are determined by the direction of the auricular surfaces, the ligaments, the muscles acting on the joint, and the symphysis pubis.

The movement that occurs is a rotation of the sacrum (or ilia) around the axis of the shortest and strongest part of the posterior interosseous sacroiliac ligament, which is situated in the angle between the posterosuperior and posteroinferior limbs of the auricular surfaces. When rotation of the upper end of the sacrum occurs in a forward direction the promontory of the sacrum will move in an anteroinferior direction, narrowing the anteroposterior diameter of the pelvic inlet, widening the anteroposterior diameter of the pelvic outlet and tightening the sacrotuberous and sacrospinous ligaments. On backward rotation of the upper end of the sacrum, the reverse movements will occur together with a widening of the anteroposterior diameter of the pelvic inlet, a narrowing of the anteroposterior diameter of the pelvic outlet and a relaxing of the sacrotuberous and sacrospinous ligaments. During the above movement the long posterior sacroiliac ligaments will tighten and restrict this backward rotation of the sacrum on the ilia.

In addition, because the auricular surfaces of the sacrum are nearer the median plane inferiorly than they are superiorly, forward rotation of the sacrum will result in a slight widening of the symphysis pubis, while backward rotation of the sacrum will result in the symphysis pubis being compressed.

When a rotation force is applied to the hip bones in opposite directions such as in extending one thigh while flexing the other thigh, e.g. in stepping up on to a high stool, the extended thigh anchors the hip bone on that side through the iliofemoral and ischiofemoral ligaments and the rectus femoris muscle, while the flexed thigh through the pull of the hamstring muscles rotates the ilium in a backward direction. In addition, the sacrum will move with the ilium on the flexed side because the pull of the hamstring muscles is transmitted to it via the sacrotuberous and sacrospinous ligaments. The result of the above facts will be that rotation of the sacrum in a backward direction will occur at the sacroiliac joint on the extended side only.

While these movements at the sacroiliac joints are small in extent, especially in males, they are quite definite. They are increased when jumping from a height, and in females especially towards the end of pregnancy and for up to three months after pregnancy, owing to the action of the hormone relaxin.

In 1971 Le Corre described the amount of rotation that he had been able to detect at the sacroiliac joint. He inserted long needles and measured the angulation. Movement amounted to only 0.25 mm.

# TESTING THE SACROILIAC JOINT

The finding that directs immediate attention to the sacroiliac joint as a possible cause of pain in the buttock and/or thigh is the unusual discovery that no lumbar movement affects the gluteal symptoms. Rarely, in acute arthritis, the lumbar movements do increase the pain a little, since at the extreme of any lumbar movement an added stress falls on the sacroiliac ligaments. This does not confuse; for, if such an indirect strain on the joints hurts, much more severe pain is set up as soon as the sacroiliac joints are directly tested.

Three methods exist whereby tension can be exerted on sacroiliac ligaments without affecting the lumbar spine.

## Stretching the Anterior Sacroiliac Ligaments

The patient lies on his back. The examiner places his hands on the anterior superior spine of each ilium and presses downwards and laterally. Crossing the arms increases the lateral component of the strain on the ligaments. Such pressure applies the patient's sacrum to the couch, of course, and may prove uncomfortable *centrally*. This the patient can identify as due to pressure on the skin, and is quite different from his deep-seated *unilateral* ache. The pelvis must not be allowed to rock, since the lumbar spine then moves. The examiner's hands cause discomfort anteriorly, and it must be made quite clear to the patient that what is sought is not local pain but aggravation of the gluteal symptom. The response to this test is positive *only if it is stated to evoke unilateral gluteal or posterior crural pain.*

Stretching the anterior ligaments in the manner described is the most delicate test for the sacroiliac joint. It is interesting to note that patients recovering from a flare may say that all pain ceased some days before. They walk and bend about painlessly; yet for a week or ten days after subjective recovery, straining the joint in this way still evokes the remembered discomfort. It is thus clear that this test applies more stress to the sacroiliac ligaments than do ordinary daily activities. Hence, if a patient has symptoms referable to the joint, this manoeuvre will elicit them.

Two other ways exist of stretching the anterior ligaments indirectly: forcing lateral rotation at the hip joint and resisted adduction of the thighs. The patient, by squeezing the examiner's hand between his knees, exerts an equally strong distraction force at the sacroiliac joints.

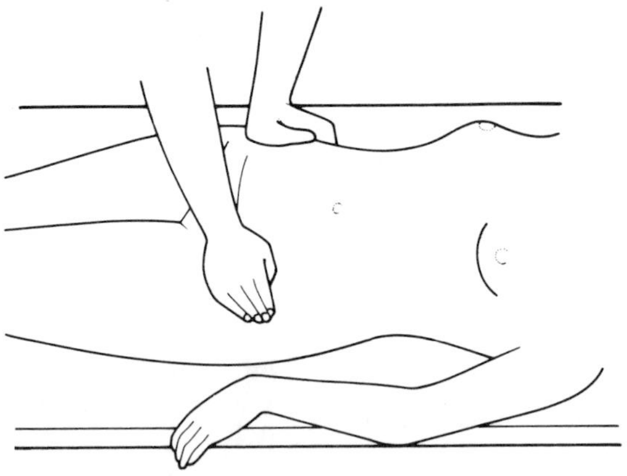

**Fig. 95.** Stretching the anterior sacroiliac joints. The patient lies supine and the examiner applies increasing pressure to the anterior superior spines of the ilia in a downward and outward direction. The pressure must be exerted evenly so that the lumbar region does not move.

When ankylosing spondylitis is more advanced and reaches the lumbar spine, testing the sacroiliac joint ceases to hurt. They are by now painlessly fixed. In, say, acute lumbago, this test is sure to appear positive; for the slightest jar transmitted to the lumbar spinal joints must prove most painful; hence, the support of a cushion or of the patient's forearm under the back may be required to stabilize the lumbar joints. In any case, in lumbago far greater pain is elicited when the lumbar movements are examined.

## Stretching the Posterior Sacroiliac Ligaments

The patient lies on his side and the uppermost part of the iliac crest is pressed towards the floor. If the pressure is applied well forward along the bone, the posterior ligaments bear the greater stress (Fig. 96). This test is much less delicate and gives rise to pain only in severe cases; indeed, in half of all patients, no discomfort is caused thus. Its advantage lies in the fact that the sacrum is not in contact with the couch, thereby obviating confusion between pain due to pressure of the couch on the skin and that due to stretching the ligaments.

Two other ways exist of indirectly stretching the posterior sacroiliac ligaments: forcing full medial rotation at the hip and adducting the flexed thigh across to the other side of the body. The latter clearly does apply tension there, but also stretches the gluteal muscles and hip joint

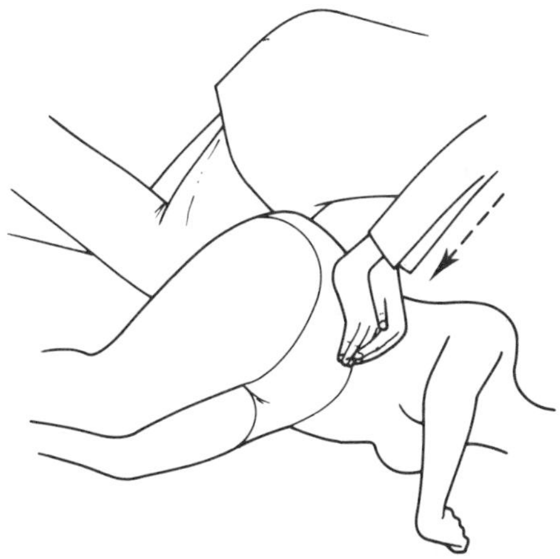

**Fig. 96.** Stretching the posterior sacroiliac ligaments. The patient lies on the painless side while the examiner exerts pressure towards the floor on the anterolateral part of the iliac crest.

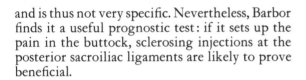

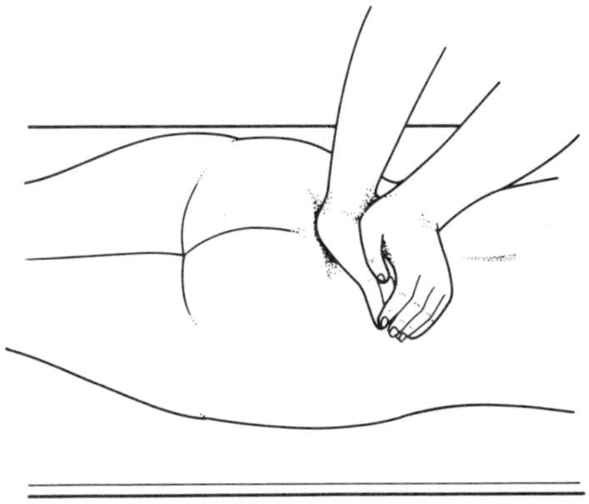

**Fig. 97.** Attempted forward luxation of the sacrum. The heel of the examiner's hand presses on the centre of the patient's sacrum.

and is thus not very specific. Nevertheless, Barbor finds it a useful prognostic test: if it sets up the pain in the buttock, sclerosing injections at the posterior sacroiliac ligaments are likely to prove beneficial.

### Forward Pressure on the Sacrum

This is a repetition in reverse of the first test for the sacroiliac ligaments (Fig. 97). The patient lies prone and the sacrum is pressed smartly forwards while the pelvis stays motionless, supported on the couch. It has the advantage that the examiner can compare the amount of pain—felt in the buttock, not where his hand rests—produced when passive extension of the lumbar spine and forward luxation of the sacrum are attempted in turn. If a lumbar lesion is causing pain in the buttock, this will be evoked only by the extension strain applied to the lumbar spine. If the lesion is sacroiliac, although transmitted stress usually results in slight gluteal aching when the lumbar spine is pushed towards the couch, much more severe pain is set up when the sacrum is pressed upon. Illouz and Coste (1964) confirmed the value of this method of eliciting pain from the sacroiliac ligaments; they called it 'the sign of the tripod'.

During any of these movements, a slight local click may be felt in adolescent boys and in women of childbearing age; it does not hurt. If, instead of a click, a snap is felt as if an adhesion had parted, the radiograph nearly always shows 'osteitis condensans'.

### Other Tests

Osteopaths have many other 'tests' for the sacroiliac joints. Maigne (1972) describes a joke he played on his manipulative colleagues. His patient was a girl aged 30 who had 'congenital fusion of the sacroiliac joints'. He offered her for examination by ten participants at the meeting. He recounts how they came forward with ten different diagnoses: 'left anterior sacrum', 'right anterior sacrum', 'posterior sacrum on both sides', etc. He draws the modest conclusion that, since the tests were 'very positive', they cannot be 'good tests'.

## CONFIRMATION

### Negative Component

Examination of the lumbar spine and lower limbs reveals no disorder contradicting the ascription of the symptoms to the sacroiliac joint. Straight-leg raising is not limited; there are no neurological signs; the arteries are patent; there is no palpable mass in the buttock; and so on. Each rotation of the hip may prove painful *at full range*; this is a consistent finding, since forcing these movements stretches the sacroiliac ligaments. In psychoneurosis, strong pressure on bony points is often strongly resented; hence the examination must include the lower limb in order to reveal the inconsistencies that indicate the presence of pain caused emotionally.

## Tenderness 'Over the Joint'

Tenderness 'over the sacroiliac joint' usually implies tenderness of the upper sacral extent of the sacrospinalis muscle. A glance at Fig. 98 which shows the relations of the sacroiliac joint, should finally dispose of the idea that tenderness of any structure within reach of the human finger denotes tenderness of the sacroiliac ligaments, for they lie covered by the overhang of the ilium and the sacral extent of the sacrospinalis muscle. Hence, even if the joint is at fault, tenderness will not be found. By contrast, since referred tenderness is a common finding in lumbar disc lesions, the discovery of tenderness somewhere in the region of the sacroiliac joint is then a likelihood—a positively misleading sign.

## Local Anaesthesia

This cannot be induced at the anterior sacroiliac ligaments, and injecting the whole of the posterior mass of ligaments would prove a huge task. Hence, positive confirmation by local anaesthesia is impracticable. In a sincere patient with an uninformative radiograph, it is my practice to carry out negative confirmation by inducing epidural local anaesthesia, in case, after all, a lumbar disc lesion should be responsible, especially in those cases where both the lumbar and the sacroiliac tests are stated to hurt. If, when the sacroiliac joints are tested, say, a quarter of an hour after the injection has been completed they still hurt, a lumbar disc lesion with false sacroiliac signs has been excluded.

## Radiography

This may help. In sacroiliac strain nothing is revealed. This is in keeping with the results of radiography of a skeleton pelvis (Young 1940). X-ray photographs taken with the symphysis pubis closed and forced wide open showed no detectable change at the sacroiliac joints. In the sacroiliac arthritis of early spondylitis, the radiograph showed the typical sclerosis in 86% of my cases. Sclerosis also occurs in Reiter's disease,

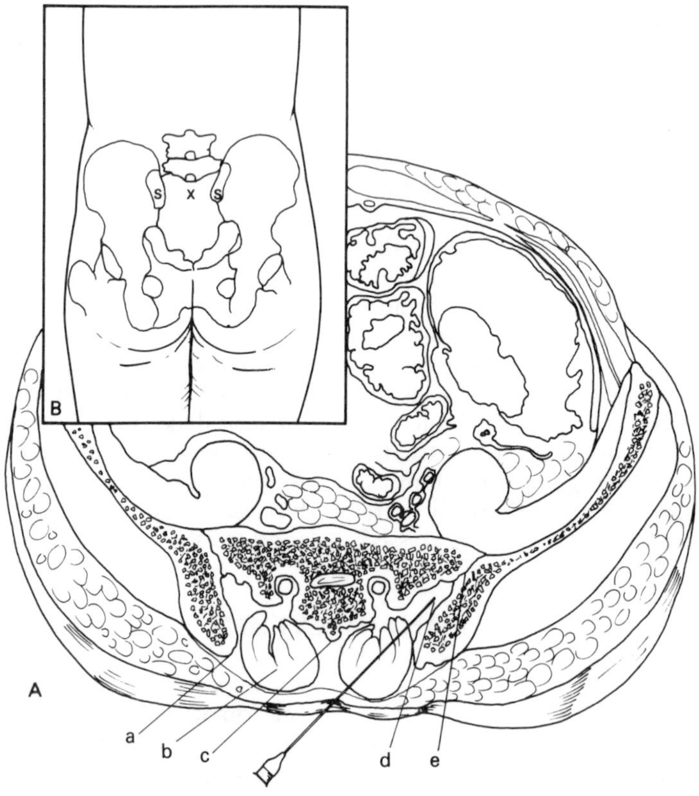


**Fig. 98.** Relations of the sacroiliac joint. Note the impossibility of eliciting tenderness at the posterior ligament by digital pressure. *a*, Posterior superior spine. *b*, Sacrospinalis muscle. *c*, Spinous process of first sacral vertebra. *d*, Interossseous sacroiliac ligament. *e*, Sacroiliac joint.

chronic rheumatoid arthritis, psoriasis, ulcerative colitis and sarcoidosis, but discomfort in the buttock is then a rarity, the sclerotic process being painless. I have met only one patient with Reiter's disease and one after colectomy for colitis, who had attacks of pain in the buttock arising from the sacroiliac joint.

In spondylitis, the iliac side of the lower part of the joint shows the sclerosis first, with blurring of the articular margin. It is often bilateral in cases of purely unilateral pain; when unilateral, it is usually on the same side as the symptoms, but not always. After many years, the joint disappears and sacrum and ilia fuse, obliterating the joint (Plate XLII/2).

It is widely believed that a diagnosis of spondylitis ankylopoetica can be made only by inspecting the radiograph, and that a normal appearance of the sacroiliac joints excludes this disease. This is not so. Clinical signs at the sacroiliac joints may precede by months or years the appearance of early sclerosis. Spondylitis spreading up the vertebral column without sclerosis ever appearing on the radiograph of the sacroiliac joints is a rarity; I have met four instances only. In one patient, whose first, symptom was increasing stiffness of the neck, one sacroiliac joint was normal, the other fused.

### Sedimentation Rate

This too may help, but much cannot be expected in difficult cases. When the disease is obvious, the erythrocyte sedimentation rate is greatly raised, perhaps to 50 mm or even 100 mm in the first hour. However, in a doubtful case, the sedimentation rate is apt to be in the region of 5 to 10 mm and thus prove of no assistance.

## LAY MANIPULATORS AND THE SACROILIAC JOINT

Lay manipulators describe a number of other tests for the sacroiliac joints, some direct, some straining the joint from a distance. I have compared the specificity of some of these tests with the three advocated above, on patients with pain arising from the sacroiliac ligaments, confirmed radiographically, in early spondylitis. The upshot has been that springing the pelvis and pressing the sacrum forwards on the iliac bones have proved the most delicate and reliable tests.

Much controversy exists among lay manipulators on what signs are and are not compatible with a sacroiliac subluxation. Some maintain that a sacroiliac subluxation can cause such and such limitation of straight-leg raising, but that greater restriction indicates a disc lesion. This leads to obvious logical difficulties, for a patient may have 10° limitation of straight-leg raising one day, 60° the next and a root palsy the day after that. I have therefore been at pains to test these movements on patients with severe degrees of active spondylitic arthritis, some bad enough hardly to be able to walk. Presumably, such arthritis would produce more advanced physical signs than a mere minor subluxation. When told that no muscle exists spanning the joint so as to maintain a subluxation in being, laymen have put forward spasm of the piriformis muscle as the agent. Were it really in spasm the thigh would be fixed in abduction.

The signs were those to be logically expected. Any movement straining the joint proved painful but was not limited. In addition to a positive result from the three tests advocated above, full trunk flexion puts a rotational strain on the joint, as does full straight-leg raising. Trunk side flexion towards the painful side increases the shearing stress on the joint. At their extremes, all passive movements of the hip stretch the joint. Coughing and resisted adduction of the thighs distract the articular surfaces. All these movements hurt at the buttock, but none was limited in range. In particular, straight-leg raising has never been found limited and no muscle spasm could ever be detected.

## SACROILIAC ARTHRITIS

Although it is well-recognized that ankylosing spondylitis begins radiologically at the sacroiliac joints, it is not widely appreciated that this can also be established by clinical examination. Spondylitis may begin as a pain in one or other buttock or thigh; if so, clinical examination shows one sacroiliac joint to be at fault. Radiography usually confirms this, but clinical signs may precede the radiological evidence by some years.

## Pathology

The ligamentous ossification in the advanced case is well-known. Ancient Egyptian mummies have been discovered showing spondylitis ankyloproctia (d'Ardois 1964). The periphery of each intervertebral joint is ossified and the facet joints are also the site of bony ankylosis. The ilia and sacrum fuse. Post-mortem studies of early cases are few but Bywaters (1968) reports that the disease starts by invasion of articular cartilage, and its localized replacement by granulation tissue. About these areas the bone is sclerotic. Pannus can be seen at the facet joints causing marginal erosion of cartilage. His conclusion on the aetiology of spondylitis is 'some change in cartilage, or some change in the body's reactions to cartilage, whereby the latter becomes an active auto-immune target, so that it gets invaded either at the margins where it joins normal connective tissue, or where the normal bony layer protecting it from marrow blood vessels becomes deficient'.

## Frequency

Between 1950 and 1965, 18 629 patients with pain in the lower back, buttock or thigh were seen by me at St Thomas's Hospital. Of these, 255 were suffering from ankylosing spondylitis, and 81 of them were in the stage of early sacroiliac involvement only (52 men and 29 women). This is probably a higher proportion than in the general run of spondylitics, for St Thomas's was known to attract the problem of obscure back trouble. In consequence, I doubtless saw an undue preponderance of patients suffering from hitherto intractable sciatica.

These patients were singled out because in every case the sacroiliac joints were tested clinically as part of the routine examination of the lower back. Probably not more than one case in ten of spondylitis ever has pain in the buttock with consequent elicitation of this symptom when the sacroiliac ligaments are stretched. Most spondylitis begins as a diffuse lumbar ache; sometimes the earlier symptoms are thoracic; in a few, painless inability to turn the neck first draws attention to the disorder. In these cases, although radiography of the sacroiliac joints shows gross sclerosis or even fusion, testing the joint clinically provokes no discomfort, since this can be elicited only in the early stage of active inflammation in the sacroiliac ligaments.

It is interesting to note that, in these 81 cases, no less than 70 showed sclerosis on the first radiograph, and in the rest it appeared on skiagrams taken later, but in two cases it took five years for this to happen. Clinical testing of the joints is, therefore, a very accurate means of deciding whether it is affected or not, more so indeed than radiography, although the two seldom fail to tally.

## Age

The age at onset of the pain in the buttock is shown in Fig. 99. The figures for men and women are virtually the same; the disorder is merely twice as common in men. Clinical arthritis can begin any time between the age of 15 and 39 and has its maximum incidence between the ages of 18 and 29. In this series, no case of sacroiliac arthritis began at or over the age of 40, but I have encountered two cases, confirmed radiologically. The first was a man of 48 who started bouts of pain in the buttock after some years of recurrent iritis; the other a woman whose gluteal pain began aged 47.

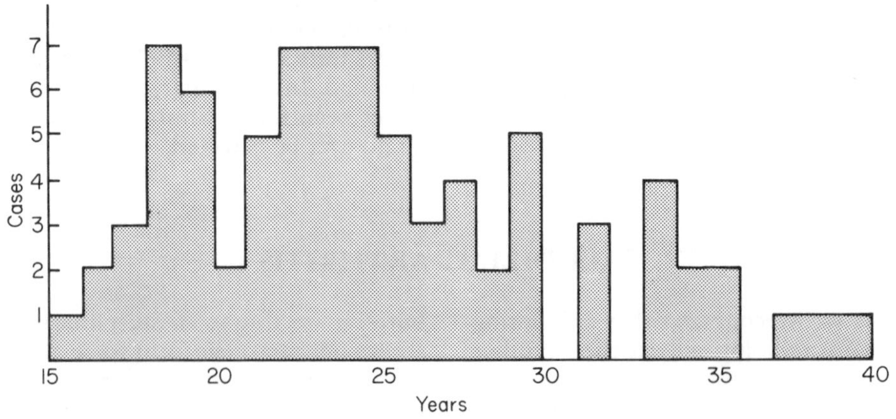


**Fig. 99.** Age at onset of sacroiliac arthritis.

## HLA–B27

Following Brewerton et al.'s (1973) discovery of the frequency of HLA–B27 in the blood of spondylitics, 78 healthy blood donors carrying the group were identified. No less than 16 were found to have pain and radiological signs of ankylosing spondylitis. A control group numbering 126 had none (Calin and Fries 1975). Moreover Carter and Fairbank (1974) had already found that the incidence in men was 30 times greater in first degree relatives than in the general population and 100 times greater in women. Those with HLA–B27 are 90 times more likely to develop ankylosing spondylitis than those without, but even so only one in five of positive reaction contracts the disease. However, spondylitis does occur in HLA–B27–negative people; hence clearly other factors are required too.

## Symptoms

The usual complaint is pain in one buttock radiating perhaps to the back of the thigh and calf. The pain never reaches the foot and there is, of course, no paraesthesia. By the time that lumbar invasion has followed involvement of sacroiliac joints, the buttock ache has largely ceased.

Since the sacroiliac ligaments are developed at the proximal extent of the first and second sacral segments, pain is referred from them in exactly the same way as it is referred from the first and second sacral nerve roots. There is therefore nothing in the nature or extent of the pain to distinguish sacroiliac arthritis from a disc protrusion compressing either of these nerve roots. Moreover, a cough usually jars the buttock or thigh in sacroiliac arthritis. Just as a momentary increase in intradural pressure jolts the nerve root, so does the same sudden increase in intra-abdominal pressure distract the ilium from the sacrum. When the ligaments joining the two bones are inflamed, this naturally hurts. This deceptive feature had led to nearly every patient being treated on the assumption that a disc lesion was present. Many had had osteopathy, which might well have been expected to increase the pain; in fact, it did not. Surprisingly enough, many patients experienced some hours' relief after manipulation, then the pain returned to its previous intensity. Only in the rare hyperacute case did osteopathy cause immediate aggravation, and even then for only a few days.

The characteristic of the pain is that it comes and goes irrespective of posture and exertion. This is the reverse of the history in disc lesions, where pain follows certain activities and subsides after their avoidance. When present, the pain can be increased by such exertion as strains the joint, but when absent the hardest work is powerless to provoke it. The pain often changes sides; it alternates and is scarcely ever bilateral, except rarely for a day or two at the changeover. The pain was recorded as alternating in 28 cases, right-sided only in 27 and left-sided only in 17. These flares are unprovoked and indeed unprovokable, and can last days, months, exceptionally years. One joint is often the main source of pain, the flares on the other side being infrequent, mild and transient.

The appearance of these patients bears no resemblance to the accepted picture of advanced spondylitis. They are cheerful, often well covered, agile in their movements and, on examination, possess a full and painless range at every spinal joint. Anaemia, iritis and trouble in the peripheral joints are as yet noticeably absent, and the clinical arthritis was found secondary to Reiter's disease and to ulcerative colitis in only one case each.

*Symptoms in Pregnancy.* By analogy with rheumatoid arthritis, it was to be expected that pregnancy would temporarily stop the symptoms, and, in fact, five of 29 female patients reported freedom from ache in the buttock for the period of the pregnancy and a month or two afterwards. However, in three others, the original attack of pain in the buttock came on during pregnancy, and two other patients experienced such a severe flare during pregnancy that they could scarcely walk, though the pre-pregnancy attacks had been quite minor.

# Prognosis

In most cases of sacroiliac arthritis, extension of the spondylitic process to the spinal joints takes place within a few years, especially in younger patients. A few patients, however, experience flares less frequently, they become less painful and last a shorter time; after five or ten years the disease appears to have burnt itself out. The sedimentation rate is of no prognostic value, nor is the presence or absence of sclerosis visible on the first film. My impression is that women do better than men, and that sacroiliitis starting in the late twenties, certainly in the thirties, follows a benign course (see Plate XLIII/2). Alternating sacroiliitis in patients in their twenties may take many years to reach the lumbar spine, flaring and subsiding for say ten years. These attacks usually cease when the process reaches the spine, but in 1978 I encountered a patient aged 47 in whom the ankylosis had reached the thoracic joints but he was still, after 17 years, having minor flares in one or other sacroiliac joint.

Since most patients eventually develop spinal arthritis but a few do not, it is unwise, when only the sacroiliac joints are affected, to draw too pessimistic a conclusion about extension to the spinal joints with final ankylosis. Naturally, a guarded long-term prognosis must be given. It is not possible to avoid extension to the spine in those in whom it is going to happen. A sound policy is to make no prognosis at all, but merely to state that the pain arises from the sacroiliac joint, which will flare on and off for at least some years; and that the patient can be kept comfortable meanwhile.

## Treatment

There are a number of very effective remedies, all of which stop pain for the time being, but none prevents recurrence or the liability to eventual extension to the spinal joints.

*Phenylbutazone.* Quite small doses suffice. If the lumbar region becomes stiff and painful after some hours in bed, a tablet of 100 mg last thing at night usually suffices. The alternative treatment is triamcinolone infiltration into the lower lumbar supraspinatus ligaments. The effect may last months and is to be preferred in those who have had a peptic ulcer or in whom the tablets cause indigestion. Dosage of 200 mg twice a day as soon as a flare starts, followed by 100 mg once or twice a day for the next week often proves enough. Flurbiprofen is stated by Calin and Grahame (1974) to be almost as effective as phenylbutazone. Methrazone, 200 mg twice or three times a day, is often successful. Prinalgin, 500 mg is worth trying.

*Indomethacin.* A 25 mg tablet two or three times a day for a few days abates a flare quickly.

*Prednisone.* A few days on 5 mg twice a day followed by one tablet a day for another few days is usually enough.

*Prostaglandin Inhibitors.* Two new drugs can be tried if phenylbutazone is not effective or is badly tolerated by the digestive tract. Both are non-steroid and act by suppressing the synthesis of prostaglandin, on whose presence the capacity for inflammation rests. They are naproxen 250 mg and ketoprofen 50 mg. Severe gastrointestinal haemorrhage has been reported.

*Intra-articular Injection of Triamcinolone.* It is not easy to get the needle into the right spot on account of the large sacral foramina into which the tip is apt to pass; the suspension then passes intrasacrally to no advantage. A needle 8 cm long is introduced at the midline at the first sacral level and thrust in at an angle of 45°. It strikes bone and the point must then be manoeuvred until it is felt to hit cartilage. Once the needle point penetrates cartilage nothing can be forced out of the syringe. The needle is then withdrawn during pressure on the piston until the suspension just begins to flow; 5 ml are now injected between the posterior ligament and the articular cartilage. It must therefore reach the right spot. After a day's soreness the pain ceases, often for months.

*X-ray Therapy.* If, rarely, systemic steroids, phenylbutazone, indomethacin and topical triamcinolone all fail, X-ray therapy should be considered. Subsidence of the pain after the third or fourth exposure takes place in four out of five cases. Exposure of 200 r three times a week for a fortnight (i.e. 1200 r in all) is average dosage. Return of pain is to be expected, in six to twelve months if the patient is young, not for some years if the patient is over 30. In a woman, the sacroiliac joints cannot be irradiated without some damage to the ovaries. A woman over, say, 30 may choose, if she already has several children, to accept the slight chance of sterilization for the relief of pain. The husband should be a party to this decision. The Medical Defence Union holds the opinion that the risks inherent in this treatment should be explained to the patient in the presence of a witness, and that she should sign a statement that she consents to the treatment knowing and accepting the risks; the witness should also sign the document. This procedure, in the Union's view, adequately safeguards the medical man concerned. The Medical Research Council's report on the hazards to man of nuclear radiation (1956) points out that the incidence of leukaemia is ten times greater in spondylitics who have received radiation than in those who have not; even so, the incidence is only 3:1000. The report is based on about 13 500 cases and the mean latent period between first exposure to X-rays and the development of leukaemia was six years. However, mount sinai hospital

# MEMORANDUM

DATE:
TO:
FROM:
SUBJECT:

08310

Sinclair (1971) investigated the cause of death in 157 cases of spondylitis all of whom had received a full course of radiotherapy years before, and in no case was leukaemia responsible. Irradiation should be avoided during pregnancy for fear of harming the fetus.

Claims have been made that X-ray treatment arrests the disease. This is not so. It abates the pain of ankylosing spondylitis but has no influence on its eventual evolution. The speed of evolution at different ages, however, is so different that the patient may have to be followed up for some years before it becomes clear that the effect of radiotherapy wears off in the end.

*Compression.* When a patient is seen scarcely able to walk because each step jars the severely inflamed ligaments, a tight binder must be applied at once and strong compression strain maintained for a week or two. This enables the patient to walk comfortably until drug treatment takes effect. Some women understandably refuse all drugs during pregnancy; if so, this is the only possible measure.

## PROSTATITIS AND SACROILIITIS

Kelly's historical research has disclosed that Rolleston quotes Musgrave as having described arthritis after non-venereal urethritis as early as 1703. He also found that Lorimer (1884) mentioned this occurrence, and that Coulson (1852) stated that arthritis can follow urethral suppuration from any cause. In fact, there appears to be some connection between sacroiliac arthritis and non-specific prostatitis; for Csonka (1958) noted that 8.6% of his patients with Reiter's syndrome suffered from sacroiliitis and 10.8% from iritis; figures from Mason et al. (1959) were 45 and 24%; 32% of Mason's (1964) cases had sacroiliitis, as had 42 of 234 of Wright and Watkinson's cases (1965). Bywaters and Ansell (1958) found that 6 of 37 patients with arthritis secondary to ulcerative colitis had radiological changes in the sacroiliac joints indistinguishable from those of ankylosing spondylitis. Mason et al. (1958) found evidence of prostatis in 33% of cases of rheumatoid arthritis, in 83% of ankylosing spondylitis and in 95% of Reiter's disease. However, this is clearly not the whole story, since women also suffer from sacroiliac arthritis. Baker et al. (1963) found sclerosis at the sacroiliac joints in 15 of 60 patients with gross psoriatic arthritis. Indeed, it looks as if a number of different stimuli can provoke sacroiliac sclerosis. But there are two important differences. Except rarely in Reiter's disease and ulcerative colitis, the patient does not suffer pain in his buttock arising from his sacroiliac joint; it is a radiological finding without a clinical counterpart. Secondly, the existence of the sacroiliac sclerosis does not imply that the disease is ankylosing spondylitis which will spread relentlessly up the spine.

In 1973 Brewerton et al. pointed out the association between HLA 27 tissue antigens and iritis, ankylosing spondylitis and Reiter's disease. They were present in 72 of 75 patients with ankylosing spondylitis and only 3 of 75 controls. First degree relatives possessed the antigen in 52% whereas it occurs in only 4% of the general population. This discovery has led to the theory that a bacterium whose structure is so like HLA that the invasion is not recognized may be responsible. The organism responsible may be Klebsiella pneumoniae (Ebringer et al. 1979).

## ANKYLOSING SPONDYLITIS

### The Usual Course

Sclerosing sacroiliac arthritis usually takes place silently, for less than 10% of patients with advanced disease can recollect having pain in the buttock or sciatica.

The first complaint is often vague discomfort and stiffness in the lower back, usually worst on waking and eased by exercise. This comes and goes, irrespective of exertion, in bouts lasting weeks or months, often with symptom-free intervals of similar length. Then the pain spreads to the thorax, tending to leave the lower lumbar levels. The patient notices that breathing has become restricted, owing to stiffness at the costovertebral joints; in the end, his respiration becomes purely diaphragmatic. Finally, the neck is involved in the ossifying process, becoming increasingly rigid. The two upper joints are affected late; hence, hyperextension here contrasts with the flattening out of the lumbar lordosis and the marked thoracocervical rounded kyphosis. The patient's face becomes pinched and haggard, the eyes hollow and the body loses its fatty covering. Microcytic anaemia is a common, and iritis an uncommon, complication. When bony ankylosis is complete, pain ceases; the pain in the trunk therefore travels upwards and comes to an end after many years.

Then the hips become affected. Until then, the patient, curved and fixed though his back is, has been able to look up by extending at the hip joints. Now this ceases to be possible and some patients are reduced to a pitiable state of crippledom (Ward 1822). The knees, shoulders and other joints are seldom affected; indeed, spondylitis is more likely to *present* as arthritis at the knee or tarsus than to lead to involvement of these joints as a late manifestation.

Happily, this sequence of events is not a certainty. The speed and extent of spread depend partly on the patient's sex and age. A few patients now aged 35 to 40 have been followed up for 10 years; radiographic evidence of sacroiliac sclerosis has appeared during this time, but the disorder has not yet spread to the lumbar spine. The younger the patient is at the onset, the worse the prognosis, and men do worse than women. When spondylitis appears before the age of 20, in either sex, severe disablement soon is very probable. Evolution of the spinal component will probably take two to seven years; the hips will be affected within another five years, treatment or no treatment. By contrast, sacroiliac arthritis coming on after the age of 25 may, even in men, go on flaring and subsiding for, say, five years before the lower lumbar joints become involved, and in women the joints may flare alternately for 10 to 15 years on end. Spread upwards may be very slow, and the thoracic spine only becomes affected by the time the patient reaches 40 or 50. The cervical spine may never fix at all; the hips usually retain full mobility indefinitely. Sclerosing sacroiliac arthritis coming on after the age of 30 is quite unimportant, except that the patient may be led mistakenly to believe that he will soon be a cripple.

Occasionally, the lumbar spine fixes, not in flexion but with its ordinary lordosis. Inspection of the patient's back then yields no information, but, directly he is asked to perform trunk movements, the fixation becomes evident and is particularly obvious on attempted side flexion. Rarely, the constitutional signs are absent; the patient is cheerful, looks well, and is amply covered. Nothing then in the patient's appearance suggests the diagnosis, but once more, side flexion of the lumbar, and probably thoracic, spine is much restricted.

Beadle (1931) has pointed out that the large lateral outcrops of bone are more marked on the left side of the lumbar spine and on the right side of the thoracic spine in right-handed spondylitics.

## Treatment

### Explanation

When a patient aged over 25 is seen at the stage of sacroiliac arthritis, little need be said to him about future disablement. Unless his job involves very heavy work, he may never become appreciably incapacitated. On the other hand, when spondylitis has already reached the lumbar spine in a man aged, say, 25, it is important to steer him towards a suitable career (unless chance has already led him to do so). It is best to state that the spine is sure ultimately to stiffen in a way that does not interfere with sedentary work; that the pain is controllable and that the disorder very seldom spreads, e.g. to the hands, thus impeding manual tasks.

When the spinal column is already stiffening, it is wise to explain that the stiffness is permanent but unimportant to a sedentary worker, whereas the pain responds to treatment, eventually disappearing altogether. The patient must be persuaded to view his disability in as cheerful a light as possible, to resign himself to avoid some pursuits, and to adopt work suited to his capacity. The question of spread to other joints, can only be answered evasively in young patients, but quite a strong negative is justified to a patient in the thirties in whom only the sacroiliac or lower lumbar joints are as yet affected.

The capacity for sedentary work is often not appreciably impaired for years. It is not deformity so much as pain keeping the patient awake and rendering his daily life miserable that upsets him. A rigid lumbothoracic spine is remarkably little inconvenience to a sedentary worker. When the disease spreads to the hip joints, however, the position is very different. Fixed flexion deformity of the thigh combined with a rigid kyphosis of the lumbar spine is a great disability.

### The Prevention of Further Deformity

This is aided by the following routine. The patient should sleep on one mattress on fracture boards, with only one pillow, and should avoid lying curled up on his side. He should lie face downwards on an unyielding couch for an hour—even for less is of some value—in the middle of his working day. If he has to sit bent over a desk for any length of time, he should make a conscious effort to pull himself up straight as often as he can remember, not less than once an hour. For the prevention of deformity this regimen is more valuable than any physiotherapy. However, this is indicated from time to time, if deformity appears to be increasing. The physiotherapist should force extension at the lumbo-thoracic spine and, if necessary, stretch out both hip joints towards extension. Total replacement of both hips is worth considering.

Osteotomy at the lower thoracic level can straighten out a gross flexion deformity of the spine.

Recumbency is no longer regarded as useful in spondylitis ankylopoetica.

## Treatment of Ligamentous Pain

Phenylbutazone is very effective and should be tried first. A mere 100 mg taken last thing at night will often abolish the severe ache waking the patient each morning. So small a dose can be continued indefinitely, but there is no need for medication during pain-free periods. The next most useful drug is indomethacin, 25 mg once to three times a day. An alternative is alclofenac 1 g three times a day. During a flare, it quickly abates the pain, and needs to be taken for a week or so as a rule. If this fails, prednisone 5 mg twice a day should be prescribed. This dose satisfies the body's daily requirement of hydrocortisone. Hence, it should not be given for too long and, when a flare subsides, it should not be dropped abruptly, but tailed off. Spinal mobilizing exercises carried out at bedtime may abate morning stiffness. Getting the patient's wife to walk up and down on his spine as he lies prone just before going to bed is another effective measure.

The patient should be informed that the pain disappears when the ankylosing process is completed. However, backache reappearing many years after ankylosis is complete suggests a fracture with pseudarthrosis.

Sharp and Purser (1957) described ten cases of spontaneous atlanto-axial dislocation in patients with advanced spondylitis, causing pressure on the spinal cord. Skull traction followed by occipitocervical arthrodesis relieved pain and caused regression in the neurological signs. Bowie and Glasgow (1961) described cauda equina lesions in spondylitis ankylopoetica leading to numbness in both lower limbs, absent ankle jerks and urinary incontinence. Laminectomy disclosed no abnormality and afforded no benefit. These lesions are thought to be connected with the arachnoid cysts and thecal diverticula that complicate spondylitis. I have encountered two cases in which straight-leg raising was so limited in lumbar spondylitis that the patient could scarcely walk; in the worse instance, the range of straight-leg raising was 5° on one side and 15° on the other.

Stretching either leg up caused no pain; it was merely impossible. Presumably, the dura mater or the dural sleeve of the lower lumbar roots had become inflamed as the result of spondylitic arachnoiditis. Certainly, it is not a purely superficial lesion, for epidural local anaesthesia did not increase the range of straight-leg raising then or afterwards, whereas a few weeks of indomethacin increased range by 30° on each side. In two other cases intractable sciatic pain had led to laminectomy being mistakenly performed at a time when the radiograph had not yet begun to show sclerosis. Each surgeon on inquiry reported that inspection during the operation showed the dura mater and nerve roots macroscopically normal.

*At the Peripheral Joints.* Triamcinolone, injected into the joint at whatever intervals prove necessary, is strongly indicated during a flare of arthritis at hip, knee, shoulder or elbow. Two large joints can be dealt with at one sitting and the injections are repeated as soon as discomfort returns. During the chronic phase, this may prove effective for many months, even years. The range of movement in joints affected for a long time does not return. Intra-articular injections at such long intervals do not provoke steroid arthropathy.

*At the Costovertebral Joints.* Sometimes one lower costovertebral joint becomes painfully included in the spondylitic process. The pattern that one would have expected in this disorder would be unilateral posterior pain on thoracic movements, on breathing and on passively springing the ribs. This occasionally proves so; surprisingly enough, more often no movement whatever affects the constant ache. Triamcinolone injected at the affected joint is most effective, but it is difficult to find the correct level.

*At the Facet Joints.* As spondylitis spreads upwards, the patient may develop *unilateral* lumbar pain, sometimes at succeeding levels. If each joint is sprung in turn as he lies prone, the culprit is identified. Triamcinolone (2 ml) should be injected into the posterior ligament and intra-articularly. This lies on a horizontal level with the tip of the transverse process, and some 2 cm from the midline. A 5 cm needle is required and can be felt traversing ligament before touching bone. Relief is immediate and lasting, but six to twelve months later the joint above may become affected and call for injection too.

The same arthritis may appear at a cervical facet joint, again causing unilateral pain. The technique of injection is the same as for an osteoarthrotic facet joint (see p. 115).

## 'LUMBAGO' IN SPONDYLITIS

A deceptive phenomenon is occasionally encountered. The patient, usually aged 30 to 35, complains that he may feel a sudden jar in his back on bending to lift a heavy weight, after which his back is painful for some weeks. He recovers, but further exertion brings on the same pain again. Naturally, a diagnosis of lumbago is made and the presence of a disc lesion appears confirmed when the X-ray appearances of his lumbar spine reveal no other cause for his symptoms. In fact, he is straining his stiffening lumbar joints, the site of the spondylitic process, perhaps fracturing an ossifying ligament. When this occurs at a low lumbar joint, nothing arouses suspicion until the range of lumbar movement is found grossly restricted for a man of his age. If, however, he identifies the site of his pain as upper lumbar, this sequence of events comes to mind at once, for he is indicating the 'forbidden area' where disc lesions are most uncommon. It is, of course, the radiograph of the sacroiliac joints, not the lumbar joints, that confirms the diagnosis.

Another possibility is the presence of a lumbar disc lesion in a patient whose disc has become invaded by the spondylitic process. Granulomatous penetration of cartilage naturally weakens it and a disc lesion may result. Alternatively a disc lesion may be caused by trauma in the ordinary way. In either of these two events there is no restriction of side flexion of the lumbar spine such as is found in a patient whose sudden pain arises from severe strain of an ossifying ligament. Lumbago in a patient with sacroiliac spondylitis causes the same attacks of temporary fixation, with pain on coughing, that occur in ordinary people, and the treatment is similar. Progression to sciatica appears not to occur. Eventual lumbar ankylosis cures the disc trouble.

## OSTEITIS CONDENSANS ILII

This is a purely radiological finding, important only because the appearance of spondylitic arthritis may be closely mimicked. Osteitis condensans occurs only in women, some of whom give a history of past minor abdominal sepsis. It is non-progressive and is essentially a sclerosis of bone without blurring of the joint margins. In the more obvious cases, the sclerosis occupies the mid-part of the joint, and is seldom confined to the lower aspect of the ilium, being more extensive upwards. Osteitis condensans bears no connection with spondylitis nor does it cause pain in the buttock. It was tempting to regard the sclerosis as a manifestation of past low-grade infection, but Gillespie and Lloyd-Roberts (1953) consider it an aseptic necrosis caused by vascular occlusion. They detected osteitis in 2.2% of 760 routine radiographs of the lumbosacral area and removed a specimen for biopsy. This showed non-inflammatory deposition of extra bone (see Plate XLIII/1).

## SACROILIAC OSTEOARTHROSIS

Radiological evidence of osteophytosis at the edges of the joint shows that the ligaments are ossifying. This entails complete stabilization of the joint. Hence, the discovery that osteoarthrosis is present at the sacroiliac joint positively excludes the joint as the source of whatever symptoms the patient may have. Taken as a disease, osteoarthrosis of the sacroiliac joints is an imaginary disorder.

## SACROILIAC GOUT

This occurs in the late stages of gout in about 10% of patients (Malawista et al. 1965). The patient, amongst his other accesses of pain, suffers recurrent discomfort at one side of his sacrum. He has had gout in his peripheral joints for years, and the X-ray photograph shows juxta-articular cysts, which Lipson and Slocumb (1965) have shown by biopsy to contain encapsulated deposits of urate.

## SPECIFIC SACROILIAC ARTHRITIS

This may be tuberculous or septic. In tuberculosis the first symptom is the swelling in the buttock; the patient does not experience appreciable pain. Fluctuation shows that a cold abscess is present and aspiration followed by inoculation of a guinea-pig shows it to be tuberculous. Testing the joint does not elicit pain, on account of the fibrous ankylosis produced by the infection.

Septic arthritis is dealt with on p. 376.

## SACROILIAC STRAIN

This occurs only in women, between the ages of 15 and 35. It is rare, and always unilateral, never alternating. It differs from the arthritis of spondylitis in that, far from coming and going for no reason, the pain in one buttock is evoked by exertion and avoided by resting the joint. It may be associated with pregnancy but as often is not. Though it is true that, as can be shown by radiography, slight relaxation of the sacroiliac ligaments occurs in some pregnant women, this is physiological. In consequence, symptoms do not arise and testing the sacroiliac joint does not set up any pain. The existence of a hormone named 'relaxin' is responsible for the ligamentous change. Luckily, no appreciable instability of the joints results and even prenatal exercises intended to increase the mobility at the sacroiliac joints prove harmless; however, they are best avoided for the sake of the lumbar spine, as nearly all of them involve trunk flexion.

Examination of women whose backache dates from pregnancy shows that the cause is very seldom sacroiliac strain but an early disc lesion—the result of 10 days in bed in 'the nursing mother's position' (see Volume II). The facile assumption that, merely because a woman's backache started during pregnancy or the puerperium, it must be due to sacroiliac strain, is not borne out by clinical examination.

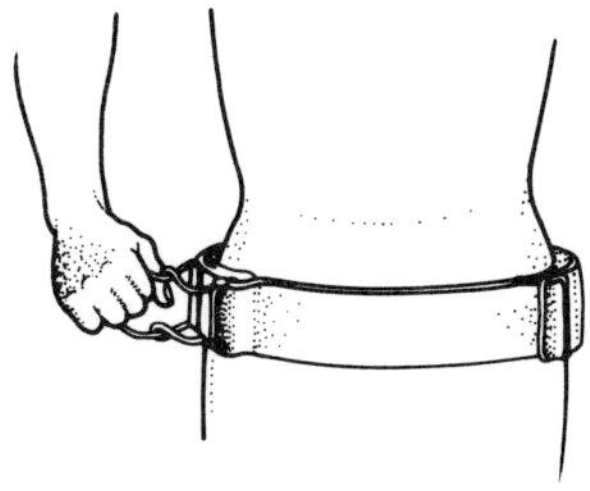

**Fig. 100.** A corrugator belt for sacroiliac strain. (*Austlid, Stockholm*).

### Treatment

The sacroiliac is like the acromioclavicular joint in that no muscle controls movement at the joint, which relies for its stability solely on its ligaments. Hence, movement plays no part in the treatment of sacroiliac strain. Mobilization of the joint, as might be expected, leads to further over-stretching and increased pain; indeed, the stresses put upon the joint merely by clinical examination temporarily aggravate the symptoms. Exercises are also harmful.

The joint requires protection. In fact, the wearing of a suitable belt for a month or two usually abolishes the symptoms, often permanently. The most suitable is the 'corrugator' (Fig. 100). This is very similar to Hilton's sacroiliac belt (1857) for preventing 'eccentric tension'. Should this fail, sclerosing injections into the posterior sacroiliac ligaments are indicated.

### Sclerosing Injections

Many are now returning to the concept of sacroiliac strain, influenced by osteopathic ideas. Before the role of the disc in lumbogluteal pain was put forward (Cyriax 1945), most backache was attributed to sacroiliac strain. This notion is now being revived in a slightly different form, and the argument runs something like this: there has been recurrent lumbar pain and the radiograph shows marked narrowing and osteophytosis at, say, the fifth lumbar level. Diminished movement at this joint must throw excessive strain on adjacent joints, i.e. the fourth lumbar joint and the sacroiliac ligaments. Hence, sacroiliac strain follows and complicates what was originally a fifth lumbar disc lesion or (as the osteopaths prefer it) a facet joint lesion.

This is not an unreasonable hypothesis, but there is considerable evidence against it. In the first place, if limited movement caused by erosion of disc substance causes sacroiliac strain, then all patients with a fifth lumbar joint fixed by sacralization would suffer much more and much earlier in life. Moreover, examination shows that (*a*) one or more lumbar movements hurt, (*b*) testing the sacroiliac joint does not hurt, and (*c*) epidural local anaesthesia (which does not deprive the sacroiliac joints of sensibility) abolishes the pain for the time being.

For these reasons, such gluteal pain ought to be regarded as referred from the lumbar spine, and if sclerosing injections are to be given, they should be used to infiltrate the lumbar ligaments not the sacroiliac. If the sacroiliac joint were to lose mobility, additional strain would be transmitted to the affected lumbar joint. Sacroiliac mobility spares the lumbar joints and must be advantageous to them, the more so if a lumbar lesion already exists.

CHAPTER 23

# THE BUTTOCK AND HIP

Most pain in the buttock has a lumbar origin. Lesions in the buttock itself, although uncommon, are often serious, some requiring urgent treatment. Their immediate clinical recognition is therefore important.

All ideas of 'gluteal fibrositis' must be discarded. Just as pressure on the dura mater in the neck sets up pain accompanied by characteristic tenderness in the upper thorax, so does the same phenomenon occur in the buttock, where pain and tenderness often result from pressure of a disc lesion on the dura mater. The lumbar spine, sacroiliac joints, buttock and hip all require examination to reach a diagnosis. If trunk extension elicits the gluteal ache, it cannot have a muscular origin. This movement relaxes the sacrospinalis and gluteal muscles, but extends the lumbar and hip joints, and puts a rotation strain on the sacroiliac joint. Gluteal pain evoked by trunk extension must, therefore, have an articular origin. It is only when gluteal pain is evoked on resisted extension of the hip that a lesion of a muscle in the buttock—a great rarity—need be considered at all.

Symmetrical collections of fat may form in the superficial tissue of the buttocks and on the outer aspect of each thigh in middle-aged women. Clinical examination shows that they do not interfere with muscle function, but their presence has misled those who rely chiefly on palpation for diagnosis, into creating a disease called 'panniculitis'. It is a myth.

## SEGMENTATION OF THE BUTTOCK

Many dermatomes meet at the buttock. The skin of the whole outer buttock is derived from the first lumbar segment, but at the inner upper quadrant the second and third dermatomes overlap the first. These two areas are separate from the second and third dermatomes along the front of the thigh. The first and second sacral segments start at mid-buttock and continue down the back of the thigh.

The muscles of the buttock are all of fourth and fifth lumbar and first sacral provenance. The gluteus medius is weak in a fifth lumbar root palsy, whereas wasted glutei accompany only a sacral root palsy. Hence, this appears to be the way the myotomes are composed.

In theory, pain in the buttock can result from any lesion situated in a tissue derived from the first, second or third lumbar or upper two sacral segments. In fact, fourth and fifth lumbar disc protrusions provide the commonest cause of pain in the buttock, in spite of the absence there of the relevant dermatomes. Pain of second lumbar origin spreads from the buttock down the front of the thigh to the patella. Symptoms of third lumbar provenance again can spread from the buttock to the front of the thigh and down the leg to just above the ankle anteriorly. Such a distribution is common to a third lumbar disc lesion and arthritis at the hip. Pain radiating from the buttock to the outer thigh indicates a lesion in a tissue derived from the fourth or fifth lumbar segment, usually a disc protrusion but sometimes gluteal bursitis. If it is projected along the back of the thigh, the first and second sacral segments are identified; pressure on these two nerve roots is usually responsible, but sacroiliac arthritis is a possibility.

## MAJOR LESIONS IN THE BUTTOCK

These possess in common an arresting pattern of physical signs that draws immediate attention to the buttock. Passive hip flexion with the knee held extended (i.e. straight-leg raising) is slightly limited and painful. Passive hip flexion, this time with the knee flexed too, is again limited and more painful. Further examination reveals a non-capsular pattern of limitation of movement at the hip joint. The deductions to be drawn are as follows. Straight-leg raising is painful; the lesion is, therefore, connected with the tissues lying behind the hip joint. Hip flexion with the knee bent is also limited; hence, neither the sciatic nerve and its roots, nor the hamstring muscles, are at fault. Were the hip joint itself affected, straight-leg raising should not be painful (except in such gross arthritis that less than 90° flexion range had resulted). The only structure left is the buttock. Thus, when passing from testing straight-leg raising to testing the passive movements at the hip joint, the *sign of the buttock* emerges at once.

There is nothing characteristic about the pain. It is felt in the buttock and spreads down the back of the thigh to the knee or calf; naturally, a disc lesion is suspected. Trunk flexion is limited, since the patient has pain when tension falls on the tissues of the buttock; the other lumbar movements are of full range. It is only when the patient is examined supine on the couch that the typical combination of signs emerges. This naturally leads to careful examination of the passive and resisted hip-movements. A non-capsular pattern emerges on passive testing, medial rotation nearly always proving of full range. Moreover, the characteristic feel of a hip joint at its extreme of range is replaced by the patient's asking the examiner, because of increasing pain, not to force a movement which the latter can clearly feel not yet to have reached its full amplitude. The resisted movements often hurt, since they too alter tensions in the buttock. Inspection as the patient lies prone may reveal that the affected buttock is larger than its fellow and palpation may disclose a tumour.

The patient's temperature is noted; a rectal examination is performed and a radiograph secured without delay.

## The Sign of the Buttock

When the sign of the buttock emerges on examination, the various possibilities are:

### Osteomyelitis of the Upper Femur

The symptoms and signs are very marked and the sign of the buttock obtrudes. Straight-leg raising and hip flexion are both considerably limited and cause intense pain. Rotation at the hip is restricted by pain with the characteristic empty end-feel.

Fulminating infection with high fever is correctly attributed at once; it is only cases with a gradual onset that are mistaken for a disc lesion and reach the orthopaedic physician. Sciatic pain is indeed present, but the patient walks in, often supported by a relative, with a far worse limp than is ever seen in a disc lesion; it resembles that of the iliac metastases or advanced arthritis at the hip. Sooner or later fever appears and the upper part of the shaft of the femur becomes very tender. The radiograph is negative at this stage. Antibiotics are given at once, and the patient transferred to surgical care.

### Chronic Septic Sacroiliac Arthritis

The symptoms and signs are very like those of osteomyelitis of the upper femur. In addition to 'the sign of the buttock', testing the sacroiliac joint is most painful. The femur is not tender. It is only some months later, when local new bone formation begins to show that the exact position of the abscess becomes clear. Rest and antibiotic therapy are indicated at once.

### Ischiorectal Abscess

Occasionally, an ischiorectal abscess points towards the buttock instead of pointing towards the rectum. The patient limps badly, preferring not to put his foot to the ground at all. The hip is fixed in considerable flexion; further flexion is limited; so is straight-leg raising. Fever is present and rectal examination reveals the cause.

### Septic Bursitis

Septic bursitis gives rise to the characteristic 'sign of the buttock'. When the patient is first seen his pain at rest may not be severe and he may not yet feel ill; but either he hobbles in with a gait suggesting an arthritic hip, or he lies in bed unable to put that leg to the ground or rest that buttock on the mattress. Such major disablement contrasts with the minor degree of discomfort; much greater pain would have been required to secure such disablement had a disc lesion, for example, been present. The temperature is between 37.2° and 37.8°C; the next day it is a little higher. Rectal examination and the radiograph reveal no abnormality. Palpation may reveal a vague area of tenderness just behind and above the greater trochanter. Rarely, a swelling is encountered lying posterolaterally at the upper end of the femoral shaft, level with the lesser trochanter. Rest in bed and antibiotics are required. Recurrence some years later is not uncommon.

Very occasionally the swelling results from acute, often haemorrhagic, bursitis due to a fall on the outer side of the hip. Pain is slight; the patient walks well. Aspiration suffices.

### Rheumatic Fever with Bursitis

In adults, recrudescence of rheumatic fever may lead to pain in the buttock and thigh; examination shows the characteristic 'sign of the buttock'. Fever is present and the patient dyspnoeic at rest. Admission to hospital for the cardiac condition is called for in any case, and the lesion in the buttock, presumably a rheumatic bursitis, clears up in the course of three or four weeks as the result of the rest in bed.

### Neoplasm at Upper Femur

Metastases at upper femur give rise to a very similar picture, but without fever. If, as is common, the erosion of bone lies close to the lesser trochanter, resisted flexion of the hip is very weak and also painful. The patient cannot bear weight on the affected limb and often attends in a wheelchair.

### Iliac Neoplasm

Primary and secondary neoplasm occur at the ilium deep to the gluteal muscles. The patient can scarcely hobble with assistance. The 'sign of the buttock' is present. Marked wasting of the quadriceps and hamstring muscles contrasts with an almost full range of movement at the hip joint. If movement is limited, the capsular pattern and the capsular feel are both absent and the intensity of the pain quite out of keeping with the minor limitation of movement. The radiograph is diagnostic.

### Fractured Sacrum

The history is of a fall on the buttocks. Sacral pain results which the patient ascribes to local bruising; he often continues to get about. The symptoms continue, tending at first to become worse. During the first week or so, when the lower limbs are examined, the 'sign of the buttock' is found on both sides. The sacrum is swollen and tender superficially (which might be due to soft tissue bruising) but equally tender when the anterior aspect of the bone is palpated per rectum. A sacral haematoma often forms.

The radiograph confirms the diagnosis. Although the patient will be more comfortable in bed, bony union without deformity takes place whether he rests or not. It is thus reasonable to leave it to the patient to make his own choice. Subsidence of symptoms takes about two months. A haematoma may be aspirated.

## MINOR LESIONS ABOUT THE HIP

These do not give rise to the 'sign of the buttock', straight-leg raising being of full range and very seldom even uncomfortable.

A minor lesion at the hip is suggested when a patient complains of pain in the buttock and testing the lumbar and sacroiliac joints draws a blank. If so, the main symptom should be pain brought on or increased by walking. The passive movements reveal a full range of movement at the hip, but some are found to hurt, others not, in a non-capsular manner, e.g. full lateral rotation hurts, full medial does not: the reverse of the situation in arthritis. This finding strongly suggests bursitis. Very early arthritis is usually symptomless, but, if it does set up pain at the extreme of range, the capsular pattern is retained. The end-feel in arthritis is hard, in bursitis soft; hence, the sensation imparted to the hand is most helpful in diagnosis.

Unfortunately, the significance of the passive hip movements is often ambiguous: for full flexion may squeeze the psoas bursa painfully, as well as stretch the hip joint and the structures lying behind it. Again full passive abduction may squeeze tissues lying between the greater trochanter and the blade of the ilium.

If then, the pattern for bursitis emerges, the main diagnostic aid is the position of the pain and its area of reference. If these are felt at the front of the thigh, the psoas bursa is incriminated; if posterolaterally, one of the gluteal bursae.

To make matters yet more complicated, one or two resisted movements usually hurt in bursitis. In the buttock, pain on a resisted movement should not be taken as suggesting a muscle lesion; it indicates instead tenderness of a bursa, painfully squeezed when an adjacent muscle contracts. The buttock is the only area in the body where this situation obtains, and in fact muscle lesions in the buttock are almost unknown. Indeed, the only resisted movements which imply trouble in the muscle itself are: (*a*) flexion, in psoas muscle strain, and (*b*) lateral rotation, when the tendon of the quadratus femoris is affected. In neither of these lesions do any of the passive hip movements hurt.

Since the passive movements often have an equivocal significance, and the common cause of pain on a resisted movement is not a muscle lesion but compression of a nearby tender bursa, diagnosis at the buttock is extremely difficult. It is the most awkward area in the whole body. The situation is aggravated by the fact that the tissues apt to become painful all lie so deeply that palpation for tenderness is futile.

## Psoas Bursitis

The psoas bursa is developed from the second and third lumbar segments. The pain is therefore felt in the groin or within the upper thigh anteriorly, and is referred along the front of the thigh to the patellar area.

The passive hip movements reproduce the pain, and adduction in flexion, by squeezing the bursa, is usually the most painful movement. Passive lateral rotation usually hurts; medial does not, and the capsular end-feel is absent. The resisted hip movements do not hurt, nor does resisted extension of the knee as the patient lies prone, thus showing that the tendon of the rectus femoris muscle is not strained. In psoas bursitis, resisted flexion of the hip does not hurt; this hurts in a lesion of the psoas muscle, of the tendon of the rectus femoris and in obturator hernia.

The main diagnostic difficulty lies between psoas bursitis and a loose body in the hip joint without osteoarthrosis. In the latter case, intermittent pain and sudden twinges are a prominent feature.

The diagnosis is always uncertain, and is not established until local anaesthesia has been induced at the front of the hip joint and found to abolish the signs for the time being. It is often curative as well. If not, triamcinolone is injected in the spot identified by the local anaesthesia.

It should be remembered that painful weakness of the psoas muscle is present in malignant invasion of the belly itself retroperitoneally, and in metastases at the upper femur. In the latter case, marked restriction of range at the hip joint is also found, with an empty end-feel. Since methysergide has been found so successful in preventing severe migraine, pain in the back, groins and anterior thighs has resulted from the retroperitoneal fibrosis that may ensue. This starts after one to four years and the main effect is ureteric obstruction causing hydronephrosis. This possibility should be remembered in obscure pain in the groins unaltered by any hip movement. The pyelogram shows the ureters displaced medially.

Weakness and pain when the psoas muscles are tested are a common complaint in psychoneurosis, in combination then with all sorts of other inconsistencies.

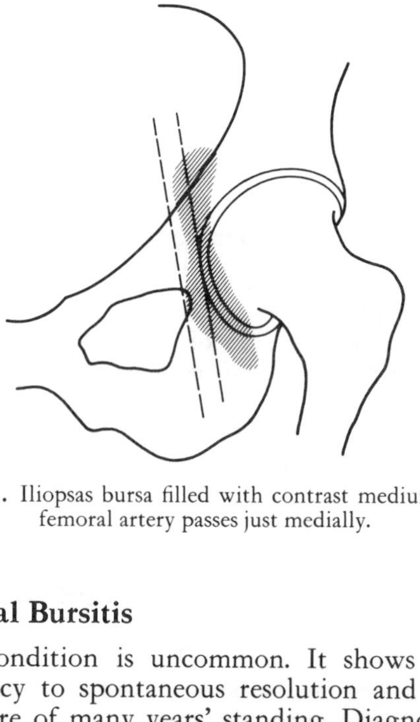

**Fig. 101.** Iliopsas bursa filled with contrast medium. The femoral artery passes just medially.

## Gluteal Bursitis

The condition is uncommon. It shows little tendency to spontaneous resolution and most cases are of many years' standing. Diagnosis is complicated. The pain is felt at the lateral or posterior trochanteric area and is referred to the outer thigh and, sometimes, outer leg. Some of the passive hip movements hurt at full range in a non-capsular way, and the arthritic end-feel is absent. The twinges typical of a loose body in the hip are not mentioned. This combination of signs suggests gluteal bursitis.

Further localization now depends on finding which accessory movements affect the pain. For example, full passive abduction squeezes a tender structure lying between the greater trochanter and the blade of the ilium. A tender bursa is often painfully squeezed when an adjacent muscle contracts. Indeed, the cause of pain on a resisted hip movement is not a lesion of the muscle itself but compression of a nearby bursa. Hence, it is the responses to the resisted movements that help to indicate in relation to which muscle the affected bursa lies; for palpation affords little assistance.

Diagnosis and treatment are pursued together. The likeliest spot is chosen, usually above the trochanter, and infiltrated with 50 ml of 0.5% procaine solution. After some minutes, whichever movements had been found painful are tested again. If relief is not secured, a further diagnostic injection is given at each attendance until the right area is finally reached. If, as is usual, one or two correctly placed injections of procaine prove curative, this is all that need be done, although the patient may need several injections before the necessary accuracy in siting the fluid has been achieved. If the immediate result of the injection shows that it has been correctly placed, but no lasting benefit is reported at the patient's next attendance, 5 ml of triamcinolone suspension must be injected into the area already identified by the local anaesthesia.

Intractable cases are rare, and operative exploration of the buttock seldom reveals anything definite or effects a cure. Hence, if conservative treatment fails, it is usually best, since the symptoms are never severe, to admit defeat.

## Ischial Bursitis

Weaver's bottom is uncommon nowadays. Indeed, gluteal pain coming on after sitting for some time, especially in a soft chair, and easing soon after the patient is upright again, is much more often due to a nuclear self-reducing protrusion at a low lumbar level. However, in bursitis the pain comes on as soon as the ischium touches the chair, especially if this is hard, and ceases the moment the patient stands up.

Ischial bursitis is brought to mind when the history indicates that a tender tissue lies between the ischium and the chair, and testing the lumbar and sacroiliac joints, the hip joint and the tissues about it is completely negative. The only finding is tenderness at, or just above, the ischial tuberosity. Local anaesthesia is induced here and the patient asked to sit once more. If there is now no discomfort, the diagnosis is confirmed, but it is not usual for the injection to give continuing benefit. At his next attendance, the tender spot is infiltrated with 5 ml of triamcinolone suspension. Should this fail, excision is indicated.

## Haemorrhagic Psoas Bursitis

This is an interesting rarity. The patient states that he jarred his thigh, slipping. Within a minute, the front of the upper thigh became painful and he found he could not flex the hip joint. Examination shows 90° limitation of passive flexion at the hip joint, all the other movements being of full range. There is no pain or weakness on any resisted movement. It is clear that a space-occupying lesion has suddenly appeared at the front of the hip joint, i.e. the psoas bursa is tensely filled with blood. These patients may be suspected of malingering; for under anaesthesia, a full range of flexion may well be obtained, the limitation returning as soon as the patient recovers.

Aspiration confirms the diagnosis and cures the patient; failing that, spontaneous cure takes three or four months.

## Claudication in the Buttock

This is a rare condition, the original description of which was given in the 1954 edition of this book. Unless the suggestion contained in the history is noted, the disorder may be most puzzling; for the pain is felt at mid-buttock just where symptoms due to a low lumbar disc lesion are so often experienced.

The patient states that after walking for 50 or 100 yards he gets such pain in his buttock that he has to stop. Occasionally, he complains that the limb goes numb rather than hurts, thus suggesting some neurological disorder. He stands still and the pain (or numbness) goes. After a minute or two, he walks on and can cover the same distance before the symptom comes on again.

Examination is essentially negative. The movements of the lumbar spine, the hip joint, and testing the buttock and thigh muscles against resistance— none of them hurts. Pulsation in the arterial tree of the limb is adequate, unless the block has occurred in the common iliac as opposed to the internal iliac artery. Then the diagnosis is less likely to be missed, since all the arteries of the limb are pulseless and, in lesions of the external iliac artery, after walking the leg and foot go objectively cold. If an epidural injection is given it does not affect the symptom.

When this condition is suspected, the patient should be asked to lie prone. His hip on the affected side is passively extended; this proves painless. He should then be told fully to extend his hip, and actively to keep his lower limb off the couch for several minutes. The result of this sustained gluteal contraction is the recognized pain in the buttock. When maintenance of active extension at the hip joint hurts, but passive extension does not, the cause must be muscular ischaemia. Bonney (1956) confirmed these views and described 10 cases of gluteal claudication, in some of which prolonged fruitless treatment had been directed to the lumbar spine.

This diagnosis can sometimes be confirmed by radiography, which may show a dense unilateral calcification of the internal iliac artery.

No treatment is effective except operative recanalization of the artery. Percutaneous transluminal angioplasty (Dacie 1981) involves placing a balloon catheter at the arterial stenosis and stretching the atheromatous plaque until it splits. Fresh intima forms healing the gap.

### Tuberculous Abscess

A cold abscess may form in the buttock in tuberculosis of the fifth lumbar vertebra or the sacroiliac joint. A painless fluctuant swelling forms, which should be aspirated and the fluid examined for tuberculosis. When the lumbar vertebra is affected, marked limitation of range is present on lumbar movements, together with a small kyphos. When the sacroiliac joint is at fault, testing the joint causes no pain; for fibrosis takes place as fast as does erosion. Nor does the abscess cause limitation of, or pain on, hip movements, passive or resisted.

## PSYCHOGENIC PAIN

It so happens that 90° limitation of flexion at the hip joints is a common finding in psychoneurotic patients complaining of pain in the lower back or thigh. If such a finding is combined with the discovery of a full range of rotation at the joint, one gross inconsistency has been detected. Another sign may be fixation of the hip in medial rotation; in arthritis fixation in lateral rotation is invariable. However in view of the matter set out in the first paragraph (bursitis) above, minor unusual signs at the hip joint should be ascribed to psychological causes only with caution. Most patients oblige by offering a multiplicity of signs indicating, as it were, that the lumbar region, the sacroiliac and knee joints and the muscles in the thigh are affected as well. It is important to test all muscles and joints in detail, and to perform a number of movements twice, e.g. first standing and then lying down; or first lying supine, then lying prone, to see if the responses tally.

## THE HIP JOINT

### Referred Pain

The hip joint is formed largely from the third lumbar segment. Hence, pain is referred from the groin, down the front of the thigh to the knee, and thence down the front of the leg to just above the ankle (see Figs 18 and 20). Since the upper inner quadrant of the buttock represents part of the third lumbar dermatome, arthrosis at the hip often also hurts here; rarely, the only pain is there and the patient very deceptively complains only of unilateral backache. At times the crural component is absent, the patient complaining solely of an anterior pain at the knee, spreading perhaps along the front of the tibia. Rarely, the hip joint is developed chiefly within the fourth lumbar segment; if so, the pain spreads along the fourth dermatome to the outer side of the mid-thigh and of the leg. In such cases, the fourth lumbar pain of sciatica is reproduced.

Pain felt only at the front of the thigh occupies the area of the second and third dermatomes; hence, its source should be sought at these levels of the lumbar spine, at the hip joint, at the anterior and inner muscles of the thigh, and at the knee. If the pain spreads down the front of the tibia as well, only the structures forming part of the third lumbar segment need be considered.

### Examination

Since most pains in the buttock stem from the lumbar spine, and pain in the thigh is as often referred thither as of local origin, the lumbar spine and sacroiliac joints must be examined before the hip. Moreover, it is when the patient stands for the lumbar examination that the best moment arises for noting any fixation of the thigh in adduction and flexion. Now too, it is appropriate to inquire whether raising the heel on the affected side alters the pain.

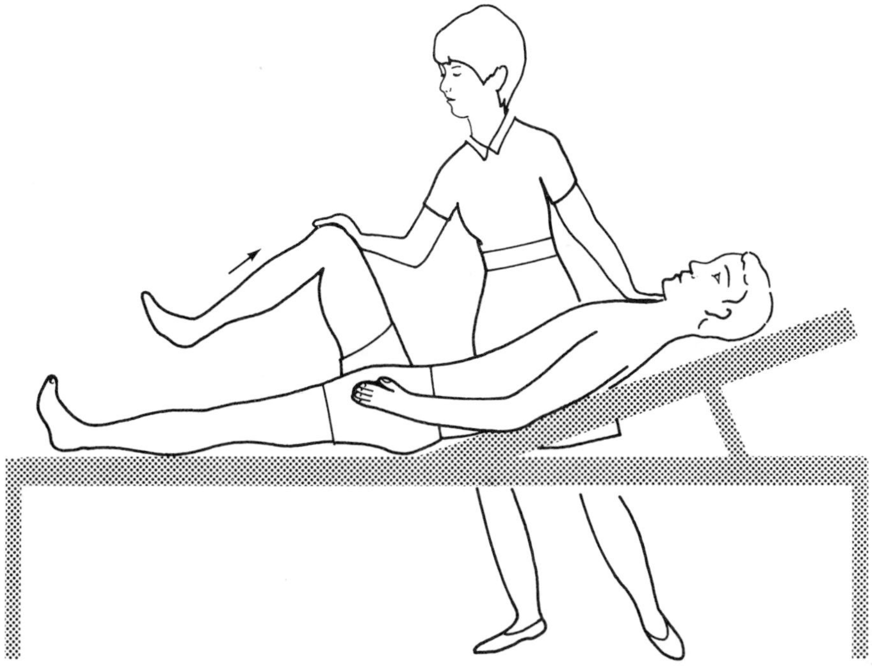

**Fig. 102.** Resisted flexion at hip. The thigh is lifted to the vertical and the examiner resists, her hand on his knee, while the knee is pressed towards the head. In this position, the upper quadriceps is thrown out of action and the psoas tested alone.

Bending backwards while standing extends both the lumbar spine and the hip joint. Hence pain in the thigh brought on by this movement cannot be ascribed to a lumbar structure unless full extension of the hip is later shown to be painless as the patient lies prone. Care must then be taken to press on the buttock with one hand when the other extends the thigh, so as to exclude the lumbar spine from the test.

Examination of the hip joint begins by noting the range, painfulness or not and end-feel of flexion, lateral rotation and medial rotation while the patient lies supine, and extension (and medial rotation again) while the patient lies prone. If, as in bursitis, it is important to know whether full passive abduction is painful or not, an assistant abducts the other leg first. Passive adduction is tested after raising up the good leg so as to get it out of the way.

The resisted movements follow. Supine: flexion, extension, adduction and abduction at the hip; prone: both rotations (with the knee flexed to a right angle); flexion and extension at the knee. In fact, muscle lesions at the upper thigh are far outnumbered in the middle-aged by lesions of the hip joint; in children, this tendency is even more pronounced and nearly all the pain felt to spread down from the front of the thigh towards the knee originates from the hip joint itself. It is chiefly young adults who during sport or athletics sprain a muscle in the thigh.

The end-feel is a great help in diagnosis at the hip, particularly when bursitis or a loose body in a normal hip joint is a possibility. The extreme of passive flexion and both rotations has a very hard feel in arthrosis, quite different from the soft end-feel of bursitis or an impacted loose body in a joint not yet arthrotic. In these two disorders, the capsular pattern is absent, lateral rotation usually hurting, medial rotation not, so that two clear findings—non-capsular pattern, soft end-feel—combine to inform the examiner that, although pain is elicited at the extremes of range, arthrosis is absent. A soft end-feel replaces a hard one when swift erosion of the femoral head occurs in osteoarthrosis.

The range of movement at most individuals' hip joint is: flexion until the thigh touches the trunk (although the last 45° of this apparent hip movement take place by the pelvis flexing at the lumbar joints); extension 15 to 30° beyond the anatomical position; 60° of medial rotation, 90° of lateral rotation, 45° of abduction and 30° of adduction. The typical pattern of capsular limitation of movement in gross arthritis is as follows: (*a*) fixed in slight adduction (i.e. 50 to 55° limitation of abduction); (*b*) no range of medial rotation; (*c*) 90° limitation of flexion; (*d*)

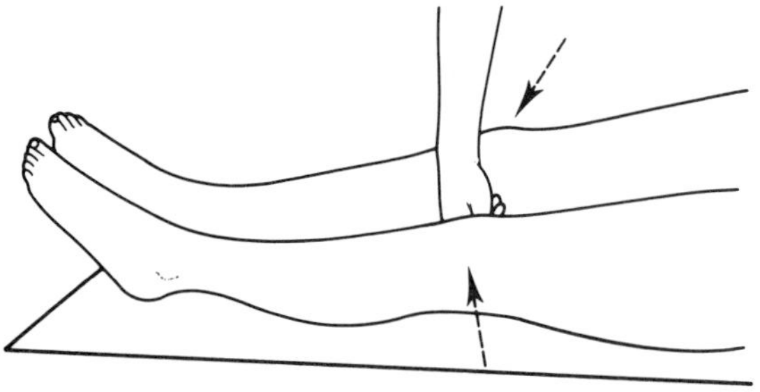

**Fig. 103.** Resisted adduction at the hips. The patient squeezes the examiner's hand between his knees.

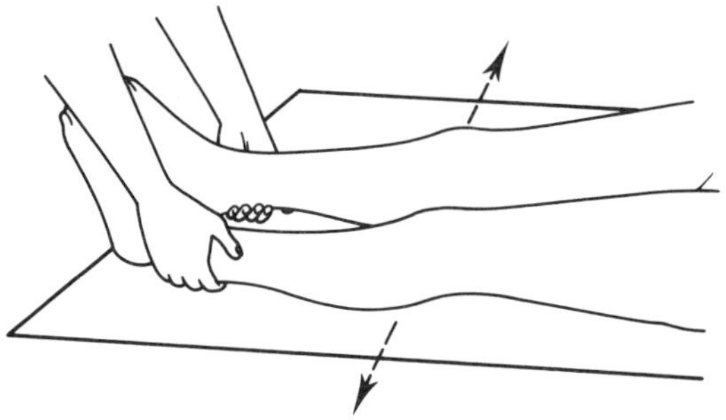

**Fig. 104.** Resisted abduction at the hips. The examiner faces the patient and resists the abduction movement by holding the ankles together.

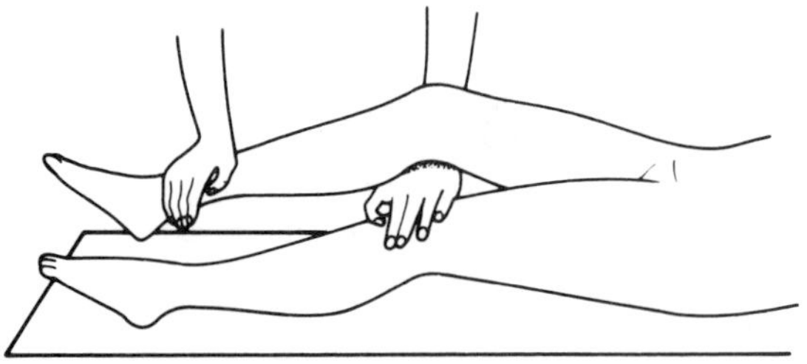

**Fig. 105.** Resisted extension at the hip. The examiner resists the downward pressure at the patient's ankle.

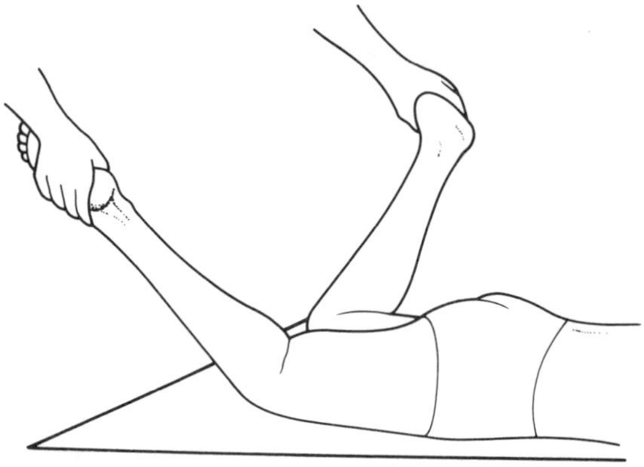

**Fig. 106.** Passive medial rotation at the hips. The patient lies face downwards, his knees together. The examiner rotates the thighs by pressing the feet apart. The buttocks must be kept level. A small amount of limitation of medial rotation can now be ascertained. Detection is often important, for this is the first movement to become restricted at the onset of arthritis.

10 to 30° limitation of extension; (*e*) full lateral rotation. In very early arthrosis, medial rotation is the first movement to become measurably restricted; slight limitation of flexion soon follows. In arthrosis, medial rotation is the most painful passive movement.

## Lesions of the Hip Joint in Children

These are nearly all serious and differential diagnosis rests largely on the radiographic appearances. Hence any child found limping or complaining of even a slight ache in the thigh or knee, who shows the slightest limitation of movement at the hip joint, should be put to bed immediately and not allowed up until the result of the X-ray examination is known. This is vital; otherwise, for example, a slipping epiphysis may slip completely and life-long deformity result.

### Pseudocoxalgia (Perthes' Disease)

This may be unilateral or bilateral and affects boys aged 4 to 12. It is a manifestation of osteochondrosis—a disorder of ischaemic aetiology. It is at this age as Trueta discovered (1957), that the blood supply of the femoral head is at its most vulnerable. He showed that, from birth to 8 years old, no blood reaches the epiphysis along the ligamentum teres. It is only then that vessels grow in through it and restore an adequate circulation (Hyrth 1846). Trueta found that the arteries to the metaphysis diminished after birth and had largely disappeared at the age of 4, leaving the lateral epiphyseal vessels the only source of blood to the femoral head.

The symptoms are trivial, perhaps an ache in the knee, but the parents have noticed a limp. Examination reveals marked limitation of movement at the hip joint. The radiograph shows flattening of the upper surface of the femoral head and a widening of the epiphyseal line. As a result, the femoral head no longer fits the acetabulum, and although prolonged recumbency leads to resolution of the arthrosis and a good range of movement for the time being, osteoarthrosis is very apt to supervene during the patient's late twenties or early thirties. Catterall (1971) has studied prognosis. He states that, if the epiphysis is only partly affected, the prognosis is good at all ages. Greater involvement carries a good prognosis only if the child is under 4 years old. Prolonged fixation in abduction and medial rotation improves the end-result, but in the severe case the outlook is bad, treatment or no treatment. Osteoarthrosis is apt to supervene during the patient's twenties owing to incongruence between the acetabulum and the head of the femur. Catterall's latest paper (1977) sets out clear radiographic criteria of what to expect, what to do and what not to do.

## Tuberculosis of the Hip

This may be difficult to distinguish from pseudocoxalgia. Clinically, the hip is found fixed in flexion, adduction and lateral rotation; muscle wasting is considerable. The patient is seldom over 10 years of age. Generalized rarefaction and a diminished joint space seen on the radiograph suggest this infection.

## Slipped Epiphysis

Since this may be bilateral, but more advanced on one side, the X-ray photograph should include the whole pelvis. For unknown reasons, the epiphyseal junction softens, whereupon weight-bearing results in a gradual downward slipping of the head on the neck of the femur. The disorder arises between the ages of 12 and 17, and examination merely reveals the capsular pattern at the hip joint with pain on passive movement, but not against resistance. The radiograph reveals the situation.

## Transitory Arthritis

This occurs in children under 10 years old and is probably the result of over-use. After a few weeks in bed the child recovers and Monty (1962) found that follow-up an average of five years later showed neither clinical nor radiological sequelae. However, other observers have found transient arthritis to carry a 10% chance of the development of Perthes' disease later. Hence, if the radiograph shows the periarticular tissues to be swollen (Mayall 1965) aspiration is the logical measure. This prevents the circulation at the epiphysis from being cut off and thus saves bone from the avascular necrosis that initiates Perthes' disease. Kemp (1973) found that, if swelling of the soft tissues at the acetabular notch displaced the femoral head laterally by 2 mm, the condition resolved spontaneously in four to six months, but if radiography showed it to be 4 mm or more, irreversible change had supervened. These cases should therefore be splinted in abduction, so as to keep the affected part continuously under cover of the curved acetabulum.

## Coxa Vara

This is usually bilateral and results from any disorder causing softening of bone. Rarely, the deformity is congenital. The range of abduction is markedly limited; the other movements may be of full range. The radiograph is diagnostic.

## Haemophilia

The hip is a very uncommon site for intra-articular bleeding, but after several episodes thinning of cartilage with juxta-articular cysts form, and by his teens the boy may have developed permanent limitation of movement at the joint.

## Congenital Dislocation

In Great Britain, the incidence is 12 per 10 000 girls and two per 10 000 boys, and it is 10 times commoner in breech presentation. It is bilateral in 10 to 25% of cases and there is then no shortening of one leg or asymmetry of the folds in the thigh to draw attention to the dislocation. There is about 5% chance of a second child being affected. Since early treatment (i.e. begun well before the child begins to walk) is so successful and avoids the later supervention of osteoarthrosis, it is important to make the diagnosis as soon after birth as possible. To this end the baby is examined as follows (Ortolani 1937). The baby lies on her back with the knees flexed and the thighs at right angles to the trunk. The examiner's thumbs are placed at the inner aspect of her knees; his fingers along the outer thigh. The knees are now pushed apart, and on the dislocated side resistance to abduction is felt at 45°. If this resistance is overcome by continued pressure towards abduction and lateral rotation, a sudden thud is felt as the head of the femur rides over the edge of the acetabulum and comes to lie in its socket. Full abduction is now free. If the thighs are now brought back to adduction again, during slight posteriorly directed pressure on the upper part of the femur, the hip redislocates.

Barlow (1962) tests the baby's hip by grasping the uppermost femur between fingers and thumb. Pressure directed anteriorly then posteriorly can then be felt to move the head of the femur in and out of the acetabulum if the joint is unstable.

These tests afford the diagnosis before the X-ray picture reveals the displacement. In due course, the epiphysis is shown radiologically to lie above the acetabulum and to be about half the size of the one on the normal side.

### Trapped Ligamentum Teres

Hamberg (1973) described cases to me, always in children aged 8 to 12, in which sudden pain in the groin was provoked by a twist of the limb. The child would fall to the ground and find himself unable to get up again because of severe pain on weight-bearing. Examination of the hip while the child was lying revealed no abnormality, but the child could not stand up. In one instance, the first diagnosis was appendicitis. A smart pull and jerk to the limb would elicit a click whereupon walking became painless at once. Goodley (1973) described such a case in a girl of 9, bedridden for five months. Cineradiography disclosed that manual traction on the femur on the normal side showed the head of the femur to shift not straight downwards but outwards, then downwards on the painful side. This suggested a swollen tissue at the acetabular fossa, i.e. contusion with trapping of the ligamentum teres. This girl too was put right by manipulation during traction.

I have not met with a case myself.

## Arthritis in Adults

The capsular pattern is present; the resisted movements do not hurt. The following conditions occur:

### Osteoarthrosis

This is revealed by osteophyte formation and a diminished joint space, especially superiorly, visible on the radiograph. If it comes on before the age of 40, it is usually the result of a severe sprain, fracture or previous disease of the hip, usually pseudocoxalgia. Limitation of movement is often quite considerable before appreciable symptoms begin.

The careful studies of Harrison et al. (1953) have shown that degeneration of cartilage at the femoral head is already present by the age of 14. It usually begins in the area of articular cartilage not subjected to pressure. Ossification of cartilage at points of instability then supervenes and increased vascularity is noted at these non-pressure areas. In due course, the whole head of the femur becomes riddled with new, dilated blood vessels. Cysts appear in the bone formed by fibrous masses with vascular walls. The head of the bone tends to flatten. It is their view that the trouble in osteoarthrosis is 'not the degeneration of the cartilage, but the vigorous and persistent attempts to repair: attempts which aggravate the already disordered function of the joint, not only by osteophyte formation but also by hypervascularity which weakens the structure of the bone beyond the point where it can carry its load'. In their view daily use is desirable; this preserves rather than erodes cartilage. The latest (1972) view of the Biomechanics Unit at Imperial College on the pathogenesis of osteoarthrosis is that the primary defect lies in the capacity to sustain a load. As the mucopolysaccharide content of cartilage dwindles, its mechanical strength becomes impaired. Now, the fatigue phenomenon may lead to excessive polysaccharide motility. Loss of tensile strength ensues. Cartilage begins to wear away. Localized areas of collapse then prevent even distribution of load throughout the surfaces in contact. Subchondral trabecular bone then suffers fatigue fractures; osteoarthrosis results.

There is a favourable and an unfavourable type of osteoarthrosis at the hip. The very slow progressive type is often bilateral and is characterized by the formation of a large collar of osteophytes all round the lateral edge of the femoral head, making it U-shaped instead of round (Plate XLIV/1). Cartilage between acetabulum and femoral head is reasonably well preserved. In more progressive osteoarthrosis, there is no joint space at the upper surface of the femoral head, and the adjacent part of the acetabulum; sclerosis of bone is seen there. The erosion is confined to the weight-bearing aspect and osteophyte formation is inconspicuous. This is the type that may well come to operation.

It is remarkable how little index to the severity of the symptoms is afforded by the radiographic appearances. Erosion of cartilage and osteophyte formation of equal degrees may be accompanied by a good deal of movement and little pain, a good deal of movement and much pain, little movement and little pain, and little movement and much pain. Outward subluxation of the head of the femur with localized erosion of cartilage superiorly is often accompanied by an almost full range of movement and much pain.

Limitation of extension at the hip leads to low backache. No longer being able to extend at the hip, the patient moves his whole pelvis instead, hyperextending the lower lumbar joints at every step. It is no use treating this backache with a corset, for the movement is essential to the patient's gait.

## Loose Body in the Hip Joint

There are three types, but it is a diagnosis which is seldom made since it is very exceptional for the loose body to contain an osseous nucleus which is X-ray opaque. The condition is not rare, merely unsuspected and, therefore, unrecognized.

The symptoms are clearly indicative of momentary subluxation of a loose body. The patient complains that, as he walks, he is suddenly halted by a severe twinge felt shooting down the front of the thigh from the groin to the knee. The leg tends to let him down at this moment. The twinge may be repeated at each step or at many weeks' intervals. The painful twinge that makes the leg momentarily give way under the patient is quite different from the painless weakness, again causing the leg to let him down, of the patient with a weak quadriceps, usually the result of a third lumbar disc lesion causing a root palsy.

*Osteochondrosis Dissecans.* I have met with only one case. Vague symptoms began at the age of 13, when slight articular signs led to X-ray examination which showed bilateral osteochondritis at the medial aspect of the femoral head by the epiphyseal line. By the time the patient was 20, he had for a year suffered from recurrent attacks of internal derangement at the right hip. They lasted up to two days and made walking impossible. During an attack, slight limitation of movement was present; between attacks, the joint was clinically normal.

The mechanism of this type of internal derangement was obscure to me until R. H. Young, who had operated on such a case, explained that it was a question of the loose fragment becoming tilted within its cave and suddenly forming a projection against the acetabulum.

Manipulation proved of little help, but a day or two in bed has so far brought about reduction.

*Loose Fragment without Osteoarthrosis.* This condition is rare. A small piece, presumably of exfoliated articular cartilage, becomes loose in the joint, presumably as the result of past trauma. It would seem to lie harmlessly inside the capsule about the neck of the femur for long periods at a time, but then to move and become nipped at the acetabular edge. When this happens, a severe twinge is felt with giving way of the limb. The patient has to stand on only the good leg for some moments; he then puts weight on his bad leg and finds it sound again. The twinge may be repeated a few steps later, or not again for some months. Those who suffer many twinges a day are severely disabled and, since at any moment they may become rooted to the spot, become understandably afraid of crossing the road.

Examination shows a full range of movement at the hip joint, with some discomfort on, as a rule, full flexion and full lateral rotation. This would correspond with psoas bursitis, but in this disorder there are never any twinges. It is thus the history that supplies the differential diagnosis.

*Loose Fragment with Osteoarthrosis.* A loose body may form secondarily to osteoarthrosis; alternatively, a loose body that keeps subluxating may set up osteoarthrosis later.

These are the commonest cases. Since the radiograph shows the osteoarthrosis and not the loose body, the condition is missed. This is an important error; for the loose body can often be shifted to a position within the joint whence it no longer subluxates. If so, the patient, instead of suffering repeated twinges which make walking very difficult, merely suffers some discomfort after a long walk. In such cases, manipulative reduction affords several years' great relief.

## Rheumatoid Arthritis

Monarticular rheumatoid arthritis at the hip is very uncommon. Considerable aching in the thigh on exertion with slight limitation of movement of the capsular pattern results. In the early case, X-ray shows no abnormality at the hip or the sacroiliac joint. Later on, the loss of joint space is not, as in osteoarthrosis, localized at the upper part of the joint, but generalized, often more marked at the medial part of the joint line. The acetabulum may begin to protrude, with simultaneous erosion of the femoral head.

## Spondylitic Arthritis

In ankylosing spondylitis after the spine has

stiffened, the arthritis often spreads to the hip joints. This progresses, by flares and subsidences, until the joints become almost or quite fixed in flexion. Although the radiograph of the hip joints reveals nothing at first, sacroiliac arthritis, later fusion, is clearly visible.

### Osteitis Deformans

If the hip joints are affected early in the disease, there may as yet be no palpable thickening of the femora or tibiae, nor increase in the size of the skull. In such cases, only the radiograph of the pelvis discloses the true state of affairs.

### Acetabular Protrusion

The signs are the same as in bilateral osteoarthrosis but all abduction is lost early, and, in contrast to other forms of non-specific arthrosis, adduction is also limited.

### Chondrocalcinosis

This is uncommon at the hip and only one case has come my way. Surprisingly, extension at the hip was 10° limited and reproduced the pain down the front of the thigh, but flexion and rotation were full and painless.

### Arthritis

Rare cases are encountered in middle-aged persons who experience aching in the upper thigh on exertion, associated with *slight* limitation of movement at the hip joint. It continues unchanged for months. The radiograph reveals nothing. Treatment by stretching out the capsule of the joint is quickly curative and there is no tendency to recurrence within five years. The nature of this type of arthritis is obscure.

### Other Lesions

Pain felt only on full passive rotation occurs in sacroiliac arthritis, tendinitis of the rectus femoris, gluteal and psoas bursitis, obturator hernia and invasion of the shaft of the femur or the pubic bone by neoplasm.

### Hysteria

The hip shares with the shoulder and intervertebral joints an enhanced liability to fixation for psychological reasons. The patient walks in with a marked limp, often leaning on a thick stick. Inspection of gait reveals the limb fixed in medial rotation instead of the lateral rotation of organic disease. Examination begins at the lumbar spine and goes on to the toes; it reveals multiple inconsistencies. The commonest are: inability to use the psoas muscle when it is tested with the patient supine; 90° limitation of passive hip flexion accompanied by a full range of passive rotations.

## Treatment

### Osteoarthrosis

Osteoarthrosis at the hip joint is very difficult to alleviate. Full relief from symptoms is seldom attained even temporarily. Cure, even prevention of further aggravation, is impossible.

In the early stage, capsular stretching by the physiotherapist under heat analgesia is indicated. The joint is heated by short-wave diathermy and movement gradually forced (see Volume II). A month's treatment twice a week is often followed by many months' ease. In particular, pain at night can often be abolished. In the end, however, stretching ceases to be effective. Triamcinolone or silicone injected into the joint then becomes the treatment of choice (see below).

Later, a raised heel (to compensate for the apparent shortening and to enable the patient to walk without trying to extend his hip so far) and a walking-stick are required.

If the pain is severe, and also disturbs sleep, operation is indicated, unless the patient is unwilling or too aged, in which case he must use a crutch. Arthroplasty is the operation of choice. When unilateral osteoarthrosis comes on in early middle age, arthrodesis should be considered, for the life of a prosthesis is about 10 years, and repeated operation is a disagreeable prospect. The time to operate is when pain compels the patient to ask for surgical interference.

A number of treatments have been tried; none are fully successful. They are:

*Intra-articular Triamcinolone.* There is often an element of overuse as the cause of pain in osteoarthrosis, or the patient may have tripped, straining the stiff joint. Triamcinolone can then be employed to abate such traumatic inflammation although it does not increase the range of movement.

The patient lies on his good side with the lower hip flexed. The painful hip is extended and the thigh allowed to adduct until the knee touches the couch. The edge of the trochanter is identified and a needle 12 cm long introduced just above it and pointing vertically downwards. The needle clears the upper surface of the trochanter and is aimed at the junction of the head and the neck of the femur. After the needle has traversed the muscles, the resistance offered by the thick capsule can be felt. The point then strikes bone; 5 ml of triamcinolone are injected. Further injections should be avoided for fear of inducing a steroid arthropathy, and silicone should be substituted.

Chandler and Wright (1958) reported a case of osteoarthrosis of the hip given a monthly injection of only 50 mg hydrocortisone on 18 occasions. As a result, the joint became painless but completely disorganized, the head of the femur disappearing with the development of 5 cm shortening. The authors liken the condition to a Charcot's arthropathy. So far, this has not occurred in any of my cases, but it is clear that repeated injections at short intervals may prove dangerous. Sweetnam et al. (1960) reported a case of cortisone arthropathy at the hip in a patient in whom the drug had been taken orally only. Views on the dangers of steroid therapy were challenged by Isdale (1962). He surveyed 600 patients who had their hips X-rayed, and found 27 with bone absorption. One of three with marked destruction and eight of twelve with moderate absorption had never had any steroid treatment. He concluded that little statistical evidence existed of harm from steroid therapy, and to discontinue it would be a mistake. Sutton et al. (1963) considered that steroid therapy enhanced the likelihood of arthropathy and described cases in which the joints became affected, though the disease being treated was non-articular, e.g. eczema.

Another cause of iatrogenic bone collapse has recently been pointed out by Murray and Jacobson (1971) who found that changes similar to those caused by steroid therapy could result from prolonged use of the phenylbutazone group of drugs. Plate XLVI shows swift erosion of the femoral head occurring in a patient taking no drugs at all. However, Bell (1824) had already published a drawing (Plate 3) showing complete erosion of the upper part of the femoral head more than a century before any such drugs existed.

*Intrathecal Alcohol.* Since the capsule of the hip joint is so largely developed from the third lumbar segment, it seemed probable that, if the posterior root of the third lumbar nerve were destroyed by an intrathecal injection of alcohol, the pain of osteoarthrosis of the hip might cease. Cases with clear third lumbar reference were chosen; J. D. Laycock kindly performed the injection. The patient lay on the unaffected side with a cushion so arranged at the loin that the third lumbar vertebra formed the top of a lumbar convexity. Alcohol (0.5 ml) was introduced at the third lumbar interspace. Numbness and tingling along the front of the thigh were noted by the patient. However, no improvement followed in six cases thus treated.

*Denervation.* The obturator nerve and the nerve to the quadratus femoris muscle carry most of the sensory fibres to the hip joint. These can be removed. This operation is more favoured on the continent of Europe than in England. The result is usually disappointing. Herfort and Nickerson (1959) reported excellent results continuing for up to four years in 15 patients with advanced arthritis of hip or knee in whom they carried out an extensive sympathetic denervation.

*Intra-articular Injection of Silicone.* After reading Helal and Karadi's (1968) paper on silicone as an intra-articular lubricant, I used their method with 200 centistoke oil, but the results were disappointing. In 1971, Wright et al. confirmed this lack of benefit in a controlled trial on osteoarthrosis of the knee, using 300 centistoke oil. While I was in New Zealand in 1970, Ongley showed me patients whom he had treated up to two years previously in this way. He had injected 25 ml of silicone oil of 10 000 centistoke viscosity into osteoarthrotic hips.

Ongley and Wright had carried out a series of animal experiments based on the fact that synovial fluid contains a highly polymerized mucin—hyaluronic acid—as the lubricant. They took the view that a viscous oil could be substituted for it, as long as it was inert, insoluble, non-toxic and would retain its viscosity in contact with human tissue. They found from experiments on animals that dimethyl polysiloxane fulfilled these criteria best, and I have followed his lead. The high-viscosity (12 000 centistoke) silicone oil is now manufactured in England and we had a pressure syringe made and arranged for a refill and sterilizing service with J. R. Fennell, 66 Old Pasture Road, Camberley, Surrey.

The preferred viscosity of Jointsil is 12 000 centistoke. Much lower viscosities had not afforded good results and a considerably higher viscosity would make injection difficult even with a mechanical syringe. As it is, it is quite hard work screwing the plunger onwards.

The filled syringe is delivered in a sealed plastic cover, in which it has been sterilized by gamma rays. With it 16 gauge Luer-lock sterile needles are supplied, 12 cm long for the hip joint.

Ongley advises 25 ml of oil intra-articularly. This seemed more than a hip joint could be expected to contain, so I injected 20 ml of the oil mixed with 5 ml of contrast medium into the hip joint of a cadaver (see Plate XLVII*a*) and none leaked out of the joint. A further 15 ml were then introduced and extravasation then resulted (see Plate XLVII*b*). The joint was then exposed and the distension could be seen and felt, but even then the tension on the capsule was not extreme.

This injection raised great hopes but later experience showed that, even when relief was obtained, it did not last beyond twelve months. I have therefore abandoned this measure for the hip, but still use it at knee and thumb.

*Operation.* McMurray's intertrochanteric osteotomy has the advantage of diminishing pain while maintaining a useful range of movement at the hip joint, and thus preventing the lumbar pain that so often complicates fixation of the hip in considerable flexion. It is indicated in the painful hip with good mobility. The period of rest in bed is seldom more than a month and weight-bearing is possible after three months. The altered angulation of the neck on the shaft of the femur presents a new area of uneroded cartilage to the acetabulum. Charnley's plastic acetabulum supporting a steel prosthesis inserted into the uppermost femur gives excellent results, and necessitates only a week or two in bed. It lasts about 10 years; then the plastic socket may wear out. The older the patient is, therefore, the better. This is probably the best and most widely practised of all contemporary operations on the hip.

### Loose Body in the Hip Joint

Manipulative reduction during traction should be attempted at once. It does not always succeed, but if the loose fragment of cartilage can be moved to a position within the joint whence it stops subluxating, great benefit results, and many patients have been afforded up to several years' relief. By cineradiography, Goodley (1973) showed that the head of the femur descended 1 cm after a few moments' manual traction in a girl of 9. On account of the defect at the acetabular fossa atmospheric pressure does not interfere with the distraction of the joint surfaces. If the symptoms return, the manipulation should be repeated (see Volume II).

Removal is possible only if the loose fragment contains an osseous nucleus and its position is visible.

### Other Disorders

In *monarticular rheumatoid arthritis,* triamcinolone injected into the joint is effective. Forcing movement is contraindicated. *Spondylitic arthritis* is also best treated during a flare by intra-articular injection of triamcinolone. When the arthritis is subsiding, gentle stretching out by the physiotherapist is indicated. Fixation is best treated by arthroplasty. The joint nearly always fixes again in the end. Nothing can be done for *osteitis deformans* except to prescribe butazolidine and sodium etidronate. *Acetabular protrusion* is treated on lines similar to osteoarthrosis, i.e. by stretching the joints out in the early stages and operation if necessary, later on. The pain originating from the posterior aspect of the capsule of the pseudarthrosis resulting from long-standing *congenital dislocation* can, surprisingly enough, often be permanently relieved by one or two local anaesthetic infiltrations.

*Mobilization of the Hip under Anaesthesia.* This is not to be undertaken lightly. Though relief lasting for some time may be obtained in younger patients with deformity due to a past pseudocoxalgia or protrusio acetabuli, in elderly patients with osteoarthrosis the neck of the femur may break. At best, only evanescent relief follows.

## MUSCLE LESIONS ABOUT THE HIP

These are all uncommon. It must be remembered that, when several resisted hip movements hurt, the likely cause is gluteal bursitis.

### Adductor Muscles

The patient is asked to lie supine and to squeeze the physician's closed fist between his knees. If resisted adduction hurts at the inner upper thigh, the upper extent of the adductor muscle is strained, most often at the musculotendinous junction, sometimes at the tenoperiosteal junction. Tenderness identifies the exact site of the lesion. This is known as *rider's sprain,* and is uncommon except in athletes. Massage is curative at either site; triamcinolone is effective at the tendon and local anaesthesia helps, especially in recent cases, at the upper belly.

Pain on resisted adduction is also elicited in fracture or neoplastic invasion of the os pubis. Fracture may follow a fall, or may be a stress fracture coming on without injury. If, therefore, no tenderness of the adductor muscles can be found in a case of pain on resisted adduction, an X-ray photograph should be taken of the pubic bone. Union is established in six to eight weeks. If resisted adduction of the thigh hurts in the buttock, the examiner must remember that this movement distracts the ilium from the sacrum and is painful in lesions of the sacroiliac joint.

## The Psoas Muscle

Strain here is uncommon, but a pleasure to meet, for it responds well to massage, but continues for years otherwise.

Pain arising from the psoas muscle may not be elicited when flexion is resisted as the patient lies with his thigh flat on the couch, since the upper part of the quadriceps muscle then shares the work with the psoas. Weakness is also obscured for the same reason. The hip must be bent to a right angle before the movement is tested. Even if a hip is already osteoarthrotic, psoas strain may complicate the joint lesion; hence, the resisted movements must be examined. In difficult cases, the induction of local anaesthesia diagnostically is indicated. It may of itself afford some degree of relief, but the consistently effective treatment is deep massage. Luckily, it seems that it is always the lower part of the muscle that becomes strained; the affected fibres lie immediately below the inguinal ligament, just medial to the inner edge or sartorius, where they are accessible to the physiotherapist's finger on deep palpation.

An obturator hernia interferes with the pelvic course of the psoas muscle, pressing on it from behind. Resisted flexion, therefore, hurts in the iliac fossa. If the patient lies in the Trendelenburg position for 10 minutes, the pain on resisted flexion ceases. This test appears to be pathognomonic.

Slight discomfort on resisted flexion may be felt in tendinitis of the rectus femoris or in partial rupture at the upper extent of the quadriceps muscle. If so, resisted extension of the knee, tested with the patient prone so as to maintain extension at the hip, evokes the pain more readily. For this reason, resisted flexion and extension at the knee are always included in the examination of the muscles about the hip.

*Painful Weakness.* Weakness accompanied by increased pain when the psoas muscle contracts is found in three conditions: (*a*) Traction-fracture of the lesser trochanter. This occurs in schoolboys. The onset is not sudden. Weakness *and* pain are elicited when the resisted flexion movement is tested. The patient is put to bed in a half-sitting position for two or three weeks. When walking no longer hurts, he can be allowed up. (*b*) Abdominal neoplasm infiltrating the psoas muscle. (*c*) Metastases at the upper femur. The weakness may be gross, and is associated with pain, and with marked limitation of movement at the hip joint.

*Painless Weakness.* Weakness, without increased pain when the muscle is tested, occurs in two other conditions. (*a*) Paresis of the psoas muscle provides the main sign in a second lumbar root palsy and forms the less obvious part of a third lumbar root palsy. (*b*) Neoplasm, benign or malignant, at the second lumbar level naturally leads to weakness, usually bilateral.

## Sartorius Muscle

'Cricket leg' was thought to be caused by rupture of the sartorius muscle, but in fact some fibres of the quadriceps have ruptured at mid-thigh.

The only lesion of the sartorius muscle is traction fracture of the anterior superior spine of the ilium. The boy is aged 15 to 18 and, while running, feels a painful click in his groin and uppermost thigh. He now finds walking painful and running impossible.

A full range of painless passive movement is present at the hip joint, but resisted flexion and lateral rotation hurt. Resisted extension at the knee also causes some discomfort. Tenderness is localized to the anterior superior spine of the ilium and the uppermost 2 cm of the sartorius muscle. Radiography shows the separation at the iliac spine. Spontaneous recovery takes two or three weeks. If the youngster wants to run, local anaesthesia can be induced just before the race.

## Gluteal Muscle

Lesions of these muscles appear not to occur, apart from direct bruising. In such cases, spontaneous recovery seldom takes longer than some days. Obstruction of the internal iliac artery leads to claudicational pain, reproduced by maintained contraction of the gluteal muscles.

*Weakness* of abduction accompanied by pain in a schoolboy suggests a traction fracture of the greater trochanter. Painless weakness occurs in congenital dislocation of the hip, when the greater trochanter has risen so high that contraction of the gluteus medius muscle has become ineffective. As the patient walks, the result is a characteristic dipping of the pelvis towards the leg that is off the ground—the Trendelenburg gait. The gluteus medius weakens in a fifth lumbar, and the gluteus maximus in a first sacral, root palsy.

## The Iliotibial Fascia

'Contracture' of the iliotibial band is no longer regarded as causing symptoms.

Sprain occurs only in dancers and athletes, and causes pain in the trochanteric region. Bursitis underlying the iliotibial band gives rise to identical symptoms but there is no trauma. If the band has become strained the characteristic signs are: (*a*) Pain on trunk side flexion towards the painless side, increased if the patient stands with his legs crossed before he bends sideways. (*b*) Pain on full passive adduction at the hip. (*c*) No pain on any other passive hip movement. (*d*) No pain on resisted abduction at the hip, or when the other resisted movements are tested. If the diagnosis is in doubt, local anaesthesia should be induced at the painful spot just behind and above the greater trochanter. A few sessions of massage are curative. In bursitis, local anaesthesia is usually effective alone; if it is not, triamcinolone must be substituted.

## Quadriceps and Hamstring Muscles

Partial rupture from indirect violence with, often, the formation of a haematoma is common in athletes. During some strenuous movement the patient feels something give way; he supplies the diagnosis correctly himself. Although the pain is not severe at the time, that evening and next morning the pain and disablement are considerable. Direct trauma, e.g. a kick on the thigh, may be responsible.

Resisted flexion and extension of the knee are examined with the patient lying prone, the hip being thus kept extended. Pain felt in the groin on resisted extension shows some part of the upper quadriceps muscle to be at fault. This used to be termed 'cricket leg' and mistakenly ascribed to rupture of the sartorius muscle. If the rupture is at all extensive and a haematoma is present, passive knee flexion is limited so long as the patient stays prone. When he is turned to lie supine, a full range of knee flexion is revealed. This is due to the quadriceps muscle being released above as fast as it is tautened below when the hip joint and knee joint are flexed simultaneously. Tenderness, distension of the muscle by effused blood and, sometimes, fluctuation demonstrates the site of the lesion. A third lumbar disc lesion is the only other condition in which the range of knee flexion alters according to whether the hip is kept extended or flexed. Both are instances of extra-articular limitation of movement with the sign dependent on the constant length phenomenon. By contrast, if the quadriceps muscle has become adherent to the mid-shaft of a fractured femur, the amount of flexion at the knee does not alter with the position of the hip.

Tendinitis of the rectus femoris shows itself by pain felt at the groin on resisted extension at the knee coupled with pain on full passive flexion of the hip, especially flexion in adduction. This implies that the lesion in the muscle lies in a position where it can be pinched.

When resisted flexion at the knee hurts at the back of the thigh, the hamstring muscles are at fault. If the sprain is tendinous and lies at the ischium, straight-leg raising is of full range. If a haematoma is present after a rupture in the belly, straight-leg raising is limited, though hip flexion with the knee bent is of full range—the constant length phenomenon again.

In either case, treatment consists of aspiration of the haematoma; the immediate induction of local anaesthesia (at least 50 ml); prolonged deep massage, begun the day after the injury, to the whole area of the tear and to the hardish swelling on either side due to infiltration of the belly with blood. Voluntary movement without weight-bearing is encouraged from the outset and faradism is of real value. It should be given with the knee kept passively fully flexed (for the hamstrings) or the knee held passively fully extended and the hip flexed (for the quadriceps). Full broadening of the muscles is then attained without pull on the healing breach. Progress is slow after a fair-sized rupture, especially towards the end. In sprinters, a recurrence is quite common unless to early a return to racing is prevented by continuing treatment for a fortnight after the patient has recovered clinically.

*Painless Weakness.* If this affects the quadriceps muscle and is unilateral, a lesion of the third lumbar nerve root is present. If the weakness is bilateral, localized myopathy or myositis should be suspected. Painful weakness characterizes a partial muscle rupture or a fractured patella.

Painless weakness of the hamstring muscles characterizes lesions of the first and second sacral roots, usually due to a disc lesion.

CHAPTER 24

# THE KNEE

Although a large variety of conditions arise in the knee, an exact diagnosis can be made with greater certainty than at any other joint. This is because different symptoms characterize different lesions, and because the greater part of the joint with its ligaments and tendons is accessible to direct palpation.

## EXAMINATION OF THE KNEE

Examination of the knee has to be conducted in the light of the history, for, by itself, the clinical state of the knee is often not characteristic of any one disorder. When diagnosis at the knee proves impossible, it is well to remember that a small cartilaginous loose body is commonplace at and after middle age, and may cause symptoms and signs that defy interpretation. Minor articular signs, particularly when associated with pain localized to one part of the knee, should suggest this probability.

### Pain Referred to the Knee

Lesions of the knee joint give rise to pain felt accurately at the knee, often at some particular part of the joint. An impacted loose body complicating osteoarthrosis is the only disorder of the knee that is apt to cause pain referred up the thigh and down the leg; even so, it is usually quite clear to the patient that the symptoms stem from the knee.

*The front of the knee* represents the second and third lumbar segments. Hence, the origin of pain referred to this area should be sought within these segments. The diagnostic point in the history, when pain is referred to the knee, is the indefinite area of which the patient complains. He may point to the whole suprapatellar area, and may have noted an ache running up the front or inner thigh towards the groin. The two principal structures apt to give rise to referred anterior crural pain are the hip joint and the third lumbar nerve root. In a third lumbar disc lesion the pain usually begins in the buttock, later affecting the front of the thigh; it is not aggravated by exertion or walking but a cough often hurts. Such a history exculpates the knee. When the hip joint is at fault, the pain is diffuse, although often worst at the knee; it is aggravated by walking and the patient may describe twinges which make the knee suddenly let him down. Only the extent of the pain then makes the examiner cautious, but later discovery of a normal knee on clinical examination naturally focuses attention on the hip: a joint also subject to internal derangement. A common error is to have an X-ray photograph taken of an elderly person's knee because pain is felt there, to find it osteoarthrotic (a fair certainty) and regard this as diagnostic. Many osteoarthrotic hips are missed this way.

*The back of the knee* is developed from the first and second sacral segments. Disorders of the knee itself very seldom cause posterior pain only. Hence the source of pain felt there is most often pressure on the first sacral nerve root as the result of a fifth lumbar disc lesion. Primary posterolateral protrusions at this level occasionally begin with pain only at the back of the knee, nothing being felt in the buttock at first. However, the patient may notice that sitting or coughing hurts his knee, whereas walking does not. A lesion of the lower part of the hamstring muscles or the upper part of the calf, whether ischaemic or due to a minor rupture, causes pain correctly attributed by the patient to the back of his knee.

### History

A detailed history is essential. A short list follows of the more important points that must be ascertained.

What is the age and occupation of the patient? What was he doing when the pain first appeared? In what position was his body and his leg, and what forces were acting on his knee at the time? Alternatively, did the pain come on for no apparent reason? Did the knee give way? If so, did the knee lock? If so, did it lock in extension or flexion? If so, how did it become unlocked? On which side of the knee was the pain or was it right inside, or was it all over? Did the pain change from one side of the knee to the other? Did it spread; if so, where to? Was the patient able to walk? Did the joint swell; if so, how quickly? For how long was he disabled? Were there recurrences; if so, what brought them on? How did they progress? What is the effect of going up and down stairs; is going down more troublesome than up? Are there sudden twinges? Does the knee click? Does it grate? Does it feel as if it might give way; if so, does the patient actually fall? What treatment has he had, and with what effect? Inquiry is made of the existence of arthritis elsewhere.

## Inspection

Diffuse swelling and the adoption of a flexed position of the knee suggest advanced arthritis, with fluid in the joint or synovial thickening, sometimes both. Limitation of extension coming on suddenly suggests displacement of part of a meniscus. The speed with which an effusion appears after an injury is significant: if it appears in a few minutes, it is haemorrhagic; if in some hours, it is probably serous. Localized swellings are usually caused by a cyst of the lateral meniscus or by bursae, especially the pre-patellar and the semi-membranosus.

Muscular wasting is noted, but has no great diagnostic value unless it is extreme, when it suggests severe arthritis. Reddening of the skin suggests sepsis or gout.

The alignment of the tibia on the femur is noted. A genu valgum deformity in a child may be due to rickets or to a valgus position of the heel from inversion of the forefoot, but it often comes on apparently without cause and disappears with growth. Knock-knee persisting after the age of ten should be treated by a year or two's stapling of the condyle. Some degree of genu varum is normal in babies. Its development in an elderly patient suggests osteitis deformans. A tiny patella characterizes the patella–nail syndrome.

## Palpation of the Stationary Joint

### Site of Tenderness

Since nearly all the tissues at the knee lie superficially, palpation lends great accuracy to diagnosis, and follows the clinical examination. Tenderness is always sought along the structure thus identified, provided that history and physical signs indicate that it lies within finger's reach.

### Heat

Heat means that the lesion, whatever it may be, is in the active stage; localized heat naturally has a strong diagnostic value. The joint should be palpated again at the end of the examination of movements, for it may have been rendered warm merely by the minor stresses entailed. The discovery of heat indicates: (*a*) recent injury or operation, (*b*) blood in the joint, (*c*) bacterial, rheumatoid, spondylitic, gonorrhoeal or Reiter's arthritis, (*d*) a loose body impacted with an osteoarthrotic joint, (*e*) gout, (*f*) fracture, or (*g*) osteitis deformans.

### Fluid

Fluid in the knee joint ('water on the knee') is sometimes dignified by the term 'synovitis'. Intra-articular effusion is a sign common to many disorders, traumatic, inflammatory and crystalline. Synovitis of the knee is a statement of fact, never a diagnosis. Testing for fluid in the knee joint can be done in two ways.

*Patellar Tap.* Unless the joint is very full, the suprapatellar pouch is first emptied by manual pressure with the palm of the hand. Fluid, if present, is thus forced downwards, lifting the patella off the femur. The patella can now be felt to hit the femur with a palpable tap as it is pushed smartly backwards by the examiner's hand. In the normal knee, the cartilaginous surfaces of patella and femur are already in contact and thus cannot be made to click against each other.

*Eliciting Fluctuation.* This is a more delicate test and should therefore always be preferred to the above manoeuvre. The examiner places his thumb to one side of the patella, and one of his fingers to the other. With the palm of his other hand over the whole suprapatellar pouch, he presses backwards. If fluid lies in the suprapatellar pouch, it is squeezed down towards the lower part of the joint and thus pushes apart the fingers of the examiner's other hand. Even the presence of only a little fluid can be detected in this way. By this method—but not by eliciting patellar tap—experience enables the examiner to tell blood from clear fluid. Blood fluctuates *en bloc* like a jelly moving, whereas a clear effusion runs up and down piecemeal.

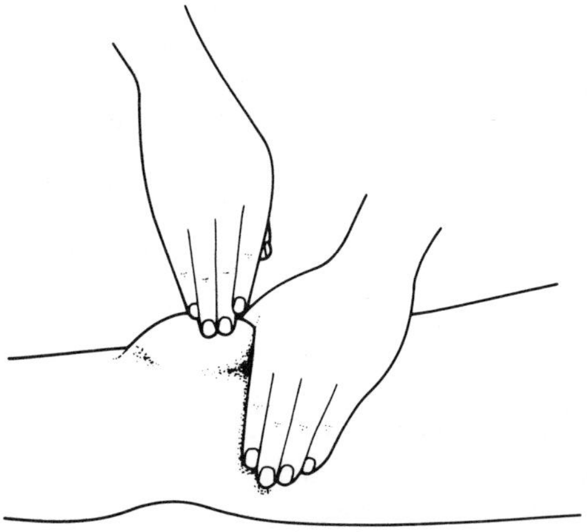

**Fig. 107.** Patellar tap. One test for fluid in the knee joint. If the patella is raised from the femur by fluid it can be felt to tap against the bone when jerked downwards by the examiner's finger. Unless the joint contains a good deal of fluid, the suprapatellar pouch must first be emptied by the pressure of the examiner's other hand.

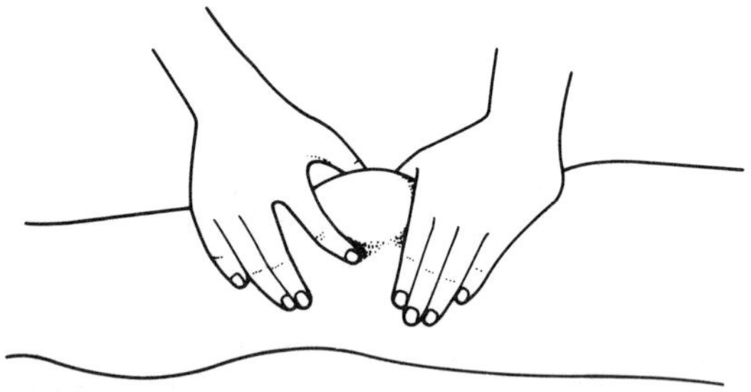

**Fig. 108.** Eliciting fluctuation. A more delicate test for fluid in the knee joint. The examiner lays one hand flat on the suprapatella pouch. Pressure here forces fluid into the lower part of the joint. If fluid is present, the fingers of the other hand, lying to each side of the patella, are forced apart as pressure is applied.

Whenever the question arises of blood in the knee joint—common after direct trauma—diagnostic aspiration is indicated immediately. If blood is present, it is all aspirated, since this is the important therapeutic measure. If the fluid turns out to be clear, there is no point in emptying the joint, since the treatment of a clear effusion is to deal with the cause.

If an effusion has developed without adequate trauma in a boy, and aspiration proves that it consists of blood, the cooperation of the pathologist should be sought and antihaemophilic globulin administered at once. This prevents the knee filling again.

## Synovial Thickening

Whether the synovial membrane is thickened or not is difficult to estimate at times; yet it may be a vital clinical finding. The examiner's finger should seek the reflexion of the membrane, where it overlies each condyle of the femur (Fig. 109), about 2 cm posterior to the medial and lateral edges of the patella. He rolls this edge under his finger, carefully comparing the two knees. Synovial swelling indicates bacterial, rheumatoid or inflammatory arthritis (e.g. gout, tuberculosis, gonorrhoea, Reiter's disease, ulcerative colitis, ankylosing spondylitis). Warmth and fluid without synovial swelling suggest traumatic arthritis (including that secondary to impaction of a small loose body), recent injury, fracture or operation, or blood in the joint. Localized warmth felt after the examination of the joint, not present at first,

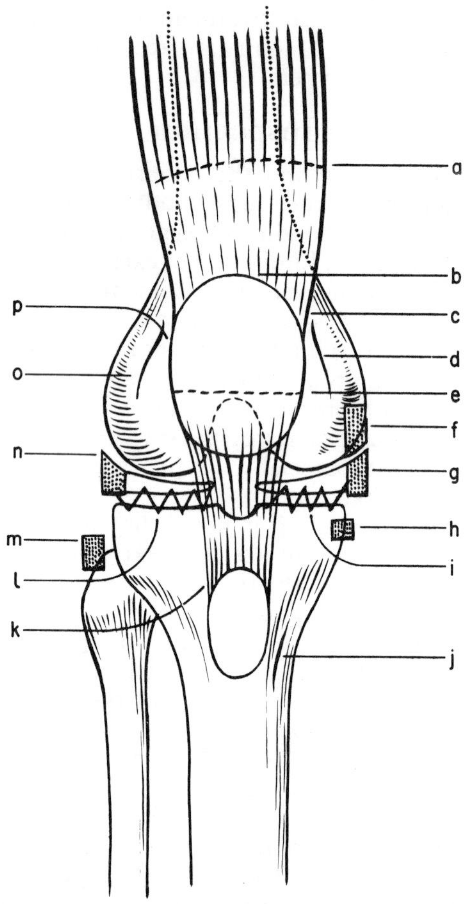


**Fig. 109.** Points of tenderness at the knee. *a*, Musculotendinous junction. *b*, Insertion of suprapatellar tendon. *c*, Quadriceps expansion. *d*, Synovial reflexion. *e*, Usual site of transverse patellar fracture. *f*, Medial collateral ligament (upper end). *g*, Medial collateral ligament: joint line. *h*, Semimembranosus tendon. *i*, Medial coronary ligament. *j*, Insertion of semitendinosus muscle. *k*, Infrapatellar tendon. *l*, Lateral coronary ligament. *m*, Biceps tendon. *n*, Lateral collateral ligament. *o*, Synovial reflexion. *p*, Quadriceps expansion.

characterizes an impacted loose body complicating osteoarthrosis.

### Other Findings

Palpation clearly reveals osteophytes of any size. Bony deformity may be seen and felt, e.g. upper tibial fracture, or the enlargement of the patella that results from an old stellate fracture or osteitis deformans. The bony expansion caused by neoplasm or chronic osteomyelitis can be palpated. When osteitis deformans affects the tibia, the sharp anterior edge is eventually lost and the front of the leg may be warm. Prominence of the tibial tuberosity left after Schlatter's disease has no significance in adult life. Syphilitic periostitis is very rare; traumatic periostitis not uncommon. A prepatellar bursa is most easily felt when the tissues at the front of the patella are pinched up. Calcified areas in the suprapatellar pouch may form palpable thickenings.

Intra-articular loose bodies should be sought if the patient mentions severe momentary twinges or locking. The patient or the doctor may feel the loose body move; hence the German name 'Gelenkenmaus'.

A cyst of the lateral meniscus can be felt by palpation along the joint-line during extension. When the knee is flexed, the small projection disappears.

## Palpation of the Moving Joint

This discloses the state of the opposed surfaces of articular cartilage. It may reveal fine crepitus, some degree of which is normal in all middle-aged individuals. Coarse crepitus indicates marked fragmentation of the surface of articular cartilage. If bone is felt creaking against bone, cartilage has been completely eroded.

In patellar–femoral osteoarthrosis, when the patient is examined lying down, the patella is not kept strongly enough applied to the front of the femur by muscular action for the marked crepitus characteristic of this condition to be felt. Hence the knee must be palpated while the patient stands, squats and comes up again, by the examiner's hand applied to the front of the knee. A number of other manoeuvres are appropriate if evidence of a ruptured meniscus is sought.

## Diagnostic Movements at the Knee

### Passive Movements

*The primary movements* are two: flexion and extension. As at the elbow, it is only in advanced arthritis that the range of rotation also becomes restricted. The capsular pattern is great limitation of flexion and slight limitation of extension. For example 5° limitation of extension would correspond with 45° to 60° limitation of flexion; 10° limitation of extension to 90° limitation of flexion.

*The secondary movements* are six: they test the ligaments for pain on stretching and for laxity. *Varus* strain tests the lateral ligament; *valgus* strains the medial ligament. In a minor sprain, pain may be better elicited if the valgus strain is applied with the knee held just short of full extension. Pain and laxity are both noted.

*Lateral rotation* is painful in medial coronary sprain and is of excessive range if the medial collateral ligament is lengthened. The converse applies to passive *medial rotation.* Rotation is not possible with the knee fully extended; hence Hughston et al. (1976) advise testing in 30° of flexion, but a clear assessment is difficult, since the thigh is apt to rotate. However, an accurate estimate can be arrived at when the patient lies prone and is examined with his knee flexed to a right angle. Now, the thigh cannot rotate, and it is easy to see how far the foot twists round and to compare the two sides, rather than just watching the tibia.

*Anterior pressure* on the tibia (draw sign) tests the anterior cruciate ligament. The patient lies supine, his knee flexed to a right angle. The examiner places one hand on the patella, the other at the back of the upper tibia, and draws the latter forwards with a strong jerk. Range and painfulness are both noted. *Posterior pressure* tests the posterior cruciate ligament likewise (see Figs 113, 114).

*A painful* arc is not often encountered at the knee, but it can occur with an impacted loose body. More seldom it indicates a torn meniscus,

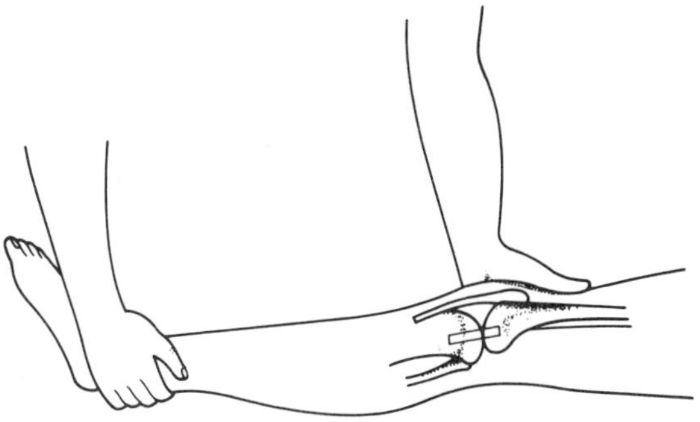

**Fig. 110.** The application of valgus strain. The knee is forced medially and the ankle laterally; as a result the inner aspect of the knee is stretched.

localized erosion of the articular edge of the femur as the patella rides over the defect, and post-traumatic irregularity of the edge of the patella.

*Shearing strain* may be applied when the knee is held bent to a right angle, the femur and tibia being pressed sideways in opposite directions. This may evoke pain when a loose body or a torn meniscus is present, and forcing the tibia laterally on the femur often elicits pain from a painful posterior cruciate ligament.

Trickey (1976) divides the knee into medial and lateral compartments. The medial extends medially from the patella to the posterior cruciate ligament and the lateral laterally to this ligament. In each compartment is a capsular ligament attached to the meniscus and divided into meniscotibial and meniscofemoral parts. The posterior third of the medial ligament is thick and called the posterior oblique ligament; this is supported by the horizontal aponeurosis of the semimembranosus tendon. On the lateral side the capsular ligament is reinforced by the arcuate ligament and the aponeurosis of the popliteus muscle.

The posterior cruciate ligament provides the axis about which the knee moves both in extension-flexion and in rotation. It is attached to the back of the tibia and to the medial femoral condyle. He points out that when lateral stability of the ligament is to be assessed, ordinary valgus strain is not enough. It should be repeated in 30° flexion of the knee. For the anterior draw test, the examiner sits on the foot and pulls the tibia forwards in full rotation each way as well as in the neutral position.

## Resisted Movements

These are best examined as the patient lies prone (see Fig. 83) but may for convenience be tested supine (Fig. 111). The primary movements are flexion and extension. Pain on a resisted muscular contraction is noted, likewise weakness, likewise the two together. If extension is painful, a lesion of the quadriceps muscle is present; if it is painful and weak, a fractured patella or a major rupture of the belly is the cause; if it is weak but the muscular contraction does not hurt, a third lumbar root palsy is suggested. If flexion is painful, medial and lateral rotation are tested against resistance while the knee is held passively flexed; this test distinguishes between the biceps and the upper tibiofibular joint (lateral rotator) and the semimembranosus, semitendinosus and popliteus muscles (all medial rotators). If it is the popliteus, the pain is felt at the back of the joint whereas the semimembranosus and semitendinosus hurt anteromedially.

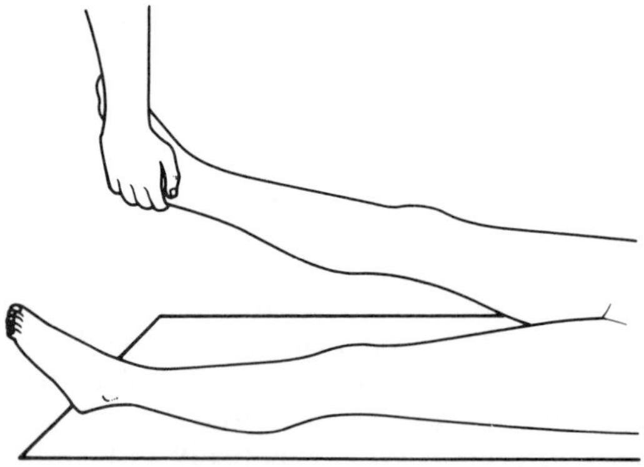

**Fig. 111.** Resisted extension of the knee. The examiner passes his forearm under the knee and supports his hand on the other knee. The patient's flexed knee rests on his lower forearm. The extension movement is resisted by the examiner's other hand at the ankle.

## Summary

For the proper examination of the knee, 12 tests are carried out while the patient lies supine on the couch.

*The Joint.* Two passive movements. Flexion and extension. Painful, painless; full range, limited range. Capsular or non-capsular pattern.

*The Ligaments.* Six passive movements. Valgus strain and lateral rotation for the medial ligament; varus strain and medial rotation for the lateral ligament; pulling the tibia forwards for the anterior cruciate ligament; pushing the tibia backwards for the posterior cruciate ligament. Painful, painless; full range, excessive range.

*The Muscles.* Two resisted movements. Resisted extension for the patella, its tendons and the quadriceps muscle. Resisted flexion for the hamstring muscles.

*Palpation.* For heat, fluid or synovial thickening. For tenderness.

# DISORDERS OF THE KNEE JOINT

The following conditions occur at the knee. The history taken together with the physical signs forms a series of characteristic patterns, though neither taken alone may be of itself diagnostic.

## Ligamentous Sprain

### Medial Collateral Ligament

The patient falls awkwardly while skiing or strains the inner side of his knee on the football field. A strong valgus strain is imposed on his knee; he feels a sudden pain or crack at the inner side of the knee. At first he can walk, but he becomes increasingly disabled and half-an-hour later is hobbling only with assistance. Some hours later, the knee is swollen and the pain is worse. He has to spend some days in bed. He limps about in great discomfort for several weeks. Then the pain and swelling slowly subside; after two or three months he has largely recovered.

In the acute stage, which lasts up to a fortnight, the knee is full of fluid, hot to the touch, and extension is about 5° limited, flexion 90° limited. An acute traumatic arthritis is present, obscuring all other signs. But the patient knows that he sprained the inner side of the joint and localized tenderness is easily found at some point along the ligament.

In the subacute stage, which lasts four to six weeks in the untreated case, the limitation of movement at the knee slowly diminishes. The knee remains warm, more so at the inner side. Testing the ligament by applying valgus strain is now possible and elicits pain, whereas varus strain does not. If the ligament was overstretched and is now permanently lengthened, an excessive range of valgus movement exists. Hughston et al. (1976) point out that lesser degrees of instability due to minor overstretching of the tibial collateral ligament are not disclosed by applying valgus strain in full extension. They advise repeating the test in 30° of flexion. Assessing the range of rotation of the tibia by watching how far the foot turns is preferable, the patient lying prone. If adhesions consolidate themselves because healing is allowed to take place without adequate movement at the knee, the chronic stage is reached.

The medial collateral ligament is nearly always damaged at the point where it crosses the joint line and is attached to the medial meniscus. Nevertheless, its whole extent must be palpated. The lower part of the tibial attachment is scarcely ever affected; the lesion lies, in order of frequency: (1) at the joint line; (2) at the femoral origin; (3) at the edge of the tibial condyle. Puzzling signs are found when the lesion lies high up on the femoral condyle. When this motionless part of the ligament suffers contusion, there may be little or no restriction of movement, yet the knee hurts and is warm, contains fluid and valgus strain is painful. Palpation reveals the reason for the small degree of limitation.

*Complete Rupture.* This is concealed for the first few days by the acute traumatic arthritis which prevents full extension of the knee and thus the assessment of valgus mobility in full extension. In slight flexion, the sign is not easy to assess, and some degree of valgus instability is consistent with full recovery and a functionally stable knee afterwards.

As soon as the arthritis is subsiding, valgus strain is found, in complete rupture, to cause no pain as the inner condyles of femur and tibia separate; then a click is felt as the bones come together again. In such a case, an excessive, but again painless, range of lateral rotation is also detected. As soon as the state of the joint allows these two signs to be established, operative suture is indicated in those patients, e.g. professional footballers, for whom any instability is a serious matter. Ordinary individuals suffer no inconvenience and get well enough to return to tennis and skiing without the operation. They may complain of a feeling of instability when the tibia is fully rotated laterally while the knee is slightly flexed, when the inner tibial condyle subluxes momentarily forwards.

### Lateral Collateral Ligament

This is very seldom sprained. If it is, the articular signs are less severe, owing to the less intimate attachment of this ligament at the joint compared with the medial ligament. Hence the knee is warm, contains fluid, but the range of movement is almost full from the outset. The patient knows that he sprained the outer side of his knee and varus strain hurts. Palpation of the ligament discloses the site of the lesion.

### Coronary Ligament

The patient describes a rotation strain, usually at football. He stands on one foot and, wishing to kick to one side, twists his femur on his stationary tibia. He feels an immediate pain in his knee, localized to the inner or the outer side. He may fall to the ground but gets up again almost at once and may even be able to go on playing. That evening the knee is painful and swollen; the next day he hobbles with difficulty. The sprain resolves very slowly, usually (unless treated) taking at least three months to recover.

The coronary ligament attaches the meniscus to the edge of the tibial condyle. In extension at the knee, the menisci are forced forwards, thus stretching the ligament. Whatever the degree of flexion, the semilunar cartilage lies in the neutral position, undisturbed. Hence extension is characteristically the really painful movement in coronary sprain.

Medial rotation tends to stretch the lateral coronary ligament; lateral rotation the medial coronary ligament; hence one or other of these passive movements is painful but not limited.

Examination soon after the accident shows the knee to be warm and filling with fluid, extension being 5° limited whereas flexion is painful and scarcely limited. By next day traumatic arthritis has supervened, and the capsular pattern, now with marked limitation of flexion, appears, but not so severely as in strain of the medial collateral ligament. The passive rotation movements remain of full range, the one towards the painless side hurting.

The history of a rotation sprain is clear, and the pain is at one side of the knee only. Applying varus and valgus strain does not hurt; this excludes the collateral ligaments. It follows that one or other of the coronary ligaments has been strained. Tenderness is sought with the knee well bent and the appropriate coronary ligament is found tender, whereas the collateral ligament is not. It is well to remember that the part of the coronary ligament that lies behind the collateral ligament may be strained. Hence search for tenderness must include the extent behind the medial ligament—the posterior oblique ligament—and that behind the lateral ligament—the arcuate ligament.

After a time, the traumatic arthritis subsides; later a full range of extension returns but the warmth and fluid persists for several months in the absence of adequate treatment.

## Cruciate Ligaments

*Recent Injury.* The history is of a sprain but not in any characteristic direction unless it is a dashboard injury with the tibia forced backward on the femur. During extension, a small degree of lateral rotation of the tibia on the femur takes place, relaxing the anterior cruciate ligament enough to allow full extension to be reached. Hence a sprain of the anterior ligament may be caused by a hyperextension strain combined with force towards medial rotation. Examination shows a warm and swollen knee containing fluid, with a full range of movement in each direction, all extremes hurting; for the cruciate ligaments limit rotation as well as extension (the anterior is then taut) and flexion (the posterior is taut). Valgus and varus strains cause no pain, but when the tibia is rocked backwards (stretching the posterior cruciate ligament) and forwards (stretching the anterior ligament) one or other of these movements is painful (Figs 113, 114).

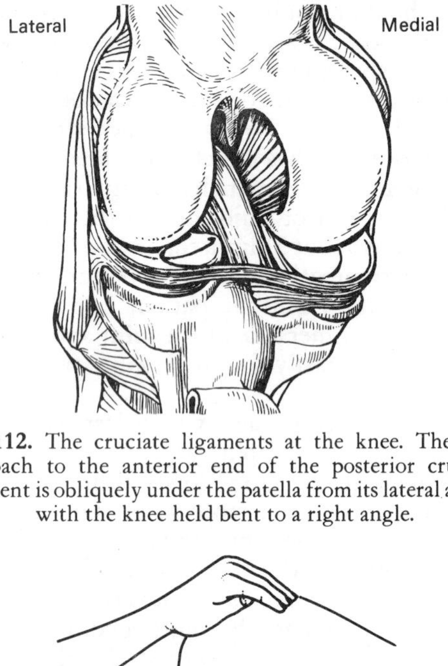


**Fig. 112.** The cruciate ligaments at the knee. The best approach to the anterior end of the posterior cruciate ligament is obliquely under the patella from its lateral aspect with the knee held bent to a right angle.

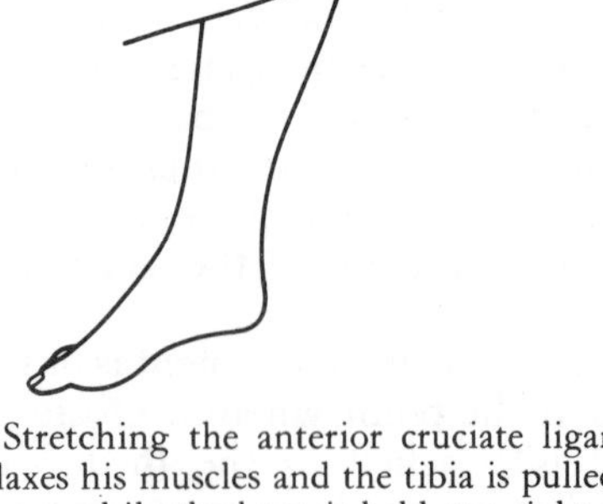

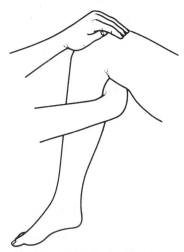

**Fig. 113.** Stretching the anterior cruciate ligament. The patient relaxes his muscles and the tibia is pulled forwards on the femur, while the knee is held at a right angle. The examiner sits on the forefoot.

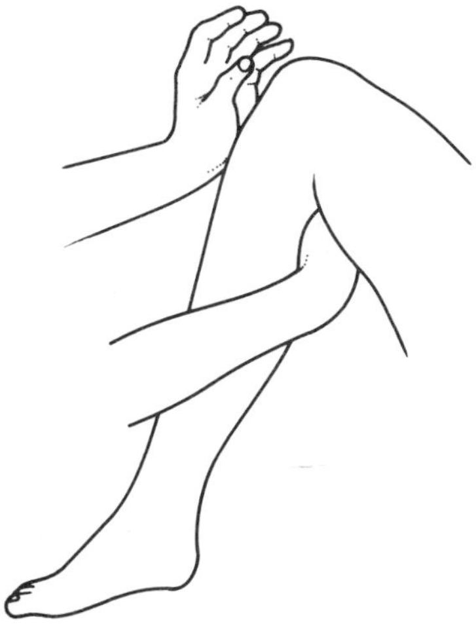

**Fig. 114.** Stretching the posterior cruciate ligament. The knee is held passively at a right angle and the tibia is pushed backwards on the femur.

The posterior cruciate ligament provides the axis about which the knee moves, dividing the knee into two compartments (Hughston et al. 1976). When it has been strained, forcing the tibia laterally on the femur with the joint at a right angle stretches it painfully. After a severe injury permanent lenghthening is common; if so, an excessive range of anteroposterior movement of the tibia on the femur is detected when the two sides are compared. No tenderness can be elicited: for no part of either ligament lies within finger's reach. Adhesions cannot form about the cruciate ligaments; the trouble is instability due to laxity. Manipulation is therefore futile.

Spontaneous recovery is slow; it often takes six to twelve months. An occasional patient fails to recover at all and, say a year later, is still unable to run, let alone play football. Chronic strain at the periosteoligamentous junction can continue for years.

*Permanent Lenghthening.* The history is now most misleading, for it simulates closely that of a ruptured meniscus.

The patient states that he suffered a severe injury to his knee a year or more ago; ever since, he has had to be careful of his knee. If he twists on it, the knee appears to him to 'go out' with a click and he has to stand on the other leg and give his leg a shake; there is another click and all is well. Actual subluxation of the tibia on the femur by rotation during weight-bearing is being described. Only when the cruciate ligaments are tested during examination of the knee does the nature of the disorder become obvious.

## Post-traumatic Adhesions

A common history is that of a sprain of some part of the knee, followed by swelling, which has been treated by a few days', possibly weeks', rest in bed and then by gradually increasing use. After a time the knee has become quite adequate for ordinary walking, but hurts at one small spot when the patient takes vigorous exercise, and is apt to become stiff after he has kept it still for any length of time, e.g. sitting. It is clear that abnormally adherent scars have been allowed to form about the torn structure during the period of healing. Quiet use of the knee does not pull at these adhesions; exertion does. Thus vigorous exercise of the knee each time sprains anew the ligament whose mobility remains impaired. Each time, after a few days, the pain and swelling subside and the knee gives no more trouble until exerted again.

As a rule the adhesions lie at the mid-part of the medial collateral ligament. The signs are: full extension hurts at the inner side; flexion is 5 or 10° limited; full lateral rotation hurts; full medial rotation is painless. The knee is not warm and there is no fluid in the joint unless the patient is seen on the day of, or soon after, some exertion. The resisted movements are painless. Valgus strain hurts; testing the lateral ligament causes no pain and stretching the cruciate ligaments sets up no discomfort either. Tenderness is sought and found at some part of the medial ligament, usually at the joint line.

If a full range of movement is found, and localized discomfort together with a history of a former sprain nevertheless suggest adhesion about a ligament, tenderness should be sought at the femoral origin of the medial collateral ligament if valgus strain hurts, but at the coronary ligament if it is painless.

### Stieda–Pellegrini's Disease

After an apparently ordinary sprain of the inner side of the knee, in due course the range of movement is found not to be increasing but actually to have diminished. Examination reveals the lesion to lie at the medial collateral ligament at its upper extent. By a month after the injury, radiography shows a linear shadow along the whole inner side of the medial femoral condyle. The periosteum has been torn up by the ligamentous pull at the time of the accident, and bone grows until it reaches the raised periosteum once more. Recovery in slight cases takes six months, in more severe cases up to a year. Treatment is useless.

## Torn Meniscus

The characteristic features are (*a*) locking *in flexion*, and (*b*) manipulative *unlocking*. The first injury leading to rupture of the meniscus nearly always takes place between the ages of 16 and 30. If a child, nearly always a girl, say, aged 12, has signs of cartilage trouble, the condition to be suspected is a congenital discoid meniscus, more often the lateral. Cartilage trouble at the knee occurs at any age; the earliest age at which Young has performed excision and found a ruptured meniscus was 9 months. If a patient is aged over 30 when he first fractures his meniscus, the crack is sometimes posterior or horizontal. Indeed, Hadfield (1966) explored 21 knees in patients over 40 who had persistent symptoms and found that 14 had a meniscus split horizontally forming a sliding tear.

During flexion–extension, the menisci move with the tibia, but when the femur is rotated on the tibia with the knee flexed, they move with the femur. It is therefore this movement that most strongly strains the coronary ligaments and the tissue of the meniscus itself. Hence tearing of a meniscus is caused by a strong rotation strain with the knee slightly bent. Thus, in the course of violent exertion, very often a game of football, the knee is severely twisted, usually in an attempt by the player to kick sideways, turning his whole body while the knee is fixed by the foot on the ground. It is this rotation strain of body on leg that fractures the intra-articular meniscus of the knee on which the player is standing. He feels a click and a sudden agonizing pain in the joint, which gives way under him, making him fall to the ground. A minute later when, recovering, he tries to move his knee, he finds that he can bend it a little but not straighten it. Then, or later, either he or the trainer forces it, and, with a click, full extension is regained. The knee then swells and is painful for a few days. Later still when the patient has recovered, he finds that he is apt, if twisting on his knee once more, to feel something 'go out' painfully in his joint; whereupon the leg gives way under him and he falls with the knee locked again in a semi-flexed position. He then kicks his leg straight or has it manipulated and suddenly the obstruction slips away and his knee becomes servicable one more. Occasionally, the layman's attempt at immediate reduction proves too painful; if so medical attention and general anaesthesia are required.

The side of the knee on which the patient felt the pain indicates which meniscus was torn; the medial meniscus is much the more commonly torn of the two (various surgeons give the proportion as three, five or seven to one).

The reason for the preponderance of medial meniscal tears was elucidated by Seedhom (1976). He showed that the medial meniscus was anchored by a coronary ligament 4–5 mm long whereas that for the lateral meniscus was 2 cm long anteriorly, 1.3 cm posteriorly. The medial meniscus was attached strongly to the tibial collateral ligament, the lateral had no attachment to the fibular ligament, the tendon of popliteus intervening. In consequence the lateral meniscus possessed a play of 10 mm, the medial only 2 mm. Such a difference in mobility clearly makes damage to the medial meniscus much more likely.

If a lesion of the lateral meniscus is present, it should be recalled that rupture is only twice as common as cyst formation. Cyst at the medial meniscus is a great rarity.

In posterior meniscal cracks occurring for the first time between the ages of 30 and 45, the history is less dramatic. The patient states that if he twists on his knee quickly he occasionally feels something go out at the back of the joint with a click; he kicks his knee out straight, the knee clicks again and is at once fit for use. In these cases, locking of sufficient degree to require reduction by another person or eventual excision is uncommon. Middle-aged patients describe an even slighter disorder when the crack merely causes a bifid posterior extremity to the meniscus. The patient says that rotation in flexion during weight-bearing (i.e. movement while squatting) gives rise to an uncomfortable click, remedied as he stands up by another click.

In middle age and later, the meniscus may crack horizontally. This is the result of degeneration within the interior of the meniscus, whereby the upper and lower surfaces come to slide on each other and eventually become detached. The tag that forms can then become displaced and form a visible and palpable projection at the joint line. Digital pressure often suffices for reduction. If the tag gets twisted round the edge of the meniscus, the free end lying on the superior surface, reduction by manipulation becomes impossible; excision is then the only remedy.

Calcification of the meniscus occurs in pseudogout as the result of deposition of crystals of calcium pyrophosphate, but does not itself cause symptoms, which are due to recurrent attacks of crystal synovitis.

As the knee straightens, the fact that the curve of the femoral condyles follows a spiral comes into play. In extension, the anterior cruciate, the collateral and the posterior aspect of the joint capsule all become taut. When all the slack in the ligaments has been taken up, the femur and tibia are strongly approximated, extension beyond 180° being prevented. At this point, there is no room for a displaced tissue lying between the two bones. Extension of the knee must therefore be limited if a fragment of meniscus intervenes at the joint surfaces.

The coronary ligament holds the meniscus in place; force sufficient to rupture the cartilage must sprain the ligament first. Indeed, coronary strain leading to rupture of the meniscus is analogous to sprain of the fibular collateral ligament preceding Pott's fracture. When the meniscus splits, the coronary ligament holds the rim in place—the handle of the bucket—but the rest of the meniscus slips across the dome of the femoral condyle to rest on the other side, i.e. displaced towards the centre of the joint (Fig. 115). Here the displaced portion gets in the way and prevents the painless approximation of the articular surfaces that accompanies extension, but it does not interfere with flexion, since in this position the ligaments are relaxed.

*Rupture with Displacement.* The patient's gait is characteristic. He hops into the room on one leg, the knee on the affected side held flexed and the limb medially rotated, the foot plantiflexed with the toes just touching the ground.

On examination the knee is warm, full of fluid, and when extension is attempted a springy block is felt limiting this movement by 5 or 10°. Flexion is somewhat limited by the traumatic arthritis. Rotation away from the affected side hurts but towards it does not. However much the joint is cajoled, the springy block prevents full extension. A posterior tear with displacement in middle age may just allow full, but very painful, extension.

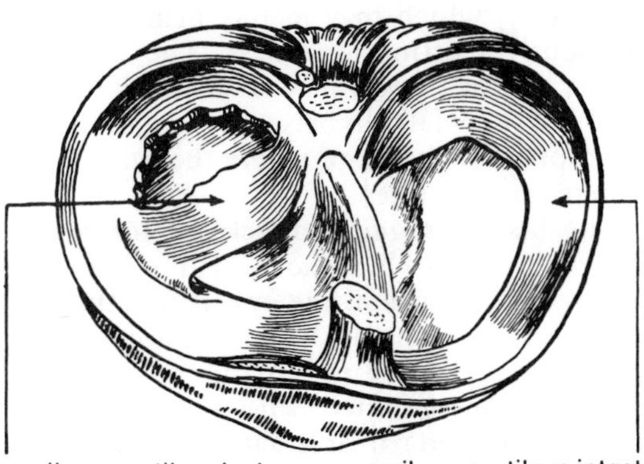
semilunar cartilage broken
displaced fragment
semilunar cartilage intact

**Fig. 115.** Torn cartilage at the knee. A view from the front, showing a tear with displacement of part of the medial meniscus. the lateral meniscus is intact.

The patient knows which side of his knee he has hurt, thus indicating which meniscus has been torn. Cartilage possesses no nerves; hence it cannot itself be tender. The tenderness on the joint line in meniscal tears is dependent on the coincident sprain of the coronary ligament. It is best sought by pressure from above downwards on the edge of the tibial condyle while the knee is kept flexed—the same position as for massage to the coronary ligament (see Volume II). In posterior cracks, no tenderness can be elicited. Intra-articular cartilage has no access to blood; hence the fracture cannot unite, however long the broken surfaces remain in apposition. Thus, once the meniscus has ruptured and the loose part has shifted, recurrence is the rule.

*Rupture without Displacement.* If the patient is seen some time after reduction of internal derangement at the knee, this may appear normal. This history is often strongly suggestive, and the following tests can be used to elicit signs of a ruptured meniscus. (1) The knee is fully flexed and the knee rotated quickly to and fro. A telltale click may be felt as the examiner's thumb presses first to one side of the infrapatellar tendon then the other, on the joint line. (2) The knee is flexed and held fully rotated in one direction. It is then slowly extended while the pressure maintaining rotation continues. As extension proceeds, the possible range of rotation diminishes and a click may be felt as the leg approaches the neutral position at almost full extension. (3) The knee is held at a right angle. The examiner interlocks his fingers and places the heel of one hand on one side of the upper tibia, the heel of the other hand on the other side of the lower femur (Fig. 116). He then applies a strong shearing strain, as if to move the femur sideways on the tibia. He tries first one way, then the other. This manoeuvre may displace the loose part of the meniscus to the other side of the femoral dome, with a loud click; simultaneously, the full range of passive extension at the knee is lost. Manipulative reduction follows. (4) The knee is held well flexed. The examiner passes his flexed fingertip from above downwards over the joint line. He may be able to hook the rim of the meniscus and pull it downwards; then it jumps back into place again with a click. (5) When the meniscus is split horizontally, a tag of cartilage may protrude at the joint line. It can be pushed back into place by the examiner with a palpable

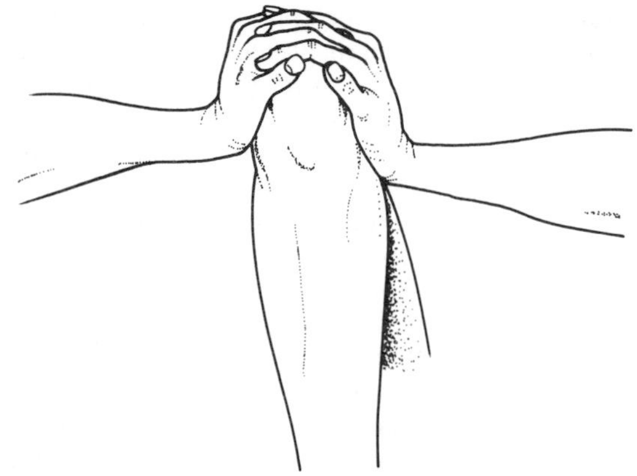

**Fig. 116.** Side pressure at the knee. A strong shearing stress is applied, first in one direction, then in the other. As the femur and tibia move against each other, a torn cartilage may subluxate. This is an accessory test for meniscal tear.

click; the patient has often learnt to do this himself. The discomfort on full extension and the painful arc that are often present in such cases then cease.

These tests, particularly the last two, are repeatable at will. Hence in doubtful cases, they are most useful since they can be demonstrated to a surgeon undecided about operation. If all these tests are negative, the patient should be sent back to full athletics, to ascertain if recurrence is thus provoked or not. If it is, the patient is asked to return at once, so that his knee can be examined again during the acute phase.

It is unwise to let the knee of a young person suffer repeated attacks of internal derangement owing to a torn meniscus. These frequent traumas set up an intractable osteoarthrosis which becomes troublesome by middle age. However, Jackson (1968) has shown that removal does not wholly prevent osteoarthrosis later. In a review of 640 knees 5 to 19 years after the operation, he found osteoarthrosis five times as common as in his controls, and 20 to 30 years later, four times as common. He attributed this change to loss of the meniscus itself—a concept confirmed by Seedhom (1976). He pointed out that the function of the menisci was to provide concave surfaces to distribute the load when the rounded femoral condyles bore on the flat tibial plateau. Without menisci, the pressure on the articulating surfaces was three times greater; no wonder the joint wore out fast. Many surgeons nowadays remove only the loose fragment leaving the edge of the meniscus attached to the coronary ligament intact. This remnant supports the curve of the femur and, it is hoped, will prevent the pressure at only one point that makes the joint wear out. Removal via the operating arthroscope bit by bit, is much less damaging to the joint and requires only two days in bed afterwards (Dandy 1978).

I make two suggestions to orthopaedic surgeons to shorten the period of disability after meniscectomy. (1) To soak the cut surface of the coronary ligament with a steroid suspension before the wound is closed. Since the traumatic arthritis after intervention must stem from the ligamentous damage, it should prove possible to minimize it by this means. (2) To make the skin incision 1 cm above or below the joint line. By drawing the wound slightly up or down, it should be possible to apply hydrocortisone ointment to the skin directly over the coronary remnants and drive the steroid in by phonophoresis, without interfering with healing of the wound.

*Arthroscopy.* This was first carried out by Bircher (1921). Bedford et al. describe the technique and provide colour plates of what is seen. In their second 100 cases the findings on arthroscopy were different from those at operation in only 6% (1979).

## Cyst of the Meniscus

The patient complains of intermittent pain at the joint line, almost always at the lateral aspect, since a cyst of the medial meniscus is very rare. Alternatively, he may complain of attacks of frank internal derangement. Since the cyst must weaken the meniscus and impair its mobility, at least half of all cystic menisci have already ruptured.

There is often a history of injury some months previously, which may merely bring to light a previously existing weakness. The alternative theory is that trauma may result in the implantation of synovial cells between the meniscus and the capsule of the joint, where the ectopic focus secretes and enlarges.

The history suggests attacks of internal derangement and, when the joint line is palpated during full extension, the cyst is felt there as a small, hard swelling. If the knee is now bent, the little tumour disappears. Had the cyst lain outside the joint, unconnected with the meniscus, it would have been palpable with the knee flexed.

Since cartilage is avascular and cannot heal, a puncture hole made in the meniscus forms a permanent vent. Since the cysts are often multiple, the needle should be thrust in in several different directions, fanwise. This manoeuvre is curative unless the cartilage is also fractured. If so, excision is required.

## Torsion of the Infrapatellar Pad of Fat

This mimics a cyst of the meniscus. I have encountered only one case—a man of 52 who had had a painful knee for two months. Examination showed a small projection at the anterolateral aspect of the joint line. Exploration unexpectedly showed a pedunculated offshoot from the infrapatellar pad of fat instead of a meniscal cyst.

## Loose Body in Young Persons

Loose bodies, often multiple, form in the knee joint of young people as the result of osteochondrosis dissecans, chondromalacia patellae or chip-fractures. The loose bodies have an osseous nucleus and thus show on the radiograph. In osteochondrosis dissecans, the gap at the inner femoral condyle whence the loose body arose is also revealed.

The history is that of momentary locking *in extension*. The knee neither gives way nor does it have to be manipulatively unlocked after the attack; hence there is little resemblance to the sequence of events in meniscal tears. The patient says that, from time to time as he walks along, the knee suddenly locks and tends to pitch him forwards on to his face, since it is fixed straight just when he expects to bend it. He is halted in mid-stride by pain within the joint; he may fall. When he tries to flex his knee again, he finds he can move it quite well, and walks on. The knee aches and swells a little for a few days. The pain may vary in position if, as often happens, the loose body moves to another part of the joint. Pain shifting from one side of the knee to the other can be due only to a loose body. Rarely the loose fragment is a foreign body.

For a week or two after an attack of internal derangement, the knee is warm and contains fluid, and clinical examination reveals no localized lesion, merely a subsiding traumatic arthritis. Occasionally, a loose body can be felt moving about in the suprapatellar pouch. In chondromalacia patellae, when the patella is pushed to one side and its posterior aspect palpated, the gap whence the loose body arose may be felt.

## Loose Body Pressing on the Tibial Nerve

On rare occasions a loose body lying at the back of the knee joint impinges against the tibial nerve. The patient complains of attacks suggesting internal derangement at the knee and also of intermittent numbness of the posterior two-thirds of the sole of the foot and the adjacent surfaces of the big and second toes. Vague aching may be felt in the thigh.

The symptoms are abolished by manipulative reduction at the knee.

## Loose Body Complicating Osteoarthrosis

Whereas minor degrees of osteoarthrosis of the knee cause no symptoms, the fact that crepitating osteoarthrosis is present means that articular cartilage is roughened. A small piece may flake off; it would be interesting to know if the loose body originates from a meniscus or the articular cartilage itself. Such a loose fragment usually occupies a harmless position at the back of the joint; however, it may move and come to lie impacted between the articular surfaces. The history is typical.

A middle-aged or elderly patient states that for no apparent reason swelling and *localized* pain has arisen at one knee. He may wake up with it, or as he is walking along suddenly find that each step hurts. If, as commonly happens, the loose fragment lies at the inner side of the knee, it occupies space there, between the femur and tibia. When the articular surfaces are approximated as the knee approaches full extension, they are held apart by the presence of the displaced fragment. This overstretches the medial collateral ligament. Clinical examination reveals chronic strain of the ligament but inquiry makes it clear that no such injury has occurred. The deduction is that the ligament has been strained by an intrinsic, not extrinsic, factor. If a sprain exists but has not resulted from external force, it can arise only from within the joint. All patients, especially middle-aged, who have a sprained ligament or a traumatic arthritis in the absence of any history of injury, should at once be regarded as suffering from this type of internal derangement. It is quite a common condition, recognizable only clinically but the diagnostic principle is clear and simple—a sprain without a sprain. This view has since been corroborated by Helfet (1963) who states that 'most traumatic arthritis of the knee in middle-aged and elderly people is due to minor derangements of the menisci. . . .'

The pain is usually at the inner side of the joint, sometimes at the outer side, sometimes felt 'right inside'—never all over. If it moves from one side of the joint to the other, the diagnosis is obvious. Sometimes the pain spreads up the outer side of the thigh and down the leg in a way suggesting a sciatic distribution. The patient is afraid to go downstairs and does so a step at a time for fear of a sudden twinge which makes the knee suddenly give way. Such twinges and the same feeling of instability are experienced less often during ordinary walking; they indicate momentary subluxations of the loose body.

The signs vary with the position of the loose fragment and may be difficult to interpret. The knee is often warm to the touch, and warmer on the painful aspect of the joint than elsewhere. Osteoarthrosis is a cold degeneration of a joint; the mere presence of warmth proves that uncomplicated osteoarthrosis is not a sufficient diagnosis. If the joint is not warm, the examination proceeds. At the end, the palpation is repeated and it is often then noted that the minor stresses imposed on the joint merely by examining its range of movement have given rise to local warmth, lasting only a minute or two. Fluid is often present in the joint, whether it is warm or not. The following possible findings suggest an impacted cartilaginous body. (1) Non-capsular pattern. Naturally if extension is, say, 5° limited but flexion of full range, a block and not arthritis is present in the joint. Again, if extension is full and painless, but flexion markedly limited by an articular lesion, internal derangement is suspected at once. Such obvious non-capsular findings are uncommon, but were the signs that originally drew my attention to his hitherto undescribed condition. (2) Flexion at the knee is slightly limited, but it is localized pain, not the supervention of muscle spasm that limits range. In other words, the movement does not come to a characteristic hard stop; it feels as if it will go farther; the limiting factor is pain. (3) Varus strain hurts at the inner side of the joint. A space-occupying lesion lies medially. (4) Localized pain at the extreme of range, warmth, fluid in the joint, no synovial thickening—these are the signs of a sprained knee, and indeed, the medial collateral ligament is usually very tender at the joint line. The conclusion is that this ligament is being strained. It is; but if the cause is not external violence, it must lie within the joint. This inference is correct; a small cartilaginous body has suddenly displaced itself towards the inner side of the joint and, every time the endeavour is made to extend the knee, the ligament is strained by the existence of a space-occupying body between tibia and femur.

At this age, some X-ray evidence of osteoarthrosis is bound to be seen at both knees, and the loose body, being almost always composed entirely of cartilage, does not show. If it has an osseous nucleus, the correct diagnosis is, of course, made. The most elementary error is thus to ignore the sudden onset, the fluid, warmth and localized pain and tenderness, and regard the patient as suffering from osteoarthrosis of the knee, because that is what the radiograph shows. A more reasonable error is to make a diagnosis of medial ligament strain complicating osteoarthrosis. This is factually correct, but omits to specify the actual cause and leads to futile treatment of the secondary phenomenon—the ligamentous strain.

Some authorities describe 'acute episodes' punctuating the progress of what they call 'osteoarthrosis'. The actual cause is this type of minor recurrent internal derangement. The loose body sets up no symptoms as long as it lies at the back of the joint, where there is plenty of room for it. If it moves anteriorly it engages between the articular surfaces and pain results. This phenomenon may continue for several years; yet manipulative reduction may well prove possible in one session.

## Monarticular Rheumatoid Arthritis

The patient complains of the gradual onset of unprovoked swelling in one or both knees, at first painless. Then the knee begins to ache all over. If the patient is under 40, the diagnosis suggests itself. A Brodie's abscess close to the joint may simulate this type of arthritis but is excluded by radiography.

Palpation of the joint reveals diffuse warmth, fluid and, sooner or later, synovial thickening. In the early case, these marked local signs contrast strongly with the discovery of a full and virtually painless range of movement at the knee. In any other disorder, such pronounced signs at the knee itself would have implied markedly restricted movement. Later on, limitation of movement of the capsular pattern supervenes. If the presence of fluid interferes with palpation of the synovial edge, the joint should be aspirated and palpated again.

Inflammatory arthritis may complicate subacute gonorrhoea, gout, ankylosing spondylitis, ulcerative colitis, Reiter's disease (non-specific urethritis) or psoriasis and is the first joint affected as a rule in pseudogout. It may also herald spondylitis, the sacroiliac joints becoming affected only some years later.

If the arthritis attacks one or more toes as well, and the knee is not improved by intra-articular triamcinolone, Reitér's disease is very probably present. If a middle-aged woman is found to have arthritis in both knees together with swelling of the hands and ankles, sarcoidosis should be suspected. Far more often, however, the arthritis is not secondary to any other disease, thus belonging to the rheumatoid group. *Villous arthritis* is merely another name for advanced arthritis with great synovial thickening. In cases of doubt, Henry (1977) advises arthroscopic removal of biopsy material.

In middle-aged patients, the distinction between monarticular rheumatoid arthritis and osteoarthritis with an impacted loose body may prove very difficult. In either case, the joint is warm and contains fluid, but in rheumatoid arthritis the pain and warmth are equal all over the joint. The radiograph naturally shows osteophyte formation, as in any patient of that age, and is thus actively misleading. In rheumatoid arthritis affecting one large joint, the sedimentation rate is seldom raised—another misleading finding. Rheumatoid arthritis does not cause sudden twinges, but secondary wasting of the quadriceps muscle may make the patient complain that the knee feels weak, and that stairs are difficult for him. However, in a loose body, the onset is sudden, the pain is localized and twinges a prominent feature. After recovery, both disorders are apt to recur.

The only certain criterion is synovial thickening, a slight degree of which is most difficult to be sure about, particularly when the patient is a middle aged woman whose subcutaneous tissues are already somewhat thickened. Since treatment is on entirely different lines in the two cases, the distinction is vital.

## Haemarthrosis

Occasionally, the patient is an adolescent youth with a minor tendency to haemophilia. If so, suspicion is aroused by the triviality or absence of causative trauma. Blood often fills the joint, in either sex, after direct contusion without fracture; or it may come on, apparently spontaneously, in the elderly, presumably as the result of rupture of an intra-articular vein.

The patient states that the knee suddenly became very painful and swollen, filling up in a few minutes. The speed of appearance of the effusion and the severe pain by far exceed that caused by clear fluid; for blood fills the joint rapidly and is a strong irritant. About half of all haemophiliac articular effusions occur at the knee.

In severe cases the patient walks in on crutches, his knee bent up, unable to put foot to ground. The knee is hot and distended to its utmost with fluid. Examination reveals 45° limitation of extension, 90° limitation of flexion. This limitation of movement is unaltered after some weeks in bed. Aspiration reveals the cause of the trouble at once. If haemophilia is suspected, a vial of Russell viper venom for local application should be at hand in case oozing from the skin puncture proves troublesome.

In less marked haemarthrosis, the patient can hobble along, but palpation of the joint shows it to be warm and very tense with fluid, far more so than when the effusion is clear. Examination shows considerable limitation of movement of the capsular pattern and aspiration confirms the diagnosis.

## Intra-articular Adhesion

This is a rare and remarkable condition. After what appears an unexceptional sprain or operation at the inner side of the knee (e.g. the removal of an osteoma at the medial femoral condyle), the knee progressively stiffens almost painlessly, in spite of vigorous physiotherapy. The patient complains of inability to flex the knee, e.g. in walking upstairs; this increases as the days go by, but there is hardly any discomfort. After say, a fortnight, the knee retains 90° of flexion range; after a month, only 45°.

This uncommon disorder is brought to mind when, after an injury, the joint is cold, not swollen, devoid of intra-articular fluid, and yet on examination has a full range of extension and 90 to 135° limitation of flexion. The discrepancy between such gross limitation of movement and the absence of local articular signs is diagnostic. The radiograph does not reveal a Stieda–Pellegrini shadow. No amount of forcing while the patient lies supine is effective. However, if the patient is turned to lie prone and the knee forced towards flexion (see Volume II) there is a loud sound as of tearing silk and full flexion is achieved at once.

## Subsynovial Haematoma

This is the result of a severe blow on the front of the thigh, just above the knee, followed by pain, swelling and disablement.

The knee is swollen and warm; if aspirated the fluid is often blood-stained. Extension is of full range and only slightly painful; flexion on the other hand is at least 90° limited. Resisted extension is painless. These findings indicate a localized articular lesion affecting the front only of the joint; palpation reveals a haematoma lying between the femur and the suprapatellar pouch. During the first few days, aspiration, not of the fluid in the joint, but by passing the needle backwards till it reaches bone, confirms this diagnosis. Later, the blood coagulates and cannot be withdrawn.

## Posterior Capsular Lesions

### Capsular Strain

The patient describes a severe hyperextension sprain of the knee from which he has never fully recovered, the joint swelling and aching for several days after exercise. The pain is behind or all over the knee, not on one side only as in a ligamentous injury.

If there has been recent exertion, the knee is warm and contains fluid. Examination shows that only full passive extension hurts. Stretching the anterior cruciate ligament is painless. Occasionally, the radiograph shows one or two linear calcified streaks at the posterior aspect of the joint.

### Capsular Rupture

Long-standing rheumatoid arthritis of the knee with chronic distension of the joint with fluid weakens the posterior ligaments, which may rupture during exertion (Baker 1877). The fluid now extravasates into the upper calf, causing sudden pain at the back of the knee. The venous return is impeded and the foot becomes very oedematous in a manner suggesting venous thrombosis. The sudden onset and the swelling at the popliteal space and upper calf should lead to immediate aspiration of the swelling (if it is fluctuant) or via the knee joint itself (if fluctuation in the calf cannot be detected).

## Osteoarthrosis

Although minor degrees of osteophyte formation do not give rise to symptoms unless a loose body forms and moves, gross osteoarthrosis causes pain as soon as articular cartilage wears through. This is apt to happen if the patient suffered repeatedly from attacks of internal derangement due to a torn meniscus that was never excised. Even if it is removed, the load-bearing of the meniscus ceases and the pressure of the curved femoral surface on the flat tibial condyle is exerted over 1 sq. cm instead of 6 sq. cm (Seedom 1980). Hence the joint is very apt to wear out prematurely. Alternatively, a marked valgus deformity has been present since youth, the result of rickets or an old mal-united fracture, and shearing strain on the joint has worn both the meniscus and the layer of articular cartilage through (on the outer side in genu valgum). Alternatively, the knee is often affected in osteitis deformans.

Osteoarthrosis of the knee is considered very common. It is not; it is rare, but is frequently mistakenly diagnosed. What incorrectly receives this label is monarticular rheumatoid arthritis or an impacted loose body, when either occurs in a middle-aged or elderly patient with osteophytes misleadingly visible radiologically: a normal phenomenon at that age.

In uncomplicated osteoarthrosis, the characteristic features are a cold joint, devoid of synovial thickening, and a hard and painless end-feel. Osteophytes can often be seen and palpated. Extension is a few degrees limited, the movement ending abruptly by bone hitting bone. Flexion may be 60 or 90° limited, the movement again coming to a sudden dead stop. An attempt to increase range is not so much painful as felt to be futile owing to bony contact. In gross osteoarthrosis, marked limitation of movement of the capsular pattern combines with the intermittent creaking of bone against bone. The same signs without any discomfort indicate a neurogenic arthropathy, nearly always tabetic.

## Chondrocalcinosis

Pseudogout is brought to mind when recurrent attacks of pain and limited movement come on suddenly without apparent cause, lasting one to four weeks. This is too long for palindromic rheumatism and too short a duration for the other types of rheumatoid arthritis or gout itself (untreated). Examination of aspirated fluid reveals crystals of pyrophosphate rather than urates. McCarty et al. (1962) showed that both sodium urate and calcium pyrophosphate crystals caused acute arthritis when injected into the knee joint. Attacks of pseudogout also occur in patients with chronic renal failure who are kept alive by intermittent dialysis (Caner & Decker 1964), since uric acid dialyses less readily than urea. Their analysis showed that the knee contained calcium and phosphates with negligible amounts of urates. Sooner or later, linear calcification of articular cartilage or meniscus makes its appearance radiographically and settles the diagnosis.

### Neurogenic Arthropathy

Painless severe disorganization of the knee joint with huge osteophytes whose engagement caused gross limitation of movement was not uncommon early this century as the result of tertiary syphilis. The tabetic gait and lack of discomfort were characteristic. Such cases no longer present themselves in this country.

## UPPER TIBIOFIBULAR JOINT

This joint is examined at the same time as the knee. It is seldom affected, but a blow may strain the ligaments holding the head of the fibula to the tibia. A spontaneously appearing lesion is rare.

The patient complains of localized pain at the outer side of the knee, just below the joint line. On examination the knee joint is normal, but when resisted flexion and lateral rotation are tested, contraction of the biceps elicits the pain by pulling the fibula backwards, especially if the movement is carried out with the knee at a right angle. When the biceps tendon is examined for tenderness, none is found. This rare disorder is then brought to mind, and the tibiofibular ligament—usually the anterior—is tender. One infiltration of triamcinolone is usually curative.

## DISORDERS OF QUADRICEPS MECHANISM

### Recurrent Dislocation of the Patella

If an accurate history is not obtained, dislocation of the patella is easily mistaken for meniscal trouble at the knee; for both are a type of internal derangement. However, the condition begins in childhood, between the ages of 8 and 15, i.e. before the age of rupture of a meniscus. The youngster complains that the knee suddenly and painfully gives way; he falls to the ground and feels that something is out of place at his knee; he straightens his leg, there is a loud click and his knee is serviceable once more. The knee swells and hurts afterwards for some days. Sooner or later, the incident recurs.

Examination may show a genu valgum deformity or poor development of the lateral condyle of the femur. With rare exceptions, the dislocation is outwards. The disorder is distinguished by the following tests: (*a*) the infrapatellar tendon is elongated and the patella correspondingly hypermobile; (*b*) for some weeks after an attack, tenderness is present at the medial aspect of the patella; (*c*) the patella is pushed laterally with the leg in full extension. As the patella approaches the position where it will slip over the lateral femoral condyle, the patient suddenly contracts his quadriceps muscle and brings the patella back. If the patella were not apt to dislocate, the patient would have no fear of such pressure and thus would not use the quadriceps muscle to avert displacement.

### Patellar–Femoral Arthrosis

In young patients, the knee is merely stated to ache anteriorly walking upstairs, after a long walk or skiing. Elderly patients complain of the same anterior ache but also say that the knee grates loudly. Walking upstairs hurts more than on the flat.

Erosion of the cartilage at the medial edge of the patella may start before the age of 20, and has been shown present in three-quarters of individuals by the age of 30.

Examination on the couch reveals nothing since this tests only the unaffected tibiofemoral joint; even moving the patella up and down against the femur does not cause more than a commonplace feeling of roughness. The patellar–femoral joint must be examined during weight-bearing, when the pull of the quadriceps applies the patella strongly to the femoral condyles. Hence, it is only when the patient is asked to stand and bend his knees that the familiar pain is brought on and the examiner's hand placed on the patella feels the marked crepitus.

If this sign is found in young patients without a history of trauma, the cause is chondromalacia patellae; if it follows an injury, flake fracture of the articular surface of the patella is probably responsible. In either case, loose bodies may form; then it is attacks of internal derangement that bring the disorder to light. If the loose body present in the joint has no osseous centre, X-rays reveal no abnormality.

If crepitus is found in middle age, osteoarthrosis affecting the patellar–condylar joint is present. An old stellate fracture leads to enlargement of the whole patella and incongruity of the opposed joint surfaces. Naturally, localized osteoarthrosis soon supervenes.

## Lesions of the Quadriceps Bellies

The patient makes a correct diagnosis himself, stating that while running or jumping he was brought up short by feeling something give way painfully at the front of his thigh. Afterwards he could walk only slowly and with a limp.

In quadriceps rupture the hip joint is normal. The knee joint is normal too except that flexion is slightly or greatly restricted, depending on the size of the rupture. If the patient is asked to lie prone (thus keeping his hip extended) marked limitation of knee flexion is found when the two sides are compared; for the upper end of the muscle remains taut in his position. Resisted extension of the knee hurts but is not weak. The tender area and the haematoma are palpable, usually at mid-thigh. This condition has been called 'cricket-leg' and mistakenly attributed to rupture of the sartorius muscle.

Major rupture occurs just above the suprapatellar tendon and may amount to complete separation. The swelling just above the knee is obvious, and palpation reveals the gap in the muscle. Resisted extension is very weak as well as painful; sometimes the patient cannot voluntarily straighten the knee against the mere resistance of the weight of the leg.

*Adherence.* When the belly of the quadriceps muscle has become adherent to the mid-shaft of the femur at the site of a fracture, limitation of flexion at the knee to 90° is a commonplace. The other knee movements are of full range—i.e. the extra-articular type of limitation of movement is present.

*Weakness of the Quadriceps Muscles.* If both muscles are weak and wasted, but there is no pain on resisted extension of the knee, the rest of the nervous system must be examined. If no other abnormality is found, the diagnoses to be considered are:

1. Spinal tumour or metastases at the third lumbar level.
2. Myopathy.
3. Myositis.

The electromyogram is helpful and if myositis is suspected biopsy should be undertaken. In myositis and sarcoidosis, granulomatous foci are seen, and in the former case treatment by cortisone arrests the disease.

## Lesions about the Patella

### Fracture

A patient with a fractured patella may walk in complaining merely of pain in the knee following either a fall on to the front of his knee (stellate fracture) or indirect violence (transverse fracture). If the capsule enclosing the patella is not ruptured, displacement is avoided and disability is often deceptively slight.

The knee is warm to the touch and is tense with blood. The passive movements hurt and are much limited by the haemarthrosis. Resisted extension is markedly weak as well as painful. This association of articular with quadriceps signs shows that the lesion partly involves the joint, and partly that section of the quadriceps mechanism overlying the knee, in other words, the patella. Local tenderness and radiography are confirmative.

### Tendinitis

This occurs at three sites: at the suprapatellar tendon, at the quadriceps expansion to either side of the patella, and at the infrapatellar tendon. The history is merely of pain at the front of the knee on walking, especially upstairs. It is uncommon except in athletes, ballet dancers and the one-legged; the latter are very apt to strain the patellar mechanism as they step downstairs.

The knee joint is normal; only resisted extension is uncomfortable. Palpation reveals the site of the lesion. The tendons are always affected at the tenoperiosteal junction and the same applies to the quadriceps expansion which becomes strained only at its insertion at the edge of the patella.

### Apophysitis

Boys aged 10 to 15 may develop osteochondrosis of the tibial tuberosity (Schlatter's disease) or, rarely, of the lower epiphysis of the patella. In either case, local pain elicited by a resisted extension movement is the only positive finding; the site of tenderness is distinctive. The age of the patient should lead to radiography. Spontaneous recovery often takes two years.

## Strained Iliotibial Band

This lesion appears confined to athletes. While running, he notices an increasing pain at the outer side of his knee, and usually has to drop out of the race. He rests a week, then runs again. This time the pain comes on sooner and is more severe; the next day, walking hurts. Thereafter, he cannot run fast or far.

Examination reveals no lesion of the knee joint or its ligaments, but discomfort is felt when extension and lateral rotation are carried out against resistance. Resisted flexion is painless. The tender spot is found at and just below the joint line, between the infrapatellar tendon and the fibular collateral ligament.

# DISORDERS OF MUSCLE

## Hamstrings

When the knee joint is normal but resisted flexion of the knee hurts in the thigh, the fault lies in the hamstrings. If it affects the muscle bellies and is of any severity, straight-leg raising is limited. Pain also on resisted lateral rotation incriminates the biceps muscle. The area of induration of muscle suffused with blood is tender and swollen. If the pain is at the knee, the bicipital tendon close to the head of the fibula may be at fault. Should resisted medial rotation hurt at the knee, strain of the semimembranosus tendon at the groove on the tibia is a possibility.

It must not be forgotten that there exist two disorders in which resisted flexion of the knee hurts without any disorder of the hamstring muscles. In each, the resisted movement hurts if the knee is (as is usual) bent to a right angle for this test. If the resisted movement is carried out with the knee almost fully extended, no pain is evoked.

### Posterior Cruciate Ligament

Contraction of the hamstrings pulls the tibia backwards on the femur, painfully straining the posterior cruciate ligament. The pain, however, is felt within the knee joint, and articular signs are present.

### Upper Tibiofibular Joint

If the biceps muscle contracts while the knee is bent, the head of the fibula is drawn backwards, straining the ligaments that attach it to the tibia. Tenderness is absent at the biceps tendon but present at the upper tibiofibular ligament.

## Strained Popliteus Muscle

The patient sprains the back of his knee in an undistinctive way; the position of pain suggests a lesion of the posterior cruciate ligament. Indeed, ligamentous strain is closely simulated by popliteus tendinitis. When an individual squats, the femur is prevented from sliding forwards not only by the posterior cruciate ligaments, but also by contraction of the popliteus muscle. Hence tendinitis here gives rise to pain felt on full flexion during weight-bearing; a movement that might well be regarded as stretching an inert structure only, since the knee is moved passively.

Examination shows that the knee joint itself is normal, but that resisted flexion and resisted medial rotation hurt posteriorly. The semimembranosus and semitendinosus tendons are not tender; only the popliteus remains.

Tenderness is sought along the muscle from the emergence of the tendon under the lateral ligament of the knee, at and just above the joint line, to the back of the upper tibia.

The tendon responds well to massage or triamcinolone, the belly to deep massage only.

# BURSITIS AT THE KNEE

Prepatellar bursitis causes pain felt at the front of the knee, chiefly on kneeling. The knee and its muscles are normal. Pinching up the tissues between patella and skin reveals a fluctuant swelling. Local heat without redness suggests haemorrhage into the bursa; if so the swelling is very tense and aspiration reveals blood. Marked local heat with thickening of the bursal wall, both disappearing within a month, characterizes chondrocalcinosis. The aspirated fluid should be tested for pyrophosphate crystals. Local heat accompanied by reddening of the skin implies a septic bursitis. Bilateral bursitis is said to be an occasional manifestation of tertiary syphilis.

The semimembranosus bursa seldom communicates with the joint. A bulging bursa does not give rise to symptoms, though a swelling at the back of the knee and pain felt there invite the patient to associate the two. In case of doubt, it should be aspirated and the patient thus shown that emptying the bursa does not alter the pain. The knee should be re-examined at once while the bursa, which soon fills up again, is empty.

## THE RADIOGRAPH

Radiography is not often informative at the knee joint; indeed, as elsewhere, its value is largely negative. Evidence of osteophyte formation, unless gross, affords no guarantee that the symptoms are due to osteoarthrosis. Careful post-mortem and radiological research in normal subjects (Bennett et al. 1942) showed that superficial fraying of the articular cartilage begins at the knee joint during a person's twenties. Roughening and splitting at the weight-bearing areas follow, but extensive erosion has to occur before the radiological appearances alter. Lipping, they found, appears during most people's forties. It is clear from these painstaking observations no less than from clinical experience that, except in gross disease, the clinical examination of the knee, not the inspection of the radiograph, alone decides the presence or absence of arthritis. If arthritis is present clinically, the radiograph may assist the attempt to determine the type of joint lesion present. Even here its value is limited, for in early rheumatoid and inflammatory arthritis the appearances are normal. Alternatively, such arthritis may come on at an age when osteophyte formation is already visible; the radiograph is then misleading. Later on, arthritis is shown as a general decalcification of the bone ends; finally, secondary disorganization of the joint with osteophyte formation is seen, but the lesion remains clinically rheumatoid.

Erosion of cartilage is shown as a thinning of the joint line. Ossification and calcification in capsule or ligament may be relevant findings. Meniscal deposits in pseudogout show well. Loose bodies within the joint are visible on the radiograph only if they contain bone or are foreign, e.g. glass. Fractures, osteochondrosis dissecans, abscess in the bone, tuberculous disease, neoplasm and osteitis deformans are clearly seen.

In soft tissue lesions, or in rupture or cyst formation of a meniscus, the radiographic appearances are normal. Air arthrography can disclose the split in a meniscus or an otherwise invisible loose body. The Stieda–Pellegrini shadow takes 3 to 4 weeks to appear. In doubtful cases arthroscopy is useful.

## TREATMENT AT THE KNEE

Nearly all lesions at the knee respond well to treatment. Accurate diagnosis with accurate physiotherapy gives the happiest results.

### Arthritis

Early osteoarthrosis causes no symptoms to speak of unless a small fragment of cartilage becomes impacted between the articular surfaces. If osteoarthrosis is gross enough itself to cause symptoms, no conservative treatment helps. Osteotomy of the tibia just below the knee joint relieves pain lastingly in a high proportion of cases, probably by abating the intraosseous venous congestion that so often causes nocturnal pain. Alternatively, hinge-arthroplasty may be required.

Monarticular rheumatoid arthritis often clears up after two or three intra-articular injections of 5 ml of triamcinolone suspension, not only in the early case, but even after some years' increasing trouble. Working in Mexico, Gil and Katona's (1971) endoscopic colour photographs show clearly the subsidence of inflammation within the knee after a steroid injection into it. If triamcinolone is ineffective in what appears a monarticular rheumatoid case, Reiter's disease should be considered.

The arthritis that heralds or complicates spondylitis ankylopoetica, psoriasis or lupus erythematosus responds well to triamcinolone. Pseudogout is best treated by an immediate intra-articular injection of triamcinolone. Phenylbutazone (200 mg four times a day during the acute phase) is prescribed.

In advanced villous arthritis, X-ray therapy or synovectomy should be considered if steroid injection fails. Reiter's arthritis is intractable, although tetracycline is usually given for the urethritis.

Considerable doubt on the reputed dangers of intra-articular steroid injections into weight-bearing joints has been thrown by Balch et al.'s observations. They examined 65 cases of osteoarthritis and rheumatoid arthritis at the knee which has received a minimum of 15 and a maximum of 167 monthly injections during 4 to 15 years. In 15 there was no change, and of these 3 had had over 100, another 3 over 50 injections into the joint. In 38 deterioration was minimal to moderate, in 10 marked, and in 2 gross. The 2 with gross aggravation had received over 80 injections each in the course of 7 years. It would seem, therefore, that the perils of steroid injections at least into the knee joint have been much exaggerated.

## Ligamentous Sprain

The principle of treatment is the attainment of healing in the presence of adequate movement. This is achieved by methods differing according to the time that has elapsed since the accident.

### Acute Stage

During the first few days after a sprain, triamcinolone injection is the treatment of choice and shortens the acute phase by aborting excessive local reaction to injury. The site of the tear should be infiltrated with 1 or 2 ml of suspension of triamcinolone as soon as the patient is seen. A thin needle 2 cm long suffices. The patient walks away. A few days later he should attend for the treatment suited to subacute sprain. However, many athletes refuse steroid infiltrations for fear of interference with firm union, and thus (possibly rightly) prefer massage. This is the alternative: deep friction, as from the first day, applied to the site of the rupture. This disengages any fibrils tethering the ligament to bone, without interfering with union of scar tissue longitudinally placed. So early on, no adhesions have formed, so that only a minute's friction is required to move the ligament adequately. But it may well take the physiotherapist some time, and recourse to gentle massage first, to enable the patient to accept such pressure as enables her actually to reach the ligament. No endeavour is made to straighten the knee, since the collateral ligaments are taut in extension, stretching the healing breach is clearly a disadvantage. For the first week, therefore, passive movements are avoided. In fact Burri et al. (1978) advise that for the first week the knee should not be allowed to straighten the last 20°, nor flex the last 60°. Research into the effect of zinc sulphate orally ought to be instituted.

### Subacute Stage

If several days have elapsed since the accident, deep massage should be given at once to the site of the minor tear in the ligament. This is essential in the coronary ligaments, for they do not span the joint. Hence, adequate movement cannot be imparted to the tibiomeniscal joint by merely moving the knee—the wrong joint—and recovery takes months if this method is adopted alone. But it is quite simple to move the ligament by drawing the finger to and fro across it (see Volume II); indeed, this way of maintaining or restoring mobility is the essential measure in coronary sprain. Similar considerations apply to the tibial collateral ligament when traumatic arthritis prevents flexion at the knee joint; the ligament cannot therefore be put through its full range. Thus unwanted scars soon bind the ligament down. Friction imitates the normal behaviour of the ligament, moving it to and fro over the bone at a time when the bone cannot be adequately moved to and fro under the ligament. The formation of adhesions is thus prevented by the movement imparted by the physiotherapist's finger. In either case the friction is followed by gentle forcing of movement to the point of discomfort but not of pain. Deep massage allows a large increase in movement to be obtained almost painlessly each day. The patient repeats the movements actively and is taught to walk slowly and carefully without a limp. Treatment should be continued until the range of movement at the knee is full and without discomfort.

Treatment which omits friction to the site of the tear usually takes months instead of weeks.

### Chronic Stage

This stage is never reached if the patient receives adequate treatment early on. The principle of treatment is to restore a full range of movement to the ligament by rupturing scar tissue binding it abnormally to bone. Deep friction to the affected part of the ligament moves it to and fro; forcing movement by a sharp jerk completes the mobilization. General anaesthesia is scarcely ever necessary. When the uppermost (non-mobile) part of the medial collateral ligament is affected, localized deep friction without forcing suffices. The sequence of events is illustrated in Fig. 117. Intra-articular adhesion is treated by a special manipulation (see Volume II).

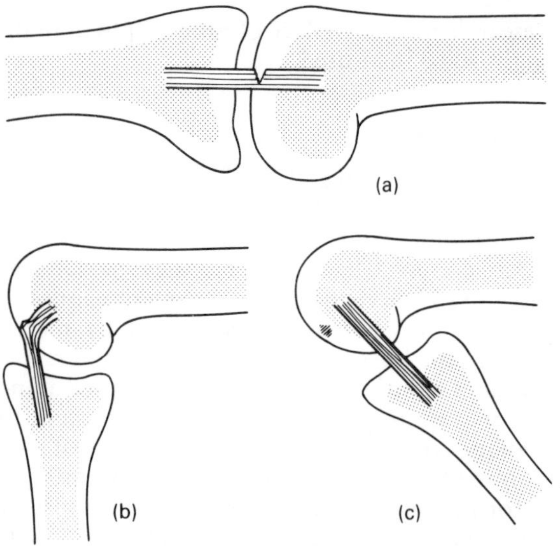


**Fig. 117.** Chronic strain of the medial collateral ligament. *a*, The patient rests with the knee held in extension. An adherent scar forms at the site of the tear, binding the ligament to the bone and restricting mobility. *b*, Limitation of flexion results from scarring. As flexion proceeds the ligament becomes progressively deformed and overstretched. *c*, Forcing full flexion at the knee frees the ligament from its abnormal attachment and a full range of movement is restored to the joint.

When the posterior cruciate ligament is the site of chronic strain, the lesion usually lies at the posterior attachment to the tibia. Infiltration with 2 ml of triamcinolone suspension must, therefore, be aimed at this point. The patient lies prone and the level of the joint line identified. A needle 5 cm long is inserted from one or other side, so as to avoid the popliteal artery. The centre of the back of the tibia is palpated with the tip of the needle, which is moved upwards until resistance is lost as it penetrates the knee joint. The needle is then moved back to the previous point, just below the articular edge of the tibia, and the infiltration given here (see Volume II). One well-placed injection is curative.

Chronic strain of the anterior cruciate ligament is rare and more difficult to treat, since the lesion may lie at either end of this ligament. If the patient feels the pain posteriorly, the medial aspect of the lateral condyle should be infiltrated by a posterior oblique approach. If he feels it right inside the knee, the anterior attachment just in front of the tibial spine should be injected. To this end, the knee is bent to a right angle and the needle inserted just below the lower pole of the patella and aimed at the centre of the upper surface of the tibia. In a difficult case, first one and then the other approach may have to be made (see Volume II).

### Lengthening of Ligaments

If this has occurred, permanent disability results. After sprain of the cruciate ligaments, the knee should be spared all strains until the traumatic arthritis subsides; this takes at least six months unless the ligaments can be correctly infiltrated with triamcinolone. If permanent lengthening results in sufficient disability, an operation depressing the tibial spine and thus indirectly shortening the ligament is indicated. Alternatively, the middle third of the patellar tendon and patella itself can be used to replace the lengthened ligament (Jones 1963). In Moscow, Mironova et al. (1970) replace a torn anterior ligament with a plastic band passed through tunnels drilled in tibia and femur, and knotted. In minor cases exercises to strengthen the quadriceps muscle help to stabilize the joint. Lengthening of the medial collateral ligament gives rise to an increased range of movement towards valgus at the knee, but remarkably little disability; surgical treatment is seldom required. Surgery has nothing to offer in Stieda–Pellegrini's disease; the treatment is expectant.

## Effusion

### Haemorrhage

Blood in the joint must be aspirated at once, and the remaining blood-tinged synovial effusion aspirated a few days later. Blood stays in the knee joint for months, causing severe arthritis owing to its strongly irritant effect on synovial membrane. It is also important to remove it at once on account of its erosive action on articular cartilage. In haemophilia, the presence of blood tends to dilate the blood vessels with which it lies in contact, thus leading to increased tendency to bleed; this enhances the liability to disintegration of cartilage. Hence aspiration should be carried out as soon as the patient is seen, in consultation with the haematologist. The cryoprecipitate method of preparing antihaemophilic globulin by freezing and thawing results in a much greater concentration of the missing factor than was previously possible. Out-patient injection of 20 ml of this precipitate replaces the large infusions that used to call for in-patient treatment.

A subperiosteal haematoma lying under the suprapatellar pouch should also be aspirated, to obviate months of disablement otherwise. If, as is apt to happen in the late case, the blood is no longer fluid, deep effleurage should be given all over the suprapatellar pouch for an hour daily for as many weeks as proves necessary, otherwise limitation of flexion can continue for more than a year.

### Clear Fluid

This designates the presence of an articular lesion at the knee and is a sign common to many disorders; it is a result, not a cause. 'Synovitis' at the knee is thus a symptom, not a diagnosis, and no reasonable treatment can be based on a diagnosis of 'synovitis of the knee'. Aspiration of a clear effusion is a waste of time; it is tapped only when a needle is inserted to discover whether an effusion is of blood or synovial fluid. The treatment of a clear effusion is to discover its cause (e.g. a sprained ligament, rheumatoid arthritis, internal derangement, gout) and to deal with that.

An effusion into the prepatellar bursa makes it impossible for the patient to kneel. It should therefore be aspirated at once. If due to haemorrhage it seldom returns. If a prepatellar bursa keeps filling up, and the provision of a soft rubber kneeling mat is ineffective, it should be excised.

## Intra-articular Displacement

The immediate measure is to reduce the displacement.

### Ruptured Meniscus

In the usual bucket-handle tear, it is the more deeply placed fragment that becomes displaced towards the centre of the joint, the superficial piece remaining in place on account of its continued attachment to the coronary ligament. Manipulative reduction (Hey 1803) is required. This is designed to allow the luxated fragment to slip back, over the dome of the femoral condyle, towards its proper bed. General anaesthesia is usually necessary, but it is often worth trying first without, especially in recurrent cases (see Volume II). An early record of manipulative reduction was in 1829 when a young American in Newport displaced the semilunar cartilage in his knee. All the doctors he consulted were agreed on the diagnosis and that nothing could be done but a bonesetter called John Sweet cured the condition by a twist towards lateral rotation and full flexion.

Splintage and conservative treatment after reduction are useless, since cartilage, having no blood supply, cannot unite; the after-treatment is that of an acute coronary sprain.

### Recurrent Displacement of Meniscus

Bonesetters, in particular the late Sir Herbert Barker, claim to cure this condition. Very occasionally they appear to succeed, but not by causing the fractured surfaces to join; this is impossible. Really forcible manipulation may complete the rupture in the meniscus and force the loosened half into the intercondylar notch. In this position, it no longer interferes with the articulating surfaces and if it stays there the patient has no more trouble; he is 'cured'. But this happy result is obtained so rarely that manipulation for recurrent meniscal dislocation is scarcely worth while. What bonesetters do in fact cure is chronic pain, i.e. adherent scars, at the tibial collateral ligament, and for the late stage of this condition forced movement is indubitably the correct treatment. The question is one of diagnosis. It is clearly undesirable and time-wasting to manipulate a joint repeatedly when there is every chance that it will finally require operation. Recurrent dislocation of either meniscus must be treated by excision (Annandale 1879).

Recognition of the importance of the meniscus as a load-spreading device has led to the revival of the operation, once regarded as obsolete, for removing only the torn part. This was first advocated by Robert Jones in 1909. Bonnin (1956) discussed the indications for partial meniscectomy and found the subsequent traumatic arthritis and the period of convalescence much diminished. An increasing number of surgeons have corroborated this view. Their results have thrown into prominence Dandy's (1978) method of closed removal via two puncture incisions under arthroscopic control. The patients spent only a day or two in hospital and were back at work in ten days. Bourne's (1980) experiments have shown that if only the loose central fragment of meniscus is removed, leaving the rim attached by the coronary ligament, no increase in weight-bearing stress on the tibia follows. Care should be taken not to confuse lengthening of the medial ligament with a torn meniscus. If the patient complains of instability of the knee when he flexes it in lateral rotation of the tibia, but of little pain, the range of lateral rotation on the two sides should be compared during prone-lying knee flexion. If excessive lateral rotation range caused by anterior movement of the inner condyle of the tibia is demonstrated, removal of the meniscus is apt to increase the disability.

Cyst formation at the meniscus can be treated by acupuncture; if the cyst contains fluid, cure may follow, since any puncture hole in cartilage remains patent indefinitely. Should this simple treatment fail, the meniscus should be excised, since many cystic menisci are also torn.

### Loose Bodies

The one or more loose bodies that are found in young person's knees should be removed as soon as possible, since the more attacks of internal derangement the knee suffers, the sooner osteoarthrosis is likely to set in.

Having an osseous centre, their position is revealed by the radiograph; since they may move, this should be taken immediately before the operation.

*Impacted Loose Body complicating Osteoarthrosis.* Such loose bodies are not suited to excision for a variety of reasons. They are usually wholly cartilaginous, and are thus not revealed by radiography. Being so small, it is doubtful if air arthrography would disclose them. The patient is old and the degenerate state of his joint precludes exploration. Manipulative disimpaction must, therefore, be carried out as often as the loose body moves and causes symptoms. Manipulation as for a dislocated semilunar cartilage is unsuccessful, because this type of loose body does not move unless the joint surfaces have been separated first. Thus the principle governing manipulation for this sort of displacement is performance during (*a*) ligamentous relaxation (i.e. in flexion) and (*b*) strong traction (see Volume II).

Recurrence is apt to follow kneeling or keeping the knee well bent for some time and the patient should be warned against this.

## Patellar Lesions

In patellar–femoral osteoarthrosis, the eroded bones present two rough surfaces and movement is naturally painful. These surfaces can be lubricated by silicone oil, which provides the only effective conservative treatment. The oil is very viscous, 12 000 centistoke, and cannot be expelled from an ordinary syringe via the usual bore needle. The piston has a screw-thread and a 14 gauge needle with a Luer lock is required (see Volume II); 10 ml are injected. This treatment was elaborated after experiments on rabbits had shown the oil to be wholly inert and to provoke no tissue reaction whatever (Helal & Karadi 1968), but they used a 200 centistoke oil, whereas a 50-times higher rating is to be preferred.

Operative removal of the patella is an effective treatment but some patients complain afterwards of permanent weakness. I find it difficult to believe that vertical excision of the central one-third of the patella would not prove successful. Union should proceed during ambulation, since weight-bearing would force the cut bony surfaces together. The edges of the narrowed bone would no longer reach the margins of the intercondylar notch where the femoral erosion is often located. Deliss (1977) obtained very good results in half the young men he operated on by coronal osteotomy. Recurrent dislocation is treated by operation in which the infrapatellar tendon is shortened and the tuberosity re-sited medially but this should be postponed until the epiphysis has closed at 14–15 years old, for fear of interfering with bone growth.

The tendons above and below the patella and the iliotibial band at the tibia recover with triamcinolone or deep massage. The quadriceps expansion responds only to deep massage, given by a special technique (see Volume II).

Fractured patella without separation requires aspiration of the haemarthrosis; with separation, the tear in the quadriceps expansion on either side should be sutured, and/or the patella wired. It is safe to wait a few days until the haemarthrosis has been dealt with and the traumatic arthritis has subsided.

## Tendons

A localized lesion is best infiltrated with triamcinolone. When the lesion is extensive, deep massage is preferred. If this cures, well and good; if a small point remains, this can be infiltrated. Tendons are nearly always strained at their tenoperiosteal junction; hence, the treatment—whether massage or injection—should be directed to this point (see Volume II). The quadriceps expansion at each side of the patella responds only to friction.

## Muscles

Major rupture requires operative suture. In minor rupture, as soon as the patient is seen, the lesion is infiltrated with 50 ml of 0.5% procaine solution. The next day, deep massage, then faradism, are given. Before the muscle is stimulated electrically, a posture is selected that fully relaxes it. For the hamstrings, full extension at the hip and full flexion at the knee must be maintained; for the quadriceps, considerable flexion at the hip and full extension at the knee. The contraction cannot now exert any tension on the healing breach and full broadening out of the belly is ensured.

The tendency to recurrence is considerable if the patient goes back to athletics too soon. Especially after a lesion of the hamstrings, the patient should continue treatment for a week after he is clinically well, and should not run hard for a month after the accident. Zinc sulphate may well prove to hasten union in these cases (see p. 15).

## Genu Valgum

If this persists beyond the age of 10, and the medial malleoli lie 5 cm apart or more, stapling the medial femoral epiphysis should be undertaken without delay. Correction takes about a year, whereupon the staple is removed.

After growth of bone has ceased, prophylactic supracondylar osteotomy is indicated. Even if no symptoms have yet arisen, by middle age, years of weight-bearing concentrated on the outer condyle of femur and tibia will lead to complete erosion of the meniscus and of articular cartilage there. Loss of tissue leads to gross arthritis with increase in the deformity and to pain from elongation of the medial ligament at the inner side and to bone impinging against bone at the outer side of the knee. If this has already occurred, some relief can be gained by throwing as much of the patient's body weight as possible on to the inner side of the knee. To this end he wears heels with a 0.5 cm inner wedge. Arthroplasty may be called for.

## Tibial Pseudarthrosis

The tibial shaft may never unite after a fracture. Pseudarthrosis is treated by a pulsed electromagnetic field. Three months' daily treatment secured union in nine out of ten cases (Bassett et al. 1981).

CHAPTER 25

# THE LEG AND THE ANKLE

The conditions that affect the leg are very simple. Diagnosis is seldom difficult. The only disorder which commonly gives rise to pain in the calf only without local cause is primary posterolateral protrusion of nuclear substance at the fifth lumbar level. The root pain is constant and remains unaltered by, e.g. standing on tiptoe. This finding naturally suggests that the pain is referred to the calf from a lesion at the proximal end of the first and second sacral segments.

Two conditions at the calf give rise to a characteristic history. Intermittent claudication presents as pain in the calf coming on after the individual has walked a certain distance, disappearing as soon as he rests and recurring as soon as he has again walked for the critical distance. In 'tennis leg' the pain in the calf comes on abruptly as the patient rises vigorously on tip-toe. Usually during a game of tennis, he feels a sudden pain resembling the lash of a whip at mid-calf and at once finds that pain prevents his putting one heel to the ground and that he has to hobble on tiptoe.

There are two other disorders that give rise to no physical signs at all—'growing pains' and angiokeratoma corporis.

## 'Growing Pains'

The common site for 'growing pains' is the legs; characteristically they are felt in the muscles, not the joints. Earlier this century, such symptoms in children were regarded as evidence of a rheumatic tendency involving the danger of myocarditis. They are common between the ages of 6 and 11—not the period of maximum speed of growth—and do not interfere with growth. Paediatricians' estimates of frequency vary from 4 to 20% of all children.

In a series of 213 patients, Naish and Apley (1951) found only two with organic disease, in only one of whom it was in the limb itself. Most authorities nowadays regard 'growing pains' as a psychogenic manifestation. If examination reveals the same multiple inconsistencies as adults offer, alternatively no physical signs and a normal sedimentation rate, these symptoms should lead to a domestic assessment.

## Angiokeratoma Corporis

This rare disease is brought to mind when a complaint is made of severe pains in hands and feet, spreading to forearms and calves as from earliest childhood. They have never stopped the patient doing anything and are not related to exertion or posture. Examination of the limbs reveals nothing, but inspection of the lower trunk reveals myriads of tiny dark pinpoint spots. These start to show about the age of 10; until then nothing suggests this diagnosis. Skin biopsy and the discovery of the characteristic corneal opacities settle the diagnosis. One such male patient with this disease had developed osteoarthrosis of the hips by the age of 46 but few reach that age, owing to increasing deposits of abnormal lipid in the small blood vessels throughout the body, especially in the kidney owing to deficiency of the enzyme alphagalactosidease A.

## GAIT

This should be observed as the patient walks in. In children who fall easily, a minor degree of spastic diplegia may be present. Various minor deviations of the lower limbs from the normal are often invoked to explain the child's instability—an idea that only watching the gait corrects.

## THE BONES

Inspection reveals the shape of the bones; palpation discloses the nature of their surface, sometimes warmth. Unilateral genu valgum or varum is pathological but bilateral deformity is normal.

Both tibiae are curved inward at birth, as a result of the ordinary intrauterine position. This bowing becomes gradually obliterated and by the age of 2 the tibia has straightened. Now knock knees replace the previous bow legs. This developmental genu valgum reaches its maximum at about 4 years of age and it is not until the age of 6 that the legs are once more as aligned as at the age of 2. If the distance between the malleoli with the legs extended is less than 5 cm, no treatment is called for. If it is between 5 and 10 cm, an inner wedge to the heel and sole is advocated by Sharrard (1976).

In almost every child, a slight *outward rotation* in the course of the tibia comes on during growth. This makes the midline of the foot point slightly laterally to the sagittal axis of the knee. In consequence, adults 'turn their feet out'. However, this twist may become exaggerated. If it is towards lateral rotation, the youngster is bad at games; for, when the foot is not kept in line with the direction in which the individual moves, he loses a few centimetres at every stride he takes. Short calf muscles, especially when associated with a plantaris deformity of the forefoot, prevent use of the foot in the sagittal plane, and the child tends to turn his foot more and more outwards; lateral rotation is forced on the growing tibia which, in due course, becomes shaped that way.

Occasionally the twist is reversed and during growth for no clear reason the tibia grows towards *inward rotation.* This is called 'pigeon-toes', but it is a misnomer, since the deformity arises not at the foot but in the course of the tibia.

Genu valgum in children persisting after the age of 6 is often the result of congenital inversion of the forefoot (Plate XLVIII). Nowadays, genu valgum due to vitamin D deficiency is almost as rare as renal rickets.

A varus deformity of the tibia with rounding of its anterior edge occurs in osteitis deformans. The front of the leg is often warm. The patient is elderly and the bowing is of recent onset. Radiography confirms the diagnosis.

Traumatic periostitis of the subcutaneous surface of the tibia may prove rather obstinate, the patient presenting himself after he has forgotten the blow. He will, however, indicate the right place, where tenderness of the periosteum together with irregularity of its surface will be found. Sometimes fluctuation from effused blood can be elicited. Post-traumatic osteoporosis occurs, the foot becoming a deep purple when dependent. Syphilitic periostitis of the tibia is very rare nowadays. In dermatomyositis atrophic glossy skin becomes attached to hard and immobile muscles, contracture of which prevents movement at the ankle joint.

### Treatment

If the child is suffering from rickets, this must, of course, be treated. Apart from that, the tibia vara of babies and genu valgum of young children should be left to correct itself. If the genu valgum is secondary to inversion of the forefoot, this must be energetically treated at once. If genu valgum persists after the age of 10, it should not be allowed to continue; for arthritis of the knee with gross erosion of the lateral tibial and femoral condyles ensues in middle age. The medial femoral epiphysis should be stapled at about the age of 10. If the patient is seen later, after bone growth has ceased, femoral osteotomy is required. Rotation in the course of the tibia can be corrected only by osteoclasis, which is best postponed until the child is at least 8 years old. The subsidence of traumatic periostitis is hastened by deep effleurage. Blood is absorbed very slowly from under the periosteum and is apt to leave thickening that remains tender for months. Aspiration is therefore indicated if fluctuation can be elicited. In osteitis deformans, severe pain warrants etidronate therapy.

## THE MUSCLES AND TENDONS

### Painful Plantiflexor Muscles

The muscles are examined next. First the patient stands and is asked to rise on tiptoe. Then he lies supine and dorsiflexion, eversion and inversion are tested against resistance. Note is made whether the movement is painful or painless, strong or weak.

If rising on tiptoe hurts, the calf muscles are at fault. In such cases, the following test distinguishes between the soleus and gastrocnemius muscles. The patient lies prone and plantiflexion of the foot is resisted, first with his knee fully extended, then while flexed to a right angle. Bending the knee relaxes the femoral extremity of the gastrocnemius muscle but does not alter the strain on the soleus muscle; hence, abolition of pain when the movement is tested during knee flexion incriminates the gastrocnemius muscle. This is the likelihood, nearly all minor ruptures occurring in the belly of this muscle.

If the upper calf is swollen after a severe strain during athletics or a direct blow, a haematoma should be sought and, if fluctuant, aspirated. When, however, the upper calf is swollen, in the absence of an injury, in a patient with long-standing rheumatoid arthritis at the knee, posterior capsular rupture with extravasation of synovial fluid into the upper calf has taken place (described by Baker in 1877 as a chronic synovial cyst). Tait et al. (1965) have shown by arthrography that the fluid escapes between the semimembranosus and semitendinosus tendons on one side and the quadriceps muscle laterally. If so, the venous return from the foot is much embarrassed and the foot becomes oedematous in a manner suggesting venous thrombosis. The diagnosis can be confirmed by contrast arthrography and aspiration is required at once.

## Tennis Leg

This disorder has for years been regarded as a ruptured plantaris tendon, but the physical signs present at once show this ascription to be false; the lesion almost always lies in the gastrocnemius muscle. The patient describes sudden pain in the calf and hobbles in, tiptoeing on the affected side. Examination reveals pain on plantiflexion against resistance but no weakness. Dorsiflexion at the ankle is markedly restricted, owing to localized spasm of the muscle about the ruptured fibres. Bending the knee increases the range of dorsiflexion obtainable at the ankle; an instance of the constant length phenomenon. Were the plantaris tendon ruptured, the foot could not be fixed in plantiflexion nor would resisted plantiflexion be painful. Palpation of the calf reveals either (*a*) a tender area in the gastrocnemius muscle, usually some 5 cm above the musculotendinous junction and rather to the inner side of the belly, or (*b*) in more severe cases, a palpable gap in much the same situation about 1 cm wide.

As soon as the patient is seen, whether it is the same day or some weeks later, local anaesthesia should be induced at the site of the partial rupture. The exact spot is difficult to find; for gentle pressure over the site of a lesion in the deeper part of the muscle naturally does not disclose tenderness, whereas strong pressure is apt to hurt throughout the belly. It is thus best to locate the spot approximately and then use 50 ml of 0.5% procaine solution for the infiltration. The pain ceases and a much greater range of dorsiflexion of the foot becomes possible within a few minutes of a successful injection. This must *not* be tested with the patient standing, since this may lead to further tearing. The patient is taught to move his foot up and down as he lies on the couch, restoring the range actively without the strain of weight-bearing falling on the muscle. While he lies there practising this movement, a cork platform should be made and fitted into the shoe. The extent of muscle above and below the breach can contract and relax normally, but the midpart is in spasm about the tear; hence, the muscle is shortened for the time being. A raised heel enables him to use the unaffected parts of the muscle without straining the healing breach. The first day he may need a rise of 3 to 4 cm and at each attendance the thickness of the platform is revised; its height is reduced until after, say, a week it becomes unnecessary.

The next and following days, the patient attends for deep massage to the area of the lesion, and, if he is an athlete, faradism to the muscle while the knee is held fully flexed and the foot plantiflexed. The muscle then moves fully without any strain falling on it at the extreme of contraction. When this treatment is instituted during the first few days after the accident, patients can expect to be playing tennis again at the end of 10 days; without immediate active treatment, the disability lasts for six weeks to six months or more. Rest and over-exertion, as in all muscular injuries, are both equally harmful. In chronic cases, scarring should be broken up by deep massage and mobility increased by the same faradism with the muscle held in the shortened position. When a palpable gap exists in the muscle belly, tiptoe exercises during weight-bearing should be avoided for three weeks.

## Tendinitis of the Tendo Achillis

The patient complains of pain at the heel, felt only during movement, and present ever since some unaccustomed exertion, perhaps in heelless shoes. He states that rising on tiptoe hurts at the back of the heel.

If, as is common, the lesion is a tendinitis, no movement hurts except resisted plantiflexion of the foot. The site of the lesion is usually at mid-tendon. Occasionally, the strain occurs level with the upper border of the calcaneus; if so, full plantiflexion of the foot squeezes the affected part of the tendon against the posterior aspect of the tibia; hence this movement hurts slightly too. Strain may rarely affect the musculotendinous junction; the site of tenderness is diagnostic.

The tendon is carefully palpated and it will be found that the lesion lies always at the inner or outer or both aspects of the tendon, sometimes on the anterior surface and scarcely ever on the posterior surface. Since the effective treatment for this disorder is deep transverse massage (and massage acts where it is applied and not elsewhere), if the anterior tenderness is not sought and treated, the commonplace is massage inadequately given. My experience with triamcinolone is disappearing; the lesion may be too extensive for thorough infiltration, and even a successful injection is often followed by relapse a few weeks or months later. Recovery after friction is nearly always permanent: an important matter to athletes. When a small enlargement of the tendon forms after a partial rupture, the localized projection is palpable. The disability is often slight, but in my experience no treatment avails.

*Athletes and Steroid Injections.* Rupture of the Achilles tendon after steroid infiltration has been described at intervals over the past 20 years. In this instance, the rupture is the result of mistaken technique; for in tendinitis here the suspension should be introduced along the surface, not into its substance. However, in tendinitis at the shoulder or knee, the suspension is indeed injected into the tendon itself, as a dozen or so droplets along the tenoperiosteal junction. Rupture has not supervened so far in any of my cases, since one small injection, not repeated, suffices. However, larger amounts injected several times might well weaken a tendon. Wrenn et al. (1954) showed that in animals receiving steroids the strength of a tendon repair after division and suture was almost halved. Hence, many athletes nowadays refuse steroid injections. As a result, the deep friction techniques that we introduced 40 years ago (see Volume II) have lately come back into favour.

## Tenovaginitis of the Tendo Achillis

This takes three forms, rheumatoid, gouty and xanthomatous.

*Rheumatoid, Gouty or Chondrocalcinotic Tenovaginitis.* The contrast between the slight symptoms and the marked signs is striking. The patient complains mainly of pain when his heel catches against an object. Examination shows that rising on tiptoe is scarcely uncomfortable. Yet the tendon is warm to the touch, swollen and very tender. There is no crepitus. In pseudogout, from time to time, a tender localized swelling forms, lasting about a month and causing no interference with function. Erosion of bone visible radiographically at the calcanean insertion of the tendo Achillis has been described in rheumatoid disease. Infiltration with triamcinolone is very successful in rheumatoid cases, and butazolidine or indomethacin is indicated in gout or chondrocalcinosis.

*Xanthomatous Tenovaginitis.* The tendo Achillis is a fairly common site for xanthomatosis. Both heels hurt during walking. Both tendons can be seen to be thickened and palpation reveals enlargement and a diffuse nodularity. The diagnosis becomes clear when similar nodules are seen and felt at the extensor tendons on the dorsum of both hands. Occasionally, similar swellings form on the tendons crossing the dorsum of the foot, and quite large deposits may form on the bone at the upper part of the ulna and tibia.

Clofibrate 0.5 g thrice daily should be given for some years and regression has been reported (Roper 1964); doubtless Bengal Gram will now be tried too.

## Intermittent Claudication

Claudication is, of course, merely a local manifestation of a general condition and the cerebral and coronary arteries are naturally apt to be affected too, particularly if the patient is diabetic. Women are seldom affected by claudication in the calf. The name was first used in 1831 by a veterinary surgeon called Bouley to designate a form of limping in horses, and Charcot described a case in 1858.

The phenomenon is dependent on the anatomical fact that two long arteries supply the gastrocnemius muscle. They follow its whole length, without forming anastomoses. This is a different pattern of blood supply from: (*a*) the soleus muscle, which receives a number of branches entering at intervals all the way down; (*b*) the tibialis anterior and extensor hallucis bellies which are supplied by a series of anastomotic loops derived from a succession of vessels (Blomfield). Owing to this exceptional arrangement of its nutrient arteries, the gastrocnemius muscle is more susceptible than others to ischaemia as the result of arteriosclerosis. Claudication in early middle age suggests endarteritis obliterans; in youth, coarctation of the aorta or an aberrant slip of muscle compressing the artery.

The history is characteristic. An elderly patient reports that pain in one calf is brought on by exertion and relieved by rest. A similar history may be given by a patient with the mushroom phenomenon, but standing still does not then relieve his pain; he must sit down. In very early claudication, the patient finds that walking some hundred yards brings the pain on, but that walking on farther, no less than resting, abolishes the pain. In the former event, continuation of the stimulus to vasodilatation has clearly enhanced the flow sufficiently to prevent the products of muscular metabolism from remaining at a painful level. Later, the symptoms can no longer be abolished by walking on; the patient is forced to rest each hundred yards or so to let the metabolites reach a concentration below the threshold of pain. He can then walk on another similar distance. Sooner or later, pain at night is apt to appear, relieved by allowing the limb to cool outside the bedclothes. When the muscles become warm, their metabolic requirement rises, just as it does during walking, to the point at which the possible arterial flow becomes inadequate. Pain at rest suggests that gangrene will come on within three to six months (Martin 1960).

Claudication is usually felt unilaterally. If the state of his arteries enables a man to walk, say, 100 yards with his left leg and 110 yards with his right, he never gets to the point of experiencing right-sided claudication. The fact of an arterial block and its approximate level can be ascertained by ultrasound, since transmission of such waves through a moving tissue (in this case, blood) alters the frequency (Strandness et al. 1966). Angiography singles out the exact site of obstruction.

If the anterior tibial artery is narrowed—a rarity—the intermittent claudication is felt at the front instead of the back of the leg. Ischaemia of the muscles of the sole is a not uncommon cause of elderly patients' 'foot strain'.

If plantiflexion is tested against resistance as the patient lies on the couch, neither weakness nor pain is elicited. If he is asked to plantiflex and dorsiflex his foot quickly and repeatedly, the familiar pain is brought on. Dependent, the foot is a dusky red. If it blanches on elevating the limb, the distal extent of the arteries of the leg and foot is shown to be patent. If not, the whole arterial tree is affected and gangrene must be anticipated. Pulsation in the dorsalis pedis, posterior tibial and popliteal arteries is absent on both sides. If the femoral arteries do not pulsate either, aortic occlusion or coarctation should be considered and aortography performed.

Vasodilator and anticoagulant drugs, Buerger's exercises and physiotherapy are all valueless. Indeed, vasodilator drugs are harmful, since they dilate arteries that are not diseased elsewhere in the body, thus diminishing blood pressure generally and reducing the flow through the sclerotic arteries. Smoking should be forbidden and great care taken of the skin of the feet. A raised heel gives the muscles rather less to do and the adoption of a steady slow pace brings requirement and supply closer to equilibrium. If the symptoms warrant, the gastrocnemius may be divided at its insertion into the tendo Achillis. This leaves the soleus muscle, with its satisfactory arrangement of arteries, intact and is to be preferred to mere tenotomy of the tendo Achillis. Crushing the motor nerve to the gastrocnemius is an alternative (Reid et al. 1963) via incision in the popliteal fossa. The late results of division of the tendo Achillis for claudication were reported by Powis et al. (1971). Only half the patients improved immediately and by two years later the figure was 17%.

Sympathectomy warms the foot but seldom increases the walking distance materially, but varicose or ischaemic ulcers often heal quickly after the operation.

The treatment of choice is the restoration of a patent artery by surgery. Cockett began in 1952 with grafting but now (Cockett & Maurice 1963) performs a rebore. If the femoral pulse is absent, the operation has an excellent result; if the femoral pulse is present and the popliteal absent, and the arteriogram shows the sural arteries to be patent, operation is again indicated. If the occlusion lies at or distal to the popliteal bifurcation, the condition is clearly insusceptible to arterial surgery. Figures from Glasgow (Watt et al. 1974) show that patency is retained five years later in two-thirds of all cases operated on.

*Venous Claudication.* Those who suffer from permanent obstruction to the venous return from a lower limb develop what Cockett et al. (1967) termed venous claudication. Exertion increases the venous pressure in the affected leg, thus exerting backpressure against the arterial flow. Discomfort in the calf after walking some way results.

### Ischaemic Contracture

A young man, after unaccustomed exercise, reports an ache and swelling in the calf some hours later. Walking is uncomfortable and increases the swelling.

Examination shows that rising on tiptoe is not difficult and is scarcely uncomfortable. The calf is diffusely swollen, and the skin over it is red and warm to the touch. Passive dorsiflexion of the foot is severely limited by loss of elasticity of the calf muscles. Palpation reveals uniform tenderness of the whole calf muscle without any localized tender area. The arteries at the ankle pulsate.

Treatment consists of a raised heel and a minimum of walking for three weeks. Lack of resolution or a recurrence calls for division of the fascia covering the gastrocnemius, lest contracture of the Volkmann type supervene.

### Nocturnal Cramp

This wakens elderly patients and can be most troublesome. It has some connection with disc lesions for it often follows sciatica and occurs on the affected side only. In other cases, no cause is discernible. It may be a most troublesome sequel to section of the posterior root at the fifth lumbar or first sacral level (Sicard & Leca 1954). The patient can sometimes precipitate an attack of cramp in the calf by stretching his leg out fully. Patients describe a ball of contracted muscle that travels along the belly, and mention various positions in which the limb is fixed during the attack; a common one is extension at the knee, plantiflexion at the ankle and extension at the toes. Such a position involves coordination between several groups of muscles and must therefore be initiated centrally. I regard cramp, therefore, as caused by an epilepsy of the anterior horn cells of the spinal cord.

Quinine diminishes the excitability of a skeletal muscle both by increasing its refractory period (Harvey 1939) and by diminishing the excitability of the motor end-plate; 300 mg taken at bed-time should be continued for some months, after which it may be found that the tendency has passed and there is no relapse. If it does, the patient should try out for himself the minimum dose that prevents the cramp; often as little as 10 mg suffices. Should quinine fail, carisoprodol 0.5 g taken last thing at night should be tried; it can be continued indefinitely. It relaxes skeletal muscle and has a central analgesic effect as well. An alternative is phenoxybenzamine, 10 mg. If the attacks of cramp follow sciatica, residual bruising of the nerve root may be the focus whence the attack originates. Epidural local anaesthesia is then often successful in mitigating or abolishing the attacks. If deep-vein thrombosis has occurred, by 5 to 10 years later, only one-third of 130 legs was symptom-free (Browse et al. 1980).

### Prevention of Venous Thrombosis

As soon as he comes to after the anaesthesia the patient should exercise his calf muscles by moving his foot up and down repeatedly. An electrical device has been evolved (Sabri et al. 1971) whereby the foot is alternately dorsiflexed and plantiflexed passively during the operation. They found this method to reduce the incidence of early venous thrombosis by 77%. Hills et al. (1972) used intermittent pneumatic compression and confirmed the finding of very significant reduction of thrombosis, except in patients with cancer.

## Weak Plantiflexor Muscles

Painless weakness is best detected by asking the patient to stand on each leg in turn and rise on tiptoe. Apart from upper motor neurone lesions, peroneal atrophy and direct injury to the sciatic nerve, the common cause of weakness unaccompanied by increase in pain when the calf muscles contract is a fifth lumbar disc lesion causing a first and second sacral root palsy.

### Rupture of the Tendo Achillis

This simple condition usually remains undiagnosed until too late, cursory examination resulting in its being dismissed as some sort of sprained ankle. The patient states that while playing, say, squash, his foot suddenly hurt and gave way. The pain was momentary, but he found at once that he could only hobble on a flat foot. He limped home and, when examined as he lay on a couch, active plantiflexion was found not to be lost. Since the plantaris, flexor longus hallucis and digitorum muscles all remain intact, the supine patient can just voluntarily plantiflex his foot. Had the movement been tested against the slightest resistance, gross weakness would have been revealed. The pain in the calf and fixed equinus of a patient with a minor tear in his gastrocnemius muscle contrast with the absence of pain, inability to plantiflex strongly and excessive dorsiflexion range at the ankle characterizing rupture of the tendo Achillis. When the patient lies prone, the defect in the tendon is easy to feel; a 1–2 cm gap is palpable at, or slightly above, the middle of the tendon.

If the rupture is discovered within 10 days of the accident, contracture of the calf muscles is not yet too great to prevent operative suture.

After this period has elapsed, spontaneous organization of the haematoma with eventual fibrous repair should be awaited. This takes several months during which the patient should make no effort to rise on tiptoe. The thickened tissues at each side of the enlarged tendon should be massaged twice a week, even for two or three months in long-standing cases. Alleviation, not cure, may be expected. For the rest of his life, the tendon remains twice its original width; the fibrous swelling at the point of rupture never disappears and some residual disability is permanent. This may amount merely to some aching towards the end of a round of golf, but other patients are permanently unable to run, or to walk any distance without pain.

## Short Plantiflexor Muscles

Shortening forms part of a talipes equinovarus deformity in babies. If the equinus position of a baby's feet can be overcome by strong resistance, diplegia is present. In some children the calf muscles are short as an isolated phenomenon; if so, it usually escapes detection. In due course the mother complains of the child's gait, mentioning his feet, not his calves. She notices that the youngster turns his feet out too much, stands tilted backwards and runs conspicuously slower than his schoolfellows. She is right. Inability to bear weight properly on the heel because of equinus, forces the lad to twist his foot into lateral rotation; hence, when he runs, instead of landing on his heel and taking off from the forefoot held in line with the movement of the body, he takes off from a foot oblique to this line. Hence he may lose several centimetres of forward movement at each step. Moreover, standing on his heels involves his remaining tilted slightly backwards; he is not properly poised above his centre of gravity. In consequence, muscular force in excess of the minimum has to be expended during standing; the child therefore complains that prolonged standing is tiring. If, as is common, a plantaris deformity of the forefoot complicates the short calf muscles, he cannot bear adequate weight on his heels and mid-tarsal hypermobility and, later, painful strain results.

On examination dorsiflexion at the ankle joint is painlessly limited to the horizontal line—what is often well described as equinus to 90°—since the calf muscles will not stretch farther.

In children, the treatment is temporarily to provide the shoe with a raised heel to protect the mid-tarsal joint, and to teach the following exercises. For stretching the soleus muscles: the child should perform a knee-flexion exercise barefoot, keeping the heel on the ground. For stretching the gastrocnemius muscle: the patient stands with the foot fully dorsiflexed at the ankle by pressure against a wall, the heel remaining on the ground; he should then lean forward vigorously keeping the knee in full extension. When the calf muscles have lengthened, which takes some months of hard work, the raised heel on the shoe can be discarded.

In adults, the process of stretching out the calf muscles is too tedious, and shortening can be adequately compensated by raising the heel of the shoe and increasing the obliquity of its upper surface. Elongation of the tendo Achillis by subcutaneous tenotomy followed by six weeks' immobilization in a plaster cast is the alternative.

## The Dorsiflexor Muscles

The strength of dorsiflexion on the two sides is compared; pain on this movement is noted. Normal dorsiflexor muscles easily overcome the examiner's resistance. This movement elicits pain in lesions affecting the anterior tibial and extensor longus hallucis and digitorum muscles. A resisted extension movement of the hallux and then of the toes picks out the offending muscle.

Myosynovitis of the tibialis anterior muscle is an interesting condition, with only one other parallel in the body—myosynovitis with crepitus of the bellies of the abductor longus and the extensores pollicis muscles in the forearm. It is an uncommon disorder except in army service, when recruits march unaccustomed distances in boots. The resisted dorsiflexion movement hurts above the front of the ankle; further testing shows the long extensor muscles of the digits to be unaffected, and palpation fails to reveal any tenderness of the anterior tibial tendon itself. If the examiner now puts his finger on the outer aspect of the junction of the middle with the lower third of the tibia, crepitus on movement is felt at the musculotendinous junction of the anterior tibial muscle close to the bone.

At the ankle, tenosynovitis (sometimes with crepitus) of the extensor longus hallucis or digitorum is a rarity and is an uncommon sequel to a sprained ankle. Shortening of these muscles complicates a pes cavus deformity, eventually fixing the toes in the clawed position.

Weakness of the muscles dorsiflexing the foot is a common finding in upper motor neurone lesions, anterior poliomyelitis and lumbar disc lesions at the fourth level.

The extensor hallucis muscle may develop ischaemic contracture or become adherent after a fracture at mid-tibia; the constant length phenomenon results. In these cases, each time the foot is plantiflexed, the big toe has to extend; it is forced against the upper of the shoe and becomes extremely sore. Tenotomy under local anaesthesia level with the first metatarsophalangeal joint gives permanent relief.

Lesions of the bellies of these muscles respond well to both local anaesthesia and deep massage. Their tendons respond to deep massage and to triamcinolone.

## Tight Fascial Compartment

Symptoms superficially resembling intermittent claudication result from a tight fascial compartment for the dorsiflexor muscles in the leg. In minor cases, the patient states that, after walking say half a mile, he becomes unable to dorsiflex his foot voluntarily, and has to stump along flexing his knee to get his foot off the ground. Alternatively, he may develop a drop-foot after kicking a football about for 10 minutes. The weakness is devoid of discomfort. After a short rest, the muscle recovers. In these cases examination in the resting state reveals nothing, and the arteries at the ankle pulsate normally. After the causative exertion, the tibialis anterior muscle is found temporarily paralysed, the pulses still remaining palpable.

The cause is a tight fascial compartment (Horn 1945). The contents of the anterior tibial compartment lie in an inelastic space. The bellies of the anterior tibial, extensor hallucis and digitorum muscles are confined by the tibia, fibula, interosseous membrane and superficial fascia. The normal increase in bulk due to increased blood flow during exertion may cause such swelling that the lumen of the anterior tibial artery is temporarily occluded. The muscle is therefore temporarily paralysed; in Horn's patient this was accompanied by the extensor muscles to all toes. If, however, the minute vessels in the belly itself gradually become silted up with cells (Harman 1948), the disorder may become irreversible. The swelling may also trap the superficial peroneal nerve at its exit through the fascial foramen at mid-leg and cause pins and needles at the inner four toes.

Severe cases are encountered. A healthy young man develops pain at the front of the mid-leg after some exertion; within a few hours it is intense. Redness and oedema of the skin now appear over the belly of the tibialis anterior muscle. If the fascia is not divided at once, ischaemic necrosis may ensure, contracture or even complete paralysis resulting. If so, the power to dorsiflex foot and toes is permanently lost.

The anterior tibial syndrome may also result from thrombosis or embolism of the anterior tibial artery in older patients. This is quite a different condition, caused by primary arterial occlusion, not a tight fascia. Watson (1955) gives a good review of the literature and describes two cases caused by arterial disease; Freedman and Knowles (1959) describe five more such cases.

Treatment consists in removal of the fascia at the front of the tibial belly; if necrosis is impending, the operation is urgent.

## The Evertor Muscles

If resisted eversion of the foot hurts, the peroneal muscles are affected. Tendinitis here occurs anywhere from the lower fibula to the cuboid and fifth metatarsal base; the site of tenderness defines the position of the lesion. Peroneal tendinitis is one cause of continued disability after a sprained ankle. Since the pain is at the outer side of the ankle, it is naturally ascribed to post-traumatic adhesions and the foot is mobilized and exercised in a way that unintentionally makes the condition worse. Testing the resisted movements gives the clue at once.

The peroneal tendons may get loose in their groove on the posterior surface of the fibula and slip forwards over the malleolus, thus giving rise to a 'snapping ankle'. This is usually not painful or much of a disability; when the foot is plantiflexed the tendons jump back again. Mucocele of the peroneal tendons results in swelling leading eventually to considerable aching. The glairy fluid can be made to fluctuate from above to below the malleolus. Ganglia occur in connection with these tendons, above as well as below the ankle.

Spasm of the peroneal muscles results, not from intrinsic defect, but from arthritis of the talocalcanean and mid-tarsal joints, which are thereby fixed in valgus and abduction respectively. Hence the term 'spasmodic pes planus' is a misnomer.

Weakness of the peroneal muscles is caused mainly by upper motor neurone lesions, peroneal atrophy and disc protrusions at the fifth lumbar level. Unreadiness to bring them into play results in recurrent varus sprain at the ankle.

Peroneal tendinitis responds excellently to massage; the lesion is seldom localized enough for an injection of a steroid (see Volume II). Mucocele has been treated merely by puncture of the tendon sheath with a tenotomy knife followed by digital expression of 30 to 60 ml of mucus. This procedure has to be repeated about once a year.

## Tight Peroneal Fascia

Overuse engorgement of the peroneal bellies in the presence of a tight fascia has been described but I have never seen such a case. There is constant pain, the muscle belly is stone hard and compression of the common peroneal nerve leads to paralysis of dorsiflexion and eversion of the foot, accompanied by numbness. Unless the fascia is divided without delay, the foot-drop is apt to prove permanent.

## The Invertor Muscles

These are the anterior and posterior tibial muscles. If a resisted inversion movement hurts, and dorsiflexion does not, the posterior tibial muscle is at fault. The tendon is palpated throughout its extent until the site of the lesion is found.

A posterior tibial tendinitis caused by ordinary overuse recovers with a few sessions of massage. However, in older patients it may result from years of overuse, secondary to a valgus deformity at the heel, especially if the cause is fixed inversion of the forefoot. The pain goes on indefinitely. It is curable only by a combined approach: a support to correct the lack of parallel between hindfoot and forefoot (Fig. 133) combined with massage to the affected extent of tendon (see Volume II). Neither measure suffices alone.

*'Shin-soreness'.* Athletes use this word for pain in the leg caused by running. Examination shows that the usual cause is a lesion of the posterior tibial or peroneal muscles at the musculotendinous junction. It is an overuse phenomenon, responding perfectly to deep massage. Rarely, the radiograph reveals a stress fracture.

# THE NERVES OF THE LEG

## Saphenous and Deep Peroneal Nerves

The saphenous nerve may suffer compression at its exit from the deep fascia just below the inner condyle of the tibia. In addition to paraesthesia at the inner ankle and along the medial border of the foot, ill-defined aching is felt along the subcutaneous border of the tibia.

Either nerve may suffer direct contusion at the point where its terminal part crosses the front of the ankle joint. If so, after the blow, the patient complains of pins and needles at the dorsum of the distal part of the foot, especially at the adjacent borders of the big and second toe in the case of the deep peroneal nerve. If the saphenous nerve has suffered contusion at the front of the ankle, the inner aspect of the dorsum of the foot as far as the superomedial aspect of the hallux tingles; sharp neuralgic twinges may be felt when the nerve is stretched by flexion of the hallux. Hirschfeld called this the 'tarsal tunnel syndrome' and found procaine curative. Whichever nerve is affected, combined plantiflexion and inversion of the foot stretch the bruised nerve and bring on or accentuate the tingling. The tender extent of the nerve usually lies level with the ankle joint. Lam (1962) has described another lesion as the 'tarsal tunnel syndrome'. The patient complained of pins and needles along the medial border of the foot and two and a half inner toes. Operation showed the peroneal nerve to be caught up by a slip of the flexor retinaculum, division of which was curative. Contusion of the medial terminal branch of the deep peroneal nerve occurs at the ankle; the dorsum of the outer foot and three outer toes become paraesthetic. In such a case, inversion of the foot during plantiflexion causes a twinge of pins and needles.

The superficial peroneal nerve issues from the deep fascia at the junction of the middle and lower third of the leg; it is compressed there when the tibialis anterior swells inside a tight fascia, also idiopathically, in a manner similar to meralgia paraesthetica. It divides into two branches, one supplying the inner three toes, the other the outer three toes; hence, in this case the dorsum of the whole foot and all the toes tingle.

Treatment consists of a diagnostic injection of procaine, which is always required to make sure the correct area of nerve has been found. Should this fail therapeutically but show that the right spot has been chosen, triamcinolone is substituted.

### Common Peroneal Nerve

This nerve is exposed to a blow or to sustained pressure at the point where it winds round the lateral aspect of the neck of the fibula. It can be compressed by sitting with the legs crossed or by keeping the knee pressed against, e.g. the side of a desk. Since the nerve supplies the tibialis anterior, extensor hallucis and peroneal muscles, drop-foot results and the outer foot and calf go numb.

Spontaneous recovery may take a month or two. How to avoid the causative posture is explained to the patient.

### Tibial Nerve

This is compressed by sitting with the knees half-crossed, the patella of the nether knee squeezing the tibial nerve against the posterior aspect of the tibia. There is seldom appreciable weakness but the heel and sole may remain numb for a couple of months. The causative posture must be avoided.

## THE ANKLE JOINT

This is a simple joint allowing two movements in only one plane: plantiflexion and dorsiflexion. The range of dorsiflexion is limited by the length of the calf muscles. These are at their most extensible in babies in whom the dorsum of the foot can often be laid against the leg with ease. Plantiflexion is limited by the engagement of the heel, via the tendo Achillis, against the back of the tibia. The talus is held in place by the tibiofibular mortice, which in turn depends on the inferior tibiofibular ligament for its effectiveness.

### Examination

There are five movements required: two primary for the joint and three accessory for ligaments.

For the joint: the range of plantiflexion and dorsiflexion is ascertained, compared with the other side and the production or not of pain noted. The end-feel has particular diagnostic importance. Both extremes are soft at a normal joint, since compression of the insertion of the tendo Achillis against the back of the tibia, and full stretching of the calf muscles, can have nothing abrupt about them. In arthritis, the joint itself is felt to come to a dead stop with a hard end-feel.

For the ligaments: the deltoid ligament is stretched by a combined eversion and plantiflexion movement, and the anterior fasciculus of the lateral ligament by inversion during plantiflexion. The inferior tibiofibular ligament is stretched by a strong varus movement applied to the talus via the calcaneus. Hence, varus at the heel is vigorously forced when a sprung mortice is suspected.

The *capsular pattern* is rather more limitation of plantiflexion than of dorsiflexion. However, in patients with a short calf muscle, this may limit dorsiflexion before the extreme of the possible articular range is reached, thus disguising the hard restriction of dorsiflexion. In such a case, a clinical diagnosis of arthritis at the ankle joint rests on the discovery of limited plantiflexion with a hard end-feel.

### Equinus

Limitation of dorsiflexion as an isolated finding designates short calf muscles and often complicates a pes cavus deformity, thus rendering the plantaris posture of the forefoot more unfortunate than ever. Equinus at the ankle joint may result in mid-tarsal strain in children and adults. Since they cannot dorsiflex at the ankle joint, they are forced to carry out this movement at the next available joint—the mid-tarsal. Since, too, the child with fixed equinus can best get his heel to the ground by rotating the limb laterally, he tends to turn his feet out more and more, thus gradually developing a considerable outward rotation deformity in the course of the tibial shaft.

In a child, an equinus deformity that disappears on strong pressure characterizes cerebral diplegia.

In children treatment consists of stretching the soleus and gastrocnemius muscles out separately—the first by active knee flexion exercises with the heel flat on the ground; the second by placing the fully dorsiflexed foot against a wall and then leaning forwards with the knee fully extended. It may take months.

Adults should have the heel raised and the obliquity of its upper surface increased, or the tendo Achillis lengthened by subcutaneous tenotomy.

## Arthritis at the Ankle

This is present when both dorsiflexion and plantiflexion are limited. In early cases, plantiflexion may be found limited alone, if the calf muscles are too short to allow the foot to reach the extreme of dorsiflexion range at the ankle joint.

The rheumatoid conditions, which so often affect the other tarsal joints, conspicuously avoid the ankle joint. Psoriatic arthritis is less uncommon at this joint; it responds very well to intra-articular triamcinolone. The only common condition is osteoarthrosis, almost always the result of mal-union of a tibiofibular fracture. If a shearing strain is put on the joint by mal-union with angulation at the fracture, osteoarthrosis will certainly supervene.

Repeated severe sprains, e.g. in rugby footballers, may in the end set up osteoarthrosis, sometimes with ligamentous ossification visible on the radiograph. Osteoarthrosis shows up well on the radiograph.

In osteoarthrosis, conservative treatment is seldom satisfactory. In early cases, intra-articular triamcinolone may help; mobilization under anaesthesia may bring several months' relief. Fitting the patient's shoes with a higher heel enables him to walk without fully dorsiflexing his foot, thus avoiding the painful extreme of movement. If the symptoms warrant, arthrodesis is most satisfactory and should be performed without delay, since the condition goes on getting worse indefinitely.

Limitation of movement without arthritis occurs after the ankle has been immobilized for months in the treatment of tibiofibular fractures. In such cases, strong daily forcing, supplemented by the patient's active exertions, in due course restores an adequate range of movement.

## Loose Body in Ankle Joint

The patient complains that, some time after a severe sprain of the ankle, he has suffered bouts of twinges at the ankle, usually on pointing the foot to go downstairs. Severe momentary pain prevents his stepping on to that foot; he gives it a shake and the disability ceases, only to be repeated some time later.

Examination and radiography reveal nothing, since the subluxation is momentary only and the fragment cartilaginous, merely showing that no other cause for the twinges is present. Differential diagnosis is difficult between momentary internal derangement at the ankle joint and a sprung tibiofibular mortice, a ruptured calcaneofibular ligament or a loose body in the talocalcanean joint. Treatment is difficult too, for the attempt must be made to shift the loose fragment to a position within the joint whence it does not subluxate (see Volume II). Since no displacement exists at the time of the manipulation, the usual clinical criteria that help guide the manipulator towards the correct way to deal with internal derangement are absent. Should manipulation fail, a Root's shoe should be tried, since the anterior wedge to the heel enables the patient to walk without full plantiflexion ever being reached.

## Unstable Mortice

The patient states that some years previously he sprained his ankle severely. He recovered in due course, but then found that he could no longer rely on his foot which has turned over easily ever since, often with a click and momentary severe pain within the ankle. After some moments, he walks on again; the ankle merely feels sore for a day or two afterwards. The cause is permanent lengthening of the inferior tibiofibular ligament.

When the ankle joint is examined, nothing is detected at first, but when valgus and varus movements are tested at the talocalcanean joint, the click is reproduced at the ankle when varus is forced hard and excessive range of varus movement demonstrated. If this movement is repeated with the examiner's fingers palpating the two malleoli, they can be felt to move apart, and if a radiograph is taken while strong varus pressure is exerted at the heel, the increased distance apart of the lower ends of tibia and fibula can be seen.

The bones must be wired together again, but it is not unknown for the wire to break in the end. It is therefore well worth trying the effect of ligamentous sclerosis first.

Measurements are taken from the anteroposterior X-ray photograph. The distance from the tip of the lateral malleolus to the articular surface of the tibia is ascertained (2 to 3 cm) and the respective widths of the tibia and fibula (about 5 and 2 cm). The patient lies prone and these two lines drawn at right angles. A 2 ml syringe is filled with sclerosant solution and fitted with a thin needle 4 cm long. It is thrust vertically downwards a few millimetres above the intersection of these two lines and is felt to penetrate ligament at about 3 cm. If it hits bone without traversing ligament first, the point is too far to one or the other side of the tibiofibular joint. A series of intraligamentous infiltrations follows. The same two lines can be drawn to cross each other anteriorly and the injection repeated from in front, the tendons of the extensor digitorum being held apart manually.

## Sprain of the Anterior Tibiotalar Ligament

This is an uncommon injury and is caused by a pure plantiflexion stress. Chronic aching often results, which may last many years, but is never severe and only prevents vigorous use. Examination shows that full passive plantiflexion hurts at the front of the ankle; all other movements are painless. Palpation involves pushing the tendons aside and searching for the tender spot at the thin sheet of tissue joining the talus and the tibia. Massage is extremely effective. Manipulation is harmful. A steroid injection is seldom helpful, since the structure is too thin to be easily identified as the tip of the needle pierces it.

## Sprain of the Posterior Talofibular Ligament

Sprain of the posterior fasciculus of the fibular collateral ligament is rare. Pole-vaulters are prone to this condition. The diagnosis is made with some difficulty; for the only painful movement is apt to be passive eversion of the foot, which compresses the tender ligament between the tip of the fibula and the everted calcaneus. If then the movement intended to stretch the deltoid ligament hurts at the *outer* side of the heel, this lesion is recalled.

One injection of triamcinolone into the tender ligament gives lasting relief.

## Anterior Periostitis

This disorder, the reverse phenomenon of dancer's heel, is a rarity. It is caused by a dorsiflexion strain that forces the neck of the talus against the anterior margin of the tibia. The ballet dancer lands flat on her foot, then bends her knee and feels an immediate pain at the front of the ankle. Examination shows full passive dorsiflexion to hurt at the front of the ankle, i.e. something is pinched. Passive plantiflexion does not hurt, thus exculpating the anterior ligament.

An injection of triamcinolone is curative and the dancer is fit to perform two days later. Prophylaxis consists of slightly raising the heel of the ballet shoe.

## Jumper's Sprain

An athlete, landing on his heel as he takes off to jump, may force his foot into dorsiflexion and eversion. As a result, the superolateral aspect of the anterior margin of the calcaneus hits against the edge of the fibula, producing a traumatic periostitis there. After that, every time he takes off the pain reappears, felt clearly at the outer side of the ankle.

Examination reveals nothing, since the ligaments and muscles are not affected. Forcing the everted foot into dorsiflexion is the only way to reproduce the pain. Palpation reveals localized tenderness at the anteroinferior surface of the fibula, but no corresponding tenderness on the calcaneus.

Although one or two injections of triamcinolone bring relief, the athlete must avoid repeating the same trauma, if necessary by wearing a 0.5 cm inner wedge within his shoe.

# SPRAINED ANKLE

'Sprained ankle' is the general name for a variety of traumatic lesions occurring at what the patient calls his ankle. Several conditions may legitimately be described under this heading; each may exist alone, but combined lesions predominate. Moreover, one structure may recover, leaving chronic disability due to another.

The talus is slightly wedge-shaped, larger anteriorly. Hence in dorsiflexion the bone is gripped in the tibiofibular mortice; force applied to it is likely to cause a fracture or lengthening of the inferior tibiofibular ligament. In plantiflexion, the bone does not fit closely in the mortice and force can produce enough movement to sprain ligaments. Strong inversion during forced plantiflexion is the way an ankle becomes sprained.

Sprained ankle may be classified according as

the causative stress is towards varus or valgus, according to the tissue damaged and according to the length of time that has elapsed since the accident.

## Varus Sprain

This is as common as valgus sprain is uncommon. The stresses imposed on the tarsus by a varus sprain are: (*a*) plantiflexion at the ankle joint, stretching its outer side and the extensor longus digitorum muscle; (*b*) varus at the talocalcanean joint, stretching the fibulocalcanean ligament and the peroneal tendons; (*c*) medial rotation and adduction at the mid-tarsal joint, stretching the ligament at the outer aspect of the calcaneo-cuboid joint. Exceptionally the cubo-fifth-metatarsal or cubonavicular joints suffer as well. Thus, injury to one or more of these structures may correctly be described by the patient as a sprained ankle.

### Examination

This must include:

1. Five passive movements at the ankle joint.
2. Two passive movements at the talocalcanean joint.
3. Six passive movements at the mid-tarsal joint.
4. The four resisted movements—dorsiflexion, plantiflexion, inversion, eversion.

The site of the lesion is deduced from the pattern that emerges when these passive and resisted movements are tested. Once the site of the sprain has been outlined by this examination, tenderness of the appropriate structure is sought. In recent severe cases, gross oedema often gives rise to such generalized tenderness that palpation yields no information; if so, the diagnosis is arrived at purely by inference from a study of the response to these movements. The affected sites, in order of descending frequency, are: (*a*) the fibular origin of the anterior talofibular ligament; (*b*) the fibular origin of the calcaneofibular ligament; (*c*) the talar insertion of the anterior talofibular ligament; (*d*) the lateral fibres of the calcaneocuboid ligament; (*e*) the peroneal tendons; (*f*) the anterior talotibial ligament; and (*g*) the tendon of the extensor longus digitorum. The commonest lesion is a combined sprain of the fibular collateral ligament and the capsule of the calcaneocuboid joint.

If examination shows the tendons to be affected as much as, or more than, the ligaments, the customary treatment of a sprained ankle by early ambulation is inadvisable. The patient should rest as much as he can for a few days until massage has cleared up the tendinous strain.

### Treatment

This depends on the time that has elapsed since the accident.

*Acute Stage.* During the first 24 hours after a ligamentous sprain, immediate injection of triamcinolone is indicated. The necessity for accurate diagnosis is now obvious, since infiltration has to be performed at some definite point. Deep effleurage is a great aid to precision; for, after the physiotherapist has removed most of the oedema, tenderness is elicited and bony points defined much more easily. If a haematoma of any size has formed, this is aspirated immediately before the injection. The 2 ml of triamcinolone give little latitude in the choice of where to inject. Strapping may be applied to prevent recurrence of the swelling and for the moral support that it gives the patient. The patient walks out and attends the following day for the treatment described below as appropriate to the subacute stage. The sooner after the injury the infiltration is made, the more spectacular the results. In tendinitis, at this stage, the lesion is too diffuse for injection of a steroid to be practicable. Massage is given daily to the tendon over all its affected extent.

*Subacute Stage.* Massage is used to move the ligament in imitation of its normal behaviour, followed by gentle passive movements, which become stronger as recovery advances. Massage consists in the first place of effleurage to reduce oedema. There follows a very few minutes' deep friction to the actual site of the tear in each ligament. This eases the pain further, disperses local effusion and moves the affected structure to and fro over subjacent bone. Movement is then increased passively in each direction, the range of each affected joint being gently forced to the point of discomfort but not of pain. The movements at the ankle, talocalcanean and mid-tarsal joints are each performed to the limit of the possible range. Unless the physiotherapist is unthinkably rough, no danger of overstretching the sprained ligaments results from these movements, since an excessive range is adequately prevented by observing the patient's reaction. The main difficulty is to get him to realize how much greater the painless range is than he believes. Active movements follow the passive movements at once; they further the effect of the friction in preventing scar tissue from forming abnormal adherence. Finally, the patient departs, walking slowly and carefully with proper heel-and-toe gait. Walking with the foot held stiffly has no therapeutic value.

If a tendon is affected alone, no treatment is required other than deep massage and the avoidance of such exertion as causes pain.

*Chronic Stage.* The foot is quite adequate for ordinary purposes but is apt to swell and ache after vigorous or prolonged use. This means that scars were allowed to form abnormal attachments as the result of healing in the absence of enough movement; alternatively, the ligamentous sprain has recovered leaving a chronic tendinitis.

The treatment of adhesions about a ligament is naturally their manipulative rupture. This is quite easy and very seldom requires anaesthesia. One sharp twist (see Volume II) stretching out the talofibular and calcaneocuboid ligaments suffices. There is a tiny crack, and the patient is cured. No after-treatment is necessary.

Chronic tendinitis requires deep massage to the affected part of the tendon. Until well, the patient should avoid such exertion as causes pain. If a small stretch of tendon remains refractory to friction, an injection of triamcinolone suspension is given there.

### Recurrent Varus Sprain

The patient states that his ankle turns over easily; it lacks stability and is thus subjected to a succession of minor sprains. If the examiner can reproduce the sprain at will, with an audible click as varus is forced at the heel, the inferior tibiofibular ligament has been overstretched. If not, the cause appears to lie in delayed contraction of the peroneal muscles.

The recent case should be treated on the lines suggested above, but the sprain in recurrent trouble is seldom severe. The patient is usually a girl in her teens, and on examination the peroneal muscles are not weak; when the ankle starts turning over, they are merely brought into play too slowly to prevent the sprain (Cyriax 1954). Freeman's (1972) demonstration of the nervous discharges on movement of the ankle joint confirmed this view. It would seem that, as time goes on, the reflex becomes more rapid. Meanwhile, repetition is best prevented by floating out the heel of the patient's shoes (Fig. 118). Alternatively, the reflex arc can be speeded up by coordination exercises on his wobble-board (Freeman et al. 1965).

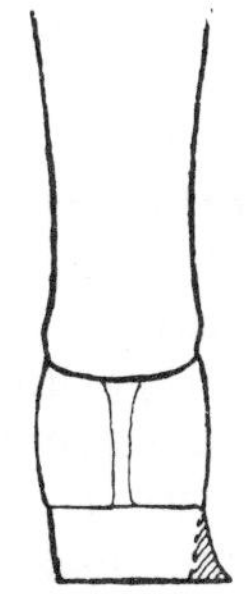

**Fig. 118.** Heel floated 1 cm at its outer side. For recurrent varus sprain of the ankle.

If the peroneal muscles are weak, it must be remembered that at times the first complaint in an upper motor neurone lesion may be recurrent varus sprain at the ankle. Sciatica leading to a fifth lumbar root palsy naturally leaves the patient liable to sprain his ankle for the duration of the peroneal weakness. In peroneal atrophy the ankle is seldom sprained, curiously enough.

## Valgus Sprain

When this rare condition is encountered, the foot should be examined in an endeavour to discover why the stress took the unusual direction. Usually the patient already stands with a valgus deformity of his heel and abduction of the forefoot. Hence, every time he puts his foot to the ground, he overstretches the damaged tibionavicular or tibiocalcanean ligaments. For this reason, sprains of the anterior and middle fasciculi of the deltoid ligament are apt to go on hurting for many months, even years, since the patient strains the ligament anew at every step.

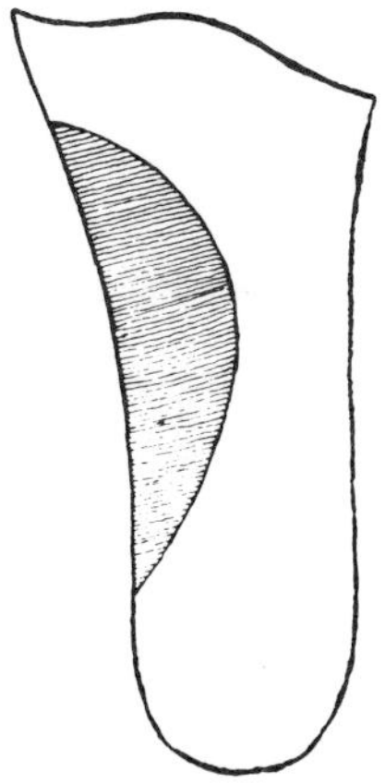

**Fig. 119.** Valgus support. The thickness (1 to 2 cm) lies at the inner side of the mid-tarsal joint.

Treatment is twofold. The heel and forefoot must be so supported that strain during weight-bearing is removed from the affected fasciculus. To this end a support is prescribed—thick at the inner aspect of its calcanean and mid-tarsal extent (Fig. 119). When this is fitted, the calcaneus assumes the neutral position during weight-bearing (thus relaxing the tibiocalcanean ligament) and the cessation of abduction of the forefoot spares the tibionavicular ligament. Triamcinolone suspension injected into the affected areas of ligament now hastens cure, but is ineffective unless the support is fitted first. Massage is useless and manipulation is harmful.

The posterior tibial tendon is often also affected. If a resisted inversion movement hurts, the affected area of tendon must be given massage. If a localized extent of tendon remains troublesome, it is infiltrated with triamcinolone suspension.

CHAPTER 26

# THE FOOT

The patient can usually point fairly accurately to the site of a lesion in the foot. Pain is hardly ever referred to the foot only; but pain in the foot unaltered by standing or walking does raise this possibility.

## EXAMINATION

Excluding the toes, the examination involves 13 passive movements and four against resistance. It comprises (1) inspection; (2) testing the five passive movements at the ankle joint; (3) testing the two passive movements at the talocalcanean joint; (4) testing the six passive movements at the mid-tarsal joint while the heel and ankle joints are held still; (5) testing the passive movements at the metatarsophalangeal and interphalangeal joints; (6) testing the resisted movements; (7) feeling for pulsation at the posterior tibial and dorsalis pedis arteries.

After the foot has been examined with the patient lying, it should be inspected again while the patient stands. The general posture of the foot, and the changes in shape caused by weight-bearing, are noted. If the examination standing is conducted first, the physician does not yet know what is wrong with the foot and he cannot therefore yet assess the bearing of any alterations in shape and colour he may see. If the foot becomes red on dependency, arterial narrowing enough to cause claudication is probable. If the foot goes a deep purple, Sudeck's post-traumatic osteoporosis is the cause. If so, the ankle, talocalcanean and mid-tarsal joints all display limited movement, sometimes the toes as well. The toenails stop growing. Arterial pulsation is present and the radiograph diagnostic. Metastasis at the second lumbar level gives rise to warm feet owing to interference with the sympathetic nerves. This occurs in one foot only in para-vertebral retroperitoneal tumour.

It is quite possible for a foot to hurt and yet to appear normal on clinical examination. This implies that the momentary stress imposed by manual testing of various movements does not suffice to evoke pain. This is particularly apt to occur in athletes and ballet dancers who get pain after, say, 15 minutes exertion, i.e. after strain far greater and more prolonged than any examiner can impose on the foot by mere clinical testing. In such cases, inspection of the shape of the foot, and of the changes it undergoes when bearing weight, shows where this undue strain falls and by corollary where it must be diminished. Inspection of the patient's worn shoes is often a help in showing where he bears most weight. Moreover, it reveals whether they suit his foot or not.

In angiokeratoma corporis, pain in hands and feet, particularly in the calves is present. They do not stop the patient doing anything and are not altered by rest or activity. Examination reveals nothing at first. In one case the pains started at the age of 4 and were bad enough to wake a perfectly sensible married girl of 25 at night reducing her to tears. Taking a contraceptive pill so increased her pain that she had to stop. Skin biopsy and the presence of corneal opacities clinched the diagnosis.

## THE HEEL

### Traumatic Periostitis and Fracture

Blows on either side of the calcaneus may set up a traumatic periostitis at its subcutaneous surface; subsidence of the swelling and pain is hastened by deep effleurage. Minor flaking or cracks are uncommon and require no treatment. More severe fractures give rise to local pain and tenderness associated with bruising at the anterior part of the sole and require up to two months' complete avoidance of weight-bearing. Fractures involving the articular surface of the calcaneus with the talus set up a painful and intractable osteoarthrosis. Arthrodesis is better performed early than late; for disabling symptoms continue for many years, sometimes indefinitely. Osteitis deformans may attack the calcaneus.

## Subcutaneous Nodules

Posteriorly, nodules may form in the subcutaneous fascia. When these get pinched between the calcaneus and the back of the shoe, severe momentary pain results. On examination, tender nodules the size of a small pea can be felt slipping to and fro under the finger. No conservative treatment avails except the provision of shoes with a gap posteriorly. Division of the nodules by subcutaneous tenotomy under local anaesthesia gives results as good as excision.

## Plantar Fasciitis

### Overstrain

The patient complains of pain at the inner aspect of the sole of one or both heels when walking and standing, quickly relieved by avoiding weight-bearing. The most characteristic symptom is severe pain at the heel on first getting up to walk after sitting. During standing, the normal shape of the foot is partly maintained by the muscles; prolonged weight-bearing may tire them. Should they prove unequal to the burden, strain, soon becoming painful, then falls on the plantar fascia instead.

Examination of the joints and muscles of the foot proves negative. Tenderness is sought and found at the inner part of the front of the calcaneus, at the origin of the plantar fascia. Various other spots are palpated first, to ensure that psychogenic symptoms are detected.

Patients with Dupuytren's contracture at the palm sometimes develop similar swellings, but without contracture, in the plantar fascia. They cause no symptoms.

### Calcanean Spur

Continued overstrain of the fascia may result in the periosteum being pulled away at its origin from the calcaneous.

Since periosteum is the limiting membrane of bone, the gap becomes filled by new growth of bone as also occurs in osteophyte formation at the lumbar joints. The fact that the patient has, or did at one time have, strain on his plantar fascia now becomes visible on radiography. The presence of a calcanean spur on the X-ray photograph cannot determine whether the patient has symptoms or not. Spurs may develop painlessly; painful plantar fasciitis may not be associated with a visible spur. Once a spur has formed, it is permanent; hence radiography may disclose spurs, the pain from which ceased years previously. If history and clinical examination show painful strain to exist at the origin of the plantar fascia, radiography is of no particular assistance.

Treatment is very simple, spur or no spur; it consists in taking the strain off the plantar fascia. The less the angle between hindfoot and forefoot, the more the fascia is relaxed. Hence, all that need be done is to stand the patient on wooden platforms of different thickness, until the minimum height of heel that abolishes the symptoms is found. Provided the upper surface of the heel of the shoe remains horizontal, the higher the heel the more must the forefoot drop towards plantaris when he stands (Fig. 120). This shortens the distance from metatarsus to heel and relieves the fascia from strain. Thus, a height of heel can be found that affords immediate relief. The short flexor muscles in the sole are now energetically treated with faradism and exercises. The soreness leaves the fascia very slowly and it is often six months before a patient can resume his ordinary shoes.

Occasionally, return to ordinary shoes provokes pain again each time it is attempted. In a woman, this is not of much account, but a man may not wish to wear a raised heel indefinitely. If so, the heel of his shoe should be wedged

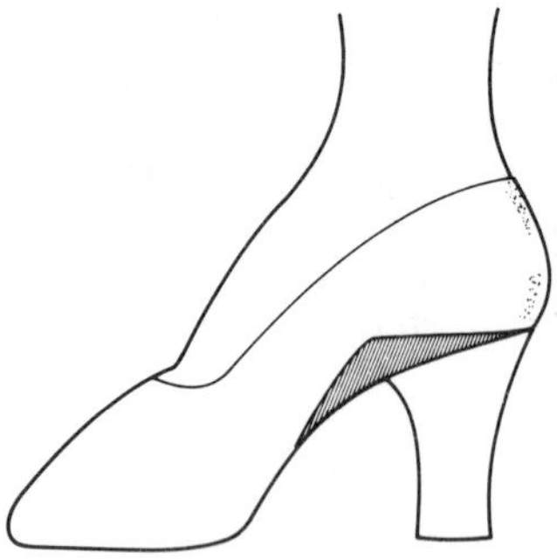

**Fig. 120.** Platform. The upper surface of the heel of the shoe is rendered horizontal by a wedge, thicker anteriorly. The plantar fascia is relaxed, because the forefoot drops into greater plantaris.

anteriorly. Shoes thus designed are on sale in England and the USA by Roots. If this does not suffice, triamcinolone may be injected into the fascial origin and the patient warned of two days' considerable after-pain. The plantar skin is too thick to be capable of surface sterilization; hence the puncture must be made in the thin skin at the inner side of the heel. Alternatively, tenotomy of the fascial origin at the calcaneus under local anaesthesia is required, followed by a couple of days in bed. Exercises for the short flexor muscles are carried out from the outset. It is a very successful little operation.

### Superficial Plantar Fasciitis

The pain is felt all over the posterior part of the sole, usually bilaterally. Curiously enough, the pain may be constant, felt even in bed, although worse during weight-bearing.

Examination shows the whole inferior surface of the heel to be uniformly tender, including the centimetre around the edge of the heel that does not touch the ground.

The only effective treatment is an injection of 10 ml of 0.5% procaine between the superficial plantar fascia and the surface of the calcaneum. The solution diffuses over the whole area forming a large tense swelling. The patient walks away and is usually pain-free by some days later, even after months or years of hitherto intractable symptoms.

### Venereal Fasciitis

*Gonorrhoea.* This disease is no longer seen in Britain. The pain is in both heels and is constant, unrelieved when the patient rests. The patient, if he is honest, admits to a recent attack of gonorrhoea. A few days in bed should be advised to avoid strain on the fascia while the primary infection is being energetically treated.

*Reiter's Disease.* When plantar fasciitis is present with disease of joints as well, the association with non-gonococcal urethritis should be recalled. Mason (1964) states that plantar fasciitis occurs in 20% of all such cases, and is characterized by a fluffy appearance of the spur, designating periostitis. Csonka (1958) also reported that 21.6% of patients with non-gonococcal urethritis develop plantar fasciitis.

## TENDINOUS LESIONS

These will merely be enumerated, having been considered in the previous chapter.

Tenosynovitis of the tendo Achillis from overuse.

Tenovaginitis of the tendo Achillis due to rheumatoid disease, gout, xanthomatosis or chondrocalcinosis.

Rupture of the tendo Achillis.

Tenosynovitis of the peroneal and posterior tibial tendons. Mucocele of these tendons.

## BURSITIS

A bursa is normally present between the tendo Achillis and the tibia. If it becomes tender, pain is elicited when it is squeezed between the tendon and the tibia at the extreme of passive plantiflexion at the ankle. Bursitis is distinguished from lesions of the tendon itself by the fact that rising on tiptoe is painless. Usually one or two injections of triamcinolone are curative.

Another bursa may form at the centre of the inferior aspect of the calcaneus. It lies superficial to the mid-part of the origin of the plantar fascia. A heel support scooped out centrally is required, i.e. shaped like a horse-shoe.

An adventitious bursa may form between the skin and the posterior aspect of the calcaneus in women who wear shoes too incurved at their upper edge posteriorly. The back of the shoe must be altered and a rubber pad can be introduced at the lower half of the back of the calcaneus, keeping the upper half away from the shoe. Excision is seldom necessary.

# LESIONS OF THE FIBULOCALCANEAN LIGAMENT

## Sprain

This is one of the possible lesions in a sprained ankle. The varus movement at the talocalcanean joint is of full range and painful; the valgus movement full and painless. Tenderness is sought along the ligament. Triamcinolone is injected at once; a few days later friction is given to this point in the standard way.

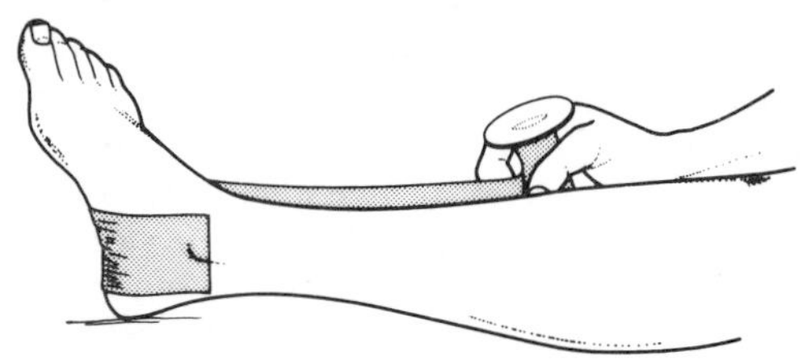

**Fig. 121.** Strapping for the protection of the fibulocalcanean ligament. The strapping begins at the medial malleolus and holds the heel in full valgus by firm application at the outer side of the lower leg.

## Rupture

This is signalled when an excessive range of varus movement is found on testing the talocalcanean joint. Strapping (Fig. 121) is applied holding the joint in valgus and kept on for a month. By then, union will have occurred. Associated lesions are dealt with in the ordinary way, but varus movements must be avoided.

If a recent rupture passes unnoticed, permanent lengthening of the ligament results for which the patient must wear a floated heel (see Fig. 118) indefinitely. Alternatively, a new ligament can be formed by fixing the tendon of the peroneus brevis through holes bored in the neck of the talus and the lower end of the fibula.

# LESIONS OF THE TALOCALCANEAN JOINT

The joint allows movement in only two directions—varus and valgus. The capsular pattern consists of increasing limitation of varus range and ultimate fixation in valgus.

## Talipes Equinovarus

A varus position of the calcaneus on the talus forms part of the club-foot deformity. Correction and the maintenance of correction by Denis-Browne splintage should be instituted as soon after birth as possible.

## Immobilizational Stiffness

Marked limitation of movement results from the immobilization imposed on the tarsal joints by the treatment in plaster of some tibiofibular fractures. The joint is stiff, but there is no muscle spasm when the joint is forced.

Mobilization of the joint is technically difficult; for there is no lever. Whether performed manually or under anaesthesia by means of a Thomas's wrench, the small size of the calcaneus affords very little purchase. Many months' repeated forcing by the physiotherapist eventually brings its reward. Restoration of a full range is not essential; a slightly limited range is compatible with good function.

## Osteoarthrosis

This follows fractures of the calcaneus involving the surface articulating with the talus. Whatever treatment, or none at all, is given to such a fracture, persistent pain is apt to result, curable only by arthrodesis. Some patients largely recover in the course of three or four years, after which no further improvement can be expected. One-third of all unoperated cases are still in pain after 12 years.

## Loose Body in the Joint

This is suggested by a history of twinges. The discomfort is produced by movement at the talocalcanean joint, and not at the ankle joint. Alternatively, the patient may complain of bouts of painful fixation at his heel and, if he attends during an attack the heel will be found fixed in valgus by muscle spasm.

Manipulative reduction must be attempted (see Volume II) but seldom proves permanent.

## Subacute Traumatic Arthritis

Recovery after a sprained ankle is unduly delayed by pain in the heel and mid-foot. Examination shows limitation of varus movement at the talocalcanean joint maintained by muscle spasm.

The mid-tarsal joint is usually also affected. Local warmth is often detectable if the patient has recently walked a distance.

This condition is often mistaken for post-traumatic adhesions; for there is chronic pain after an injury and the radiograph shows that the bones are not damaged. If the limitation of movement at the talocalcanean joint is missed, such patients may well be treated by mobilization under anaesthesia for supposed adhesions, which leads to aggravation for one to two months. Patients in whom a subacute traumatic arthritis has been exacerbated by manipulation are often regarded as hysterics, but in psychological disorders the heel is fixed in varus, not valgus.

Treatment consists of one or two injections of triamcinolone into the joint. Since the heel is held in valgus, the simpler approach is at the inner side. The lower edge of the medial malleolus is identified, and 2 cm below lies the prominence of the sustentaculum tali. The needle is inserted at this level and passes to about 1 cm before striking bone. The point of the needle is then manoeuvred up and down slightly until the spot is found where resistance ceases and the needle passes another 1 cm and lies intra-articularly; 1 ml of the suspension is injected into each of the two compartments of the joint (see Volume II). This treatment seldom fails, but if it does, several months immobilization in plaster is indicated.

## Monarticular Rheumatoid Arthritis

There is no history of injury and the disorder is often bilateral. In addition to the limitation of movement towards varus by muscle spasm, local heat and synovial thickening are palpable. The mid-tarsal joint is usually also affected. It is a rheumatoid manifestation, often accompanied by the typical changes in other joints. In young men, Reiter's disease and ankylosing spondylitis are possible alternative causes; in elderly men, gout should not be forgotten. In rheumatoid arthritis, triamcinolone injected into the joint destroys the pain within a day and, even if the range does not increase, the patient can by this means be kept comfortable for many months, even years.

## Dancer's Heel

During their training, ballet dancers develop hypermobility towards plantiflexion at the ankle joint as the result of work *sur les pointes.* Consequently, bruising of the periosteum at the back of the lower tibia may be caused from repeated pressure by the upper edge of the posterior surface of the calcaneus. Athletes may bruise the periosteum in the same way; less often, one plantiflexion strain may have this result.

The pain is felt at the back of the heel and is reproduced by full passive plantiflexion at the ankle, which presses the calcaneus against the area of traumatic periostitis.

About two injections of triamcinolone stop the tenderness, but the dancer must have the mechanism of the disorder explained, so that she takes care not to repeat the causative trauma by repeatedly over-pointing the foot again.

A similar condition occurs in soccer players. When the ball is kicked from underneath, the foot may suddenly be forced into full plantiflexion, whereupon the impact of the upper surface of the calcaneus bruises the lower edge of the tibia. The pain may last several years, but is permanently relieved by a few sessions of deep friction. This was shown to me by F. Harris in 1974.

## Calcanean Apophysitis (Osgood)

Between the ages of 6 and 12 years, apophysitis may occur, often bilaterally. The bone is slightly tender and the radiographic appearances characteristic. I have seen a child in whom a piece of radiotranslucent glass lying against the periosteum gave rise to what at first appeared to be an apophysitis. Spontaneous recovery occurs in a year or two, often with the development of a slight permanent prominence at the posterior aspect of the calcaneus.

# THE MID-TARSAL JOINT

The talonavicular and calcaneocuboid joints comprise the mid-tarsal joint. Movement is possible in six directions: dorsiflexion and plantiflexion, adduction and abduction, lateral and medial rotation. On account of the obliquity of the joint surfaces, dorsiflexion at the mid-tarsal joint is accompanied by abduction of the forefoot with consequent stretching—often painful—of the calcaneonavicular ligament. Hence excessive dorsiflexion strains on the mid-tarsal joint should be avoided.

When movement at the mid-tarsal joint is

tested, the heel must be pulled down and held still. This precaution prevents movement at the ankle and talocalcanean joints from complicating the clinical picture. The capsular pattern is increasing limitation of adduction and medial rotation owing to peroneal spasm.

Five different conditions affect the mid-tarsal joint.

## Mid-tarsal Strain

If power in the musculature of the sole becomes insufficient to maintain a sufficient degree of plantaris of the forefoot during weight-bearing, the mid-tarsal ligaments become painfully strained. This is particularly likely to occur in patients who already have an over-arched foot or an equinus deformity at the ankle. In such cases, weight-bearing dorsiflexes, and therefore abducts, the forefoot at the mid-tarsal joint. At first the plantiflexion–dorsiflexion range of movement increases and the foot becomes wobbly; later on discomfort (mid-tarsal strain) appears, pain occurring at the extremes of passive range, especially rotation. Later, the inner side of the foot becomes prominent owing to the abduction of the forefoot on the hindfoot and painful overstretching of the calcaneonavicular (spring) ligament results.

Treatment consists of three measures: (1) raising the heel of the shoe, so as to allow the forefoot to adopt a more plantigrade position during weight-bearing; (2) exercises (faradic and resisted) to the short flexor muscles in the sole so that they become adequate to take the strain and thus relieve tension on the ligament; (3) mobilization of the mid-tarsal joint, to ensure that the full range of movement can be achieved painlessly. Although the range of movement at the joint is excessive, repeated strains, followed by healing of minor ligamentous ruptures, will have led to the formation of adhesions and consequent discomfort at the extremes of range. This is the only example in the body of manipulation being required at a joint which already possesses an excessive range of movement. Faradism to the short flexor muscles and exercises follow.

Marked persistent tenderness of the calcaneonavicular ligament calls for infiltration with triamcinolone suspension.

## Mid-tarsal Osteoarthrosis

Unless gross and the result of fracture or of an old navicular apophysitis (Kohler), osteoarthrosis causes no symptoms. It results in osteophytes

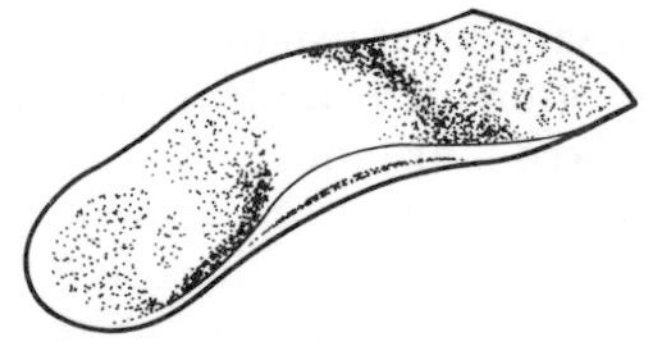

**Fig. 122.** A steel support. This is accurately moulded to the sole of the foot and prevents as far as possible all movement at the tarsal joints.

visible and palpable at the dorsum of the foot and equally visible on the radiograph. Osteoarthrosis at the mid-tarsal joint is largely a misnomer, based on mistaken deduction from radiological appearances. If the ligaments are strained—whether osteoarthrosis shows on the radiograph or not—the treatment for mid-tarsal strain applies. If gross disturbance of the anatomy of the foot has really led to marked osteoarthrosis causing symptoms, a steel support moulded accurately to the sole of the foot (Fig. 122) minimizes movement as far as possible at the disorganized joints. Arthrodesis is a last resort.

## Mid-tarsal Ligamentous Contracture

After immobilization in plaster for fractures of the lower leg, middle-aged patients may complain months or some years later that, although they can walk short distances in comfort, they cannot run or ski without immediate pain. Limitation of movement at the mid-tarsal joint has become permanent owing to ligamentous contracture. This has proved resistant even to mobilization under anaesthesia, which has already been carried out, usually several times, without benefit.

Examination discloses considerable limitation of movement at the mid-tarsal joint, without muscle spasm. This indicates structural contracture. The shortened ligaments on the dorsum of the foot are tender.

After all the tender ligaments have been adequately infiltrated with triamcinolone suspension, pain ceases, usually permanently, although there is no increase in the range of movement. The foot does not become quite normal, but running and skiing once more become possible with, at most, slight discomfort.

## Subacute Arthritis in Adolescence (Spasmodic Pes Planus)

This disorder has for years been known as 'spasmodic pes planus' because the sign that first

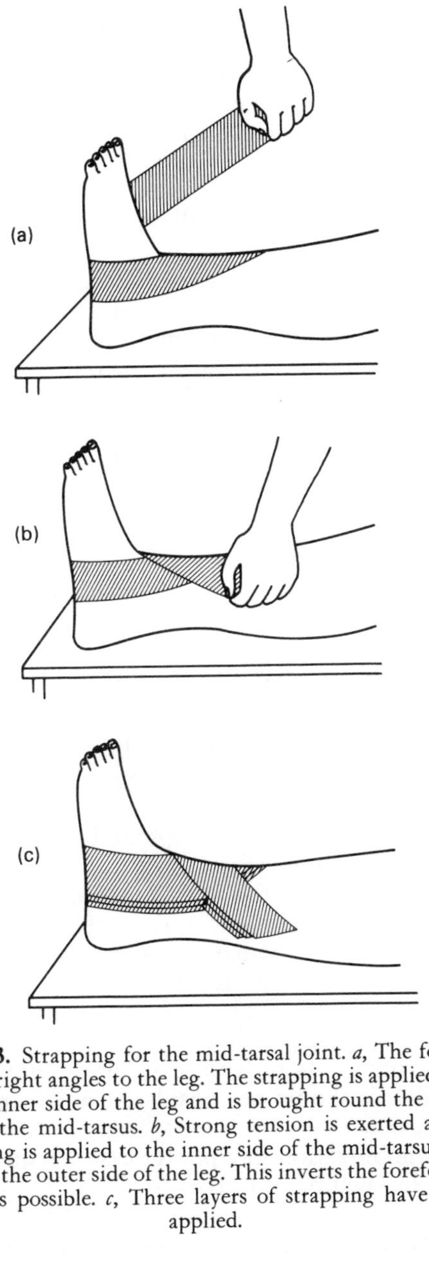


**Fig. 123.** Strapping for the mid-tarsal joint. *a*, The foot is held at right angles to the leg. The strapping is applied first to the inner side of the leg and is brought round the outer side of the mid-tarsus. *b*, Strong tension is exerted as the strapping is applied to the inner side of the mid-tarsus and fixed to the outer side of the leg. This inverts the forefoot as much as possible. *c*, Three layers of strapping have been applied.

drew attention to the condition was spasm of the peroneal muscles. The name originated with a past generation of orthopaedic surgeons, but muscle spasm is never primary. In this instance, the spasm results from arthritis, and is not intermittent, but continuous. The name is misleading and should be abandoned.

This overuse arthritis occurs almost exclusively in boys between the ages of 12 and 16. The talocalcanean and mid-tarsal joints of both feet are affected together. Little or no pain results; the patient's mother is the person who usually complains. The boy stumps in with a clumsy gait and is found either to have a long thin foot or to be overweight and have some degree of pes cavus—in other words, a foot so shaped as to be easily overstrained.

The condition is not common except in districts where a large number of factories exist and boys fresh from school are put to work (e.g. at a lathe) that entails standing all day. Such overuse is the aetiological factor. On examination, valgus deformity of the heel and abduction deformity of the forefoot are seen to be maintained by spasm of the peroneal and extensor longus digitorum muscles. When the patient stands, the tendons are seen as a prominent tight band behind and below the lateral malleolus. Passive inversion at the heel and tarsus is prevented by muscle spasm. A mere valgus position of the heel and abduction of the forefoot during weight-bearing do not suggest this uncommon condition; the diagnosis is justified only when muscle spasm restricts movement at, or long-standing spasm has led to contracture fixing, these two joints. The radiograph reveals no abnormality.

Untreated, the slight symptoms cease at the end of two years and the foot becomes permanently but painlessly fixed in the deformed position. An ungainly gait results; that is all. No troubles ensue in later life.

## Conservative Treatment

*Early Case.* Movement at the joint has not been entirely lost and the patient experiences discomfort on standing for some time but walking is painless and in the absence of weight-bearing there is no aching. The essence of treatment is relief from weight-bearing and support for the joint.

The lad therefore requires (*a*) a sedentary job, (*b*) a bicycle, (*c*) a wedge on the heels of his shoes and (*d*) strapping of the joint. He is told never to stand for one instant if he can help it. If he sits at home, sits at work and travels everywhere on a bicycle, weight-bearing is almost completely avoided. Nevertheless he remains able to get about satisfactorily.

The heels of his shoes are fitted with inner wedges; these tend towards a varus position of the calcaneus. Non-elastic strapping is applied freshly each week to support the affected joint. The strapping should be put on while the foot is held at a right angle and as far over towards varus as possible. First the strapping is fixed to the inner aspect of the lower leg, then carried round the mid-tarsus, then fixed to the outer aspect of the lower leg during strong traction (Fig. 123). The patient is kept under observation and in the course of 6 to 12 months usually regains a full range of movement and loses his deformity. Recurrence is improbable.

*Late Case.* There is no movement at the talocalcanean joint which is fixed by peroneal spasm in the position of valgus; little or no movement is possible at the mid-tarsal joint.

The leg and foot should be encased from below the knee to the toes in a plaster cast while the foot is held in the varus position. In most cases, this position can be attained by blocking the peroneal nerve at the point where it winds round the neck of the fibula. The nerve trunk is identified by palpation and local anaesthesia induced. Paralysis of the peroneal and extensor longus digitorum muscles results and the bar to varus movement is thus abolished. The plaster cast is kept on for six weeks, when it is removed and the measures indicated for the early case instituted.

*Fixation.* If paralysis of the evertor muscles does not permit movement towards varus, structural contracture of the ligaments about the talocalcanean and mid-tarsal joints has occurred. The decision must now be taken whether to allow the deformity to continue in the knowledge that it will remain as a fixed deformity, painless but unsightly, or to perform arthrodesis. This leads to fixation in a good position, but is scarcely worth while.

## Pseudarthrosis of a Talocalcanean Bridge

A different type of fixation in valgus results from arthrosis that may appear in adolescence at the defect between the two halves of a talocalcanean bridge. Such a painful pseudarthrosis is associated with lipping of the upper edge of the talus and later of the adjacent edge of the navicular too (Harris & Beath 1948). Gross restriction at both the talocalcanean and mid-tarsal joints results, causing a pain which may prove relievable only by arthrodesis.

## Subacute Arthritis in Middle Age

The patients are usually stout women. The muscular spasm and limitation of movement are less pronounced than in adolescence. Overuse is a much commoner cause than an isolated sprain. Cases that have persisted for two or three years are not uncommon; without treatment the condition appears to continue indefinitely without much alteration. Examination reveals that muscular spasm partly restricts an inversion movement at the talocalcanean and mid-tarsal joints, usually unilaterally. The radiological appearances are normal. If only one joint is affected, it can be successfully infiltrated with triamcinolone. If the lesion is too diffuse, affecting many of the tarsal joints, treatment by rest, tilting the heel and strapping in the varus position nearly always leads to eventual subsidence of the arthritis. Usually six months of this modified rest are required and for some years afterwards the patient should guard against renewed overuse. Mobilization under anaesthesia is contra-indicated.

## Monarticular Rheumatoid Arthritis

Arthritis, usually bilateral, sets in for no apparent reason at the talocalcanean and mid-tarsal joints. If the arthritis is at all severe, the patient can scarcely hobble a few steps and attends in a wheelchair. Sleep is disturbed.

In severe cases, the foot is markedly oedematous, warm to the touch and movement at these two joints is very much restricted. If the oedema allows, synovial swelling is palpable at the dorsum of the foot. The usual cause is a rheumatoid type of disorder, but in young men gonorrhoea, Reiter's disease and ankylosing spondylitis should be considered, and in elderly men, gout.

Immobilization in a plaster cast is required at once in rheumatoid arthritis. This is followed within a few days by complete relief from pain, the patient being able to walk short distances without discomfort. He can return to sedentary work. The plaster cast has to be kept on for at least a year. In practice the patient requests its removal or it becomes loose after some months; in either case the pain returns and another cast has to be applied. Recovery usually takes one or two years. If not, rather than allow the patient to continue indefinitely in pain, arthrodesis is recommended.

Triamcinolone, so useful when one joint can be accurately infiltrated, is scarcely practicable in acute polyarthritis, especially as the inferior ligaments are difficult to locate precisely.

## THE CUNEO-FIRST-METATARSAL JOINT

### Osteoarthrosis

Goodfellow's (1965) research on hallux rigidus showed that this resulted from a previous osteochondrosis. It is thus highly probable that the cause of bilateral osteoarthrosis at the cuneo-first-metatarsal joint also appearing in adolescence is also a past osteochondrosis.

The onset is usually insidious. The patient, usually a girl, finds that if she wears shoes that lace tightly across the dorsum of her foot, localized pain arises at the site of a small bilateral projection. Palpation reveals this to be an osteophyte at the cuneo-first-metatarsal joint; radiography confirms this. By the age of 16, the osteophytes may have become quite large, and in a man wearing laced shoes is a sufficient embarrassment for removal to be requested.

Rarely, the onset is sudden, both joints becoming tender and swollen for about a week. After this severe phase has subsided, the girl finds she has a small prominence, previously absent on each foot.

The condition is harmless. Recurrent pain is due to pressure of a lace-up shoe squeezing the skin against the osteophytes. In men, or for cosmetic reasons in girls, the bony prominences can be chiselled away.

If the arthritis is acute, a few days' rest is advised, with weight-bearing only in a high-heeled court shoe, no part of which touches the joint. Spontaneous recovery from the pain is a certainty. Avoiding pressure on the now prominent joint and wearing a heel high enough to make the plantiflexion deformity innocuous keep the patient's foot comfortable. A felt ring round the bony outcrop enables the girl to wear lace-up shoes.

It is important that the patient should not be told without adequate explanation that she has 'arthritis' in her feet. This is alarming to patient and parents, who, when the onset is so early in life, naturally envisage eventual crippledom.

Osteoarthrosis of the cuneo-first-metatarsal joint may lead to fixation of the joint with considerable plantaris deformity. This may in turn result in metatarsalgia affecting the first metatarsophalangeal or the sesamoid-metatarsal joint. If so, a support (Fig. 124) must be prescribed to take weight off the head of the bone.

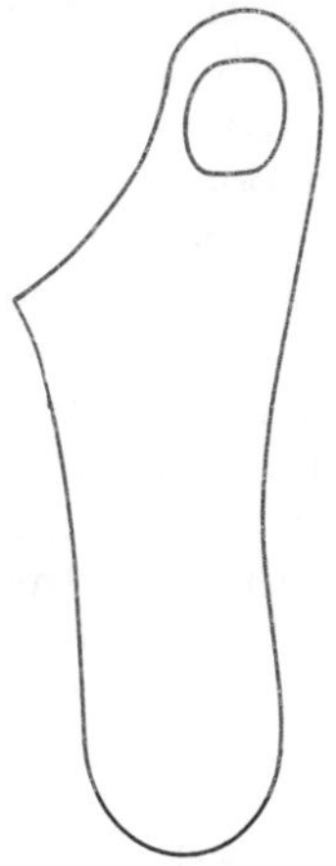

**Fig. 124.** A support for sesamoiditis. The hole in the support corresponds to the first metatarsophalangeal joint.

### Gout

This rarely attacks this joint before the big toe. Warmth, reddening of the skin and pain at night suggest the diagnosis.

### Loose Body

Athletes may complain of sudden twinges at this joint during a sprint. These are recurrent and disabling in race after race.

Examination shows that the twinges appear not to arise from the ankle or the talocalcanean joint, and that no actual subluxation of the metatarsal bone itself on the cuneiform occurs when the patient rises on tiptoe.

Sustained traction on the joint of 9 kg (20 lb) for 30 minutes two or three times a week (see Volume II) is curative; presumably internal derangement is the cause.

## CUBOID ROTATION

Some 4% of pain in athletes' feet results from fixed rotation of the cuboid bone caused by the pull of the tendon of peroneus longus. The mid-tarsal movements are of full range but lost at the outer side of the foot, where the inferior aspect of the cuboid ligaments is found tender. Treatment (Newell and Woodle 1981) consists of forcing plantiflexion of the forefoot while the manipulator's thumbs apply strong upward pressure on the bone.

## THE METATARSAL SHAFTS

### Short First Metatarsal Bone

Much is made of atavistic shortening of the first metatarsal bone. Such shortening is compatible with full painless function of the foot, and the cause of pain should be sought elsewhere.

### Marching Fracture

The feature that should bring this condition to mind at once is unilateral localized warmth and oedema lying in a circular patch over the metatarsus. The condition is a stress fracture. As a rule, there is no history of injury or of an audible crack, not even always of excessive walking.

Children are almost as liable to marching fractures as adults; my youngest patient was a six-year-old.

Examination during the first month after the pain began reveals: (*a*) local warmth; (*b*) oedema over the dorsum of the forefoot; (*c*) tenderness of the metatarsal shaft and of the interosseous muscles on each side of it. Clearly the two halves of the bone cannot move on each other without straining these muscles (cf. fractured rib). The tenderness is therefore more diffuse than is expected from the fracture as such, and it is not always easy to decide which of the metatarsal bones has broken. The fracture is most often at the neck of the second or fourth metatarsal bone but may lie anywhere along the shaft. Stress fractures appear not to occur at the first and fifth metatarsal bones.

After two or three weeks, the tumour caused by callus becomes clearly palpable, especially when the distal part of the shaft has broken. Diagnosis is then easy, and may be confirmed by radiography. Since appreciable displacement does not occur, and no callus is visible during the first two or three weeks and the tiny crack may not show on the radiograph of a recent case, it is well to wait until the third week before having X-rays taken.

Abortive cases occur, in which the periosteal reaction round the neck of the bone is indicated by a faint fusiform shadow, visible only on one side of the bone. Such an appearance suggests a partial crack not extending through the whole shaft, but the condition is nevertheless painful.

Circular elevation on the dorsum of the foot may be seen, caused by a tendency to oedema localized by a shoe with a narrow strap across the dorsum, but this is bilateral, painless, not warm and absent on waking.

Localized warmth, swelling and tenderness at the dorsum of the distal part of the foot occur in: (*a*) Gout. The recurrent history in an elderly man is suggestive; the skin over the joint is at least slightly red. (*b*) Gonorrhoea, when the rheumatoid type of response has occurred. (*c*) Rheumatoid arthritis. This is usually multiple, and the disorder has persisted for too long. A marching fracture recovers spontaneously in six weeks. (*d*) Freiburg's arthritis of the second metatarsophalangeal joint. (*e*) Sarcoidosis and Reiter's disease usually affect several metatarsophalangeal joints simultaneously, and also a large joint. (*f*) Ringworm. If a small crack exists between two toes owing to infection with the fungus, local cellulitis may occur with swelling, warmth and reddening at the dorsum of the foot. Inspection of the interdigital clefts makes the diagnosis clear. (*g*) Morton's metatarsalgia. If a patient with this disorder is seen within a few hours of an attack, the vascular reaction that follows gives rise to local warmth but no oedema. (*h*) Tuberculosis. This is a rarity at the cuneometatarsal joint. Swelling and warmth were present in the one case that I have encountered, but there was no oedema of the forefoot.

The bone is firmly enough united to be painless in six weeks, whether the fracture was partial or complete. Mal-union need not be feared. There is no necessity for the patient to stop walking during the period of union; his forefoot should merely be firmly bound to diminish movement at the fracture and to enable the other metatarsal shafts to splint the broken bone. Even so, weightbearing is bound to hurt a little; it is for the patient to do as much as he will in these circumstances.

Persistent pain after the six weeks have elapsed originates not at the fracture but at the interosseous muscles, strained by the abnormal stresses. They should be treated by deep massage (see Volume II), which brings about full recovery in four to six treatments.

## SPLAY-FOOT

When this causes symptoms, these are due to painful over-stretching of the transverse interosseus ligaments, whereby the metarsal bones are given excessive horizontal play. Other conditions, particularly weakness of the short flexor muscles of the toes, are also usually present. Such weakness should be treated energetically and the foot bound.

Localized splaying indicates a ganglion lying between two metatarsal heads. When the patient stands, an excessive interval is seen between two toes and palpation reveals that a semi-solid tumour keeps them apart. Since the tumour is thick and loculated, often composed partly of fibrolipomatous material, attempted aspiration seldom diminishes its size or the patient's symptoms. Excision is indicated.

## THE TOE JOINTS

### The First Metatarsophalangeal Joint

This joint is normally capable of 30° of flexion and 90° of extension; it is the latter movement which is important. As he walks, an individual has to extend the big toe of his hinder foot to at least 45° when his other foot goes forwards, more if high heels are worn. Hence in men osteoarthrosis remains painless until half the range of extension has been lost, whereas women suffer much earlier.

#### Arthritis in Adolescence

The cause of osteoarthrosis at the first metatarsophalangeal joint long remained obscure. Since the disorder was unprovoked, bilateral and appeared in adolescence, this suggested a constitutional factor. However, in 1965 Goodfellow presented his research into the aetiology of hallux rigidus. He showed that the cause was the same osteochondrosis dissecans as occurs at other joints during adolescence, and included in his paper radiographs and microscopical sections of excised tissue.

In a youngster aged 15 to 20, large osteophytes gradually form at the dorsum of both first metatarsophalangeal joints. Patients are nearly always male. The onset is slow and unprovoked by overuse or injury. At first, compensation is achieved in such young patients by the development of hyperextensibility at the interphalangeal joint. Within a few years the joint fixes in the neutral position and a hallux rigidus has developed; now pain at every step is inevitable due to bone being forced against bone at the dorsum of the joint. Examination shows a fixed big toe, little or no range of extension remaining, and gross dorsal osteophytes.

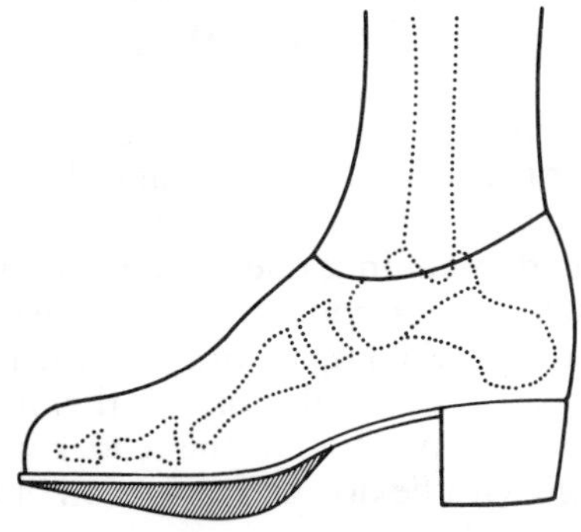

**Fig. 125.** A rocker for the relief of hallux rigidus. Instead of extending at the first metatarsophalangeal, the forefoot rocks over the thickened sole.

Conservative treatment consists in the prescription of a rocker (Fig. 125) whereby the patient can adopt a normal gait, pivoting over the rocker instead of forcing his osteoarthrotic joint towards extension. If this does not suffice, operative removal of the base of the proximal phalanx is indicated. Alternatively, a steel sole prevents movement at the metatarsophalangeal joint, but the gait is less natural.

#### Arthrosis in Middle Age

Osteoarthrosis at the first metatarsophalangeal joint also occurs between the ages of 40 and 60; this cannot be the result of osteochondrosis. Sometimes a heavy weight falling on the joint stimulates the degeneration. In men, symptoms begin when only 45° of extension range remain, but a woman, with her higher heels, gets pain when 30° range has been lost. Since aggravation is slow, no symptoms may arise for years.

The arthrosis itself causes no symptoms unless the joint is overstrained by being forced into extension with each step the patient takes. In minor cases, or if the cause was one long walk, the disorder is really a superimposed traumatic arthritis. The result of such overuse can be abolished by one intra-articular injection of triamcinolone. The pain caused by the injection is considerable for 12 hours; the patient is then comfortable, but must be careful in the future.

Good results can also be achieved by traction. The foot is fixed and a Japanese fingerstall applied to the hallux. Traction of 10 kg (20 lb) for 20 minutes on, say, six to eight occasions, is an average (see Volume II). Afterwards, recurrence must be avoided by a rocker fitted to the sole of the shoe (Fig. 125). Alternatively, a strong plate can be incorporated in the sole of the shoe, lying at the medial side and extending from the waist to the anterior edge of the sole. This impedes extension at the affected joint.

## Gout

This occurs typically at the big toe in elderly men. Monosodium urate is believed to injure leucocytes when phagocytosis of the crystals forms lyosomes. These are enclosed in an envelope which on disruption releases proteolytic enzymes which damage adjacent cells, provoking inflammation. Weissman and Rita's (1972) experiments with synthetic membranes showed that when they contained oestradiol they were not injured by urates, whereas the presence of testosterone enhanced damage. This accounts for the largely male incidence of gout.

The attacks are unprovoked, recurrent, alternate from one foot to the other and for at least some years leave the joint normal between attacks. The joint swells and becomes warm to the touch. Soon the skin becomes red, owing to the accumulation of plasma kinins in sufficient concentration to cause vasodilatation. Eisen (1966) showed that phagocytosis of the microcrystals of urates in the inflammatory effusion caused release of proteolytic enzymes activating kininogen. This change in colour should not be waited because, sepsis apart, no other condition causes spontaneous swelling and warmth of the joint. The radiograph is no help in the early case, showing nothing or perhaps, on account of the patient's age, a little osteoarthrosis—misleadingly. The punched-out areas appear only after some years.

The best drug is indomethacin (six tablets of 25 mg the first day, three the next) which aborts the attack in about 24 hours. This drug (like aspirin but unlike hydrocortisone) inhibits the synthesis of prostaglandin on which the capacity of a tissue to become inflamed depends. Butazolidine comes a close second, 200 mg four times the first day and then gradually diminishing also stops the pain in a day or two. Colchicum has been superseded except as a diagnostic medium: 0.5 mg tablets are taken hourly, and relief comes on after 24 hours, usually accompanied by diarrhoea. Since colchicine has no effect on any other form of arthritis, such a result is diagnostic. It acts by preventing the leucocytes which have ingested the urate crystals from releasing the chemotactic factors to which the inflammation in the joint is due. In the absence of drug treatment, an attack of gout in the big toe may well take a month or two to subside. Between attacks, the excretion of urates has to be enhanced by aspirin, probenecid (Benemid) 500 mg tablets, sulphinpyrazone (Anturan) (100 mg) or allopurinol (Zyloric) 100 to 200 mg.

Pseudogout also attacks the big toe. McCarty and Hollander (1961) examined the crystals in synovial fluid from gouty patients and found that, in a small proportion, the crystals were not urates but calcium pyrophosphate. These show birefringence when examined by polarized light. However, the response to butazolidine is satisfactory in these cases too. An intra-articular injection of triamcinolone is curative by the next day. Currey and Swettenham (1965) report that more than one type of crystal can often be isolated from the aspirated joint fluid in cases of calcified joint cartilage.

## Metatarsalgia at the First Joint

This is uncommon. The cause is an excessively small angle between forefoot and hindfoot, usually as the result of a pes cavus deformity or secondary to osteoarthrosis at the cuneo-first-metatarsal joint. Intra-articular triamcinolone quickly abates the traumatic arthritis. A raised heel with a horizontal upper surface prevents recurrence.

## Sesamometatarsal Lesions

Bruising of the sesamoid bone of the flexor longus hallucis may result from stepping on a pebble barefoot, for example. If so, pain at the inner aspect of the forefoot is felt at each step, and resisted flexion of the big toe hurts inferiorly. The tender spot shifts with the position of the hallux.

Alternatively, overuse may set up a traumatic arthritis at the sesamo-first-metatarsal joint. This is particularly likely in patients with a pes cavus complicated by equinus due to short calf muscles. At each step, the individual comes down too hard on his forefoot, the impact bruising the joint. In such a case, resisted flexion of the hallux is painful, but the position of the tender spot does not change with flexion and extension of the big toe.

In either case, infiltration of the correct spot with 1 ml of triamcinolone is curative. Recurrence is prevented both by fitting a mid-tarsal support and by raising the heel of the shoe, while keeping its upper surface horizontal.

## The Outer Four Metatarsophalangeal Joints

Pain at the plantar aspect of the forefoot is called metatarsalgia.

### Chronic Metatarsalgia

This affects the middle three toes and arises in the following conditions, in which an excessive proportion of the body weight falls on the forefoot. Normally the forefoot should bear only one-third of the total and that third should be distributed between the pads of the toes and the metatarsophalangeal joints. When the digital flexor muscles contract adequately, the metatarsal heads are relieved of much pressure, which falls on the flexed toes instead.

In the conditions listed below there is pain felt at the plantar aspect of the forefoot on standing and walking, relieved by rest. Although the tenderness is always spoken of as 'of the metatarsal heads', it is not the articular cartilage which is tender, but the plantar aspect of the capsule of these metatarsophalangeal joints. Since this capsulitis is essentially traumatic and due to excessive pressure, no irreversible changes have taken place and relief from bearing too much weight on the forefoot leads to full recovery.

*Pes Plantaris.* In patients with a pes plantaris deformity—especially if there is also a slight equinus—too much pressure is borne by the forefoot (Fig. 126) with the result that the plantar aspect of the capsules of the metatarsophalangeal joints, especially the second, third and fourth, develops traumatic tenderness.

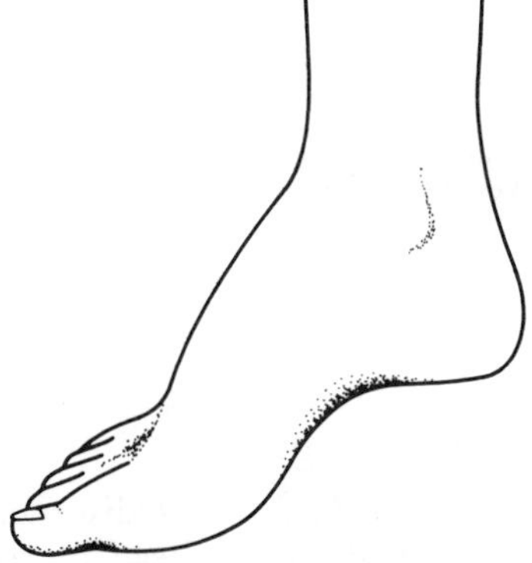

**Fig. 126.** Pes plantaris. Note the dropped forefoot without any other deformity.

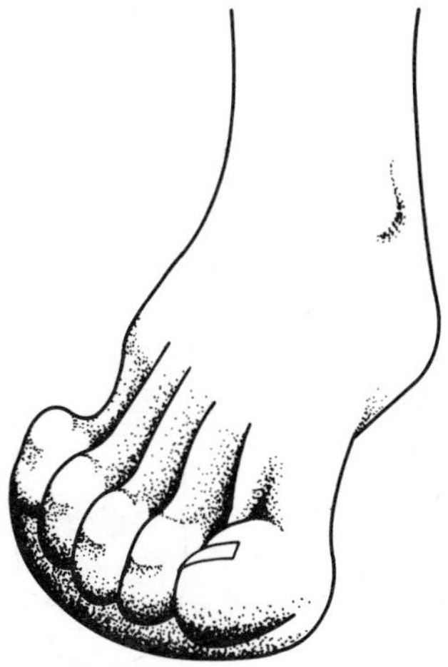

**Fig. 127.** Pes cavus. The foot is short and broad. The extensor tendons of the toes stand out, holding the toes clawed. The toes have corns and a large callosity has formed under the metatarsal heads.

*Pes Cavus.* Hyperextension at the metatarsophalangeal joints, which so often accompanies a pes cavus deformity, is caused by shortening of the extensor longus hallucis and digitorum muscles. In such a case the toes bear none of the body weight, and metatarsalgia with a large callosity under the heads of the middle three metatarsal heads is almost inevitable (Fig. 127).

*Weak Flexor Muscles.* This is a common cause of pain in the foot. If the short muscles in the sole weaken as the result of rest in bed during an illness, or are suddenly given too much to do, i.e. during an unwonted long walk, they prove inadequate. Since they cease to flex the toes properly at each step, excessive weight is repeatedly thrown on to the metatarsophalangeal joints instead; pain results.

*Results of Wearing High Heels.* In all ready-made shoes, high heels possess an oblique upper surface. The patient stands on an inclined plane, sliding down on to her forefoot all the time. High heels, the upper surface of which is horizontal, or nearly so, are free from this defect and would bring comfort to all women with a plantaris forefoot. No such ready-made shoes exist.

Treatment consists of the avoidance of excessive weight-bearing at the forefoot. Active and passive measures can be taken. The former consist

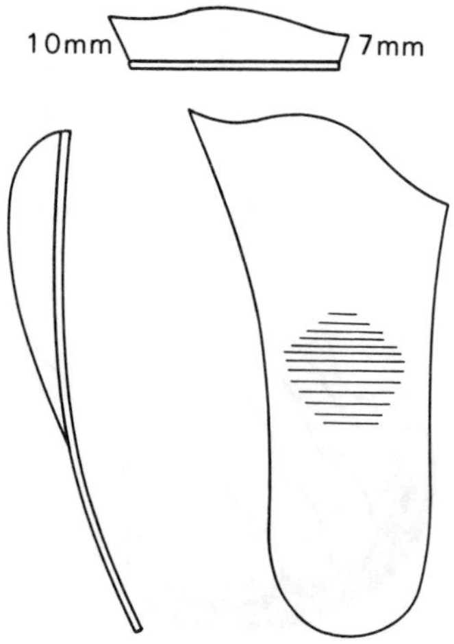


**Fig. 128.** A support for metatarsalgia. The thickness lies just behind the heads of the metatarsal bones, the shafts of which are made to bear the greater weight.

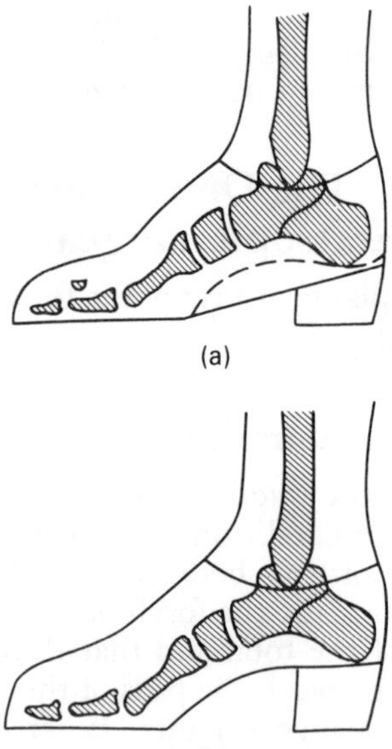


**Fig. 129.** A shoe with an oblique heel (*a*) and a horizontal heel (*b*). In (*a*) note how the central part of the sole of the foot is out of contact with the shoe and how the pressure of the heel on an inclined plane pushes the body weight on to the forefoot. In (*b*) note how the shoe fits the sole of the foot and how weight-bearing on the heel is devoid of forward stress.

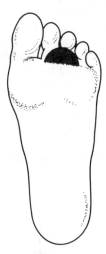

of so strengthening the short flexor muscles of the sole by faradism and exercises that the toes flex properly at every step and do not tire after standing or walking. Prophylactic foot exercises, after a long stay in bed or debilitating illness are an obvious precaution. The latter comprises a support (Fig. 128) which stops short just behind the heads of the metatarsal bones and ensures that the shafts of these bones bear more weight than the joints themselves. A heel with a horizontal upper surface hinders the foot from sliding forwards and enables more weight to be borne on the hindfoot and less on the forefoot (Fig. 129).

*Local Injury.* Traumatic arthritis at a metatarsophalangeal joint is rare. It can result both from violence applied to the toe straining the joint indirectly and from a direct blow. Limited movement results which continues for many months but responds very well to one intra-articular injection of triamcinolone. The joint is very sore for 12 hours, whereupon complete lasting relief is to be expected.

*Dancer's Metatarsalgia.* A dancer who does much tiptoe work (not *sur les pointes*) may bruise the pad of fibrous tissue in the sole lying anterior to the second, third and fourth metatarsophalangeal joints. When this happens, he must be made to bear more weight at the plantar surface of the toes. To this end his ballet shoes are fitted with a small semilunar pad (see Fig. 130) which ensures that the joints are spared as much weight as possible.

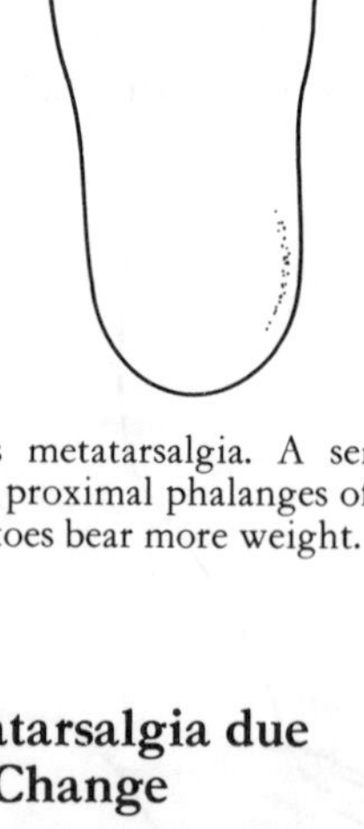

**Fig. 130.** Dancer's metatarsalgia. A semi-lunar anterior support makes the proximal phalanges of the three middle toes bear more weight.

## Chronic Metatarsalgia due to Structural Change

*Freiburg's Osteochondrosis.* This disorder was regarded as confined to the head of the second metatarsal bone, but in Hoskinson's (1974) series, five of 28 occurred at the third. It was first described by Freiburg in 1914. My youngest patient was 14 years old and had had a fortnight's pain. Examination showed localized arthritis of the second metatarsophalangeal joint. At first, local swelling and warmth are present, together with limitation of flexion and extension at this joint. So early on, Freiburg's disease is difficult to distinguish from a marching fracture. Radiography gives no immediate help, since it takes a month from the onset of pain for the characteristic radiographic change to begin to show at the head of the bone, and it often takes three weeks for a marching fracture to become visible.

Spontaneous recovery from the subacute arthritis takes a year. By that time, the joint recovers an adequate, but not full, range of movement, and the head of the bone is permanently enlarged. Palpation reveals the increase in size and a prominent ridge on the bone at the dorsal aspect of its articular edge. Metatarsalgia due to the bony enlargement may ensue. In due course, osteoarthrosis supervenes and, by the time the patient is 40 or 50, the joint may become fixed in a manner analogous to hallux rigidus.

Limitation of extension can be rendered symptomless by the provision of a rocker.

Before the fissure fracture across the head of the metatarsal head has become complete, the blood supply to the distal part can be restored by Smillie's (1967) operation. However, once the plantar isthmus of bone has given way and the fragment is fully detached it is too late.

Hoskinson (1974) noted that radiopaque loose bodies were apt to form and that their excision abolished pain, whereas removal of the metatarsal head of the base of the phalanx was not a long-term success.

*Rheumatoid Arthritis and Gout.* In advanced cases, the toes become fixed in the clawed position. Metatarsalgia inevitably results, and is largely relieved by a support.

## Pressure on Nerves at the Forefoot

Pressure on nerves here causes acute twinges of pain, but no loss of conduction is discernible. Hence the diagnosis is made largely on the history.

### Bruising of the Second Digital Nerve

This nerve passes forwards at the lateral side of the plantar aspect of the first metatarsophalangeal joint, and can easily be palpated there as a thick strand. It bifurcates just distal to the joint, supplying sensation to the adjacent borders of the first and second toes. In view of its exposed position, it is surprising that it is so seldom injured. Stepping on a sharp stone, or a puncture wound at the place where the nerve crosses the joint may be followed by persistent bruising of the nerve. Consequently, the patient gets sharp painful twinges on walking followed by a few seconds' pins and needles.

The patient should wear a thick rubber pad under the forefoot for three to six months; this may prevent the twinges. Triamcinolone suspension should be injected about the affected extent of nerve at once. A long thin needle is introduced at the dorsum of the foot, between the first and second metatarsophalangeal joints and thrust in until it is felt to impinge against the plantar skin. Its point can be felt, and steered towards the tender extent of nerve.

A neuroma requiring excision seems not to occur at the first interspace.

### Acute Metatarsalgia (Morton)

This condition was described by Morton in 1876. The history is characteristic. The patient complains that, as he walks, he is suddenly seized with agonizing pain at the outer border of his forefoot. He has to stop still and stand on his good foot; he takes his shoe off and rubs the painful area. After some minutes the pain ceases but the foot becomes warm and stays so for several hours. When the pain has gone, he is able to walk on comfortably. He may experience two attacks in a week then none for a year; recurrences are very variable and tend to become more frequent. Between attacks, there are no symptoms or physical signs.

The disorder comes on between the ages of 15 and 50, and is much commoner in women. The aetiology was first put on a firm basis by Betts (1940), who ascribed it to nipping between the bones of a fibrous swelling of the fourth digital nerve proximal to its point of division. Resection of the nerve was curative. This view has been amply confirmed. Although the fourth and fifth toes are those usually affected, an occasional case between the third and fourth toes is encountered.

Examination is wholly negative. An attempt to reproduce the attack by moving the heads of the metatarsal bones against each other during compression fails. Cutaneous analgesia at the affected toes is absent. Palpation of the sole fails to reveal the tumour on the digital nerve. The

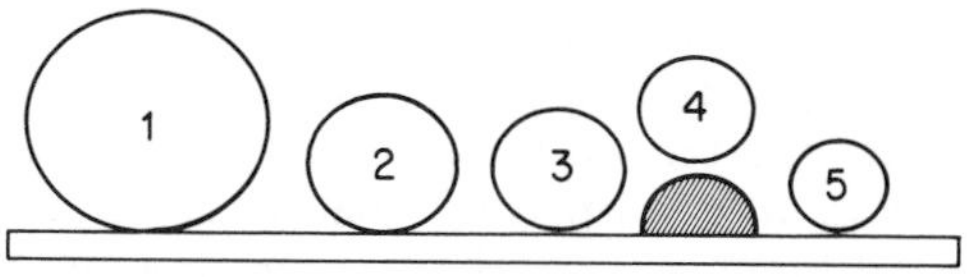


**Fig. 131.** A support for Morton's metatarsalgia. The small pad alters the alignment of the fourth metatarsal head on the fifth. Painful nipping of the digital nerve is then obviated.

diagnostic points are therefore: (*a*) the history of severe momentary bouts of pain at the outer forefoot followed by long periods of freedom, and (*b*) the absence of any discernible disorder at the foot.

Conservative treatment consists merely of altering the alignment of the metatarsal heads. If the nerve is nipped in the fourth interspace, the patient is prescribed a support elevating the head of the fourth bone (Fig. 131). This keeps the bones slightly out of line and prevents pinching. Since it is arguable whether the swelling on the nerve is the cause or the result of a series of nippings, it may well be that such a support prevents the later formation of the enlargement that aggravates the condition. Occasionally, the patient finds this support uncomfortable and may prefer one supporting the third and fifth bones. The effect is the same in respect of the alteration in position of the fourth bone in relation to its neighbours—merely down instead of up. In 1979 Guiloff described two cases of pinching of the digital nerve, of ten and fourteen years standing, cured by carbamazepine.

Should conservative treatment fail, the sole of the foot should be explored and the nerve with its neuroma excised

## THE TENDONS OF THE FOOT

Disorders of the tendons are few and obvious. A ganglion or a xanthoma may form at the dorsum of the foot in connection with a tendon.

The extensor hallucis and digitorum muscles become shortened in pes cavus, leading to clawing of the toes, i.e. fixation in extension at the metatarsophalangeal joints and flexion at the interphalangeal joints. Tenotomy under local anaesthesia may be required. Tenosynovitis of the extensor hallucis or digitorum tendons at the front of the ankle is uncommon; it leads to pain elicited by resisted extension of the big or the four little toes. Massage cures in so few sessions that a steroid injection is seldom required. In dancers, gross crepitus is often present at the flexor hallucis tendon at its course at the back of the ankle. It is due to overuse and, although this crepitus may even be audible, symptoms seldom ensue. If pain is provoked when the tendon moves, deep massage is rapidly curative. Rupture of the flexor longus hallucis at its insertion leads to a flail distal phalanx and is an appreciable disability; for the big toe keeps catching when the patient walks without shoes. Arthrodesis is indicated. Ischaemic contracture of the extensor hallucis longus after fracture is rare. In such a case, when the foot is plantiflexed, the big toe is forced into extension and is bruised against the upper of the shoe. Tenotomy under local anaesthesia is curative.

A plantaris deformity of the forefoot may induce excessive weight-bearing on the joint between the head of the first metatarsal bone and the sesamoid bone in the flexor hallucis longus tendon. Triamcinolone and a support (see Fig. 124) to relieve this bone of stress are required.

Weakness of the extensor hallucis muscle is a common result of fourth or fifth lumbar disc lesions.

## THE HALLUX

### Fractured Terminal Phalanx

Several days' severe pain results from the tense subungual haematoma that forms after fracture. Puncture of the nail with a red-hot needle allows the blood to exude and affords immediate relief; it also largely prevents subsequent sepsis.

A collodion splint should be applied and kept on for a month. In factories where workmen are apt to drop weights on their big toes, shoes with steel toe-caps should be worn to prevent this common industrial accident.

## THE TOE-NAILS

### Ingrowing Toe-nail

In this condition the two sides of the nail of the big toe press into the flesh and may cause severe pain. This can occur only if the nail is stiff and curved. When pain begins for this reason, the patient seeks relief by paring away the sides of the nail. This aggravates the condition, since the flesh is no longer held away from the sides of the nail by a full width distally.

In treatment, all that is required is to pare away the centre of the convex surface of the nail with a knife until it is quite thin and has lost its rigidity (Durlacher 1845). The edges of the nail are then no longer held pressed against the sides of the bed. Thinning is maintained until a nail of full width has grown beyond the full extent of the bed. If now the patient cuts the nail straight across, he seldom has further trouble. If he does, he must keep the nail thinned and flexible indefinitely, or submit to operation. Amputation of the whole nail bed and the distal half of the terminal phalanx gives a very good result.

### Dancer's Toe-nail

A similar condition causes dancers great trouble at the second and third toes. If a nail is stiff and curved, it forces itself into the flesh of the toe when she rises *sur les pointes*. Scraping the nail so as to keep it thin removes the disability at once.

### Onychogryphosis

Brown discoloration and great thickening of the nail occurs in onychogryphosis. Removal only leads to the growth of another identical nail. The chiropodist, by using a burr, can keep the nail thin and the patient comfortable. The alternative is amputation of the distal half of the terminal phalanx.

### Nipped Flesh

An uncommon cause of pain that may escape detection is such an excessive degree of flexion of the toes during weight-bearing that the pad of the toe at the free edge of the nail becomes nipped. A piece of felt placed under the bases of the toes prevents the toes from bending over too far.

## ISCHAEMIA OF THE FOOT

In advanced arteriosclerosis, the circulatory defect may show itself at the sole rather than in the calf muscles, particularly when the posterior tibial artery is affected. Alternatively, the nutrition of the toes may suffer. Claudication in the short flexor bellies is usually called cramp by the patient and comes on when the metabolic requirement is increased on walking or when the feet get warm in bed.

The foot, especially the toes, is a dusky red colour when the patient stands. The circulation returns slowly after an area of skin has been blanched by pressure. Elevation of the limb for a minute or less leads to rapid blanching of the foot; on dependency the redness returns equally soon. The foot feels cold both to the patient and the examiner. No pulsation is palpable at the posterior tibial or dorsalis pedis arteries, which the radiograph may show to be calcified. The patient, lying on the couch, is asked to flex his toes repeatedly as quickly as he can. This soon induces pain in intermittent claudication.

No treatment is of much avail. Sympathectomy warms the foot but seldom stops the muscles claudicating.

## DEFORMITIES OF THE FOOT

### Congenital Deformities

#### Equinus

The triple deformity of talipes equinovarus (equinus at the ankle, varus at the talocalcanean, adduction at the mid-tarsal joint) is familiar. But when one of these deformities occurs alone it may initially be overlooked. A pure equinus deformity results from short calf muscles. An equinus deformity that disappears on pressure only to reappear when this is released, may be the first sign to be noted of a cerebral diplegia.

### Metatarsus Varus

This is an uncomplicated adduction deformity of the forefoot, sometimes accompanied by a hallux varus.

### Metatarsus Inversus

This is an uncomplicated inversion deformity of the forefoot at the mid-tarsal joint, and in children is a common cause of valgus deformities at the knee and the heel (Plate XLVIII). In this condition, on walking, the outer side of the forefoot reaches the ground first. Then, as the patient's weight comes on to it, it rotates towards eversion until flat on the ground, thereby bringing the hindfoot with it and inducing a valgus deformity at the talocalcanean joint—its worst posture. The hindfoot may also carry the leg with it and throw it slightly out of the vertical. Thus a genu valgum deformity develops in due course (Fig. 132).

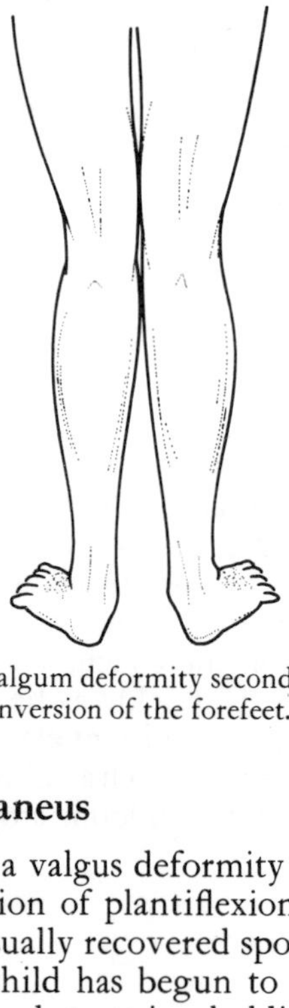

**Fig. 132.** Genu valgum deformity secondary to congenital inversion of the forefeet.

### Talipes Calcaneus

There is often a valgus deformity of the heel as well as limitation of plantiflexion range at the ankle. It has usually recovered spontaneously by the time the child has begun to stand; if not, manipulation and strapping holding the heel in varus are indicated.

### Pes Planus

The congenital variety is rare. A bony talocalcanean bridge lying just posterior to the sustentaculum tali may unite the two bones and is commoner than calcaneonavicular fusion (Harris & Beath 1948). The latter may cause no symptoms but the former is apt to set up mid-tarsal arthritis. A steel support (Fig. 122) may help.

### Hammer Toe

There is a fixed flexion deformity at the proximal interphalangeal joint with hyperextension at the distal joint. This would be symptomless but for the wearing of shoes, pressure against which causes a painful corn on the prominent joint.

## Acquired Deformities

### Pes Cavus

This deformity begins to be noticeable at the age of 8 and progresses steadily until growth ceases at about the age of 20; it then remains stationary. The foot is short, broad and thick (see Fig. 127), and the angle between the forefoot and hindfoot is abnormally small, sometimes even approaching a right angle. The toes are clawed (i.e. held in full extension at the metatarsophalangeal joints and in flexion at the interphalangeal joints) because of the increased tone, leading to structural shortening, that develops in the extensor longus hallucis and digitorum muscles as a result of an attempt to compensate for the weakness of the interosseus and lumbrical muscles. A large callosity nearly always forms under the heads of the middle three metatarsal bones because—the toes not being used in walking—they transmit excessive pressure to the underlying skin.

### Pes Plantaris

By this is meant an over-arched foot, i.e. one in which the angle between the hindfoot and the forefoot is diminished (as in cavus deformity) but the foot and toes are otherwise normal (see Fig. 126). In women, a minor degree of this condition is very common and not necessarily the result of wearing high-heeled shoes. Adolescent girls, who have worn low heels all their lives, may nevertheless develop a plantaris deformity which results in painful strain until compensated by raising the heel of the shoe.

In pes plantaris, the stress of weight-bearing first induces a greatly increased range at the mid-tarsal joint, particularly dorsiflexion–plantiflexion. Initially, there are no symptoms. Sooner or later the muscles of the sole of the foot prove unequal to the task of maintaining the plantaris position of the forefoot during weight-bearing. Excessive stress then falls upon (*a*) the ligaments at the mid-tarsal joint (mid-tarsal strain); (*b*) the plantar fascia; (*c*) the metatarsal heads (metatarsalgia). Thus, three separate lesions may develop according to where in the foot the major stress falls.

This is the type of foot that is often called 'flat'. It is not; it is over-arched, and flattens towards the normal shape only with pain.

### Pes Planus

When excessive dorsiflexion takes place at the mid-tarsal joint, two further deformities arise: valgus at the heel and abduction at the forefoot. The calcaneonavicular ligament, the mid-tarsal ligaments, and the plantar fascia are all overstretched; the first becomes painful, tender and prominent. Finally, shortening of the various joint capsules may occur, thus fixing the foot in the deformed position. The deformity is now no longer reducible and cannot profitably be treated by conservative measures. Not all flat feet hurt; those that do not should be left alone.

### Hallux Rigidus

This is the late result of an adolescent osteochondrosis at the first metatarsophalangeal joint.

### Hallux Valgus

If the upper surface of the heel of a shoe slopes downwards, the foot tends to slide forwards during weight-bearing. Since most shoes taper at the toes, the first and fifth toes are squeezed towards the midline of the foot at each step. The big toe is forced farther and farther towards valgus, and once this has begun, the pull of the flexor and extensor tendons increases the deformity. Shine (1965) found in St Helena that hallux valgus was present in only 2% of unshod islanders, but in 16% of men and 48% of women who had always worn shoes. The deformity is symptomless unless complicated by arthrosis, bursitis or pressure of the skin over the prominent bone against the upper of the shoe.

## Treatment

In the treatment of any deformity here, two alternatives exist: either to force the movement that cannot be performed until good passive and active over-correction is obtained, or to compensate for the deformity by alterations to the shoe. Exercises, supports and strapping are used to prevent relapse. Both methods may be employed together.

### Plantaris Deformity

Compensation is secured by raising the heel of the patient's shoe, while keeping its upper surface horizontal (see Fig. 129). The short muscles in the sole must be strengthened so that they can keep the forefoot in the plantaris position during weight-bearing, thus diminishing movement at the mid-tarsal joint. Furthermore, their increased power takes pressure off the metatarsophalangeal joint and tension off the plantar fascia.

### Planus Deformity

The valgus element that occurs in this condition can be corrected by giving the heel of the patient's shoe a 0.5 cm inner wedge, to push his heel over into a varus position as he takes weight. Since the abduction deformity is secondary to excessive dorsiflexion at the mid-tarsal joint, plantiflexion should be encouraged here by providing the heel of the shoe with an anterior wedge (see Fig. 129) to the heel (as long as he has no equinus deformity) and by strengthening the short flexor muscles of the sole of the foot and the tibialis anterior and posterior muscles. If these measures do not suffice, a support, thick at the inner aspect of the mid-tarsus, becomes necessary (see Fig. 119).

### Cavus Deformity

*A child* may be seen whose foot has the typical shape but no symptoms have yet arisen. The progressive nature of the deformity should be explained and the importance of maintaining full length of the extensor longus hallucis and digitorum muscles, and full strength in the small muscles of the sole, must be emphasized. To this end, the child himself, or an adult, should stretch the toes out daily, until full flexion is reached and maintained. Resisted exercises towards toe flexion follow. The heel should be kept at a height adequate to compensate for the plantaris element in the deformity. If this is done, and the child kept under observation, say, yearly until the age of 20, no symptoms need ever arise.

*In adults* with fixed deformity of the toes, division of the extensor longus tendons is an essential preliminary to reduction of the clawing. This is very simply done under local anaesthesia. There is practically no after-pain and the patient walks home immediately after the tenotomy. He must keep stretching his toes out towards flexion for the next few days to prevent the tendons uniting without lengthening. If only two tendons are cut at a time, a cradle (see Fig. 134) is applied.

Measures to strengthen the short flexor muscles of the sole by faradism and exercises are vigorously pursued daily, during which the flexion range at the metatarsophalangeal joints is maintained. A support (as for metatarsalgia) is often also required.

In advanced cases, the fitting of a thick support to raise the heel and take weight off the metatarsal heads may prove the only practicable measure. Open operation is sometimes necessary.

## Metatarsal Deformity

Forcing the mid-tarsal joint towards eversion or abduction (for metatarsus inversus and varus deformities respectively) calls for great strength, even in the treatment of children. For the forcing of an eversion movement, the hands should be clasped about the patient's forefoot (see Volume II) and a series of twists given of gradually increasing range. The ligamentous fibres limiting movement must be stretched out and broken; hence the mobilization should be continued at each session until at least one strand is heard to part. Treatment must continue for a year or two. In adults, a suitable support (Fig. 133) is required.

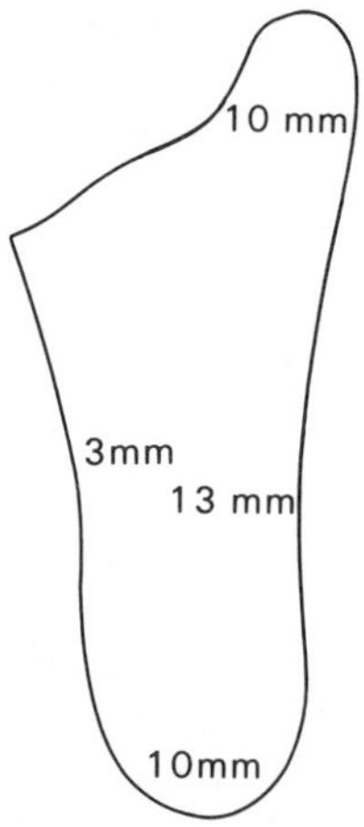


**Fig. 133.** A support for metatarsus inversus. The support is thick all along its inner side and is prolonged under the first metatarsophalangeal joint, so as to enable weight-bearing to take place while the forefoot remains inverted.

## Hammer Toe

Hammer toe can be straightened by merely breaking the plantar aspect of the capsular fibres by force; local anaesthesia suffices. The toe must be kept straight in a cradle for a week or two afterwards. A cradle consists of strapping passed under the toes on either side and over the one affected, so placed as to hold the proximal interphalangeal joint in extension (Fig. 134). If this procedure fails, arthrodesis is indicated.

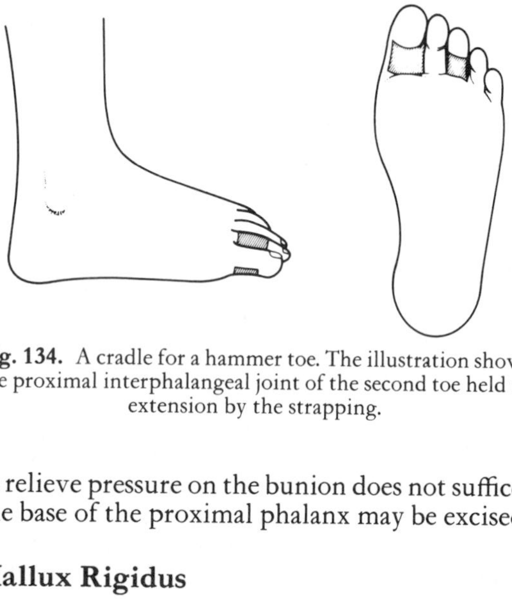

**Fig. 134.** A cradle for a hammer toe. The illustration shows the proximal interphalangeal joint of the second toe held in extension by the strapping.

## Hallux Valgus

Children should wear shoes with a straight inner border for prophylaxis. If alteration of the shoe to relieve pressure on the bunion does not suffice, the base of the proximal phalanx may be excised.

## Hallux Rigidus

A rocker or a built-in steel in the sole relieves symptoms if some extension range remains. If not, the base of the first phalanx is excised.

# SUPPORTS

The main purposes for which supports are prescribed are as follows:

## To Ensure Plantiflexion at the Mid-tarsal Joint

If the height of a heel is raised without a change in the angle of its upper surface, plantiflexion occurs at the mid-tarsal joint. The same object is achieved when the heel is kept the same height but the angle of its upper surface altered to approach more nearly the horizontal. Good plantiflexion must be ensured here in order to reduce strain in a pes planus deformity. Again, the essence in the treatment of pes plantaris deformity and of plantar fasciitis is to allow increased plantiflexion during weight-bearing (see Fig. 130).

### To Diminish Pressure on the Metatarsal Heads

A thick platform stopping short of the metatarsal heads encourages weightbearing by the whole extent of the metatarsal shafts and takes much of the weight off the metatarsophalangeal joints (see Fig. 128). A metatarsal bar, which crosses the shoe just behind the heads, makes the necks of the metatarsal bones bear the greater weight; it is much less satisfactory.

### To Diminish a Pes Planus Deformity

The inner aspect of the mid-tarsus is kept raised by a support, thick under this area (see Fig. 119).

### To Prevent Movement at the Mid-tarsal Joint

When there is a mid-tarsal arthritis, pain is elicited towards the extreme of every movement. The application of a well-fitting steel to the sole of the foot prevents movement as far as is possible.

### To Compensate for Metatarsus Inversus

This deformity may be discovered for the first time in middle age, perhaps because of a secondary posterior tibial tendinitis. The support must enable the heel to maintain the mid-position during weight-bearing; that is, it must allow the forefoot to remain inverted and yet in contact with the ground. It is therefore made like a wedge, thick at the inner and tapering to nothing at the outer border of that forefoot. It must project under the first metatarsophalangeal joint almost as far forward as the interphalangeal joint. At the heel the support is level (see Fig. 133). The alternative is an inner wedge on the sole, not the heel.

### For Sesamoiditis at the First Metatarsophalangeal Joint

A support taking the weight off the joint by providing thickness at the metatarsal neck often suffices. It should take the form of a ring, thick in front of, as well as behind, the sesamoid bone (see Fig. 124). The heel of the shoe should be raised, while keeping its upper surface horizontal to encourage weightbearing posteriorly.

### For Calcanean Bursitis

The support is 1 cm thick and made of non-porous rubber in the shape of a horseshoe.

### For Strain of the Plantar Fascia

As an alternative to raising the heel of the shoe, a heel-pad may be fitted within the shoe. It should be of hard rubber and 1 cm thick anteriorly, tapering to nothing at the back of the shoe, so that the front of the upper surface of the heel lies at a higher level than posteriorly.

### For Morton's Metatarsalgia

The alignment of the metatarsal heads is altered by raising the fourth on a small dome (see Fig. 131). Occasionally, the patient prefers the third and fifth bones raised, leaving the fourth relatively depressed (Fig. 135).

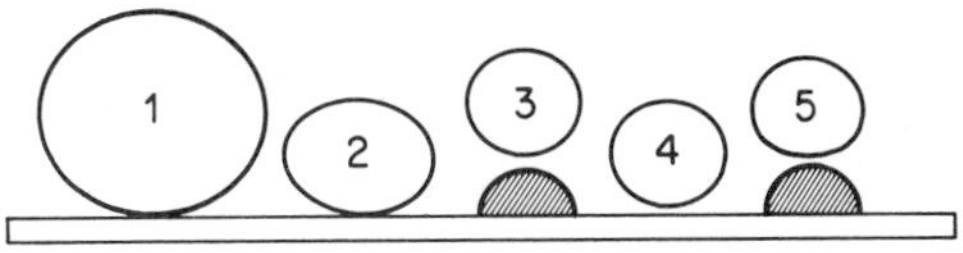


**Fig. 135.** An alternative support for Morton's metatarsalgia. Instead of raising the fourth metatarsal head (see Fig. 131) the third and fifth are supported and the fourth is allowed to sink down.

## ALTERATIONS AND ADDITIONS TO THE SHOE

### Inner Wedge

When a reducible valgus deformity at the talocalcanean joint is present, a varus position of the calcaneus during weight-bearing can be secured by an inner wedge to the heel of the shoe: 5 mm thick for adults, 3 mm for children (Fig. 136). An inner and an anterior wedge can often be advantageously combined.

### Anterior Wedge

This renders horizontal the oblique upper surface of a heel. The shoe thus becomes properly adapted to a foot with a plantaris deformity (see Fig. 120). Shoes with a horizontal heel are the most comfortable for nearly all women; it is therefore the more surprising that women's shoes always have an oblique heel—which looks no more

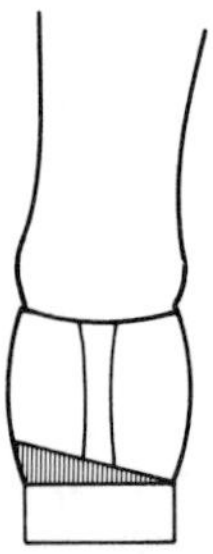

**Fig. 136.** An inner wedge for the heel of a shoe.

elegant, increases the apparent length and diameter of the foot—and hence are so shaped that the waist of the shoe is not in contact with the sole of the foot. All women with a tendency to plantaris shaping of the forefoot ought to wear horizontal heels; these have several important advantages: (*a*) the patient can take weight directly on the heel; (*b*) the waist of the shoe lies against the tarsus and some weight can be borne there; (*c*) plantiflexion at the mid-tarsal joint is assured; and (*d*) as there is no tendency for the foot to slide forward, metatarsalgia is prevented. Moreover such a shoe is more elegant.

## Raising the Heel

When a horizontal heel is to be supplied, it must be the right height. For this purpose, blocks of wood of various thicknesses are placed under the patient's heel while he is standing with forefoot on the ground. The most comfortable height is measured and the thickness of the sole of the shoe added to this figure. Hence the same height will not apply for thin and walking shoes.

When compensation for an equinus deformity is required, the heel is raised and the obliquity of its upper surface increased.

## Floated Heel

If recurrent varus sprain of the ankle is to be prevented, broadening the base of the heel on its outer side is effective (see Fig. 118).

## Rocker

A hallux rigidus deformity can be rendered symptomless and natural gait restored by a device that avoids extension of the hallux, i.e. a rocker. In theory, a ridge built into the sole of the shoe at the metatarsophalangeal joint line would best ensure this, but, as the joint itself is tender, the maximum thickness is better placed a short distance behind this point. Surgical shoe-makers usually put the projection too far back. This, or the fact that the rocker is too low, is the fault when full relief is not obtained. The patient must wear shoes with a rocker constantly and permanently (see Fig. 125). A metatarsal bar can be used as a rocker if it is put straight across the sole instead of obliquely, and *at*, rather than behind the metatarsal heads.

## Steel

In a congenital pes planus deformity nothing can be done, particularly if there is calcaneonavicular fusion, except to make an entire steel sole so that as little movement as possible occurs at all the joints of the foot (Fig. 137).

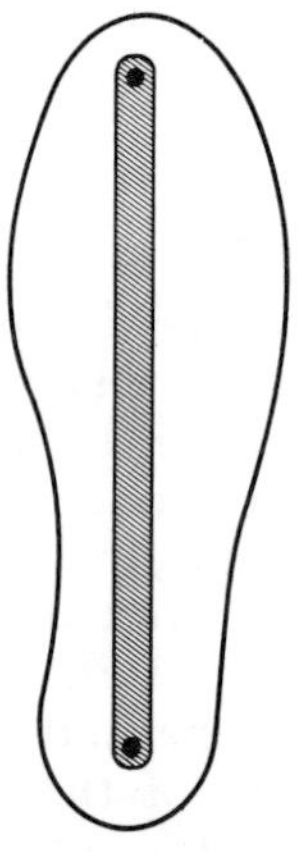

**Fig. 137.** A steel sole for preventing all movement at the tarsal joints. Useful in congenital pes planus.

## Posterior Plate

Dr David Evans has devised a plate fixed to the heel which extends posteriorly for 5 cm. It enables the patient to lean over backwards thus maintaining his lordosis without falling.

CHAPTER 27

# PSYCHOGENIC PAIN

Patients with pain devoid of organic basis naturally gravitate to the orthopaedic physician, since it is he who normally deals with patients whose symptoms give rise to few or no physical signs. If the patient is examined by the methods here described, it is difficult for imagined disorders to escape detection at the first attendance. Broadly, patients with genuine pain which is doubted are fewer than those who have partly or wholly carried off the deception.

The fact that patients with every type of obscure pain reach an orthopaedic physician for diagnosis and treatment provides him with many interesting problems. While it is no substitute for a diagnosis to regard every patient with a symptom the source of which is not immediately apparent as suffering from an imaginary disorder, much confusion results from believing too much. An open mind accepts and registers as they appear disorders not previously familiar. The difficult balance between excessive scepticism and credulity must be maintained.

Nothing is more disheartening to a physiotherapist than to treat, apparently endlessly, a patient whose malady has not been clearly defined, who never improves and never stops coming. By contrast, the short course of stimulating measures applicable to patients with psychogenic pain can be confidently—and therefore effectively—instituted when the patient's symptoms are known not to have an organic basis.

### 'Psychological Basis of Rheumatism'

Much has been written about a psychogenic basis for what has been misnamed 'rheumatic' pain. This is an inverted attitude towards the disorder present; for a pain devoid of physical cause should not be called rheumatic. It is a better attitude to discard such labels as 'fibrositis' or 'rheumatism' for patients whose complaint has no organic foundation and to substitute a diagnosis of psychogenic pain.

### Criterion of Cure

In many of the lesions discussed in this book, the patient's uncorroborated statement may provide the chief, at times the only, criterion of the results of treatment.

If a patient states that manipulation of his back has made him better or worse, it is almost useless for the doctor to offer a contrary opinion. Hence, it is important to avoid active methods of treatment unless patient and doctor are, so to speak, on the same side. If, no matter what is done, the patient (on account of his attitude of mind) will probably allege aggravation, it is essential to avoid any measure that he could credibly suggest made him worse. It may, therefore, be unwise to treat a patient who is psychoneurotic with a grievance or is enmeshed in a compensation claim, even when he clearly has a minor lesion which can be remedied easily.

When the patient's attitude appears to be more important than the minor organic lesion, the hospital social worker's view on how the patient is likely to react to treatment, even if effective, is valuable. Sometimes it is best to warn a patient, his doctor and his solicitor, before any treatment begins, that measures to achieve relief may on the one hand upset the patient's psyche or, if they prove successful, may on the other hand damage his position in law.

## EXAMINATION IN CASES OF SUSPECTED PSYCHOGENIC PAIN

A necessary preliminary to this examination is to bear in mind and face the implications of four not uncommon prejudices on the doctor's part. In Canada, Becker and Karch (1979) matched 83 control women who had no backache with a similar group with backache. They found no difference in psychological troubles between the two.

### Confusion between the Unknown and the Inconsistent

The practitioner should not assume that a condition which he has not encountered before does not exist. Indeed, his opinion is likely to be sought in just those cases of unwavering complaint which have defied elucidation. Sooner or later, one meets one of the rarer causes of pain in a patient referred for an opinion. If the patient's symptoms do not transgress the segmental boundaries, and if his responses to diagnostic movements remain the same at each examination, an organic lesion must be present. It should be remembered that, particularly in affections of a nerve root, pain may be present in the virtual absence of physical signs. If the patient's history, symptoms, progress and responses conform closely to the known patterns and to the segmentation of the limb, his story is credible. As a rule, it is only when a condition is seen for the second or third time and the similarity between patients' stories and signs—or lack of signs—becomes apparent, that the examiner is confident that he is dealing with a real entity.

### Suspicions engendered by the Patient's Manner or by the Diffuseness of his Pain

A patient who has seen several practitioners without avail naturally feels under suspicion, perhaps begins to suspect himself, and so may develop the demeanour of a suspect. According to his temperament, he may become prolix and emphatic, or sullen, or apologetic. It is not so much the way he says it, as the remarkable sequence of events and sensations that he describes which should raise the question of psychogenic pain. Even so, the extrasegmental way in which pain radiates from the dura mater must be taken into account. The presence of pain in an apparently normal limb is not a reason for suspecting the patient's veracity, but rather for considering whether and whence the pain may be referred.

### Suspicions based on the Results of Treatment

I regard it as unjustifiable to regard a patient's symptoms as devoid of organic basis unless this fact became evident at the first interview. Otherwise this attribution can become an excuse for the physician's failure. The fact that expert and apparently adequate treatment has not been followed by cure, is not evidence that the patient's ills are imaginary. Many common painful disorders are entirely unrelievable in the absence of an exact diagnosis implemented by equally exact treatment. For example, unless the doctor can inject a steroid, or the physiotherapist gives massage, accurately, a diagnosis of supraspinatus tendinitis remains purely academic.

It is important not to treat patients until the question of psychogenesis becomes clear, one way or the other. If a patient has several months' physiotherapy and then the physician gets up in Court and states that there is no organic lesion, he puts himself into a logical dilemma which opposing counsel will be quick to seize.

### Bias towards the Employer

A doctor, like any other individual, tends towards sympathy for those who come to him for help. Hence, when he sees a patient—particularly a private patient—his natural reaction is to side with him. Equally, when a doctor is retained by an insurance company, his instinct is to protect their interests. It takes a conscious effort to be perfectly impartial in these cases. Nevertheless, a dispassionate view is the essence of an examination to decide whether or not the patient's symptoms are psychogenic; and, when an organic lesion has led to excessive disablement, to assess the proportions of each factor. No medical man should feel that he is acting *for* or *against* the patient; he is there to establish certain facts, to report on his findings and to draw reasoned conclusions.

Magnuson (1932) warns against bias in industrial cases: 'the mental attitude of the examiner at the start of the examination must be as carefully analysed as the mental attitude of the patient at the time of the examination.' He too regards doctors as pure diagnosticians, not partisans in a lawsuit.

## The History

The examiner should listen to the history with care, from the time when the symptoms began. Attention should be directed to the circumstances leading up to their first appearance, and the patient should be asked to point to their exact site then, and to indicate the area to which they have since spread. Such diligence may elicit a coherent account from a patient apt to ramble or unable to explain himself well. By contrast, patients with psychogenic pain are apt to embroider, and their symptoms may be heard to come and go in the most improbable ways or to diffuse further and further as the tale continues. Radiation may be alleged which grossly transgresses the rules that referred pain keeps within one dermatome and does not cross the midline. Thus, unilateral pain may spread to both limbs, or a pectoral pain travel down to the lower abdomen.

Patients with psychogenic symptoms are disinclined to describe them; for, without necessarily being fully conscious of the fact, they are dimly aware that they do not quite know what they should say. Instead, they enlarge on the degree of suffering and disablement and embark on a long list of doctors consulted, diagnoses made and ineffective treatments received. When repeatedly brought back to the point, i.e. what the symptoms were that made them seek medical advice, they become increasingly restive. They are irritated, implying that the listener must be a very inadequate physician not to realize that such intense suffering drove the patient to seek help. When pressed to describe the exact position of the pain, its variation and spread, what makes it better or worse and so on, these questions are resented. This attitude provides a strong contrast to the patient with organic disease who is only too glad to find a doctor who listens attentively and inquisitively.

Then there are a number of sequences—what I call 'inherent likelihood'—that the experienced physician recognizes: for example, pain in the back radiating to the lower limb, the backache easing when the root pain becomes severe; the painful shoulder preventing the patient from lying on that side at night because of pain in the upper limb. Certain accounts characterize certain disorders, but in neurosis none of the recognizable patterns emerge.

It is always more difficult to be sure that there is no organic cause for a pain than that there is; hence, the ability to listen without losing patience and to adopt a sympathetic manner often repays the examiner well. Moreover, the patient who is allowed to go on talking, as well as contradicting his own earlier statements, may advance irrelevancies that afford a clue to the true origin of his symptoms.

## Inspection

Little is to be expected from inspection for, should this reveal obvious abnormality, the question of purely psychogenic symptoms hardly arises. Difficulties are encountered when a patient knows that he has a deformity, perhaps postural since adolescence or the result of past disease or fracture, and makes use of it to give colour to his story.

The mere fact that the patient can walk in and sit down shows certain muscles not to be paralysed and indicates that movement exists at the joints of the lower limbs. The patient may be well-nourished and show none of the facial expression that designates sleepless nights and severe pain.

The gait may reveal a limp or small shuffling steps or a joint held stiffly when no limitation of joint movement, loss of muscle power or impaired nervous control can later be found to account for it. Joints assume a characteristic posture when diseased, whereas psychogenic stiffness characteristically results in fixation in quite different positions, e.g. medial rotation at the hip, full extension at the knee, varus at the heel. Sometimes the wrong joint is held fixed; for example, a patient with lumbar pain may hold the neck and thoracic spine to one side, while the lumbar spine remains vertical. In true lumbar deviation, the list is seen there, with a compensating curve in the other direction above. Again, disorders of the cervical spine do not cause the scapula to be held elevated by contraction of the trapezius muscle.

## Examination of Movements

The responses on examination of patients with organic lesions form a pattern. If an unusual pattern results, one must consider whether it is impossible or conceivable. During a resisted movement, pain may be felt at a site unsuited to the muscle being tested. For example, the patient who is asked to bend his elbow and then push his wrist away from his body is having his infraspinatus muscle tested. He can therefore reasonably allege pain in the arm, but not at the wrist. A complaint of pain on all the resisted movements at the scapula, shoulder, elbow and wrist joints is self-contradictory, since it would identify the lesion as situated in a dozen different places. However, the fact that every resisted shoulder or hip movement hurts is consistent with acute internal derangement of a cervical or lumbar intervertebral joint, and, in such a case, direct examination of the neck or lumbar movements must reveal a severe disorder. If, therefore, little abnormality is detected here, the reality of the symptoms is in great doubt. Except at a few sites, and then in a known manner, limitation of movement at a joint is also accompanied by proportionate limitation in the other directions.

Pain on a resisted movement is accompanied, except in rare instances, by a full range of movement at the joint, and the extremes of such movements as neither stretch nor squeeze the affected tissue are always of full range and painless. Weakness of some resisted movement may be alleged, whereas the visible bulk of the relevant muscle shows that it is strong; or a muscle may have full power when tested in one way, but appear paralysed when tested by a different method. Alternatively, the mere fact that the patient walked in and sat down may show that the weakness is not organic. The muscles that are alleged to be weak may transgress the known patterns and, if pins and needles or numbness are present, they may occupy an inconsistent area of skin. It must be remembered that what is inconsistent or contradictory to the doctor versed in anatomy is by no means so to the patient.

Patients assume that the first act of the examiner after listening to the history is to request them to make a movement which causes pain. A part of the body, as far distant as is reasonably possible from the allegedly affected area, should be chosen; if the knee or shoulder is said to hurt, for example, trunk movements may be tried first. It is remarkable how few psychoneurotic patients possess the strength of mind to resist this invitation.

The essence of examination is to give the patient plenty of scope. If inconsistencies are to be revealed, a large number of movements must be tested so that a congruous or an incongruous pattern can emerge. Trial of a series of active, passive and resisted movements at a number of joints, accompanied by a request to be told whether each hurts or not, and if so where, is very confusing to a patient without organic disease. He cannot know, nor work out quickly in his mind, which movement he should say is painful and which not. He is, therefore, apt to guess wildly, his random answers forming a pattern inconsistent with any one lesion. Or he may say that every movement at several joints sets up pain; this is too much. Suspicion is aroused if the patient allows the examiner's tone of voice to influence his response to movements, or by a pause followed by a glance at his face that appears designed to read the answer in his countenance. More difficulty is presented when every movement is said to leave the pain unaltered, for this is a perfectly possible finding in visceral pain (since the wrong parts are being examined) or in some cases of pressure on a nerve root.

There is one remark which crops up again and again. When the series of movements is tested, ordinary patients say that such-and-such a movement hurts whereas another movement does not. The idea that any movement should be quite painless is repugnant to many neurotic patients and, instead of declaring some of the movements to be painless, they say 'not too bad'. If this phrase keeps recurring, the physician is put on his guard.

## Positive Inconsistencies

The doctor who deals with the moving parts is in a happy position when the question of psychogenic pain arises. The physician who deals with dyspepsia or debility or headache cannot go further than to sum up the patient's character and, when every test proves negative, suppose that the trouble is caused by neurosis. The orthopaedic physician bases his diagnosis on the discovery of positive inconsistencies, and thus treads on much firmer ground. It is not the fact that nothing can be found to account for a pain that enables him to decide that the symptoms possess an emotional origin; it is the contradictions that pile up as the examination proceeds. Indeed, I have found (rather to my annoyance, for everyone likes to think himself a good judge of his fellow men) that when a patient appears quite sincere while he recounts the history but examination suggests psychogenesis, the examination is the better criterion. The opposite also holds; a nervous patient may by his manner suggest neurotic symptoms and yet examination may show a neat pattern that is clearly organic.

To uncover inconsistencies, the patient must be given plenty of rope. A large number of movements must be tested, some relevant to a pain at the site described, many not. If lumbar pain is alleged, the resisted movements of the neck make a good starting point.

Inconsistencies are:

*Between* the patient's appearance and his degree of suffering.

*Between* his description of his symptoms, even taken at their face value, and his disablement. He can sit at home and walk out shopping but cannot travel to work.

*Between* the site of pain and the way it has spread. The area of radiation that is reported restricts the number of inherent likelihoods. These are later sought but may not be found present.

*Between* the site of the pain and the movements

he cannot perform. In extreme cases, pain in the back may prevent elevation of the arms above the horizontal.

*Between* the site of pain and the movements reported to hurt.

*Between* his symptoms and his posture and gait.

*Between* what he can do and the physical signs. For example, the patient who cannot abduct the arm at all, but possesses a full range of movement at the shoulder joint when it is examined passively, together with full strength in the abductor muscles tested with the arm by the patient's side, has shown that he refuses to carry out a movement that he can in fact perform.

*Between* one set of physical signs and another set. If pain in the arm is brought on by neck movements, the lesion must be cervical. Hence the shoulder, elbow and wrist movements will not exacerbate the pain (although they may demonstrate a root palsy), and vice versa.

*Between* the results of the same movement carried out in different ways or a second time. A patient who sits normally must possess 90° range of flexion at the hip and knee.

*N.B.* It is important to realize that the range of straight-leg raising is not necessarily the same as the range of trunk flexion, for, in the former case, the body weight is not borne by the joint, whereas in the latter the joint is compressed. In consequence, it is a common finding in subacute lumbago that the patient cannot bend forwards and yet has a full range of straight-leg raising. The valid comparison in this connection is between trunk-flexion and sitting up with the legs out straight; for in both cases the joint is identically squeezed. This finding is medico-legally important; hence, it must be demonstrated in the way that is fair to the patient.

*Between* a finding of limitation in one direction and the range in other directions. There are many known patterns, but the one proffered may not fit with any.

*Between* the bulk of a muscle belly and allegations of weakness.

*Between* the position in which a joint is held and the capsular pattern. For example, the hip joint does not fix in medial rotation nor the talocalcanean joint in varus.

*Between* a limp and where the pain is felt or the lesion alleged to account for it is situated.

*Between* the signs put forward and the site of alleged tenderness.

*Between* the site of tenderness at one moment and another.

*Between* the lesion possibly present and the fact that there is any tender point at all. If arthritis at the hip or shoulder is suspected, there is no relevant tenderness.

### Doubtful Cases

Naturally, difficult cases abound especially when a minor ache is elevated into a disabling disease by neurosis. If the interview with the hospital social worker also proves uninformative, the next step is to record all the patient's responses. He should then be ordered a fortnight's indifferent treatment chosen for its known lack of effect on whatever the possible lesions are, e.g. heat or faradism. At the end of this period he may state himself to be cured; this is strong evidence of absent organic lesion. If not, he should be examined again, the same movements being tried, this time in a different order. When a series of movements is tried in rapid succession at several joints, patients seldom remember at this interval of time which were and which were not originally said to hurt. Should the responses tally closely on the two occasions, his complaint should be taken seriously and detailed examination repeated in an attempt to establish the source of his pain.

It is never the mere absence of physical signs that provides a confident diagnosis of psychogenic pain. On the other hand, the patient who alleges the presence of signs that contradict each other himself supplies the evidence of his own mental state.

## Local Anaesthesia

In local anaesthesia, the examiner has another means of detecting unreal pains. The nature of the solution should not be explained; it suffices to say that the examiner wishes to give an injection. Patients anxious to make the worst of their case are often tempted into saying that the infiltration has made the pain worse. This is impossible. Again, the induction of local anaesthesia cannot fail to abolish local tenderness. It must be remembered, however, that if local anaesthesia does not remove a pain felt at the infiltrated area, this is perfectly consistent with an organic lesion situated elsewhere and referring pain to this spot.

## Radiography

Although it is a sad waste of material, this examination should not be omitted. An unexpected positive finding is a great rarity, for soft tissue lesions which alter the radiological appearances are usually advanced enough to make the clinical diagnosis easy. The presence of some trivial abnormality, e.g. an osteophyte or a diminished intervertebral joint space, must not be regarded as proving a patient's symptoms to have an organic cause.

## FINDINGS IN SUSPECTED PSYCHOGENIC PAIN

The terminology used in this book is as follows: malingering means conscious deception; neurosis, unconscious deception; and hysteria, paralysis or fixation without organic defect.

The possible findings on examination conducted on these lines fall into four main groups.

### Absence of Organic Lesion

In obvious cases the history is remarkable, the disability is out of proportion even to the alleged symptoms; the responses to diagnostic movements conflict; clear inconsistencies are detected; tenderness is severe and diffuse. If the patient appears to have an unconscious belief in the reality of his symptoms, he is regarded as suffering from a psychogenic disorder. If he does not even believe in them himself, he is termed a malingerer. If the disability depends on so intense a conviction that some part of the body is functionless that it becomes either paralysed or fixed, the label 'hysteria' is justified. Examination reveals only the absence of organic basis for the patient's pain; the study of his state of mind during this time may or may not allow an opinion on how far he believes in his own symptoms. No hard and fast line can in any case be drawn; cases at each extreme are clearly enough defined but they merge at a centre about which self-deception changes to conscious assumption. No objective test can distinguish psychoneurosis from malingering. An emphatic but cheerful description of non-organic symptoms characterizes assumed pain; bland indifference to a serious disability denotes hysteria; normal examination findings in an apathetic patient, who clearly maintains a hopeless view that he will never get better, signify endogenous depression.

### Organic Lesion with Psychogenic Overlay

These are difficult cases requiring much patience and clinical experience to disentangle. The symptoms and physical signs, though largely correct in quality, are grossly excessive in quantity. Moreover, mixed in with and obscuring the genuine factors are unbelievable complaints and alleged signs. Much time and considerable repetition of the examination may be required to enable the real lesion to emerge after it has been distinguished from the welter of unfounded symptoms. In such cases, it is often wise to convert the patient to a more reasonable frame of mind by a fortnight's indifferent treatment from a physiotherapist. She, by imparting her unemotional and commonsense attitude, can nearly always get a patient so to collect himself that, at the next examination, it is hard to believe that there could have been any difficulty in arriving at a diagnosis.

It is well to remember that psychogenic signs may over-shadow organic signs. For example, a patient with 10° limitation of abduction at the shoulder, who refuses to move his arm from his side at all, conceals a genuine sign, which only assiduity and repetition will reveal. Although the patient has brought the misdiagnosis on himself, unfairness results if such a patient is regarded as suffering from a purely psychogenic disability. Treatment by suggestion is apt to be powerless in the presence of real—however minor—pain; in contrast, relief of the genuine lesion, by depriving the patient of the basis for his malady, is sometimes curative alone. Even if it is not, he may now have become responsive to psychotherapy.

### Pain in Neurotic Patients

Another difficulty appears with the psychoneurotic patient who happens to develop a painful condition, for pain in a neurotic patient has nothing to do with pain due to neurosis. Since the perception of pain is an emotional experience mediated by the cells of the frontal lobes of the brain, heightened excitability there increases the severity of the symptoms. His excessive distress and nervous behaviour on giving his history conflict with the simple and consistent pattern that, to his own and the examiner's surprise, is discovered on examination. The hypersensitive state present must be allowed for when treatment is ordered, but there is seldom any need for treatment of his mental state with which, as long as no painful disorder has upset its balance, he has coped quite well for years.

## No Physical Signs Detected

There always remains a very small group of patients in whom no decision is possible. The history is credible and the response to movements unhelpful but constant on repetition and devoid of inconsistency. Tenderness may be absent and local anaesthesia unavailing. Sometimes, repeated examinations may enable a decision to be reached in the end; in a very few cases no decision is ever really arrived at.

Elderly patients with, for example, a minor disc lesion at an osteophytic spinal joint, may have no clear signs to explain their brachial, thoracic or sciatic pain. In due course, such signs do sometimes develop; only analogy with these cases enables an early diagnosis to be made. In other cases also of irritation of the sheath of a sciatic nerve root, the pain may be felt at, say, the calf only and, even if this possibility is kept in mind, investigation may at first reveal nothing. Paraesthesiae in one hand may be the first symptoms of protrusion of a cervical intervertebral disc, or of the thoracic outlet syndrome, or of compression in the carpal tunnel; at first, all signs may be absent. Pain in the groin or iliac fossa may be caused by dural compression at a low lumbar level, without necessarily any physical signs. When perineal pain first arises from pressure on the fourth sacral root, it is exceptional for any physical signs to exist at all.

In such cases, the fault clearly lies with the examiner rather than the patient; an examination delicate enough to detect his organic disorder does not exist. It is wise, after repeated endeavour has failed to detect the lesion, local anaesthesia has been no help, and a short course of such treatment as suggested itself has proved vain, to confess to the patient the failure to arrive at a diagnosis. In fairness, one should add that one has no doubt that the symptoms are genuine, that since clinical examinations and radiography have all failed to disclose a source, it is most unlikely to be anything serious; that he is welcome to come and be seen again, that further treatment is clearly a waste of time equally for the patient and doctor; that, should a diagnosis ever be made, or any method of treatment prove effective, he should certainly report it so that the doctor might know more next time.

# TREATMENT OF PSYCHOGENIC DISABILITY

## Hospital Practice

It is unreasonable and impractical to refer all patients with minor psychogenic trouble to the psychologist. Moreover, simple suggestion of the type that physiotherapy supplies often succeeds in dispelling symptoms, at any rate for the time being. My endeavour in these cases is to get the patient back to work with the least possible delay. The first essential is to bring the patient over to cooperate with the doctor and so enable the former to declare that he is cured without loss of the very self-esteem that the symptoms are unconsciously designed to protect. Nothing, therefore, can be more unfortunate in its results than a cursory examination followed by a brusque statement that there is nothing the matter with the patient and that he is fit to return to work at once. This engenders immediate dislike of the doctor, who is at once regarded as unsympathetic and incompetent (and rightly so; for there *is* something the matter, although not what the patient believes); indeed, this attitude is tantamount to asking the patient to admit to others and—far worse—to himself, that he is shamming: a situation that he naturally resents. Such a statement, then, only induces in the patient an added determination to prove by unwavering complaint that his disablement is genuine.

After a sympathetic hearing and a thorough examination, the patient's confidence will have been won and a pleasant relationship established. Finally the examiner confidently announces that the patient will receive a fortnight's treatment which it is hoped will put him on the road to recovery. To say that cure is certain is too strong and annoys the patient by its disparaging suggestion of a minor malady.

Full physical examination, especially the diagnostic movements, has another advantage. If detailed notes are kept, and they are lying on the table before the doctor, it dawns on the patient when he comes up for examination at the end of a fortnight that, if he states he is no better, he will be put through all these movements again. A large factor in obtaining 'cure' may be provided by the patient's unwillingness to be asked questions to which he suddenly realizes he has now forgotten the answers. This explains those cases in which the physiotherapist has, so she reports, not affected the allegations of pain; yet the patient walks into the clinic beaming, declaring he is well.

This friendly atmosphere abolishes the patient's stubbornness and readiness to take offence. The physiotherapist with her faradic battery continues in the same strain. On the one hand, she applies faradic stimulation of increasing strength to whatever area the patient alleges is painful or weak, after which the patient practises the hitherto impossible or painful movement. On the other, she too maintains a persistent pleasant and encouraging manner. Her conversation should turn on the patient's life and circumstances, and emphasize the advantages to him of getting well. The patient, swayed in the same direction by such pleasant people and such disagreeable measures, more often than not declares himself well after a week or two of such treatment. In a series, 76 of 107 patients seen in my department in 1943 and regarded as suffering from purely psychogenic symptoms declared themselves well and returned to work at the end of two or three weeks. Compensation cases were not included in this series.

Treatment should not be continued for longer than two weeks. A fortnight's stimulating physiotherapy may induce a patient to state that he is cured; if not, prolongation of treatment is merely added evidence to all of the presence of organic disease. Hence, the remaining patients must be taken off physiotherapy and the decision reached whether they should be discharged or referred for psychological investigation, or sent to an institutional rehabilitation centre. Consideration of the patient's age, work record in the past; responsibilities, apparent character and social value determine the result; obviously the investigations of the hospital social worker bear strongly on these points. This residue of patients, otherwise reasonably sound human beings, for whose relief these superficial measures have not sufficed, are troubled by deep unconscious motives that require a psychiatrist.

It may well be argued that this is a most superficial approach to a deep-seated psychological frailty and that nothing has been done to prevent recurrence of symptoms later or to build up the patient's strength of will. This is true; but even the best psychologist cannot evoke character of which the patient is constitutionally devoid. Moreover, that a psychologist should spend many hours in the attempt to build with such inferior material is a great deal to ask. Hence, the rough and ready method outlined here, since it so often results in the patient's speedy resumption of his proper activities, may be regarded as a reasonable pragmatic approach, however unsound theoretically. Of patients relieved of psychogenic symptoms, less than 10% return with further allegations during the next two years—at any rate to the same hospital.

## Private Practice

In private practice, the situation is rather different, for the patients are less suggestible, there is no hospital social worker and the physician has more time. The diagnosis, and the reasons for arriving at this conclusion, should be stated at once, and the patient asked without further ado if, in view of this finding, he would like psychiatric advice. It is explained that both pent-up tension and depression can give rise to sensations that are interpreted as painful in such states of emotional tone. It is remarkable how many patients immediately agree that this ascription is correct, even though they may have insisted on physiotherapy and osteopathy for years. With this agreement, a talk on how to avoid the now overt emotional strain follows; often simple constructive proposals can be made for patient, spouse and doctor. Some patients find the diagnosis hard to accept. If so, I ask them to see a psychiatrist and, if he considers this mistaken, offer then to examine them again. Some patients reject the diagnosis and merely leave the consulting room unconvinced. For this reason, it is always best to set out the basis for the opinion by talking to the patient in the presence of the nearest relative. The diagnosis is then communicated to the patient's family, who have usually suspected that neurosis was present, but in the absence of support have been unable to take suitable steps. Once the relations know the situation, they can direct their sympathy into more useful channels.

In children, it is best to talk to the parents alone. Psychological symptoms of the sort seen by the orthopaedic physician commonly arise in two sets of circumstances: (*a*) when the child wants to direct his parents' attention to himself, since he has concluded that they like or value a younger brother or sister more; (*b*) when a child resents his parents' decision being forced on him, particularly in the choice of a career. The situation is usually fairly simple; to discover why the child thinks his parents prefer his sibling or where the parents are being inflexible and disregarding the child's wishes about his own future. If they alter their attitude and ignore the child's complaints, symptoms gradually cease. If the parents wish to make a face-saving provision for the child, a week or two's stimulating physiotherapy may be justified.

There is one subtle device that can be used by patients with psychogenic troubles to discredit the physician who makes the diagnosis. Only by proving him incompetent can the patient hope to regain relative's sympathy. A few days after the consultation, the patient becomes 'much worse', and may be brought for a second consultation, which serves only to confirm the original opinion. The patient goes at once to a healer, masseur or lay-manipulator who naturally says that all sorts of lesions are present. He now gives 'treatment' which the patient allows this time to be effective whereas the previous endeavours of the same cultist had proved vain. The patient remains well, unwilling to risk illness again, and sings the other man's praises, while writing aggrieved letters to the physician.

## THE HOSPITAL SOCIAL WORKER

It would be absurd to send all patients with psychogenic symptoms straight to the psychologist. He would find his department overwhelmed by trivial cases. Moreover, many such patients are so weak charactered that his skill and time are inadequately rewarded, even when alleviation, often ephemeral, results. It is amply justifiable in the first place to turn such patients over to the combined efforts of the social worker and the physiotherapist.

The work of a conscientious and understanding hospital social worker supplies a vital part in the treatment of psychogenic pain; for she represents the patient's link with the outside world. She must possess aptitude and human understanding, and be the sort of person whose evident sympathy encourages confidences. She must have enough time to give special attention to those cases in which an uncertain diagnosis has been reached of pain devoid of organic basis or complicated by a neurotic overlay. Hospital social workers find some of the most interesting problems in their work with this type of case. During inquiries into domestic, workaday and financial circumstances, factors may come to light that serve to explain the alleged disability. In doubtful cases, the discovery by the social worker of the presence or absence of conscious or unconscious motives lends weight to, or detracts from, the tentative diagnosis. Her conversation also enables her to help in dividing patients into the relatively deserving and undeserving. Some patients seek relief from unpleasant situations only on severe provocation; in such cases, the social worker can get in touch with employer or Labour Exchange, visit the home or arrange for various forms of assistance or convalescence. Others allege symptoms for the most unworthy reasons; in these cases, it would be an abuse to bring such facilities to the patient's aid. She can also help in cases where the nature of the domestic background indicates that a short talk by the doctor with a member of the patient's family is desirable.

## TRAUMATIC NEURASTHENIA

This is neurosis after an accident leading to the idea of disordered function. Such cases are often sent for a medicolegal opinion. Neurosis is noticeably uncommon after severe fractures or injuries sustained at home or during games and sport, whereas after car smashes or accidents at work emotional reactions often follow, since claims for compensation then arise. It is interesting to note that in France and in the Iron Curtain countries, where compensation is payable for bodily injury but no account is taken of emotional shock, traumatic neurasthenia is almost unknown. For that reason, some authorities prefer the term 'compensation neurasthenia'.

Traumatic neurasthenia is a self-engendered disorder, at least at first: the voluntary perpetuation of the shakiness that almost everyone feels immediately after escaping from what he realizes might have been a serious accident. It is kept in being by a wish to make the most of the incident, and is further maintained by the anxieties and delays of litigation. Field (1978) puts it very neatly. They seek help '... not because they are ill, but because they are in the social role of being plaintiff. There is a world of difference between being sick and acting the role of sickness.'

Cases that come to the Courts are seldom settled until several years after the accident and, during the whole of this time, the patient has to lend colour to his claim by keeping off work, including such work as he could easily carry out, even if all his allegations were well-founded. He pesters his doctor. Moreover, solicitors like their clients to be undergoing treatment at a hospital, since this adds weight to their allegations of disablement. This policy leads to exasperation all round. Now financial loss leads to real worry over his chances of eventual reimbursement, which sets up well-grounded anxiety, augmented by the strains of protracted negotiation. These negotiations, unhappily, are not concerned with how best to speed the patient's recovery, but with reconciling different opinions on what is the matter with him, how long it may be before he recovers, and how much compensation he deserves. By now, his preoccupation may well have become very real, though it is centred on the possible result of litigation, not on the original injury; hence, a time comes when traumatic neurasthenia begins to possess a factual basis.

The insurance companies benefit from delay, and the law moves slowly. The prospect of another medical examination in six months' time, and very likely another, equally inconclusive, six months after that, and so on, engenders an exasperation that leads patients to wish for an early settlement on almost any terms. When, however, this manoeuvre fails, the doctor's efforts to prevent the case dragging on from year to year usually prove futile.

### Depression

Depression precipitated by injury is not traumatic neurasthenia. In patients liable to periods of depression, an accident may bring on such a state. Alternatively, the depressed patient who sustains, say, a fracture may, in that state of mind, decide that he will never recover, or his unavoidable absence from his business may give rise to ideas of impending financial ruin.

Such patients, when examined, do not allege a series of inconsistent signs of the neurasthenic type. Their signs are just what they ought to be, but it is clear that the construction that they put on their disorder is deeply coloured by their mood.

## Treatment

The emphasis is different according to the presence of neurosis, endogenous depression or traumatic neurasthenia.

### Neurosis

If an organic lesion is present, this should be treated with due regard to the patient's state of mind. Little should be done at a time; traction is preferable to manipulation and the induction of epidural local anaesthesia is best carried out in a nursing home, the patient staying for one night afterwards. It is well to point out to the patient that, despite his long-standing symptoms, he has remained healthy. There is thus no reason for fear or despondency. Meanwhile the psychological consultant treats the neurosis energetically.

### Endogenous Depression

The depression should be dealt with, not (at any rate at first) the minor organic trouble. Once the depression lifts, many patients disregard a slight genuine ache. This should be treated only if and when the psychologist says so, but such reference back again is quite uncommon.

### Traumatic Neurasthenia

To embark on active treatment is to court disaster. It fixes the idea of disablement in the patient's mind and persuades him that he has got the better of his doctors.

Treatment is obvious but not simple: to bring to an end the litigation that maintains it. As soon as the suit is settled, the neurasthenia ceases to serve any purpose and it abates quickly in nearly every instance. Even if the case goes against the plaintiff, however disgruntled he may feel, he nearly always sets about earning his living again, though not necessarily at his original work. Erichson (1882) says that this type of patient makes 'a good recovery, but never until the anxieties of litigation have passed away'.

Miller's (1961) classic paper on accident neurosis must be read by all interested in the subject; it is entertainingly written as well as most informative. Of 50 patients with this disorder, he found only two who had not returned to work by two years after the legal suit was concluded, whether favourably or unfavourably. He found that workmen were much more prone to neurosis than employers, and that the likelihood of neurasthenic symptoms bore an inverse proportion to the severity of the injury. However, Miller's views have been strongly refuted by Kelly (1981) who found that 44 out of 62 patients were of upper social status. Of 26 patients who had not returned to work by the time the case came up, only one returned afterwards. He found that persistent unreasonable resentment carried a bad prognosis.

### Prophylaxis

A patient's annoyance at feeling well but being

unable to go to work because of, say sciatica, does not last. After some months of inactivity, he casts around for other ways to occupy his time, often developing new hobbies and interests. His life-style changes, his urge to be a useful citizen abates and he may now become unemployable.

Swift and effective treatment of the original injury (if any) allows no time for ideas of compensation to burgeon. If no lesion is present, immediate return to work turns the individual's mind to other channels at a time when he can still be influenced.

## Financial Advice

The potential litigant has, at first, no idea of what will happen. He should be warned that it takes four to five years for the case to come up, since the insurance company's doctor will examine him, make as sanguine a prognosis as the facts allow and ask for another consultation six months hence. This policy spins the situation out until the exasperated plaintiff finally accepts a small sum. Assuming that he earns £3000 a year, he loses £15 000 in five years. He receives sick benefit of about £4000 during that period. If he loses his case, he loses £11 000. If he gets, say, £2000 damages, he loses £9000. Once he realizes this, he becomes ready to accept some small sum out of court, jettisoning his lawyers and abandoning his suit. If he favours this reversal, I offer him a fortnight's stimulating physiotherapy, so that he can allege 'cure' without loss of face.

## Courteous Inaction

If the patient insists that the case must go to court, all treatment is in vain. Nevertheless, his solicitor insists that he attend hospital, to avoid counsel averring that if he did not seek treatment his symptoms must have been very slight. By the time I see such a patient he has already had endless physiotherapy, so it is clearly logical to state that further treatment wastes his time. Treatment lends colour to the plaintiff's allegations and exasperates the staff of the department who baulk at endlessly treating a patient who never gets better and never stops coming. Moreover, the doctor who has advocated a variety of treatments finds himself logically embarrassed if he later has to appear in Court and state that in his view no organic lesion was present. I merely offer to see him again at as long an interval as he and his lawyers countenance, say two months. Even if my time is wasted, at least that of department is not. When he comes again complaining that he is no better, I give him a polite hearing, an adequate examination and agree that there has been 'no change'. This phrase allows him to depart without ill-feeling. This ritual continues but I have noted that in the long run the patient stops coming and I suspect that he tries his luck afresh at some other hospital.

## Explanation to Doctor

After the first visit, the diagnosis of traumatic neurasthenia is communicated to the family physician in a neutral way, e.g. 'no physical signs were detected to account for his symptoms, but multiple inconsistencies were revealed leading to this ascription'. There is nothing overtly censorious in this wording and, even if this letter is shown to the patient and his solicitor later as part of the evidence, no resentment is evoked.

## Domestic Disposal

No one with backache, still less with traumatic neurasthenia, should be taken on at a rehabilitation centre. He must be shifted at once to a vocational training centre. He is asked to describe his daily routine, and it soon becomes clear that he can walk and sit, let us say. He is then recommended for re-training for a job that by his own admission he can carry on, e.g. cobbler, night-watchman, shop assistant. Once he is employed again, no more need be done than now and then to lend an attentive ear to his grumbles. If some remark appears required, 'I see what you mean' or 'I understand your difficulty' are appropriate. They neither gainsay nor corroborate the allegations but the patient does not notice that.

# ENVOY

The principal element in delaying the acceptance of my policy of manipulation by physiotherapists has been apathy.

My efforts have been not so much resisted as ignored, and it has proved a very effective counter. Doctors' interest in the non-surgical aspect of orthopaedics has proved difficult to arouse; the same applies to the Minister of Health. Curiously enough, the very people who would have benefited most from the implementation of my policy reacted in the same way, and my extension to physiotherapists of tuition on the indications for, and technique of, manipulation was passed over in silence by their leaders for years. Indeed, my offer (1970) of an introductory course to all final year physiotherapy students who cared to come still stands in abeyance. Thus, methods advocated more than 2000 years ago (Hippocrates) and successfully practised throughout the world ever since (Schiötz & Cyriax 1975) seldom reach those who need them. There is surely no other branch of medicine in which the patient is forced to frequent irregular practitioners for sheer lack of medical, or medically trained, personnel. After all, there are no diabeticopaths, cardiopractors or nerve setters. Though patients do not know it, they are seeking an orthopaedic physician. But understandably enough, they have never heard of such a consultant, and so cannot press for his creation in sufficient numbers to cope with the large demand. They have to make do with whoever offers—all sorts of laymen. In my view, every orthopaedic team should contain an orthopaedic physician working daily with the orthopaedic surgeon. The same collaboration would then be created as now exists between neurologist and neurosurgeon, gastroenterologist and abdominal surgeon. Such a colleague would relieve the orthopaedic surgeon of the very work he enjoys least—the non-surgical aspect of diseases of the moving parts. This association had the happiest results during my time at hospital.

The fact that no post in orthopaedic medicine is offered at any hospital in Britain has, of course, had a strong deterrent effect on the actual recruitment of young doctors tentatively drawn towards this speciality. Applicants for training for a non-existent job have naturally not proved numerous, however vital their existence may be to the working capacity of the community. Here lies the main reason for the lack of appeal that orthopaedic medicine makes, though this is the tuition that I offered continuously at St Thomas's Hospital for 30 years. I then offered it from 1970 to 1975 at St Andrew's Hospital. Few came.

Pending the Chartered Society's reappraisal of the position, doctors must attempt to fill the educational gap. After all, at this moment, countless people are in pain and off work unnecessarily. They continue disabled, not because the way to put them right is unknown, but because there are far too few orthopaedic physicians to go round, and an equal dearth of physiotherapists trained in the accurate use of their hands. Some cheer may be gained from the statement published in *Physiotherapy* in 1976 which explained that students were 'at liberty to take up Dr Cyriax's offer themselves, and ask him to lecture to them outside school hours'.

## Orthopaedic Medical Foundation

It is a remarkable fact that the medical man who wants detailed instruction in how to examine the moving parts of the body, what inferences can be drawn, and what treatment to prescribe, has virtually nowhere to go in any country in the world. It is scarcely less remarkable that the doctor or physiotherapist who wants to learn when, when not, and how, to manipulate has really nowhere to go, either. The osteopaths offer a two-year course to state registered physiotherapists and a nine-month course to doctors, but in both instances those taking the courses become embroiled in manipulating as a near-panacea, in theories about the osteopathic lesion, the cure of diseases not connected with the spine, and so on. Furthermore, the assumption that osteopathic spinal technique is the best is based on widespread unawareness that we have devised other methods expressly for disc lesions. It must also be remembered that orthopaedic medicine embraces the whole body, not just the spine, and manipulation forms only one part of the effective treatments offered.

If just one Foundation of Orthopaedic Medicine existed in Britain, patients requiring this approach would have somewhere to go. Doctors would have a centre where the methods of examination and treatment would be on view and taught daily throughout the year. Physiotherapists wishing for a grounding in these methods would also be welcome. At any time during the last 20 years, the situation could have been resolved in this way. Interested doctors would have learnt the work; physiotherapists would understand how to localize a lesion and how to apply accurate treatment. Lay manipulators would soon have become superfluous and the abuses inherent in their practices would have ceased. Everyone would have benefited.

Readers can picture my relief when, in September 1975, the University of Rochester, New York, inaugurated the first Department of Orthopaedics (the word surgery was deleted from the previous title). Equal emphasis was to be placed on the medical and on the surgical aspect of Orthopaedics. At the reception Mrs Dorris Carlson, whose benefaction had made this innovation possible, described her personal experience of the benefits of orthopaedic medicine and congratulated Dr Evarts (who had led the new concept) and myself on the evident fruits of surgical and medical collaboration under one roof. Until that day, it looked as if the knowledge that I had so slowly garnered would be largely lost to posterity. Now, however, a department exists where both aspects of orthopaedics are dealt with together and medical students receive equal grounding in each discipline. We must hope that European universities will in due course follow suit.

Did it but know it, the Chartered Society of Physiotherapy has held lay manipulators in the hollow of its hand for the last 20 years. These men have reason to be extremely grateful to its leaders. During my time at St Thomas's, their policy of withholding tuition on manipulation from their students served to maintain the prosperity of lay manipulators only at the expense of graduates of their own society. Immediate reversal of this policy, coupled with the use of such teachers and examiners as now exist, might still swing the public round to the physiotherapists' side, though every year of further delay makes such a change of attitude more difficult. The existence of a Foundation of Orthopaedic Medicine would enable the Chartered Society of Physiotherapy to send its students for courses in this work, until it was eventually able to supply a trained teacher at each school. There are 40 schools and, in the absence of such a centre, the time-lag will prove crippling.

A Foundation of this sort could be started tomorrow. Until official backing or a wealthy benefactor comes forward, there the matter rests. Vickers (1978) mocked the 'Chartered Society of Physiotherapy', saying 'Placebo workers of the world unite; you have nothing to lose but your brains'.

## 'EMPTY AT THE TOP'

In 1979, after a silence of ten years, I went to see the Education Committee of the Chartered Society of Physiotherapy in London. I explained that it looked as if England would soon be the last country in Europe to possess no centre for teaching any orthopaedic medical work. I was assured that all students knew my work. When I asked how this was possible the answer was: 'from their teachers'. When I pointed out that no teacher of the CSP had ever been to see me about my teaching I was assured that the Committee had every faith in its teachers; I have not. When I asked if students were examined in assessment and manipulation I was assured that the answer was 'yes'. When I asked if anyone present had been to a final examination to listen, no-one had. When I pointed out that none of the examiners had ever been to see me about my work, I was told that the Committee had every confidence in its examiners. I have not.

There is no doubt in my mind that all family doctors would welcome the emergence of the manipulative physiotherapist. The addition of training in manipulation to these auxiliaries' training is long overdue and could lead to the complete replacement of the separate sorts of laymen offering different varieties of this treatment, by trained personnel working outside the Health Service. The family doctor would no longer be forced either to manipulate himself, perhaps hurriedly with unskilled assistance, or covertly to advise recourse to some layman. He would send the patient for manipulative physiotherapy; this would be faithfully carried out as a matter of course by an auxiliary fully trained in these methods and accustomed to working side by side with the medical profession. The arrangement has already been established in Norway, where a special register of those skilled in manipulation is available to doctors. They can send their patients to a physiotherapist who has, by attending a special course and passing an extra examination, obtained a postgraduate diploma.

A curious situation exists putting manipulation in an anomalous position. Since the teaching schools (other than St Thomas's until 1969) do not offer medical students a grounding in these methods, such doctors as do decide to practise it have to learn it as best they can after qualification. They have been forced to go to the London College of Osteopathy, which has now 40 medically qualified graduates, or to learn it out of Stoddard's, Maigne's or my own illustrated book.

The doctor who takes up manipulation is usually a good general practitioner. He has found that a group of his patients, in despair after ordinary medical measures have failed and after the consultants at one or more hospitals have not been able to help either, have wandered off to lay manipulators who cured a proportion of them. A minority of doctors, finding that their patients need a certain type of treatment and that it is unobtainable via the Health Service, meet the challenge and decide to carry it out themselves.

They do not know how to set about this worthy endeavour and must try and hope. A certain number have a natural aptitude, find the work interesting and rewarding and so persevere until they become competent, with little or no guidance, while carrying on as family doctors. After a time, they become known for this work, and more and more patients come to them from far and wide. In due course, they develop a part-time practice in manipulation, soon acquiring rooms in the Harley Street area. Some continue in this way; others finally shift to full-time manipulative practice. These doctors are now 'specialists' in the eyes of the public, with rooms in the accepted area, plenty of patients who praise their skill, and so on. They are not so in the eyes of the medical profession; for they do not have the academic qualifications nor the hospital appointments which normal consultants all possess, and they have no opportunity to teach medical students. Naturally, if a method of treatment is seen to be practised as a speciality almost entirely by doctors who do not conform to their colleagues' ideas of professional respectability, a slur falls on the method. But it is not these doctors' fault that the manipulative branch of medicine is empty at the top; it is so understaffed, and the disorders responding are so common, that today it cannot be entered modestly in the accepted way. The doctor cannot serve an apprenticeship (where would he find a post and a teacher?); he can only be a specialist from the start, since *any* knowledge of this branch of medicine is so far in advance of no knowledge, whatever that pressure of patients forces him to start at the top.

## BACKACHE SOCIETIES

In Britain and the USA, awareness has been growing about the universality and importance of lumbar troubles. Not only do they spoil the quality of so many people's lives, but the drag on industry from absenteeism has been calculated to cost £200 million a year. This omits huge sums expended also on medicolegal suits and compensation. These associations are to be welcomed on both humanitarian and economic grounds.

In my view their function should be twofold, as I pointed out in a memorandum submitted to the Back Pain Association in 1973 when it was first established.

First priority should be given to setting up centres all over the country where sufferers can go and receive treatment known to them to be effective but unobtainable locally. Why should a patient needing a lumbar manipulation attend consultants and hospitals for months before obtaining relief, at his own expense, from some layman in a distant town? The same applies to epidural local anaesthesia. Since this injection lastingly relieves many patients who would otherwise be subjected to laminectomy, each such case saves the Health Service many hundreds of pounds, quite apart from leaving the patient with a whole back. I do not know of any hospital in Britain, Canada or the USA where these treatments are offered on a scale even remotely proportional to the requirement.

The immediate need therefore is to establish clinics on a countrywide scale, and to staff them with orthopaedic physicians and physiotherapists trained to use their hands competently. The low cost of orthopaedic medicine makes this project entirely feasible; for apart from couches and syringes no equipment is necessary. Every orthopaedic team in every large hospital should number an orthopaedic physician and several trained physiotherapists. The running costs are so small that the saving to the country would probably amount to a hundred times the meagre outlay.

However, it seems that the public will subscribe towards research, but not towards rendering available the treatments already in existence, but not provided. Such establishment of clinics is rightly regarded as the duty of the Health Service. Since no such centres have been put up during the thirty years of my advocacy, this hope clearly rests on a delusion. Patients will still have to take their chance outside the medical sphere for one of the commonest causes of disablement known to man, sometimes with relief, sometimes without; and inevitably, occasionally with severe aggravation.

The second priority is research. This is of course important and may well lead to clearer pathological concepts and even better prophylaxis and treatment. Research could clearly be carried out concurrently or as soon as the clinics were running. But if one tiny part of the sums that the Insurance Companies and Sickness Benefit saved by the work at such clinics was devoted to research, the financial provision for scientific measures would prove more than ample.

# BIBLIOGRAPHY


Adams, C. B. T. & Logue, V. (1971) Studies in cervical spondylotic myelopathy. *Brain, 94*, 557.
Adson, A. W. (1925) Diagnosis and treatment of tumours of spinal cord. *N. W. Med., 24*, 309.
Alajounine, T. & Dutallis, P. (1928) Compression de la queue de cheval par une tumeur du disque intervertébrale. *Bull. Soc. natn. Med., 54*, 1452.
Anderson, H. G. & Dukes, C. (1925) Treatment of haemorrhoids by submucous injections of chemicals; with a description of the pathological change produced. *Br. med. J., ii*, 100.
Anderson. J. A. D. (1972) Epidemiology of back pain in different occupations. In *The Painful Back*. London: Royal College of Physicians.
Angaard, E., Arturson, G. & Jonsson, C. E. (1970) Prostaglandin in lymph from scalded tissues. *Acta physiol. scand., 80*, 46A.
Annandale, H. W. (1879) Case of loose cartilage recovered from the knee joint by a direct incision with antiseptic precautions. *Lancet, ii*, 1.
Arderne, J. (1350) Ad guttam in osse que dicetur bonschawe. *Chirurg. in Promp. parv.*, 44.
Armstrong, J. B. (1950) *Lumbar Disc Lesions*. London: Livingstone.
—— (1965) *Lumbar Disc Lesions*, 3rd ed. Edinburgh: Livingstone.
Arnold, J. (1965) Fatal thrombosis of basilar artery after chiropractice. Quoted by Ford, F. R. & Clark, D. (1956).
Aronson, H. A. & Dunsmore, R. H. (1963) Herniated upper lumbar discs. *J. Bone Jt Surg., 45A*, 311.
Asher, R. (1947) The dangers of going to bed. *Br. med. J., ii*, 967.
—— (1972) *Talking Sense*. London: Pitman.
Attall, P. (1957) Accidents graves après manipulation intempestive par un chiropracteur. *Rev. rhumat., 24*, 652.
Bailey, P. & Casamajor, L. (1911) Osteoarthritis of spine compressing cord. *J. nerv. ment. Dis., 38*, 588.
Baker, H., Golding, D. N. & Thompson, M. (1963) Psoriasis and arthritis. *Ann. intern. Med., 58*, 909.
Baker, W. M. (1877) Chronic synovial cysts. *St. Bart's Hosp. Rep.*
Balch, H. W., Gibson, J. M. C., El-Ghobarey, A. F., Bain, L. S. & Lynch, R. P. (1977) Steroid injections into knee. *Rheumatol. Rehab., 16*, 137.
Balfour, W. (1819) *Compression and Percussion*, 2nd ed. Edinburgh: Hill.
Banks, P. & McKenzie, I. (1975) Criteria for condylotomy. *Proc. R. Soc. Med., 68*, 601.
Barbor, R. (1955) Low backache. *Br. med. J., i*, 55.
—— (1964) Treatment for chronic low back pain. *Proc. IVth. int. Congr. phys. Med., Paris.*
—— (1972) Das Schultergelenk. *Man. Med., 10*, 25.
Barlow, T. G. (1962) Early diagnosis and treatment of congenital dislocation of the hip. *J. Bone Jt Surg., 44B*, 292.
Barnett, C. H. (1963) Effects of age on articular cartilage. *Res. Revs.*, 183.
Barry, P. J. & Kendall, P. H. (1962) Corticosteroid infiltration of the extradural space. *Ann. phys. Med., 6*, 267.
Bassett, C. A. L., Pawluk, R. J. & Pilla, A. (1974) Augmentation of Bone Repair by inductively coupled magnetic field. *Science, 184*, 575.
Batt, S. M. (1939) Aetiology of spondylolisthesis. *J. Bone Jt Surg., 21*, 879.
Bauer, R., Sheehan, S. & Meyer, J. S. (1961) Arteriographic study of cerebrovascular disease. II. Cerebral symptoms due to kinking, tortuosity, and compression of carotid and vertebral arteries in the neck. *Archs Neurol., Chicago., 4*, 119.
Beadle, O. A. (1931) *The Intervertebral Discs*. Medical Research Council Report 161. London: HMSO.
Bechgaard, P. (1966) Late post-traumatic headache and manipulation. *Br. med. J., i*, 1419.
Becker, L. A. & Karch, F. E. (1979) Low back pain in family practice. *J. Fam. Pract., 9*, 579.
Beckett, W. (1724) *Philosophical Transactions*. London: Innys.
Bedford, A., Aichroth, P. & Hutton, P. (1979) Arthroscopy. *J. Roy. Soc. Med., 72*, 6.
Beetham, W. P., Polley, H. F., Slocumb, C. H. & Weaver, W. I. (1965) *Physical Examination of the Joints*. Philadelphia: Saunders.
Bell, B. (1824) *Interstitial Absorption of the Thigh Bone*. Edinburgh: MacLachlan-Stewart.
Bénassy, J. & Wolinetz, E. (1957) Quadriplegie après manoeuvre de chiropraxie. *Rev. rhumat., 24*, 555.
Beneke, R. (1897) Zur Lehre von der Spondylitis deformans. *Med. Fstschr. 59 Versamml. dt. Naturforsch.*
Benn, R. T. & Wood, P. H. N. (1975) Pain in back: size of problem. *Rheumat. Rehab., 14*, 121.

Bennett, G. A., Waine, H. & Bauer, W. (1942) *Changes in the Knee Joint at Various Ages.* New York: Commonwealth Fund.
Benson, R. & Fowler, P. D. (1964) Treatment of Weber-Christian disease. *Br. med. J., ii,* 615.
Berlioz, L. V. J. (1816) *Memoires sur les Maladies Chroniques, les Evacuations Sanguines et l'Acupuncture.* Paris: Croullebois.
Bernhardt, M. (1896) Uber eine wenig bekannte Form des Beschäftigungsneuralgie. *Neurol. Zentbl., 15,* 13.
Betts, L. O. (1940) Morton's metarsalgia. *Med. J. Aust., i,* 514.
De Beurmann. (1884) Note sur un signe peu connu de la sciatique. *Archs Physiol. norm. path., 3,* 375.
Bihaug, O., Kjärschow, M. & Sjong, W. (1980) Paravertebral Provokasjonstest på Ischiaspasieuter (in the Press) Norwegian Phys. J.
Bircher, E. (1921) Arthroscopic. *Zeutral blatt für Chirurgie, 48,* 1460.
Black, R. G. (1975) Epidural and selective spinal anaesthesia. Lecture at St. Mary's Hospital, San Francisco, USA.
Blackburne, J. S. & Velikas, E. P. (1977) Spondylolisthesis in children and adults. *Proc. R. Soc. Med., 70,* 421.
Blaine, E. S. (1925) Chiropractic dislocation of atlas. *J. Am. med. Ass., 85,* 1356.
Blair, G. A. S. & Gordon, D. S. (1973) Trigeminal neuralgia and dental malocclusion. *Br. med. J., ii,* 38.
Blau, J. N. & Logue, V. (1961) Intermittent claudication of the cauda equina. *Lancet, i,* 1081.
—— & Rushworth, G. (1958) Blood vessels of the spinal cord and their response to motor activity. *Brain, 81,* 354.
Bogduk, N, Colman, R. R. S. & Winer, C. E. R. (1977) Anatomical Assessment of 'Percutaneous Rhizolysis'. *Med. J. Aust., 1,* 397.
Bohn, E., Franksson, C. & Petersen, I. (1956) Sacral rhizopathies and sacral syndromes. *Acta chir. scand.,* 216.
Boldrey, E., Maas, A. & Miller, E. R. (1956) Rôle of atlantoid compression in etiology of internal carotid thrombosis. *J. Neurosurg., 13,* 127.
Bonney, G. (1956) Arterial disease as a cause of pain in the buttock and thighs. *J. Bone Jt Surg., 38B,* 686.
Bonnin, J. G. (1956) Modern Trends in Orthopaedics. *144.* London: Butterworth.
—— (1973) Transplantation of coracoid tip. *Proc. R. Soc. Med., 66,* 755.
Boshes, L. D. (1959) Vascular accidents associated with neck manipulation. *J. Am. med. Ass., 171,* 274.
Bosman, A. H. (1972) Normal and selected abnormal motion of the spine based on cineradiography. In *The Painful Back.* London: Royal College of Physicians.
Bouchet, Pardy & Pallier, P. (1960) Surdité brutale et chiropraxie. *Ann. Otolaryngol., 77,* 951.
Boudin, G. & Barbizet, J. (1958) Des accidents nerveux de chiropraxie du rachis cervicale. *Rev. Practicien., 8,* 2235.
Bouillet, R. (1976) Traitment des lombosciatiques par injection intradiscale de chymopapaine. *Acta ortop. belge., 42,* 101.
Bourne, R. (1980) Menisci distribute Weight., *Medical Post., 16,* 29.
Bowie, E. A. & Glasgow, G. L. (1961) Cauda equina lesions associated with ankylosing spondylitis. Report of three cases. *Br. med. J., i,* 24.
Boyd, H. B. & McLeod, A. C. (1973) Tennis elbow. *J. Bone Jt Surg., 55A,* 1183.
Brackett, E. G. (1924) Low back strain. *J. Am. med. Ass., 83,* 1068.
Brain, W. R. (1954) Cervical spondylosis. *Lancet, i,* 687.
—— (1963) Some unsolved problems of cervical spondylosis. *Br. med. J., i,* 771.
—— & Wilkinson, M. (1967) *Cervical Spondylosis.* London: Heinemann.
—— Wright, A. D. & Wilkinson, M. (1947) Spontaneous compression of both median nerves in carpal tunnel: 6 cases treated surgically. *Lancet, i,* 227.
Brånemark, P. I., Goldie, I. & Lindstrom, J. (1967) Action of intra-articular prednisolone and methyl prednisolone in rabbit knee joint. *Acta orthop. scand., 38,* 247.
Breig, A. (1960) *Biomechanics of Central Nervous System.* Uppsala: Almquist & Wiksells.
—— & Troup, J. D. G. (1979) Straight-leg Raising. *Spine, 4,* 242.
Brenner, L. (1973) Subcutaneous lumbar 'rhizolysis'. *Med. J. Aust., 2,* 707.
Brewerton, D. A., Caffrey, M., Hart, F. D., James, D. C. O., Nicholls, A. & Sturrock, R. D. (1973) Ankylosing spondylitis and HLA 27. *Lancet, i,* 904.
—— Nichols, P. J. R., Logue, V., Manning, C. W. F., Martin-Jones, M., Mason, R. M., Newell, D. J. & Sandifer, P. H. (1966) Pain in the neck and arm: a multicentre trial of the effects of physiotherapy arranged by the British Association of Physical Medicine, *Br. med. J., i,* 253.
Bridges, J. B. & McLure, P. (1968) Experimental soft-tissue calcification. *Ir. J. med. Sci., 1,* 237.
Brissaud, E. (1890) Des scolioses dans les neuralgies sciatiques. *Archs Neurol., Paris, 19,* 1.
British Orthopaedic Association (1954) Low back pain. *Br. med. J., ii,* 1349.
Brodal, A. (1969) *Neurological Anatomy in Relation to Clinical Medicine,* 2nd ed. London: Oxford University Press.
Broderick, G. L. (1972) Orthopaedic medicine in general practice. *N.Z. med. J., 75,* 155.
Brodin, H. (1973) Apophyseal Cartilage. Lecture given to the British Association for Manipulative Medicine.
—— (1977) Results from lumbar spine mobilization. Congress of Manual Medicine, Copenhagen.
—— Bang, J, Bechgaard, P., Kaltenborn, F. & Schiotz, E. (1966) *Manipulation av Ryggraden.* Copenhagen: Scandinavian University Books.

Brown, M. D. & Daroff, R. B. (1977) Double blind study comparing disease to placebo. *Spine, 2,* 233.

Brown, T. (1828) Irritation of spinal nerves. *Glasg. med. J., 158.*

Browse, N. L. (1965) *Physiology and Pathology of Bed-rest.* Springfield, Ill.: Charles C. Thomas.

—— Clemensen, G. & Thomas, M. L. (1980) Is the postphlebitic leg always postphlebitic? *Br. med. J., 281,* 1167.

Brügger, A. (1960) Documenta Geigy. *Acta rheum. scand., 18.*

Brust, J. C. M. (1979) Pathology of Drop Attacks. *Neurol., 29,* 786.

Buck, J. E. & Phillips, N. (1970) Trial of chymoral in professional footballers. *Br. med. clin. Pract., 24,* 375.

Bulgen, D. Y., Hazleman, B. L. & Voak, D. (1976) HLA-B27 and frozen shoulder. *Lancet, i,* 1042.

Bull, J. W. D. & Zilkha, K. I. (1966) Rationalizing requests for X-ray films in neurology. *Br. med. J., ii,* 569.

Burke, C. L. (1964) Backache from Occiput to Coccyx. Vancouver: McDonald.

Burn, J. M., Guyer, P. B. & Langdon, L. (1973) Spread of solutions injected into epidural space. *Br. J. Anaesth., 45,* 338.

—— (1973) Spread of solutions injected into epidural space. *Br. J. Anaesth., 45,* 340.

Burnett, C. H. (1965) Effects of age on articular cartilage. *Res. Rev.*

Burri, C., Helbing, G. & Spier, W. (1973) Rehabilitation of Knee Ligament Injuries. In *The Knee.* New York: Springer.

Burton, C. V. (1978) Lumbo-sacral arachnoiditis. *Spine, 3,* 24.

Bywaters, E. G. L. (1968) Case of ankylosing spondylitis. *Br. med. J., i,* 412.

—— & Ansell, B. M. (1958) Arthritis associated with ulcerative colitis; a clinical and pathological study. *Ann. rheum. Dis., 17,* 169.

Calin, A. & Grahame, R. (1974) Trial of flurbiprofen and phenylbutazone in ankylosing spondylitis. *Br. med. J., iv,* 496.

Calvé, J. (1925) Localised affection of spine suggesting osteochondritis of vertebral body. *J. Bone Jt Surg., 7,* 41.

Calvé, J. & Galland, M. (1922) Calcification of Nucleus Pulposus. *J. de Radiol et d'Electrol., 6,* 21.

Campbell, A. M. G. & Phillips, D. G. (1960) Cervical disc lesions with neurological disorder. *Br. med. J., ii,* 481.

Campbell, D. G. & Parsons, C. M. (1944) Referred head pain and its concomitants; report of preliminary experimental investigation with implications for post-traumatic 'head' syndrome. *J. nerv. ment. Dis., 99,* 544.

Caner, J. E. & Decker, J. L. (1964) Recurrent acute arthritis in chronic renal failure treated by haemodialysis. *Am. J. Med., 36,* 571.

Capener, N. (1966) Vulnerability of the posterior interosseous nerve. *J. Bone Jt Surg., 48B,* 770.

Carp, L. (1932) Tennis elbow (epicondylitis) caused by radiohumeral bursitis; anatomic, clinical, roentgenologic and pathological aspects with suggestions as to treatment. *Ann. Surg., 24,* 905.

Carter, C. O. & Fairbank, T. J. (1974) Genetics of Locomotor Disorders. Oxford Univ. Press, 126.

Cathelin, M. F. (1901) Injection epidurale par le procédé du canal sacré. *Comp. rend. Soc. biol., 53,* 452.

Catterall, A. (1971) Prognosis in Perthes's disease. *J. Bone Jt Surg., 53B,* 37.

—— (1977) Perthes's disease. *Br. med. J., i,* 1145.

Chandler, G. N. & Wright, V. (1958) Deleterious effect of intra-articular hydrocortisone. *Lancet, ii,* 611.

Charcot, J. M. (1888) quoted by Miller, H. (1967) Three great neurologists. *Proc. R. Soc. Med., 60,* 399.

Charnley, J. (1960) Surgery of the hip joint: present and future developments. *Br. med. J., i,* 821.

Chatterton, J. (1960) Surgery of the hip joint: present and future developments. *Br. med. J., i,* 821.

Chatterton, C. C. (1949) Radiographic evidence of intermittent protrusion of intervertebral disc. *Minnesota Med., 32,* 730.

Chemonucleolysis Symposium (1969) *Clin. Orthop., 67,* 6.

Churchill, J. M. (1821) *Treatise on Acupuncturation.* London: Simpkin Marshall.

Clark, C. J. & Whitwell, J. (1961) Intraocular haemorrhage after epidural injection. *Br. med. J., ii,* 1612.

Clarke, E. & Bearn, J. G. (1972) Spiral nerve bands of Fontana. *Brain, 95,* 1.

Clercq, E. de, Decreet, H., Wildiers, J., Jonge, G. de, Drochmans, A., Descamps, J. & Somer, P. de (1980) Oral E-5 2-bromovinyl deoxymidine in severe herpes zoster. *Br. med. J., 281,* 2, 1178.

Cleveland, D. A. (1955) Use of methyl-acrylic for spinal stabilization after disc operation. *Marquette med. Rev., 20,* 62.

Cochrane, T. (1979) Working Group on Back Pain. Department of Health and Social Security.

Cockett, F. B. & Maurice, B. A. (1963) Evolution of direct arterial surgery for claudication and ischaemia of legs. A nine-year survey. *Br. med. J., i,* 353.

—— Thomas, M. L. & Negus, D. (1967) Iliac vein compression; its relation to ilio-femoral thrombosis and the post thrombotic syndrome. *Br. med. J., i,* 214.

Cohen, P. (1966) Myelomatosis treated with sodium fluoride. *J. Am. med. Ass., 198,* 583.

Cole, J. P., Lesswing, A. L. & Cole, J. R. (1968) Analysis of lumbosacral dermatomes in man. *Clin. Orthop., 61,* 241.

Collis, J. S. (1963) *Lumbar Discography.* Springfield, Ill.: Charles C. Thomas.

Conesa, H. (1976*a*) Incorporacion de la medicina ortopedica a la rehabilitacion. *Rehabilitacion, 10,* 29.

—— (1976*b*) Retraction capsular del hombro hemiplejico. *Rehabilitacion, 10,* 215.

—— & Argote, M. L. (1976) *A Visual Aid to the Examination of the Nerve-Roots.* London: Baillière Tindall.

Conlon, P. W., Isdale, I. C. & Rose, B. S. (1966) Rheumatoid arthritis of cervical spine. *Ann. rheum. Dis.*, *25*, 120.

Coomes, E. N. (1959) In *The Innervation of Muscle*, ed. C. Coërs & A. L. Woolf, pp. 74–79.

—— (1961) Comparison between epidural local anaesthesia and bed rest in sciatica. *Br. med. J.*, *i*, 20.

—— & Sharp, J. (1961) Polymyalgia rheumatica. *Lancet*, *ii*, 1328.

Coonrad, R. W. & Hooper, W. R. (1973) Tennis elbow: Course, natural history, conservative and surgical management. *J. Bone Jt Surg.*, *55A*, 1177.

Cooper, A. (1822) Treatise on Fractures and Dislocation of Joints. London: Wilkie.

Cooper, I. S. (1965) Clinical and physiologic implications of thalmic surgery for dystonia and torticollis. Bull. N.Y. Acad. Med., *41*, 870.

Cope, S. & Ryan, G. M. S. (1959) Cervical and otolith vertigo. *J. Lar. Otol.*, *73*, 113.

Corrigan, A. B. (1965) The pulled elbow. *Med. J. Aust.*, *2*, 167.

Costen, J. B. (1936) Neuralgia associated with disturbed function of tempero-mandibular joint. *J. Am. med. Ass.*, *107*, 252.

Cotugno, D. (1764) De Ischide Nervosa Commentarius. Vienna: Gräffer.

—— (1775) *Treatise on Nervous Sciatica or Nervous Hip Gout.* London: Wilkie.

Coudère, A. (1896) Etude sur un nouvel accident professional des maîtres-d'armes dû à la rupture probable et partiale du tendon epicondylien. Thèse de Bordeaux.

Coulson, W. (1852) *Diseases of Bladder and Prostate Gland*, p. 104. London: Churchill.

Cox, T. (1824) *Observations on Acute Rheumatism.* London: Cox.

Crelin, E. S. (1973) Scientific test of chiropractic theory. *Am. Sci.*, *61*, 574.

Crisp, E. J. (1948) Treatment of lumbar disc lesions by immobilization in plaster jacket. *Rheumatism*, *4*, 211.

Critchley, R. (1938) Spasmodic torticollis. *Proc. R. Soc. Med.*, *31*, 717.

Crow, N. E. & Brogden, B. G. (1959) The 'normal' lumbo-sacral spine. *Radiology*, *71*, 97.

Csonka, G. W. (1958) The course of Reiter's syndrome. *Br. med. J.*, *i*, 1088.

Currey, H. L. F. & Swettenham, K. V. (1965) Synovial fluid in gout. *Br. med. J.*, *ii*, 481.

Curtis, A. C. & Pollard, H. M. (1940) Felty's syndrome; its several features, including tissue changes, compared with other forms of rheumatoid arthritis. *Ann. intern. Med.*, *13*, 2265.

Cushing, H. (1926) The Life of Sir William Osler. Vol. 1, 177. Oxford University Press.

Cyriax, J. (1936) Pathology and treatment of tennis elbow. *J. Bone Jt Surg.*, *18*, 921.

—— (1938) Rheumatic headache. *Br. med. J.*, *ii*, 1367.

—— (1941*a*) Sacro-iliac strain. *Br. med. J.*, *ii*, 847.

—— (1941*b*) *Massage, Manipulation and Local Anaesthesia.* London: Hamilton.

—— (1942) Perineuritis. *Br. med. J.*, *i*, 578.

—— (1945) Lumbago: the mechanism of dural pain. *Lancet*, *ii*, 427.

—— (1947) Rheumatism and Soft-tissue Injuries. London: Hamilton.

—— (1948) Fibrositis. *Br. med, J.*, *ii*, 251.

—— (1949*a*) *Osteopathy and Manipulation.* London: Crosby Lockwood.

—— (1949*b*) Pressure on the nerves of the neck and upper limb. *St. Thom. Hosp. Rep.*, *5*, 67.

—— (1950*a*) Thoracic disc lesions. *St. Thom. Hosp. Rep.*, *6*, 171.

—— (1950*b*) Treatment of lumbar disc lesions. *Br. med. J.*, *ii*, 1434.

—— (1952) Zervicale bandscheibenschäden. *Medsche Welt. Stuttg.*, *2*, 489.

—— (1953) *Disc lesions.* London: Cassell.

—— (1954) *Textbook of Orthopaedic Medicine, Vol. I. Diagnosis of Soft Tissue Lesions*, 2nd ed. London: Cassell.

—— (1955*a*) Les Manipulations Vertebrales. Premières journées internationales de kinésithérapie Bruxelles.

—— (1955*b*) Spinal disc lesions: assessment after 21 years. *Br. med. J.*, *i*, 140.

—— (1956) *Hydrocortisone in Orthopaedic Medicine.* London: Cassell.

—— (1957*a*) Statistics on conservative treatment of lumbar disc lesions. *Rep. int. Congr. occup. Hlth., Helsinki*, *i*, 124.

—— (1957*b*) *The Shoulder.* London: Cassell.

—— (1958*a*) Lumbar disc lesions; conservative treatment. *S. Afr. med, J.*, *31*, 1.

—— (1958*b*) Diagnosis at the shoulder. *S. Afr. med. J.*, *32*, 62.

—— (1958*c*) Soft-tissue injuries in athletes. *Medna Sport.*, *12*, 249.

—— (1959*a*) Esame funzionale nelle lesioni delle parti non scheletriche dell'apparato locomotore. *Atti. Soc. lomb. Sci. med. biol.*, *14*, 829.

—— (1959*b*) Indications for and against manipulation. In *Die Wirbelsäule in Forschung und Praxis*, Vol. 13, 104. Oldenburg: Junghanns.

—— (1959*c*) Use and misuse of physiotherapy. *Med. Press* 505.

—— (1960) Clinical applications of massage. In *Massage, Manipulation and Traction.* ed. Licht. New Haven, Conn,: Licht.

—— (1961) Lesions Discales Lombaires. *Act. Orthop. Belg.*, *27*, 443.

Cyriax, J. (1962) *Textbook of Orthopaedic Medicine, Vol. 1. Diagnosis of Soft Tissue Lesions*, 4th ed. London: Baillière, Tindall & Cassell.
—— (1964) Pros and cons of manipulation. *Lancet, i*, 571.
—— (1966*a*) Manipulation. *Clin. med. Surg., 73*, 37.
—— (1966*b*) Manipulative surgery. In *Clinical Surgery*, ed. C. Rob & R. Smith. London: Butterworths.
—— (1968) Léze bederniko disku. *Acta chirg. orthop. czech., 35*, 188.
—— (1970) *The Slipped Disc.* London: Gower Press.
—— (1971) *Cervical Spondylosis.* London: Butterworths.
—— (1971) *The Slipped Disc.*, 2nd ed. London: Gower Press.
—— (1972) *Der Schulterschmerz und seine Behandling.* München: Schwarzeck.
—— (1973) Paper presented to the International Seminar of Orthopaedic Medicine.
—— (1975) Tratamiento del Dolor Lumbar 'Intratable'. *Revista Iberoamericana de Rehabilitation Medica, 11*, 3.
—— (1975) Orthopaedic beds. *Br. med. J., ii*, 231.
—— (1975) *Treatment of Pain by Manipulation.* NINCDS Monograph 13. Washington, D.C.: US Department of Health, Education and Welfare.
—— (1976) Spinal manipulation. *Sth. African J. Physiother., 32*, 2.
—— (1977) Osteopathy. In *Dictionary of Medical Ethics.* London: Darton, Longman & Todd.
—— (1977) Deep Massage. *Physiother., 63*, 60.
—— (1977) Osteopathy. In *Dictionary of Medical Ethics.* London: Darton, Longman & Todd.
—— (1978*a*) Lawyer's guide to lumbar disc lesions. *New Law J., 128*, 97.
—— (1978*b*) Dural Pain. *Lancet, i*, 919.
—— & Gould, J. (1953) Pain in the trunk. *Br. med. J., i*, 1077.
—— & Troisier, O. (1952) Hydrocortisone and soft-tissue lesions. *Br. med. J., ii*, 966.
Cyriax, R. J. (1912) Mechano-therapy in America. Chiropractic Naprapathy. *Gymn. J. Stockh., 117*, 171.
Dabbet, O., Freeman, D. G. & Weiss, D. G. (1970) Spinal meningeal haematoma, warfarin therapy and chiropractic adjustment. *J. Am. med. Ass., 214*, 2058.
Dacie, J. E. (1981) Percutaneous transluminal angioplasty. *Br. J. Hosp. Med., 26*, 314.
Dalseth, I. (1974) Anatomic studies of osseous cranio-vertebral joints. *Manip. Med., 12*, 130.
—— (1976) Reply to Lewit. *Manip. Med., 14*, 11.
Damany, P. (1914) Compression of cord and cauda equina by osteo-arthritis. *Presse med., 30*, 285.
Dandy, D. J. (1978) Early results of closed partial meniscectomy. *Br. med. J., ii*, 1099.
Dandy, W. E. (1929) Loose cartilage from intervertebral disc simulating tumour of spinal cord. *Archs Surg., Chicago., 19*, 660.
Darwell, J. (1829) Forms of spinal and cerebral irritation. *Midland med. surg. Reporter, 1*, 229.
Davidson, J. A. (1962) Assessment of hypnosis in pregnancy and labour. *Br. med. J., ii*, 951.
Davies, D. V., Barnett, C. H., Cochrane, W. & Palfrey, A. J. (1962) Electron microscopy of articular cartilage in the young rabbit. *Ann. rheum. Dis., 21*, 11.
Davis, P. R. (1973) Human evolution and load carriage. Lecture at Northwick Park Clinical Research Centre.
Decker, K. (1975) Early diagnosis of vertebral tumours by radiography. Lecture at Fifth Reunión sobre Patologia de la Columna Vertebral, Murcia, Spain.
Degenering, P. W. (1961) Hazards of chiropractice. *Med. Klin., 56*, 1756.
Déjerine, J. (1906) Sur la claudication intermittente de la moelle épinière. *Rev. neurol., 14*, 341.
Deliss, L. (1977) Coronal patellar osteotomy. *Proc. R. Soc. Med., 70*, 257.
Depassio, L. (1975) L'exercise illegala des thérapeutiques manuelles. Service du Prof. Guilkiet, Hospital Edouard Herriot, Lyons.
Deshayes, P. & Geoffroy, Y. (1962) Paralysie plexique superieure, accident d'une manipulation vertebrale. *Rev. Rhumat., 29*, 137.
Dillane, J. B., Fry, J. & Kalton, G. (1966) Acute back syndrome, a study from general practice. *Br. med. J., ii*, 82.
Dingle, J. T., Gordon, J. L., Hazleman, B. L., Knight, C. G., Page-Thomas, D. P., Phillips, N. C. & Shaw, I. H. (1978) Novel Treatment for Joint Inflammation. *Nature, 271*, 372.
Dodd, H. (1948) Reactions to intravenous sclerotics. *Br. med. J., ii*, 838.
Dörr, W. R. (1958) Über die Anatomie des Wirbelgelenke. *Arch. orthop. Unfallchir., 50*, 222.
Dove, C. I. (1967) History of Osteopathic Vertebral Lesion. *Brit. Osteopathic J., 3*, 1.
Doyle, L. (1970) Hypertrophic osteoarthropathy. *Br. med. J., i*, 630.
Durlacher, R. L. (1854) *Corns, Bunions and Disease of Nails.* Philadelphia: Lea & Blanchard.
Dupuytren, G. (1832) *Leçons Orales de Clinique Chirurgicale*, Vol. I. Paris: Baillière.
Easton, J. D. (1977) Chiropractic Cerebral Damage. Lecture at World Congress of Neurology. Medical Post 22 November.
Ebringer, R., Ebringer, A. & Cawdell, D. (1979) Klebsiella pneumoniae and acute anterior uveitis in ankylosing spondylitis. *Br. med. J., i*, 383.

Eccles, J. C. & Sherrington, C. S. (1930) Numbers and contraction values of individual motor units. *Proc. R. Soc. Med., 106*, 326.
Edgar, M. A. (1973) *Clinical Significance of Innervation of Lumbar Spinal Dura and Dural Root-sleeve.* London: Society for Back Pain Research.
—— & Nundy, S. (1966) Innervation of the spinal dura mater. *Neurol. Neurosurg. Psychiat., 29*, 530.
Ehret, H. (1899) Beiträg zur lehre Skoliose nach Ischirs. *Mitt. aus Greuzgeb Med. Chir., 4*, 660.
Eisen, V. (1966) Urates and kinin formation in synovial fluid. *Proc. R. Soc. Med., 59*, 302.
Elliotson, J. (1827) Acupuncture. *Med. Chir. Trans., 13*, 467.
Ellis, R. (1976) Spinal contrast radiography. Lecture at Rochester University, New York.
Ellis, W. (1973) Rubella arthritis. *Br. med. J., ii*, 549.
Elsberg, C. A. (1916) *Diagnosis and Treatment of Surgical Diseases of the Spinal Cord and Its Membranes.* Philadelphia and London: Saunders.
Erichson, J. E. C. (1863) Lectures on Railway and other Injuries of the Nervous System. London: Walton & Maberley.
—— (1882) Concussion of the Spine. London: Longmans Green, 203.
Evans, J. G. (1964) Neurogenic intermittent claudication. *Br. med. J., ii*, 985.
Eyring, E. J. (1969) Biochemistry of the intervertebral disc. *Clin. Orthop., 67*, 16.
Fahlgren, H., Jansa, S. & Lofstedt, S. (1966) Retrofaryngeal tendinit. *Lakärtigning, 63*, 3779.
Fajersztajn, J. (1901) Über das gekreuzte Ischiasphänomen; ein Beitrag zur Symptomatologie der Ischias. *Wien, klin. Wschr., 14*, 41.
Feldberg, W. (1951) Physiology of neuromuscular transmission and neuromuscular block. *Br. med. J., i*, 967.
Féré, G. (1897) Note sur l'epicondylalgie. *Revue Med., 17*, 144.
Fernström, U. (1957) Lumbar intervertebral disc degeneration with abdominal pain. *Acta chir. scand., 113*, 436.
—— (1960) Discographic study of ruptured lumbar intervertebral discs. *Acta chir. scand., 122*, 258, 1.
—— (1964) Diskprotes av metall vid lumbal diskruptur. *Nord. Med., 71*, 160.
Field, H. (1978) Compensation Neurosis. *Brit. J. Hosp. Med.*, 92.
Filitzer, D. L. & Bahnson, H. T. (1959) Low back pain due to arterial obstruction. *J. Bone Jt Surg., 41B*, 244.
Fisher, E. D. (1943) Ruptured intervertebral disc following chiropractic manipulation. *Kentucky med. J., 41*, 14.
Fisk, B. (1971) Manipulation in general practice. *N.Z. med. J., 74*, 172.
Flevell, G. (1956) Reversal of pulmonary hypertrophic osteoarthropathy by vagotomy. *Lancet, i*, 260.
Flint, M. M. (1965) Electromyographic comparison of iliacus and rectus abdominis muscles. *Phys. Ther. Rev., 45*, 248.
Floyd, W. F. & Silver, P. H. S. (1955) Function of erector spinae muscles in certain movements in man. *J. Physiol., 129*, 184.
Foerster, O. (1933) Dermatomes in man. *Brain, 56*, 1.
Fontana, F. (1781) *Différentes Experiences sur la Reproduction des Nerfs.* Florence.
Ford, F. R. (1952) Syncope, vertigo and disturbance of vision resulting from intermittent obstruction of vertebral arteries due to a defect in the odontoid process and excessive mobility of the second cervical vertebra. *Bull. Johns Hopkins Hosp., 91*, 168.
Ford, F. R. & Clark, D. (1956) Thrombosis of basilar artery with softening of cerebellum due to manipulation of neck. *Bull. Johns Hopkins Hosp., 98*, 37.
Ford, L. T. (1969) Chymopapain in lumbar and dorsal disc-lesions. *Clin. Orthop., 67*, 81.
Forestier, J. & Rotes-Querol, J. (1950) Senile ankylosing hypertosis of spine. *Ann. rheum. Dis., 9*, 321.
Forst, J. J. (1881) Contribution à l'etude clinique de la sciatique. Thése de Paris.
Francis, J. (1973) Subcutaneous lumbar 'rhizolysis'. *Med. J. Aust., 2*, 750.
Franke, F. (1910) Über Epicondylitis humeri. *Dt. med. Wschr., 36*, 13.
Freedman, B. J. & Knowles, C. H. R. (1959) Anterior tribial syndrome due to arterial embolism and thrombosis. *Br. med. J., ii*, 270.
Freeman, M. A. R. (1972) Ciba Foundation Symposium.
—— Dean, M. R. E. & Hanham, I. W. F. (1965) Aetiology and prevention of functional instability of foot. *J. Bone Jt Surg., 47B*, 678.
Freiburg, A. H. (1914) Infraction of the second metatarsal bone, a typical injury. *Surgery Gynec. Obstet., 19*, 191.
Freund, H. A., Steiner, G., Leichtentritt, B. & Price, A. E. (1942) Peripheral nerves in chronic atrophic arthritis. *Am. J. Path., 18*, 865.
Frimoyer, J. W., Hanley, E., Howe, J., Kuhlmann, D. & Matteri, R. (1978) Lumbar Disc Excision and Spine Fusion. *Spine, 3*, 1.
Frohse, F. (1908) *Muskeln des Menschlichen Armes.* Jena.
Frykholm, R. (1951*a*) Lower cervical nerve-roots and their investments. *Acta chir. scand., 101*, 457.
—— (1951*b*) Lower cervical vertebrae and intervertebral discs. Surgical anatomy and pathology. *Acta chir. scand., 101*, 345.
Garden, R. S. (1961) Tennis elbow. *J. Bone Jt Surg., 43B*, 100.

Gelch, M. M. (1978) Herniated Thoracic Disc at T 1–2 level with Horner's syndrome. *J. Neurosurg.*, *48*, 128.
Gerlach, H. L. (1884) Über die Bewegung in den Atlasgelenke unde deren Beziehungen du der Blutströmmung an den vertebral Arterien. *Beitr. Morphol*, *1*, 104.
Gibson, H. J., Kersley, G. D. & Desmarais, M. H. L. (1946) Lesions in muscle in arthritis. *Ann. rheum. Dis.*, *5*, 131.
—— —— —— (1948) Muscle histology in rheumatic and control cases. *Ann. rheum. Dis.*, *7*, 132.
Gil, J. R. & Katona, G. (1971) Utilatà clinica e terapeurica dell'artroscopia. *Gazz. sanit.*, *Milano.*, *42*, 201.
Gill, G. G., Manning, J. G. & White, H. L. (1955) Surgical treatment of spondylolisthesis without spine fusion; excision of loose lamina with decompression of nerve roots. *J. Bone Jt Surg.*, *37A*, 493.
Gill, G. G., Manning, J. G. & White, H. L. (1955) Surgical treatment of spondylisthesis. *J. Bone Jt Surg.*, *37A*, 518.
Gillespie, H. W. (1949) The significance of lumbo-sacral abnormalities. *Br. J. Radiol.*, *22*, 257, 270.
—— & Lloyd Roberts, G. (1953) Osteitis condensans. *Br. J. Radiol.*, *26*, 16.
Glorieux, P. (1937) *La Hernie Posterieure du Ménisque Intervertebral.* Paris: Masson.
Glover, J. R. (1972) The Facet Joints. Lecture at the British Association for Manipulative Medicine Symposium.
Goald, H. J. (1978) Microlumbar Discectomy. Lecture at International Association for Study of Pain. Montreal.
Goddard, M. D. & Reid, J. D. (1965) Movements induced by straight-leg raising in the lumbo-sacral roots. *J. Neurol. Neurosurg. Psychiat.*, *28*, 12.
Goldthwaite, J. (1911) The lumbo-sacral articulation. Explanation of cases of lumbago, sciatica and paraplegia. *Boston med. Surg. J.*, *164*, 365.
Goodfellow, J. (1965) Aetiology of hallux rigidus. *Proc. R. Soc. Med.*, *59*, 821.
Goodley, P. (1973) Film shown at the International Seminar on Orthopaedic Medicine, Spain.
Gowers, W. (1904) Lumbago. *Br. med. J.*, *i*, 117.
Green, D. & Joynt, R. J. (1959) Vascular accidents to the brain stem associated with neck manipulation. *J. Am. med. Ass.*, *182*, 522.
Gresham, J. L. & Miller, R. (1969) Evaluation of lumbar spine by discography. *Clin. Orthop.*, *67*, 29.
Griffin, J. E. & Touchstone, J. C. (1963) Ultrasonic movement of cortisol into pig tissues. I. Movement into skeletal muscle. *Am. J. phys. Med.*, *43*, 77.
—— —— & Liu, A. C.-Y. (1965) Ultrasonic movement of cortisol into pig tissues. II. Movement into paravertebral nerve. *Am. J. phys. Med.*, *44*, 20.
Griffiths, H. (1959) *National Dock Labour Board Educational Booklet* 2. London: HMSO.
Guillain, G. & Courtellemont (1905) L'action du muscle court supinateur dans la paralysie du nerf radial. *Press méd.*, *13*, 50.
Guiloff, R. J. (1979) Carbamazepine in Morton's Metatarsalgia. *Br. med. J.*, *ii*, 904.
Gurdjian, E. S. & Thomas, L. M. (1970) *Neckache and Backache.* Springfield, Ill.: Charles C. Thomas.
Hackett, G. S. (1956) *Joint Ligament Relaxation Treated by Fibro-osseous Proliferation.* Springfield, Ill.: Charles C. Thomas.
—— (1958) *Ligament and Tendon Relaxation.* Springfield, Ill.: Charles C. Thomas.
Hadfield, G. (1966) Immobile meniscus syndrome. *Proc. R. Soc. Med.*, *59*, 117.
Hager, W. (1885) Neuralgia femoris. *Dt. med. Wschr.*, *II*, 218.
Hakelius, A. (1970) Prognosis in sciatica. *Acta orthop. scand.*, Suppl. 2, 129.
Hamberg, J. (1973) Trapped ligamentum teres. Lecture to the International Seminar on Orthopaedic Medicine, Spain.
Hamby, W. B. & Glaser, H. T. (1959) Replacement of spinal intervertebral discs with locally polymerizing methyl methacrylate; experimental study of effects upon tissues and report of a small clinical series. *Neurosurgery*, *16*, 311.
Hamkin, B., Jonsson, N. & Landberg, T. (1964) Arteritis in polymyalgia rheumatica. *Lancet*, *i*, 397.
Hannington-Kiff, J. G. (1974) Intravenous sympathetic regional block with guanethidine. *Lancet*, *i*, 1019.
Hannington-Kiff, J. G. (1979) Relief of causalgia by regional intravenous guanethidine. *Br. med. J.*, *ii*, 367.
Hansen, K. & Schliack, H. (1962) *Segmentale Innervation.* Stuttgart: Thieme.
Harley, C. (1960) Extradural corticosteroid infiltration; a follow-up study of 50 cases. *Proc. Br. Ass. phys. Med.*, *9*, 22.
Harman, J. (1951) Angina in analgesic limb. *Br. med. J.*, *ii*, 521.
Harman, W. (1948) Significance of local vascular phenomena in ischaemic necrosis in skeletal muscle. *Am. J. Path.*, *24*, 625.
Harris, R. I. & Beath, T. (1948) Aetiology of peroneal spastic flatfoot. *J. Bone Jt Surg.*, *30B*, 624.
Harrison, E. (1820) Effect of spinal distortion on the sanguineous circulation. *Lond. med. phys. J.*, *44*, 373.
—— (1821) Observations respecting the nature and origin of the common species of disorder of the spine. *London med. phys. J.*, *45*, 106.
—— (1824) Diseases occasioned by distortion of the spinal column. *Lond. med. phys. J.*, *51*, 267.
Harrison, M. H. M., Schajowicz, F. & Trueta, J. (1953) Osteoarthritis of hip; study of nature and evolution of disease. *J. Bone Jt Surg.*, *35B*, 598.
Hart, F. D. (1969) Polymyalgia rheumatica. *Br. med. J.*, *I*, 99.

Hart, F. D. (1974) Naproxen (Naprosyn) and gastro-intestinal haemorrhage. *Br. med. J., i*, 51.
—— & Golding, J. R. (1960) Rheumatoid neuropathy. *Br. med. J., i*, 1594.
Harvey, A. M. (1939) Action of quinine on skeletal muscle. *J. Physiol, Lond., 95*, 45.
Hassler, O. (1970) Human intervertebral disc. *Acta orthop. scand., 40*, 765.
Healey, N. (1981) Rehabilitation and manual medicine. *Brit. Ass. Manip. Med.*, April 4.
Heberden, W. (1802) Commentaries on the History and Cure of Diseases. London: Payne.
Hébréard. (1817) Memoirs sur la gangrene ou mort partielle. *Memoires Soc. Med. Paris.*
Helal, B. & Karadi, B. S. (1968) Artificial lubrication of joints. *Ann. phys. Med., 9*, 334.
Helfet, A. J. (1963) *Management of Internal Derangements of the Knee.* Philadelphia: Lippincott.
Hench, P. S. & Rosenberg, E. F. (1944) Palindromic Rheumatism. *Arch. int. Med., 73*, 293.
Henderson, R. J. & Hill, D. M. (1972) Subclinical *Brucella* infection in man. *Br. med. J., ii*, 154.
Hendry, N. G. C. (1958) The hydration of the nucleus pulposus and its relation to intervertebral disc derangement. *J. Bone Jt Surg., 40B*, 132.
Henry, A. N. (1977) Arthroscopy in practice. *Br. med. J., i*, 87.
Henson, R. A. and Parsons, M. (1967) Ischaemic lesions of the spinal cord: an illustrated review. *Q. Jl. Med., 142*, 205.
Herfort, R. & Nickerson, S. H. (1959) Relief of arthritic pain and rehabilitation of chronic arthritic patient by extended sympathetic denervation. *Archs phys. Med., 40*, 133.
Herndon, R. F. (1927) Back injuries in industrial employees. *J. Bone Jt Surg., 9*, 234.
Hey, W. (1803) *Practical Observations in Surgery.* London: Cadell & Davies.
Hills, N. H., Pflug, J. J., Jeyasingh, K., Boardman, L. & Calnan, J. S. (1972) Prevention of deep vein thrombosis by pneumatic compression of calf. *Br. med J., i*, 131.
Hilton, J. (1863) *In the Influence of Mechanical and Physiological Rest in the Treatment of Accidents and Surgical Diseases.* London: Bell & Dalby.
Hilton, R. C., Ball, J. & Benn, R. T. (1976) Vertebral end-plate lesions (Schmorl's nodes). *Ann. Rheum. Dis., 35*, 127.
Hinz, P. (1968) Sektionsbefunde nach Schleudertraumen der Halswirbelsäule. *Dt. Z. Med., 64*, 204.
Hipp, E. (1961) Gefahren der chiropraktischen und osteopathischen Behandlung. *Med. Klin., 56*, 1020.
Hirsch, C. (1959) Pathology of low back pain. *J. Bone Jt Surg., 41B*, 237.
Hirschfeld, P. F. (1962) Die Konservative Behandlung des lumbalen Bandscheibenvorfalls nach der Methode Cyriax. *Dt. med. Wschr., II*, 299.
—— (1974) Bandscheibenvorfälle bei Kindern. *Kind Chirurg., 15*, 322.
Hitselberger, W. E. & Whitten, R. M. (1968) Abnormal myelograms in asymptomatic patients. *J. Neurosurg., 28*, 204.
Hockaday, J. M. & Whitty, C. W. M. (1967) Patterns of referred pain in the normal subject. *Brain, 90*, 481.
Hoffman, H. L. (1950) Epidural local anaesthesia. *Presse Med., 224*, 278.
Hohmann. (1926) Das Wesen und die Behandlung des sogenannten Tennis-Ellenbogens. *Munch. med. Wschr., 80*, 250.
Holling, H. E., Brodey, R. S. & Boland, H. C. (1961) Pulmonary osteoarthropathy. *Trans. Ass. Am. Phycns., 73*, 305.
Hood, W. P. (1871) On Bonesetting. London: Macmillan.
Hooker, W. (1849) Physician and Patients. New York: Baker & Scribner.
Hooper. J. (1973) Low back pain and manipulation: paraparesis. *Med. J. Aust., I*, 549.
Horn, C. E. (1945) Acute ischaemia of anterior tibial muscle. *J. Bone Jt Surg., 27*, 615.
Horton, B. T., Magath, T. B. & Brown, G. E. (1932) Giant-cell arteritis. *Proc. Staff Meet. Mayo Clin., 7*, 700.
Hoskinson, J. (1974) Freiberg's disease: Review of long-term results. *Proc. R. Soc. Med., 67*, 10.
Houston, J. R. (1975) Subcutaneous rhizolysis in chronic backache. *J. R. Coll. gen. Pract., 25*, 692.
Hovelacque, A. (1925) Le neuf sinu-vertebral. *Annals Anat., path., 2*, 435.
—— (1927) *Anatomie des Nerfs Craniens et Rachidiens et du Systeme Grand Sympatique.* Paris: Doin.
Huard, P. & Ormek, M. D. (1960) *Le Premier Manuscrit Chirurgical Turc.*, Paris: Dacosta.
Hudgins, W. R. (1977) Diagnostic Summary of lumbar Discography. *Spine, 2*, 305.
Hughston, J. C., Andrews, J, R., Cross, M. J. & Moschi, A. (1976) Classification of knee ligament instabilities. *J. Bone Jt Surg., 58A*, 159.
Hult, L. (1954*a*) *The Munkfors Investigation.* Copenhagen: Munksgaard.
—— (1954*b*) *Cervical, Dorsal and Lumbar Spinal Syndromes.* Copenhagen: Munksgaard.
Humphries, S. V. (1973) Personal view. *Br. med. J., ii*, 452.
Huskisson, E. C. (1975) Treatment of palindromic rheumatism by D-penicillamine. *Br. med. J., ii*, 979.
Hutchinson, J. (1890) On a peculiar form of thrombotic arteritis. *Archs Surg., Chicago, I*, 323.
Hutson, M. A. (1973) Treatment of lumbo-sacral disc disorders. *Practitioner, 210*, 415.
Hutton, S. R. (1973) Subcutaneous lumbar rhizolysis. *Med. J. Aust., 2*, 1027.
Hutton, W. C., Stott, J. R. R. & Cyron, B. M. (1977) Is spondylolysis a fatigue fracture? *Spine, 2*, 202.

Hyrtl, J. (1846) Anatomie des Hüftgelenkes. Zeitschr. der K. K. *Gesellschaft der Ärztezu Wein, 1*, 58.
Illingworth, C. (1975) Pulled elbow. *Br. med. J., i*, 672.
Illouz, G. & Coste, F. (1964) Le signe du trepied dans l'exploration clinique des sacro-iliacques. *Presse med., 72*, 1979.
Inman, V. T. & Saunders, J. B. (1942) Clinico-anatomical aspects of lumbo-sacral Region. *Radiology, 38*, 669.
Isdale, I. C. (1962) Femoral head destruction in rheumatoid arthritis and osteoarthritis. A clinical review of 27 cases. *Ann. rheum. Dis., 21*, 23.
Jackson, J. P. (1968) Degenerative changes in the knee after meniscectomy. *Br. med. J., ii*, 525.
Jayson, M. I. V., Herbert, C. M. & Barks, J. S. (1973) Intervertebral discs: nuclear morphology and bursting pressures. *Ann. rheum. Dis., 32*, 308.
—— & Nelson, M. A. (1979) Spinal stenosis and low back pain. *Rheum. Dis.*, 70.
Jeffcoate, T. N. A. (1969) Pelvic pain. *Br. med. J., ii*, 431.
Jenner, J. R. & Mathews, J. A. (1978) Study of Intradiscal Chymopapain in Treatment of Sciatica. Lecture at Society of Back Pain Research.
Jennett, W. D. (1956) Cauda equina compression caused by intervertebral discs. *J. Neurol, Neurosurg. Psychiat., 19*, 109.
—— (1974) Treatment of sciatica. *Lancet, i*, 132.
Jepson, E. M. (1961) Hypercholesterolaemic xanthomatosis. Treatment with a corn-oil diet. *Br. med. J., i*, 847.
Jirout, J. (1969) Pneumomyelography. Springfield, Ill.: Charles C. Thomas.
Johnston, A. W. (1960) Acroparaesthesia and acromegaly. *Br. med. J., i*, 1616.
Jones, K. G. (1963) Reconstruction of anterior cruciate ligament. *J. Bone Jt Surg., 45A*, 925.
Jones, R. (1909) Notes on Derangements of the Knee. *Ann. Surg., 50*, 1000.
Jones, R. A. C. & Thomson, J. L. G. (1968) Narrow lumbar canal. *J. Bone Jt Surg., 50B*, 595.
Joplin, R. J. (1935) Intervertebral disc. *Surgery Gynec. Obstet., 61*, 591.
Joseph, J. (1964) Electromyographic studies on muscle tone and the erect posture in man. *Br. J. Surg., 51*, 616.
Jowsey, J., Riggs, B. L., Kelly, P. S. & Hoffman, D. L. (1972) Effect of sodium fluoride, vitamin D and calcium in osteoporosis. *Am. J. Med., 53*, 43.
Jung, A. & Brunschwig, A. (1932) Recherches histologiques sur l'innervation des corps vertebraux. *Presse med., 17*, 136.
Jung, K. & Hassler, R. (1960) *Handbook of Physiology*. Baltimore: Williams & Wilkins.
Kahlmeter, G. (1918) Bidrag till kännedonnen om spondylitis deformans, *Svenska LäkSällsk. Handl., 44*, 169.
Kanis, J. A., Cundy, T., Bartlett, M., Smith, R., Heynen, G., Warner, G. T. & Russell, R. G. G. (1978) Is 24,25 dihydroxycholecalciferol a calcium-regulating hormone in man? *Br. med. J., i*, 1382.
Keenan, C. (1977) Warning from a Chiropractor. *Ont. med. Review, 431*.
Kellgren, J. H. (1938) Observations on referred pain arising from muscle. *Clin. Sci., 3*, 175.
—— (1939) On distribution of pain arising from deep somatic structures with charts of segmental pain areas. *Clin. Sci., 4*, 35.
Kelly, R. (1981) The post-traumatic syndrome. *J. Roy. Soc. Med., 74*, 242.
Kelsey, K. L. (1975) Epidemiological study of acute lumbar intervertebral discs. *Rheumat. Rehab., 14*, 144.
Kemp, H. B. S. (1973) Perthes' disease. *Ann. R. Coll. Surg., 5*, 18.
Kendall, B. E. (1972) Radiological investigation of pain referred to lower limb. *Br. J. Hosp. Med., 7*, 500.
Kewalremani, L. S., Krebs, M. & Saleem, A. (1981) Congress of Phys. Med.
Key, C. A. (1838) On paraplegia depending on disease of the ligaments of the spine. *Guy's Hosp. Rep., 111*, 17.
Key, J. A. (1945) Intervertebral disc lesions are the commonest cause of low back pain with or without sciatica. *Ann. Surg., 121*, 534.
Kibler, R. F. & Nathan, P. W. (1960) Relief of pain and paraesthesiae by nerve block distal to a lesion. *I. Neurol. Neurosurg. Psychiat., 23*, 91.
Kilian, H. F. (1854) De Spondylolisthesi Gravissimae Pelvangustiae Causa Detecta. Bonn.
Kinmonth, J. B. (1952) Physiology and relief of traumatic arterial spasm. *Br. med. J., i*, 59.
Kleinberg, S. (1951) *Scoliosis: Pathology, Etiology and Treatment*. London: Baillière, Tindall and Cox.
Kleinkort, J. A. & Wood, F. (1975) Phonophoresis with 1% versus 10% hydrocortisone. *Phys. Thera., 55*, 1320.
de Kleyn, A. (1939) Some remarks on vestibular nystagmus. *Confinia neurol., 2*, 257.
—— & Nieuwenhuyse (1927) Schwindelanfälle und Nystagmus bei einen bestimmten Stellung des Kopfer. *Acta oto-lar., 11*, 155.
Kocher, T. (1896) Die Verlezungen der Wirbelsäule. *Med. Chir., 1*, 415.
Koehler, A. (1905) Borderlands of normal and early pathology in skeletal radiology. Translated S. Wilk. New York and London: Grune & Stratton.
Konstam, P. G. & Blesovsky, A. (1962) Ambulant treatment of spinal tuberculosis. *Br. J. Surg., 50*, 26.
Kopell, H. P. & Thompson, W. A. L. (1963) *Peripheral Entrapment Neuropathy*. Baltimore: Williams & Wilkins.
Kovass, A. (1955) Subluxation and deformation of cervical apophyseal joints; contribution to aetiology of headache. *Acta radiol., Stockh., 43*, 1.

Krause, F. (1910) *Surgery of Brain and Spinal Cord.* London: Lewis.
Kremer, M. (1958) Sitting, standing and walking. *Br. med. J., ii*, 121.
Krueger, B. (1980) Chiropractogenic stroke. *Med. Post.*
—— & Okazaki (1980) Vertebrobasilar infarction following chiropractic cervical manipulation. *Mayo Clin. Proc. 55*, 322.
Kunkle, E. C., Muller, J. C. & Odom, G. L. (1952) Brainstem thrombosis: mechanism of injury. *Ann. intern. Med. 36*, 1329.
Lam, S. J. (1962) Tarsal tunnel syndrome. *Lancet, ii*, 1354.
Lasségue, C. (1864) Considerations sur la sciatique. *Archs gen. Med., 2*, 558.
Lazorthes, G. & Gaubert, J. (1957) L'innervazion des articulations interapophysaires vertébrales. *C. r. Ass. Anat. 95*, 488.
Leavitt, S. S., Johnson, T. L. & Beyer, R. D. (1972) Patterns in industrial back injury. *Industry. Med. Surg., 40*, 8.
Lecuyer, J. L. (1959) Congenital occipitalisation of atlas with chiropractic manipulations. *Nebraska St. med. J., 44* 548.
Lenoch, F. (1970) Disturbances of nourishment of articular cartilage. *Rev. Czech. Med., 16*, 113.
Leriche, L. H. (1972) It all hangs upon the spine. *Can. Doctor*, 39.
Leriche, R. (1924) Essai sur patologie du nerf sinu vertébrale. *Presse med., 1*, 409.
Lettin, A. W. F. & Scales, J. T. (1972) Total replacement of shoulder joint. *Proc. R. Soc. Med., 65*, 373.
Levernieux, J. (1960) *Traction Vertébrale.* Paris: Expansion Scientifique.
Lewin, T. (1966) Osteoarthritis in lumbar synovial joints. *Acta orthop. scand.*, Suppl. 73.
——, Moffett, B. & Viidik, A. (1961) Morphology of lumbar synovial intervertebral joints. *Acta Morphol. neerl.-scand., 4*, 229.
Lewis, T. (1942) *Pain.* New York: Macmillan.
Lewit, K. (1967) Beitrag zur reversiblen Gelenksblockierung. *Z. Orthop., 55*, 150.
Lichtman, A. L., McDonald, J. R., Dixon, C. F. & Mann, F. C. (1946) Talc granuloma. *Surgery Gynec. Obstet., 83*, 531.
Liddell, E. G. T. & Sherrington, C. S. (1924) Further observations on myotatic reflexes. *Proc.* R. *Soc. Med.*, 267.
Liévre, J. A. (1953) Paraplégie du aux manoeuvres d'un chiropracteur. *Rev. rheumat., 20*, 708.
Lindahl, O. (1966) Hyperalgesia of the lumbar nerve roots in sciatica. *Acta orthop. scand., 37*, 367.
Lindblom, K. (1948*a*) Diagnostic puncture of intervertebral disc. *Acta orthop. scand., 17*, 231.
—— (1948*b*) Diagnostic puncture of intervertebral discs in sciatica. *Acta orthop. scand., 20*, 315.
—— (1950) Myelography and disc puncture. *Acta radiol., 34*, 321.
—— (1952) Experimental rupture of intervertebral discs in rats' tails. *J. Bone Jt Surg., 34A*, 123.
—— & Rexed, B. (1948) Spinal Nerve injury in dorso-lateral protrusion of lumbar discs. *J. Neuro. surg., 5*, 413.
Lipson, R. L. & Slocumb, C. H. (1965) The progressive nature of gout with inadequate therapy. *Arthritis Rheum., 8*, 80.
Livingston, K. E. & Perrin, R. G. (1972) Central physiological effects of intravenous procaine. *J. Neurosurg., 37*, 188.
Livingstone, M. C. P. (1971) Spinal manipulation causing injury. *Clin. Orthop., 81*, 82.
Lora, J. & Long, D. (1976) Facet denervation in intractable back pain. *Spine, 1*, 121.
Lorimer. (1884) Discussion: The nosological relations of chronic rheumatic (rheumatoid) arthritis. *Br. med. J., ii*, 269.
Luschka, H. (1850) *Die Nerven des Menslischen Wirbelkanales.* Tübingen: Laupp.
Luyendijk, W. (1962) *Canalografie.* Leiden: Groen & Zoon.
McCall, I. W., O'Brien, J. P. & Park, W. M. (1978) Induced pain from posterior lumbar elements in normal subjects. Lecture at Society for Back Pain Research. London.
McCarthy, D. J., Halverson, P. B., Carrern, G. F., Brewer, B. J. & Kozin, F. (1981) Milwaukee shoulder. *Arth. Rheum., 24*, 464.
McCarthy, D. J. & Hollander, J. L. (1961) Identification of urate crystals in gouty synovial fluid. *Ann. intern. Med., 54*, 452.
——, Kohn, N. N. & Faires, J. S. (1962) Significance of calcium phosphate crystals in synovial fluid in pseudogout. *Ann. intern. Med., 56*, 711.
MacConnaill, M. A. & Basmajian, J. V. (1959) *Muscles and Movements.* Baltimore: Williams & Wilkins.
McCulloch, J. A. (1977) Chemonucleolysis. *J. Bone Jt Surg., 59*, 3, 45.
—— (1981) Chemonucleolysis for relief of sciatica due to herniated intervertebral disc. *Canad. Med. Assn. J., 124*, 879.
—— & Organ, L. W. (1977) Percutaneous radiofrequency lumbar rhizolysis. *Can. med. Ass. J., 116*, 30.
McCutchen, C. W. (1964) Lubrication of joints. *Br. med. J., i*, 1044.
McDonald, G. & Petrie, D. (1975) Ununited fracture of scaphoid. *Clin. Orthop., 108*, 110.
McGill, D. M. (1964) Tarsal tunnel syndrome. *Proc. R. Soc. Med., 57*, 1125.

McKay, N. N. S., Woodhouse, N. J. Y. & Clark, A. K. (1977) Post-traumatic reflex sympathetic dystrophy (Sudeck's atrophy). *Br. med. J.*, *i*, 1575.
McKee, G. K. (1937) Tennis elbow. *Br. med. J.*, *ii*, 434.
MacKenzie, R. A. (1972) Manual correction of sciatic scoliosis. *N.Z. med. J.*, *76*, 194.
—— (1981) The Lumbar Spine. Spinal Publications. Waikanae.
McKenzie, Y. (1966) Personal communication.
MacKinney, L. (1965) *Medical Illustrations in Medieval Manuscripts.* London: Wellcome.
MacRae, D. L. (1956) Asymptomatic intervertebral disc protrusion. *Acta radiol.*, *46*, 9.
Magill, H. K. & Aitken, A. P. (1954) Pulled elbow. *Surgery Gynec. Obstet.*, *98*, 753.
Magnuson, P. B. (1932) Backache from industrial standpoint. *J. Bone Jt Surg.*, *14*, 165.
Magora, A. (1972) Relations between low back pain and occupation. *Indust. Med. Surg.*, *41*, 12.
Maigne, R. (1960) *Les Manipulations Vertébrales.* Paris: Expansion Scientifique Française.
—— (1972) *Newsl. N. Am. Acad. manip. Med.*
Maitland, G. D. (1964) *Vertebral Manipulation.* London: Butterworths.
Malawista, S. E., Seegmiller, J. E., Hathaway, B.E. & Sokologg, L. (1965) Sacro-iliac gout. *J. Am. med. Ass.*, *194*, 954.
Marie, P. & Foix, C. (1913) L'atrophe isolée non-progressive des petits muscles de la main. *N. iconog. Salpetrière*, *25*, 353, 427.
Maroudas, A., Nachemson, A., Stockwell, R. & Urban, J. (1973) *In Vitro Studies of Nutrition of Intervertebral Disc.* London: Society for Back Pain Research.
Martin, J. P. (1965) Curvature of the spine in post-encephalitis parkinsonism. *J. Neurol. Neurosurg. Psychiat.*, *28*, 395.
Martin, P. (1960) Atherosclerosis of the arteries of the limbs. *Proc. R. Soc. Med.*, *53*, 31.
Masif, P. (1975) Lumbar spine biomechanics. Lecture at Reunión sobre Patologia de la Columna Vertebral, Murcia, Spain.
Mason, B. & Perry, C. B. (1965) Effect of clofibrate and androsterone on hypercholesterolaemic xanthomatosis. *Br. med. J.*, *i*, 102.
Mason, R. M. (1959) Ankylosing spondylitis. *Br. J. vener. Dis.*, *35*, 71.
—— (1964) Spondylitis. *Proc. R. Soc. Med.*, *57*, 533.
——, Murray, R. S., Oates, J. K. & Young, A. C. (1958) Prostatitis and ankylosing spondylitis. *Br. med. J.*, *i*, 748.
—— —— —— —— (1959) A comparative radiological study of Reiter's disease, rheumatoid arthritis and ankylosing spondylitis. *J. Bone Jt Surg.*, *41B*, 137.
——, Oates, J. K. & Young, A. C. (1963) Sacro-iliitis in Reiter's disease. *Br. med. J.*, *ii*, 1013.
Matheson, A. T. (1960) Cauda equina syndrome. *Br. med. J.*, *i*, 570.
Mathews, J. A. (1968) Dynamic discography: a study of lumbar traction. *Ann. phys. Med.*, *7*, 275.
—— (1977) Backache. *Br. med, J.*, *i*, 432.
Mathews, W. A. (1972) Intradural and extradural corticosteroids for sciatica. *Anaesth. Analg.*, *51*, 999.
Mathur, K. S., Kahn, M. A. & Sharma, R. D. (1968) Hypocholesterolaemic effect of Bengal gram; a long-term study in man. *Br. med. J.*, *i*, 30.
Matthews, B. F. (1952) Collagen/chondroitin sulphate ratio of human articular cartilage related to function. *Br. med. J.*, *ii*, 1295.
Mattingly, S. (1971) Rehabilitation of registered dock workers. *Proc. R. Soc. Med.*, *64*, 753.
Mauric, G. (1933) *Le Disque Intervertébral.* Paris: Masson.
Mayall, G. F. (1965) Acute synovitis of hip. *Br. med. J.*, *i*, 1613.
Mayoux, R., Girard, P. & Chappaz, P. (1951) Signes vestibulaires objectifs dans le syndrome Barré-Liéou. *Ann. oto-Lar.*, *68*, 705.
Meares, R. (1971) Natural history of spasmodic torticollis and effects of surgery. *Lancet*, *ii*, 149.
Melzack, R. (1972) Mechanisms of pathological pain. In *Scientific Foundations of Neurology*, ed. M. Crotchley, J. L. O'Leary and B. Jennett, pp. 153–165. London: Heinemann.
—— & Wall, P. D. (1964) Pain mechanisms: a new theory. *Science, N.Y.*, *150*, 971.
Mengert, W. F. (1943) Pelvic referred pain. *Sth. med. J.*, *35*, 256.
Menkin, V. (1943) Chemical basis of injury in inflammation. *Archs Path.*, *36*, 269.
—— (1956) *Biochemical Mechanisms in Inflammation.* Springfield, Ill.: Charles C. Thomas.
Mercado, L. (1599) Para el Aproueche-chemiento y Examen de los Algebristas. Madrid: Madrigal.
Mercer, W. (1959) Osteopathy. *Practitioner*, *198*, 1.
Middleton, G. S. & Teacher, J. H. (1911) Injury of the spinal cord due to rupture of an intervertebral disc during muscular effort. *Glasg. J. Med.*, *76*, 1.
Di Miglio, G., Fovino, P. & Papandrea, G. (1964) Le lombalgie da sofferenze intersomatica: sindrome apico-transversa. *Archo Ortop.*, *77*, 5.
Miller, H. (1961) Accident neurosis. *Br. med. J.*, *i*, 919.

Miller, H. (1964) Some neurological complications of surgical treatment: spinal manipulation. *Proc. R. Soc. Med. 57*, 145.

—— (1966) Polyneuritis. *Br. med. J., ii*, 1219.

Mills, G. P. (1928) Treatment of tennis elbow. *Br. med. J., i*, 12.

Mineiro, J. D. (1965) *Coluna Vertebral Humana*. Lisbon: Sociedad Industria Graphica.

Mironova, Z. S., Lavristcheva, G. I. & Bogutskaya, E. V. (1970) Alloplasty of sportsmen's ligaments. *Proc. 18th Wld Cong. Sports Med.*, 73.

Mixter, W. J. & Barr, J. S. (1934) Rupture of intervertebral disc with involvement of spinal canal. *New Engl. J Med., 211*, 210.

Moberg, E. (1967) Surgery of the rheumatoid hand. *Br. med. J., i*, 696.

Mondor, H. (1939) Tronculite sous-cutanée subaiguë de la paroi thoracique antèro-lateral. *Mem. Acad. Chir., 65*, 1271.

Monro, A. (1688) *Description of All Bursae Mucosae of Human Body*. Edinburgh: Elliott.

Montgomery, W. W., Peroue, P. M. & Schall, L. A. (1955) Arthritis of cricoarytenoid joint. *Ann. Otol. Rhinol. Lar., 64*, 1025.

Monty, C. P. (1962) Prognosis of 'observation hip' in children. *Archs Dis. Childh., 37*, 539.

Moore, R. (1978) Bleeding gastric erosion after oral zinc sulphate. *Br. med. J., i*, 754.

de Moragas, J. M. & Kierland, R. R. (1957) Outcome in patients with herpes zoster. *Archs Derm., Chicago., 75*, 193.

Morgan, F. P. & King, T. (1957) Instability of lumbar vertebrae as a cause of back pain. *J. Bone Jt Surg., 39B*, 6.

Morris, H. (1882) Rider's sprain. *Lancet, ii*, 557.

Morrison, L. R., Short, C. L., Ludwig, A. O. & Schwar, R. S. (1947) Neuromuscular system in rheumatoid arthritis; electromyographic and historical observations. *Am. J. Sci., 214*, 33.

Morton, T. G. (1876) Peculiar painful affection of fourth metatarsophalangeal articulation. *Am. J. med. Sci., 71*, 37.

Murray, D. G. (1964) Experimentally induced Arthritis using intra-articular Papain. *Arth. & Rheum., 7*, 211.

Murray, I. P. & Simpson, J. A. (1958) Acroparaesthesia in myxoedema; a clinical and electromyographic study. *Lancet, i*, 1360.

Murray, R. O. & Jacobson, H. G. (1971) *Radiology of Skeletal Disorders*, Edinburgh: Livingstone.

Nachemson, A. (1960) Measurement of intradiscal pressure. *Acta orthop. scand.*, Suppl. 43, 1.

—— (1962) Some mechanical properties of the lumbar intervertebral discs. *Bull. Hosp. Jt. Dis., N.Y., 23*, 2.

—— (1972) *The Painful Back*. London: Royal College of Physicians.

—— (1975) Review of mechanics of the lumbar disc. *Rheumat. Rehab., 14*, 129.

—— (1976) The lumbar spine. *Spine, 1*, 59.

—— & Elfström, G. (1969) Intravital dynamic pressure measurements in lumbar discs. *Scand. J. rehab. Med.*, suppl. 1.

——, Lewin, T., Maroudas, A. & Freeman, M. A. R. (1970) *In vitro* diffusion of dye through end-plates and annulus fibrosus of human intervertebral discs. *Acta orthop. scand., 41*, 589.

—— & Lind (1969) Measurement of abdominal and back muscle strength with and without low back pain. *Scand. J. rehab. Med., 1*, 60.

—— & Morris, J. M. (1963) *In vivo* measurements of intradiscal pressure. *J. Bone Jt Surg., 46A*, 1077.

Nachlas, I. W. (1934) Pseudoangina pectoris. *J. Am. med. Ass., 103*, 323.

Nagler, W. (1973) Mechanical obstruction of vertebral arteries during hyperextension of neck. *Br. J. Sports Med., 7*.

Naish, J. M. & Apley, J. (1951) Growing pains. *Archs Dis., Childh., 26*, 134.

Nelson, M. A. (1975) Lumbar intervertebral disc-lesions. *Rheumat. Rehab., 14*, 163.

Neugebauer, F. L. (1888) *History and Aetiology in Spondylolisthesis*. London: New Sydenham Society.

Neviaser, J. S. (1945) Adhesive capsulitis of shoulder; study of pathological findings in periarthritis of shoulder. *J. Bone Jt Surg., 27*, 211.

Newell, S. G. & Woodle, A. (1981) Cuboid Syndrome. *Physician and Sports medicine, 9*, 71.

Newman, J. H. & Goodfellow, J. W. (1975) Fibrillation of head of radius as one cause of tennis elbow. *Br. med. J., i*, 328.

Newman, P. H. (1968) The spine, the wood and the trees. *Proc. R. Soc. Med., 61*, 35.

—— & Stone, K. H. (1963) Aetiology of spondylolisthesis. *J. Bone Jt Surg., 45B*, 39.

Nicaige, E. (1890) Grande Chirurgie de Guy de Charliac. Paris: Alcan 518.

Nichols, P. J. R. (1960) Short-leg syndrome. *Br. med. J., i*, 1863.

—— (1965) Pain in the neck and arm. *Br. med. J., i*, 253.

Nick, J., Contamin, M. H., Nicholle, M. H., Des Lauriers, A. & Zeigler, G. (1967) Accidents neurologique dus aux manipulations vertébrales. *Soc. méd. Hop. Paris, 118*, 435.

Nicod, P. L. A. (1818) *Observations de Neuralgies Thoraciques*, Vol. 3. Paris: Migneret.

Noordenbos, W. (1959) *Pain: Problems Pertaining to the Transmission of Nerve Impulses which give rise to Pain.* Amsterdam and London: Elsevier.

Nordin, B. E. C. (1959) Osteomalacia, osteoporosis and calcium deficiency. *Clin. Orthop.*, *17*, 235.
—— (1973) Personal communication.
—— (1979) Bone loss in postmenopausal women. Mims Mag. Sept.
Norris, F. W., Gasteiger, E. L. & Chatfield, P. O. (1957) Induced and spontaneous muscle cramp. *Electroenceph. clin. Neurophysiol.*, *9*, 139.
Oates, G. D. (1960) Median-nerve palsy as complication of acute pyogenic infections of hand. *Br. med. J.*, *i*, 1618.
O'Connell, J. E. A. (1951) Protrusion of lumbar intervertebral discs. *J. Bone Jt Surg.*, *33B*, 8.
—— (1956) Cervical spondylosis. *Proc. R. Soc. Med.*, *49*, 202.
Oger, J. (1964) Accidents des manipulations vertebrales. *J. belge Med. phys.*, *19*, 56.
O'Laiore, S. A., Crockard, H. A. & Thomas, D. G. (1981) Prognosis for sphincter recovery. *Br. med. J.*, *i*, 282.
Ortolani, M. (1937) Un segno poco noto e sua importanza per la diagnosi precoce di prelussazione congenita dell'anca. *Pediatria*, *45*, 129.
Osborne, G. (1974) Spinal stenosis. *Physiotherapy*, *60*, 7.
Osgood, R. B. (1922) Radiohumeral bursitis, epicondylitis, epicondylalgia (tennis elbow). *Archs Surg., Chicago.*, *4*, 420.
Ott, V. Fl., (1953) Uberdie Spondylosis Hyperostotica. *Schweitz med. Wochens.*, *34*, 790.
Ounenhoven, R. C. (1977) Paraspinal Electromyography following Facet Rhizotomy, *Spine*, *2*, 299.
Owen, D. (1976) *The Times*, 13th May. p. 6.
Paget, J. (1860) Cases that bonesetters cure. *Br. med. J.*, *i*, 1.
—— (1877) A form of chronic inflammation of bone (osteitis deformans). *Med.-Chir. Trans.*, *60*, 37.
Pak, C., Zisman, E., Evens, R., Jowsey, J., Delea, C. S. & Bartter, F. C. (1969) Treatment of osteoporosis with calcium infusions. *Am J. Med.*, *47*, 7.
Pallis, C. A. & Scott, J. T. (1965) Peripheral neuropathy in rheumatoid arthritis. *Br. med, J.*, *i*, 1141.
Panas, P. (1878) Paralysis du Nerf cubital. *Arch. Gen. Méd.*, *2*, 5.
Paton, H. O. (1978) Traumatic Tenosynovitis of Wrist. *Br. med. J.*, *i*, 789.
Paulley, J. W. (1977) Polymyalgia arteritica. *Br. med. J.*, *i*, 1348.
Pauwels, F. (1959) New guides for the surgical treatment of osteoarthritis of the hip. *Rev. chir. Orthop.*, *45*, 681.
Pearce, J. M. S. (1974) Headache. *Br. med. J.*, *ii*, 242.
—— & Moll, J. H. (1967) Conservative treatment of natural history of acute lumbar disc lesions. *J. Neurol. Neurosurg. Psychiat.*, *30*, 13.
Peatfield, R. C. (1981) Lithium in cluster headache. *J. Roy. Soc. Med.*, *74*, 432.
Pedersen, H. E., Blunk, C. F. J. & Gardner, E. (1956) Anatomy of sinu-vertebral nerves. *J. Bone Jt Surg.*, *38A*, 377.
Penny, W. J. (1888) On bone-setting. *Br. Med. J.*, *i*, 1102.
Player, R. P. (1821) Irritation of spinal nerves. *Lond. med. phys. J.*, *47*, 301.
Polley, H. F. & Hunder, G. G. (1978) Physical Examination of Joints. 2nd ed. Philadelphia: Saunders.
Pories, W. J., Henzel, J. H., Rob, C. G. & Strain, W. H. (1967) Acceleration of wound healing by zinc sulphate given by mouth. *Lancet*, *i*, 121.
Porter, I. G. (1823) On neuralgia of the spinal nerves. *Am. J. med Sci.*, *7*, 205.
Porter, R. (1979) Spinal Stenosis. *Pain Topics*, October.
Powers, S. R., Drislane, T. M. & Iandoll, E. W. (1963) The surgical treatment of vertebral artery insufficiency. *Archs Surg., Chicago*, *86*, 60.
—— —— & Nevins, S. (1961) Intermittent vertebral artery compression: A new syndrome. *Surgery, St. Louis*, *49*, 257.
Powis, S. J. A., Skilton, J. S., Ashton, F. & Slaney, G. (1971) Achilles tenotomy in intermittent claudication. *Br. med. J.*, *ii*, 422.
Pratt-Thomas, H. R. & Bammer, H. G. (1957) Syndrome of vertebral artery compression. *Neurology*, *7*, 331.
—— & Berger, K. E. (1947) Cerebellar and spinal injuries after chiropractic manipulation. *J. Am. med. Ass.*, *133*, 600.
Pribek, R. A. (1962) Brainstem vascular accident following neck manipulation. *Wis. med. J.*, *62*, 141.
Pringle, B. (1956) Approach to intervertebral disc lesions. *Trans. Ass. ind. med. Offrs.*, *5*, 127.
De Puky, P. (1935) Physiological oscillation of the length of the body. *Acta orthop. scand.*, *6.*, 338.
Püschel, J. (1930) Wassergehalb normaler und degenerierte Zurachen Wirbelscheiben. *Beitr. path. Anat.*, *84*, 123.
Putti, V. (1927) Pathogenesis of sciatic pain. *Lancet*, *i*, 53.
de Quervain, F. (1895) Uber eine Form von chronischer Tendovaginitis. *KorrespBl. schweizer. Ärtze.*, *25*, 389.
Raaf, J. & Berglund, G. (1949) Results of operations for lumbar protruded intervertebral disc. *J. Neurol. Neurosurg, Psychiat.*, *6*, 160.
Rasmussen, G. (1977) Manipulation in the treatment of low back pain. Congress of Manual Medicine, Copenhagen.
Raynaud, M. (1888) *Local Asphyxia and Symmetrical Gangrene of the Extremities.* London: New Sydenham Society.
—— (1891) Alternirende Scoliose bei Ischias. *Dt. med. Wschr.*, *17*, 257.

Récamier, M. (1838) Extension, massage et percussion cadencée dans le traitment des contractions musculaires. *Rev. méd. fr.*, *1*, 74.

Redfield, J. T. (1971) The low-back X-ray as pre-employment screening tool in the forest products industry. *J. occup. Med.*, *13*.

Rees, W. S. (1971) Multiple bilateral subcutaneous rhizolysis of segmental nerves for intervertebral disc syndromes. *Ann. gen. Pract.*, *16*, 126.

Reeves, B. (1966) Arthrographic changes in frozen and post-traumatic stiff shoulder. *Proc.* R. *Soc. Med.*, *59*, 827.

Reid, J. D. (1958) Ascending nerve roots and tightness of dura mater. *N.Z. med. J.*, *57*, 16.

Reid, W., Watt, J. K. & Gray, T. G. (1963) Selective nerve crush in intermittent claudication. *Br. med. J.*, *i*, 1576.

Reivich, M., Holling, H. E., Roberts, B. & Toole, J. F. (1961) Reversal of bloodflow through vertebral artery. *New Engl. J. Med.*, *265*, 87B.

Remak, E. (1894) *Beschaftigungsneurosen.* Wien: Urban & Schwarzenberg.

Renton, J. (1830) Observations on acupuncturation. *Edinb. med. J.*, *34*, 100.

Rettig, A., Jackson, D. W., Wiltse, L. L. & Secrist, L. (1977) Epidural venogram. *Am. J. Sports Med.*, *5*, 158.

Riadore, J. E. (1843) *A Treatise on Irritation of the Spinal Nerves as the Source of Nervousness, Indigestion, Functional and Organical Derangement of the Principal Organs of the Body.* London: Churchill.

Ribbert, H. (1895) Über die experimentelle Erzeugung einer Ecchondrosis Physalifora. *Verh. Kongr. inn Med.*, *13*, 455.

Richard, J. (1967) Disc rupture with cauda equina syndrome due to chiropractic adjustment. *N.Y. St. J. Med.*, *67*, 2496.

Rissanen, P. M. (1960) Surgical anatomy and pathology of supraspinous and interspinous ligaments. *Acta orthop. scand.*, Suppl. 46.

Ritchie, J. H. & Fahrni, W. H. (1970) Changes in lumbar intervertebral discs. *Can. J. Surg.*, *13*, 65.

Ritter, H. G. & Tarala, R. (1978) Pneumothorax after acupuncture. *Br. med. J.*, *ii*, 602.

Rob, C. G. & Standeven, A. (1958) Arterial occlusion complicating thoracic outlet compression syndrome. *Br. med. J.*, *ii*, 709.

Roberts, G. M., Roberts, E. E., Lloyd, K. N., Burke, M. S. & Evans, D. P. (1978) Lumbar spinal manipulation on trial. Radiological assessment. *Rheumat. Rehab.*, *17*, 54.

Robertson, G. (1924) The bonesetter and his professional brother. *Practitioner*, *113*, 442.

Rodaway, H. E. (1957) Education for childbirth and its results. *J. Obstet. Gynaec. Br. Emp.*, *64*, 545.

Roholm, K. (1937) *Fluorine Intoxication.* London: Lewis.

Rolander, S. D. (1966) Motion of lumbar spine. *Acta orthop. scand.*, Suppl. 90.

Roles, N. C. & Maudsley, R. H. (1972) Radial tunnel syndrome. *J. Bone Jt. Surg.*, *54B*, 499.

Romagnoll, C. & Dalmonte, A. (1965) Semeiological contribution to sciatic pain in hernia of disc. *Gazz. sanit., Bologna*, 24.

Roper, B. W. (1964) Essential hypercholesterolaemic xanthomatosis. *Br. med. J.*, *ii*, 990.

Rose, G. A. (1965) Study of treatment of osteoporosis with fluoride therapy and high calcium intake. *Proc. roy. Soc. Med.*, *58*, 436.

Ross, E. (1962) Ergebnisse einer Reihenröntgenuntersuchung der Wirbelsäule bei 5000 Jugendlichen. *Fortschr. Röntgenstr.*, *97*, 734.

Roston, J. B. & Haines, R. W. (1947) Cracking in metacarpophalangeal joint. *J. Anat.*, *81*, 165.

Roy, D. (1976) Bones from the laboratory. *New Sci.*, *21*, 163.

Ruff, S. (1950) *Brief Acceleration: German Aviation Medicine: World War II.* Washington, D.C.: U.S. Government Printing Office.

Rugtveit, A. (1966) Disc-lesions in children. *Acta orthop. scand.*, *37*, 348.

Runge, F. (1873) Zur Genese und Behandlung des Schreibekrampfes. *Berl. klin. Wschr.*, *1*, 245.

Russe, O. (1960) Fracture of the carpal navicular. *J. Bone Jt Surg.*, *42A*, 759.

Russell, R. G. G., Preston, C., Smith, R. & Walton, R. J. (1974) Diphosphonates in Paget's disease. *Lancet*, *i*, 894.

Russell, W. R. (1959) Treatment of intractable pain. *Proc.* R. *Soc. Med.*, *52*, 983.

——, Miller, H. & O'Connell, J. E. A. (1956) Discussion on cervical spondylosis. *Proc.* R. *Soc. Med.*, *49*, 197.

Ryan, G. M. S. & Cope, S. (1955) Cervical vertigo. *Lancet*, *ii*, 1355.

Ryan, W. G., Schwartz, R. B. & Perlin, C. P. (1969) Effects of mythramycin on Paget's disease. *Ann. intern. Med.*, *70*, 549.

Ryder, H. W. (1953) Mechanism of change in cerebrospinal fluid pressure following induced change in volume of fluid space. *J. Lab. clin. Med.*, *41*, 428.

Sabri, S., Roberts, V. C. & Cotton, L. T. (1971) Prevention of postoperative deep vein thrombosis. *Br. med. J.*, *iii*, 82.

Salter, R. (1980) Continuous passive motion. *The Graduate*, *7*.

Sampson, P. (1978) Chymopapain. *J. Am. med. Ass.*, *240*, 195.

—— (1978) Russia honours chymopapain discoverers. *J. Am. med. Ass.*, *240*, 205.

Sanford, H. (1972) Ligamentous sclerosis. Lecture at the Symposium on Orthopaedic Medicine.

Scheuermann, H. (1936) Kyphosis juvenilis. *Fortschr. Röntgenstr., 53*, 1.
Schiotz, E. H. (1958) Manipulasjonsbehandling av columna under medisinskhistorisk synsvinkel. *Tidsskr. norske Laegeforen*, 359, 429, 946, 1003.
—— (1967) Personal communication.
—— & Cyriax, J. (1975) *Manipulation: Past and Present.* London: Heinemann.
Schmidt, J. (1921) Bursitis calcarea am epicondylus externus humeri. *Arch. orthip. Unfallchir., 19*, 215.
Schmorl, G. (1927) Über die anden Wirlbandscheiben verkommenden Ansdehnungs- und Zereissungsvergänge und die dadurch an ihnen und der Wirbelspongiosa hervorgerufenen Verändrungen. *Verh. dt. path. Ges., 22*, 250.
Schneider, R. C., Gosch, H. H., Taren, J. A., Ferry, J. D. & Jerva, M. J. (1972) Blood vessel trauma following head and neck injuries. *Clin. Neurosurg., 19*, 312.
Schreger, G. B. (1825) *De Bursis Mucosis Subcutaneis.* Erlangen: Palmand Enke.
Schulz, A. (1962) Faulty employment of chiropractic manoeuvres. *Med. Welt., 10*, 62.
Schultz, A. B. (1975) Reported in *Times Union*, Rochester, N.Y., 10 February.
Schultze, U. (1971) Osteochondrosis vertebralis juvenilis im Röntgenbild. *Beitr. Orthop. Traum., 4*, 205.
Schwartz, G. A., Geiger, J. K. & Spano, A. V. (1956) Posterior inferior cerebellar artery syndrome of Wallenberg after chiropractic manipulation. *Archs intern. Med., 3*, 352.
Schwarz, H. G. (1956) Anastomoses between cervical nerve roots. *J. Neurosurg., 13*, 190.
Scott, J. T. (1975) Analysis of joint fluids. *Br. J. Hosp. Med.*, 653.
Scott, P. D. & Mallinson, P. (1944) Hysterical sequelae of injuries. *Br. med. J., i*, 450.
Scott-Charlton, W. & Roebuck, D. J. (1972) Significance of primary posterior divisions of nerves in pain syndromes. *Med. J. Aust., 2*, 945.
Seedhom, B. B. (1976) Loadbearing function of menisci. *Physiotherapy, 62*, 223.
—— (1980) Can footballers play well without their cartilages? *Medisport, 2*, 98.
Séguin (1838) Torticollis: gueri par extension, massage et percussion cadencée. *Rev. méd. fr., 75*, 2.
Selby, P. J., Powles, R. L., Jameson, B., Kay, H. E. M., Watson, J. G., Thornton, R., Morgenstern, G. & Click, H. M. (1979) Parenteral acyclovir therapy for herpes virus infections in man. *Lancet, ii*, 1267.
Semmes, R. E. (1964) *Rupture of Lumbar Intervertebral Disc.* Springfield, Ill.: Charles C. Thomas.
—— & Murphy, F. (1943) Unilateral rupture of sixth cervical intervertebral disc with compression of the seventh cervical nerve-root. *J. Am. med. Ass., 121*, 1209.
Seward, G. R. (1966) Pain from dental disease. *Br. med. J., ii*, 509.
de Séze, S. (1955) Lés attitudes antalgiques dans la sciatique disco-radiculaire commune. Etude clinique et radiologique; interprètation pathogènique. *Sem. Hôp. Paris, 31*, 2291.
——, Ryckwaert, A., Welfling, J., Renier, J. C., Hubault, A., Caroit, M. & Poinsard, G. (1959) Etude sur l'epaule douloureux. *Rev. rheum., 67*, 323.
Sharp, J. & Purser, D. W. (1961) Spontaneous atlanto-axial dislocation in ankylosing spondylitis and rheumatoid arthritis. *Ann. rheum. Dis., 20*, 47.
Sharrard, W. J. W. (1976) Knock knees and bow legs. *Br. med. J., i*, 826.
Shealy, C. N. (1973) *Role of Spinal Facets in Back and Sciatic Pain.* New York: American Association for the Study of Headache.
Sheehan, E. (1977) One thousand orthopaedic cases in general practice in a rural area. *Practitioner, 218*, 580.
Shine, I. B. (1965) Hallux valgus. *Br. med. J., i*, 1648.
Shore, N. A., Shaefer, M. G. & Hoppenfeld, S. (1979) Iatrogenic TMJ difficulty. *J. Pros. Dentistry*, 541.
Sicard, A. (1901) Les injections medicamenteuses extradurales par voie sacro-coccygienne. *C. r. Seanc. Soc. Biol., 53*, 96.
—— (1954) Le chirurgien devant des douleurs du bas du dos. *Sem. Hôp. Paris, 30*, 2793.
—— & Leca, A. (1954) Place de rhachiotomie dans traitement chirurgical des sciatiques. *Presse med., 62*, 1737.
—— Boureau, M. & Leca, A. (1958) Hernies du troisème disque lombaire. *Presse méd., 66*, 1809.
Simmons, W. (1803) Bonesetting. *Med. phys. J.* London *9*, 202.
Sims-Williams, H., Jayson, M. I. V., Young, S. M. S., Baddeley, H. & Collins, E. (1978) Controlled trial of mobilisation and manipulation for patients with low back pain. *Br. med. J., ii*, 1338.
—— (1978) Controlled trial of mobilisation and manipulation for back pain. *Br. med. J., ii*, 1318.
Sinclair, R. J. G. (1971) Treatment of rheumatic disorders. *Proc. R. Soc. Med., 64*, 1031.
Smillie, I. S. (1967) Treatment of Freiburg's infarction. *Proc. R. Soc. Med., 60*, 29.
Smith, L. (1969) Chemonucleolysis. *Clin. Orthop., 67*, 72.
—— & Brown, J. E. (1967) Treatment of lumbar intervertebral disc lesions by direct injection of chymopapain. *J. Bone Jt Surg., 49A*, 502.
—— Garvin, P. J., Gesler, R. M. & Jennings, R. B. (1963) Enzyme dissolution of nucleus pulposus. *Nature, Lond., 198*, 1311.
Smith, M. J. & Wright, V. (1958) Sciatica and the invertebral disc. *J. Bone Jt Surg., 40A*, 1401.

Smith, R. A. & Estridge, M. N. (1962) Neurological complications of head and neck manipulations. *J. Am. med. Ass.*, *182*, 528.

Smith, R. L. (1969) *At your own Risk.* New York: Trident Press.

Smythe, H. A. & Moldofsky, H. (1977) Two contributions to understanding of 'fibrositis' syndrome. *Bull. Rheum. Dis.*, *28*, 928.

Snell, N. J. (1977) Iatrogenic pneumothorax. *Brit. J. clin. Pract.*, *35*, 220.

Snider, A. J. (1975) Bone engineer. *Rochester Times Union.*, Feb 10th.

Snoek, W., Weber, H. & Jorgensen, B. (1977) Double blind evaluation of extradural methyl prednisolone for herniated lumbar discs. *Acta orthop. scand.*, *48*, 635.

Soderburg, I. & Andren, L. (1956) Disc degeneration and lumbago ischias. *Acta orthop. scand.*, *25*, 137.

Somolinos d'Ardios (1964) *Historia de la Medicine.* Permaca: Peru.

Sorensen, B. F. & Hamby, W. B. (1965) Spasmodic torticollis. *J. Am. med. Ass.*, *194*, 706.

Southworth, J. D. & Bersack, S. R. (1950) Anomalies of lumbosacral vertebrae in 550 individuals without symptoms referable to low back. *Am. J. Roentgen.*, *64*, 624.

Spinner, M. (1968) Arcade of Frohse and its relation to posterior interosseous nerve paralysis. *J. Bone Jt Surg.*, *50B*, 809.

Stary, O. (1956) Pathogenesis of discogenic disease. *Rev. Czech. Med.*, *2*, 1.

—— (1959) *Nektere Otazky Patogenesy Diskogenni Nemoci.* Praha.

Stearns, M. L. (1940) Studies on development of connective tissue in transparent chambers in rabbit's ear. *Am. J. Anat.*, *67*, 55.

Steinberg, V. L. (1960) Neuropathy in rheumatoid disease. *Br. med. J.*, *i*, 1600.

—— & Parry, C. B. (1961) Electromyographic changes in rheumatoid arthritis. *Br. med. J.*, *i*, 630.

Stern, I. J. (1969) Biochemistry of chymopapain. *Clin. Orthop.*, *67*, 42.

Stevenson, T. M. (1966) Carpal tunnel syndrome. *Proc. R. Soc. Med.*, *59*, 824.

Stewart-Wynne, E. G. (1976) Iatrogenic femoral neuropathy. *Br. med. J.*, *i*, 263.

Stilwell, D. L. (1956) Nerve supply of vertebral column and its associated structures in monkey. *Anat. Rec.*, *125*, 139.

Stoddard, A. (1959) *Manual of osteopathic Technique.* London: Hutchinson.

—— (1973) Adult backache sequelae of missed Scheuermann's disease. Lecture to the British Association for Manipulative Medicine.

—— (1976) *Br. Ass. manip. Med. Newsletter*, September.

Stookey, B. (1928) Compression of Spinal Cord by Ventral Extradural Spinal Chondroma. *Arch. Neurol. Psych.*, *20*, 275.

—— (1940) Compression of spinal cord and nerve-roots by herniation of cervical nucleus pulposus. *Archs Surg., Chicago*, *40*, 417.

Strandness, D. E., McCutcheon, E. F. & Rushmen, R. F. (1966) Transcutaneous flowmeter in occlusive arterial disease. *Surgery Gynec. Obstet.*, *122*, 1039.

Strange, F. G. St. C. (1966) President's address: Debunking the disc. *Proc. R. Soc. Med.*, *59*, 952.

Sturge, W. A. (1882) Phenomena of angina pectoris. *Brain*, *5*, 492.

Sturniolo, P. (1961) Lumbago primitivo y secundario: Syndrome apico-transverso. Thesis, Faculty of Medicine, Buenos Aires.

—— (1963) Sindrome apico-transverso. *Boln Soc. Argent. Ortop.*, *3*, 782.

—— (1971) Lumbago habitual: sindrome apico-transverso. *Congr. Argent. Ortop.*, *782.*

Sudeck, P. (1900) Uber die acute Entzündliche Knockenatzophie. *Arch. klin. Chir.*, *62*, 147.

Sullivan, M. (1975) Chemonucleolysis. *Proc. R. Soc. Med.*, *68*, 480.

Sutow, W. W. & Pryde, A. W. (1956) Incidence of spina bifida occulta in relation to age. *J. Dis. Childh.*, *91*, 211.

Sutton, R. D., Benedek, T. G. & Edwards, G. A. (1963) Aseptic bone necrosis and corticosteroid therapy. *Archs intern. Med.*, *112*, 594.

Svanberg, H. (1915) Intervertebral foramina in man. *Med. Rec.*, *87*, 177.

Sweetnam, D. R., Mason, R. M. & Murray, R. O. (1960) Steroid arthropathy of the hip. *Br. med. J.*, *i*, 1392.

Swerdelow, M. & Sayle-Creer, W. S. (1970) Use of extradural injections in relief of lumbosciatic pain. *Anaesthesia*, *25*, 128, 341.

Swischuk, L. E. (1970) Beaked, notched or hooked vertebra. *Radiology*, *95*, 661.

Szechenyi, F., Csipó, L. & Kiss, E. (1978) Epidurográfiáral kimutatott, torziós extensióral reponált ágyéki porckorongsérvek. *Ideggyógyászati Szemle*, *31*, 436.

Tait, G. B., Bach, F. & Dixon, J. (1965) Acute synovial rupture. *Ann. rheum. Dis.*, *24*, 273.

Tatlow, W. F. T. & Bammer, H. G. (1957) Syndrome of vertebral artery compression. *Neurology*, *7*, 331.

Taverner, D., Cohen, S. B. & Hutchinson, B. C. (1971) Comparison of corticotrophin and prednisolone in Bell's palsy, *Br. med. J.*, *i*, 20.

Taylor, C. F. (1864) *Spinal Irritation: Cause of Backache among American Women.* New York: Wood.

Teale, T. P. (1829) *Treatise on Neuralgic Diseases, Dependent on Irritation of the Spinal Marrow.* London: Highley.

Theobald, G. W., Menzies, D. N. & Bryant, G. H. (1966) Critical electrical stimulus which causes uterine pain. *Br. med. J.*, *i*, 716.
Thompson, A. R., Plewes, L. W. & Shaw, E. G. (1951) Peritendinitis crepitans. *Br. J. indust. Med.*, *8*, 150.
—— & Felix-Davies, D. D. (1978) Response of 'idiopathic' angioneurotic oedema to tranexamic acid. *Br. med. J.*, *ii*, 608.
Thornes, R. D. (1976) Dublin trials in brucellosis. *Irish med. Times*, *10*, 6.
Tietze, A. (1921) Über eine eingenartige Hängung von Fallen mit Dystrophie der Rippenknorpel. *Berl. klin. Wschr.*, *58*, 829.
Tini, P. G., Weiser, C. & Zinn, W. M. (1977) Transitional vertebra of lumbar spine. *Rheum. & Rehab.*, *16*, 180.
Tkaczuk, H. (1968) Tensile properties of human lumbar longitudinal ligaments. *Acta orthop. scand.*, Suppl. 115.
Toakley, J. G. (1973) Subcutaneous lumbar 'rhizolysis'. *Med. J. Aust.*, *2*, 490.
Todd, T. W. & Pyle, S. I. (1928) Quantitative study of vertebral column by direct and roentgenoscopic methods. *Am. J. phys. Anthropol.*, *12*, 321.
Toglia, J. U. (1976) Acute flexion-extension injury of neck. *Neurology*, *26*, 803.
Töndury, G. (1940) Beitrag zur Kenntnis der kleinen Wirbelgelenken. *Z. anat. EntwGesch.*, *110*, 568.
Tonna, E. A. & Cronkite, E. P. (1903) Quoted by Burnett (1965).
Trickey, E. L. (1976) Ligamentous Injuries around the Knee. *Br. med. J.*, *i*, 1492.
Troisier, O. (1957) Diagnostic et therapeutique schématiques des divers syndromes douleureux de l'épaule. *Gaz. med. fr.*, *64*, 881.
—— (1958) Les capsulites de l'épaule. *Rhumatologie*, *3*, 113.
—— (1960) Les parésis musculaires des membres inferieurs dans les compression radiculaires discalis. *Ann. med. Physiques*, *ii*, 21.
—— (1962) *Lèsions des Disques Intervertébraux*. Paris: Masson.
—— (1973*a*) *Semiologie et Traitment des Algies Discales et Ligamentaires du Rachis*. Paris: Masson.
—— (1973*b*) Infiltrations dans les lombalgies. *Concours med.*, 7119.
Trowbridge, W. V. & French, J. D. (1954) False positive lumbar myelograms. *Neurol.*, *4*, 339.
Trueta, J. (1957) Normal Vascular Anatomy of Human Femoral Head during Growth. *J. Bone Jt Surg.*, *39B*, 358.
Tsaltas, T. T. (1958) Papain-induced changes in rabbit cartilage. *J. Exp. Med.*, *108*, 507.
Unander-Scharin, L. (1950) On low back pain. *Acta orthop. scand.*, Suppl. 5.
Unsworth, A., Doverson, D. & Wright, V. (1971) Cracking joints. *Ann. rheum. Dis.*, *30*, 348.
Vaino, K. (1967) Surgery of the rheumatoid hand. *Br. med. J.*, *i*, 686.
Vaishnava, H. P. & Rizvi, S. N. A. (1967) Osteomalacia in Northern India. *Br. med. J.*, *i*, 112.
Varma, S. K., Gulatia, R., Mukherjee, A. & Mohini, I. (1973) Role of traction in cervical spondylosis. *Physiotherapy*, *59*, 268.
Verbiest, H. (1954) Pathological influence of developmental narrowness of bony lumbar vertebral canal. *J. Bone Jt Surg.*, *37B*, 576.
Vernon-Roberts, B. (1975) Ageing lumbar spine. Lecture to the Society of Back Pain Research.
Vesalius (1543) *De Humani Corporis Fabrica*, vol. VII, Basel: Operinum.
Vickers, M. D. (1978) Chartered society of placutherapy. *World Med.*, *13*, 43.
Viner, N. (1925) Intractable sciatica: sacral epidural injection. *Can. med. Ass. J.*, *15*, 630.
Virchow, R. (1857) *Pathologie des Tumeurs*, vol. I, p. 447. Paris: Baillière.
Wadsworth, T. G. & Williams, J. R. (1973) Cubital tunnel external compression syndrome. *Br. med. J.*, *i*, 662.
Wahren, H. (1946) Herniated nucleus pulposus in child of twelve. *Acta orthop. scand.*, *16*, 40.
Wansbrough. (1826) Acupuncturation. *Lancet*, *xx*, 847.
Ward, L. E. & Okihiro, M. M. (1959) Palindromic Rheumatism: Follow-up Study. *Arch. Interameric. Rheum.*, *2*, 208.
Ward, T. G. (1961) Surgery of mandibular joint. *Ann. R. Coll. Surg.*, *28*, 139.
Ward, W. T. (1822) *Distortions of the Spine, Chest and Limbs*. London: Underwood.
Warr, A. C., Wilkinson, J. A., Burn, J. M. B. & Langdon, L. (1972) Chronic lumbo-sciatic syndrome treated by epidural injection and manipulation. *Practitioner*, *209*, 53.
Wasse, R. (1724) *Philosophical Transactions*. London: Innys.
Wassman, K. (1951) Kyphosis juvenilis Scheuermann—occupational disorder. *Acta orthop. scand.*, *21*, 65.
Waters, W. E. (1971) Headache and blood pressure. *Br. med. J.*, *i*, 142.
Watt, J. K., Gillespie, G., Pollack, J. G. & Reid, D. W. (1974) Arterial surgery in intermittent claudication. *Br. med. J.*, *i*, 23.
Watson, D. C. (1955) Anterior tibial syndrome following arterial embolism. *Br. med. J.*, *i*, 1412.
Weber, H. (1973) Traction in sciatica due to disc prolapse. *J. Oslo City Hosp.*, *23*, 167.
—— (1978) Lumbar disc herniation. *Ibid.* *28*, 33.
Webster, A. D. B., Loewi, G., Dourmashkin, R. D., Golding, D. N., Ward, D. J. & Asherson, G. L. (1976) Polyarthritis in adults with hypogammoglobulinaemia. *Br. med. J.*, *i*, 1314.

Weddell, G., Sinclair, D. C. & Feindel, W. H. (1948) Anatomical basis for alterations in pain sensibility. *J. Neurophysiol., 11*, 99.
Weissman, G. & Rita, G. A. (1972) Molecular basis of gouty inflammation. *Nature, Lond., 240*, 167.
Weitbrecht, J. (1742) *Syndesmologia.* St. Petersburg: Typographia Academiae Scientarum.
Weller, R. O., Bruckner, F. E. & Chamberlain, M. A. (1971) Rheumatoid neuropathy. *J. Neurol. Neurosurg. Psychiat., 33*, 592.
Weston, W. J. & Goodson, G. M. (1959) Vertebra Plana. *J. Bone Jt Surg., 41B*, 477.
Whitty, C. W. M. & Willison, R. G. (1958) Some aspects of referred pain. *Lancet, ii*, 226.
Wilkinson, M. (1964) Anatomy and pathology of cervical spondylosis. *Proc. R. Soc. Med., 57*, 159.
—— (1974) Pain in the neck. *Br. med. J., ii*, 242.
Willi, T. A. (1931) The separate neural arch. *J. Bone Jt Surg., 13*, 709.
Williams, R. W. (1978) Microlumbar discectomy. *Spine, 3*, 175.
Wilson, D. G. (1962) Manipulative treatment in general practice. *Lancet, i*, 1013.
Wiltse, L. L. (1971) Effect of common anomalies of lumbar spine on disc-degeneration and low back pain. *Orthop. Clin. N. Am., 2*, 569.
—— Widdell, E. R. & Yuan, H. A. (1975) Chymopapain chemonucleolysis in lumbar disc disease. *J. Am. med. Ass., 231*, 474.
Wing, L. W. & Hargrave-Wilson, W. (1973) Cervical vertigo. *10th Wld Congr. Oto-lar.*
Winkworth, C. L. (1883) Lawn tennis elbow. *Br. med. J., ii*, 557.
Winnie, A. P., Hartman, J. T., Meyers, H. L., Ramamurthy, S. & Barangan, V. (1972) Intradural and extradural corticosteroids for sciatica. *Anaesth. Analg., 51*, 990.
Wiseman, R. (1676) *Several Chirurgicall Treatises.* London: Flesher & Macock.
Wojtulewski, J. A., Sturrock, R. D., Branfoot, A. C. & Hart, F. D. (1973) Cricoarytenoid arthritis in ankylosing spondylitis. *Br. med. J., ii*, 145.
Wolf, B. S., Khilnani, M. & Malis, L. I. (1956) Sagittal diameter of bony cervical spinal canal and its significance in cervical spondylosis. *J. Mt. Sinai Hosp., 23*, 283.
Woltman, H. W. (1940) Median neuritis with acromegaly. *Mayo Clin. Pap., 32*, 944.
Woodhouse, N. J. Y. (1974) Clinical applications of calcitonin. *Br. J. Hosp. Med.*, 677.
Woolf, A. L. & Till, K. (1955) Pathology of the lower motor neurone in the light of new muscle biopsy techniques. *Proc. R. Soc. Med., 48*, 189.
Woolsey, C. N., Marshall, W. H. & Bard, P. (1941) Observations on cortical somatic sensory mechanism of cat and monkey. *J. Neurophysiol., 4*, 1.
Worden, R. E. & Humphrey, T. L. (1964) Effect of spinal traction on length of body. *Archs phys. Med., 45*, 318.
Worthington, B. (1980) X-rays face new challenge. *Sunday Times*, 7 September.
Wrenn, R. N., Goldner, J. L. & Markee, J. L. (1954) Effect of cortisone on healing process and tensile strength of tendons. *J. Bone Jt Surg., 36A*, 588.
Wright, V. (1971) Cracking joints. *Ann. rheum. Dis., 30*, 348.
—— Haslock, D. I., Dowson, D., Seller, P. C. & Reeves, B. (1971) Evaluation of silicone as artificial lubricant in osteoarthritis. *Br. med. J., i*, 370.
—— & Watkinson, G. (1965) Sacro-iliitis and ulcerative colitis. *Br. med. J., ii*, 675.
Wyke, B. D. (1969) *Principles of General Neurology. An Introduction to the Basic Principles of Medical and Surgical Neurology.* Amsterdam and London: Elsevier.
—— (1973) Perceptual and reflex contributions of cervical arthrokinetic receptors. Lecture to the British Association for Manipulative Medicine.
—— (1976) In *Lumbar Spine and Back Pain.* London: Sector.
—— (1980) Electromyography in back-pain diagnosis. *Pain Topics, 3*, 3.
Wynn-Parry, C. (1980) Electromyography in back-pain diagnosis. *Pain Topics, 3*, 3.
Yates, D. A. H. (1964) Indications for spinal manipulation. *Ann. phys. Med., 10*, 146.
Yoss, R. E., Corbin, K. B., MacCarty, C. S. & Love, J. G. (1957) Symptoms and signs in localisation of root involved in cervical disc protrusion. *Neurology, 7*, 673.
Young, A. C. (1967) Radiology in cervical spondylosis. In *Cervical Spondylosis.* London: Heinemann.
Young, J. (1940) Relaxation of pelvic joints in pregnancy. *J. Obstet. Gynec., 47*, 493.
Young, J. H. (1952) Personal communication.
Young, R. H. (1952) Results of surgery in sciatica and low back pain. *Lancet, i*, 245.
Zammitt, F. (1958) Undulant fever spondylitis. *Brit. J. Radiol., 31*, 683.
Zitnan, D., Sitaj, S., Huttl, S., Skrovina, B., Hanic, F., Markovic, O. & Trnavska, Z. (1963) Chondrocalcinosis articularis, I. Clinical and radiological study. *Ann. Rheum. Dis., 22*, 158.
Zizina, M. (1910) La doleur controlateral dans la sciatique. Thèse de Montpellier.
Zorab, P. A. (1966) Chest deformities. *Br. med. J., i*, 1155.
—— (1969) *Scoliosis.* London: Heinemann.

# TEACHING FACILITIES IN ORTHOPAEDIC MEDICINE

*(Corrected to January 1983)*

1. Twice a year, in early summer and late autumn, I give a four-day course in London for doctors and physiotherapists alike. Information from my Course Organizer, 206 Albany Street, London NW1, England.

2. Each year, two four-day courses are organized for me at the Orthopaedic Department of the Strong Memorial Hospital, 601 Elmwood Avenue, Rochester, NY 14642. They are for doctors and physiotherapists alike and include personal tuition for each participant. They are held in spring and autumn and similar courses are given in Canada or the USA just before and just after, when universities request it. Information is available from my Course Organizer in London some six months ahead.

3. All the year round, teaching in orthopaedic medicine is available from: Richard Ellis, MRCP, FRCS (Salisbury General Infirmary) and Michael Wright MRCP (St Andrew's Hospital, London, E3) and Olivier Troisier, MD (3 Avenue Bugeaud, 75116) at the Hospital Foch, Paris; Peter Hirschfeld, MD, and Miss E. Longton, MCSP (25 Zedernstrasse, 2807 Achim-Uesen, Germany) at the Zentral Krankenhaus, St. Jurgenstrasse, 28 Bremen; Salvador Conesa, MD, Orthopaedic Medicine Department, Hospital Arrixaca, Murcia, Spain (who also gives a six-day course for doctors once a year); Yardley MacKenzie, MRCP, at St. Luke's Hospital, Guildford, Surrey; H. Heers MD, Zentral Krankenhaus Reinkenheide, 285 Bremerhaven, West Germany; K. Krajca MD, Neurological Dept., Dubnica n/ Vahom, Czechoslovakia; Professor W. Gibson, University of Calgary Medical School, Alberta, Canada; O. Bihaug, KMI, Orthopaedic Hospital, Joerg Loerlandsgatan 2, Oslo 5, Norway.

4. In Holland, courses are given twice a year by physiotherapist, D. Winkel (33 Gebbenlaan, Delft) for doctors and physiotherapists at a series of adjoining week-ends.
   In Belgium week-end courses are given by physiotherapist R. de Coninck for doctors and physiotherapists (Peter Benoit Laan 27, 8420 deHaan).
   Week-end courses are given at my consulting rooms for final year physiotherapy students and recent graduates. They last from 10.00 a.m. till 6.00 p.m. on Saturday-Sunday. As soon as we accumulate twenty applicants from various schools, the course is given.
   Requests are dealt with by my Course Organizer.

5. A doctor or a physiotherapist can sit in on my private consultations for a few days but only one at a time, by arrangement with me.

6. Private tuition from my physiotherapy staff in London is available by arrangement with my Senior Physiotherapist.

7. Copies of audio recordings of my lectures at Rochester ($155) and audiovisual tapes ($256) are obtainable from Audio Visual Inc., 1308 de Kalb Street, Norristown, Penua, 19401, USA, and from Oliver Cyriax, 206 Albany Street, London NW1. A new illustrated manual will appear in 1983.

8. The videotape recordings of Dr. Paul Williams's and my lectures at Atlanta in 1977, together with the panel discussion afterwards are obtainable from the Department of Rehabilitation, Emory University, Atlanta, Georgia, USA.

9. The film that Hirschfeld and I made on the shoulder is obtainable from my Course Organizer. Dr Hirschfeld and Miss E. Longton, MCSP, have made three more films: the

Knee, the Ankle and the Lumbar Spine. The first two are obtainable from Chemische Fabrik von Heyden, Volkartstrasse 83, 8 München 19, West Germany.

10. Doctors in difficulties over procaine solution for epidural injections, P2G solution for ligamentous sclerosis, or a proper traction harness are invited to get in touch with my secretary. She orders and sends them out; the bill goes to the doctor.

# INDEX